—USING REPURPOSED DRUGS FOR CANCER TREATMENT—

CRACKING
CANCER
TOOLKIT

JEFFREY DACH MD

Author Contact information:
Jeffrey Dach MD
7450 Griffin Road, Suite 180/190
Davie, Florida 33314
Office Telephone 954–792–4663
Websites: www.crackingcancertoolkit.com and   www.jeffreydachmd.com

ISBN: 978-1-73242-101-1

Library of Congress Control Number: 2020922391

Editing: Edward Levy, www.edwardlevy.com
Formatting: Deborah Stocco, www.mybookdesigner.com
Cover Design: Yesna @ www.99designs.com

Dedication

This book is dedicated to the 500,000 Americans who last year died of cancer, and the 500,000 next year who won't.

Table of Contents

Note: Boldface has been added to portions of some quotations for emphasis.

Foreword by Carol Petersen, RPh, CNP

BIG-BOX BOOKSTORES AND AMAZON BRING us sources of information that used to be almost impossible to access. A book written by someone with direct personal experience is priceless. Many have turned to writing books to disseminate information that could never be heard or discussed otherwise.

In 2004 Dr. Marcia Angell, now former editor of the New England Journal of Medicine, blew the whistle on the corruption of medical science by the pharmaceutical industry in her book *The Truth About the Drug Companies: How They Deceive Us and What to Do About It.* Medical literature has sold out. Studies have been fabricated or information altered to align with a predetermined narrative. The average person has little opportunity to successfully find useful information nor the means to use that information for practical application to a health issue.

Richard Nixon's "war on cancer" has succeeded only in making the cancer industry a cancer itself upon society. Tremendous monetary gains keep the chemo, radiation, and surgery narrative the only choice. Deviation can cost careers and livelihood for practitioners and investigators.

There are cracks in the narrative, however. Dr. Jeffrey Dach found himself face to face with serious cancer challenges to family members. His training in radiology gave him a platform to launch his investigation and he worked tirelessly to find information that could change a deadly outcome. His searches cover five years of study. He investigated practitioners and scientists who might have insights. In the end, his family members had successful outcomes.

He has decided to share the information he accumulated. *Cracking Cancer Toolkit* is not a protocol or recipe for success for any particular cancer. It is, however, a gateway to learning much more about cancer than the average oncologist will relate to their patients. Knowledge is power. Reading this book and keeping it as a reference will open doors to learning new theories and potential therapies. Many therapies already exist but have been unused because of strict adherence to the narrative.

Dr. Dach presents us with the gift of translation. His writing is clear and understandable. We don't have to have a PhD or medical degree to grasp concepts that come cloaked in medical jargon. This compilation of cancer information is a great work. He sends it into the world so many more can benefit.

Carol Petersen, RPh, CNP
Carol@thewellnessbydesignproject.com

Foreword by Akbar Khan, MD

WHEN CANCER PATIENTS ASK ME for advice, I often reply: "Don't blindly trust your oncologist!" After all, oncologists complete 12 long years of university and challenging medical training, and there is the perception they must really know their job. Can we trust them with placing our lives in their hands? Paradoxically, when cancer patients do so, their lives may be in jeopardy. Some may be shocked by this statement, considering it unethical or unprofessional. Let me explain.

Cancer is a complex disease, and with few exceptions, has no generally accepted curative therapy. Despite the billions spent on cancer research, cancer specialists are still using high dose cytotoxic chemotherapy, a form of treatment decades old and of limited effectiveness, associated with severe toxicities.

One of the most promising new drug discoveries is the Checkpoint Inhibitor family of immunotherapy drugs, ipilimumab and nivolumab. In 2011, when these drugs were first approved for human use, news reports exclaimed: "**This is it! This is the cure for cancer we have all been waiting for**." Sadly, this was not to be. Even more disappointing, these drugs can actually **accelerate** cancer growth in 10–15% of cases.

How do we explain the ongoing frustration and failures in oncology? Could it be that our fundamental understanding of cancer is flawed? Perhaps it is time for a radical change in the theory of cancer. Most cancer experts accept the theory that cancer is caused by mutations in our DNA, the genetic code for the trillion cells in our bodies. And, these mutations lead to uncontrolled growth and spread of cancer cells. This is a failed theory, leading to many treatment failures. A more credible alternate theory, presented in Dr. Jeffrey Dach's book, *Cracking Cancer Toolkit*, is the theory of *Cancer as a Metabolic Disease*.

In 2009, a young lady came to me with a diagnosis of glioblastoma, one of the deadliest forms of brain cancer. She underwent neurosurgery to remove the bulk of the tumor. Following surgery, she received a course of radiation combined with low dose oral chemotherapy, the standard treatment protocol. Upon completion, the doctors offered a maintenance program of oral high dose chemotherapy, with expected survival of only 12 months, a fact this young lady was acutely aware of. As a result, the patient refused the monthly chemotherapy and instead started oral Dichloroacetate (DCA), a form of metabolic cancer therapy. DCA works by switching off the glucose usage, the energy supply in cancer cells. The patient completed a 3-month course of DCA, and follow up scans showed her cancer had completely disappeared. She remains alive and well today more than 10 year after her diagnosis, with no ongoing therapy. This dramatic case is not alone. I have witnessed many others, serving as clinical confirmation of the validity of metabolic theory of cancer, successfully applied to clinical practice today.

Patients looking for meaningful treatment solutions for their cancer diagnosis should take heart, and become an advocate for their own health. We now have access to online medical research, such as the National Library of Medicine (PubMed). In the past, this type of resource was only accessible with a personal visit to a medical library. Nowadays, this medical information is accessible from the comfort and convenience of your home computer. We now have online discussion forums with other cancer patients around the world, successfully treated or even cured with non-standard therapies. And now we have Dr. Dach's book, *Cracking Cancer Toolkit*, which explains the metabolic theory of cancer and other novel theories in a comprehensible writing style, understandable to the non-medical reader. Given how common cancer is today, this book is a valuable addition to any home library. Indeed, the knowledge you gain may save your life, or the life of a friend or family member. Happy Reading!

Akbar Khan, MD
Medicor Cancer Centres
4576 Yonge St, Suite 301
Toronto, ON Canada M2N 6N4
Telephone 416-227-0037
web site: https://medicorcancer.com/

Chapter 1

Introduction by Jeffrey Dach, MD

FOR THE TYPICAL PATIENT SITTING on the examining table at the oncology office, the cure for cancer remains as elusive as ever. Billions have been spent on the "war on cancer" with little to show for it.

Lung, colon, pancreatic, liver, brain, breast, lymphoma, myeloma, and leukemia are the common cancers treated with the traditional trio of surgery, chemotherapy, and radiation, known in the vernacular as cut, poison, and burn.

In the coming pages, you will be shocked and surprised to learn that thousands of patients are bypassing the oncologist's office and finding good outcomes on their own with a toolkit of repurposed drugs and supplements. Many enlist the assistance of the "integrative oncologist," a new and rare breed of oncologist who incorporates repurposed drugs and supplements into their protocols.

Technological Advances

Three technological advances have made this paradigm shift possible. First, the invention of the positron emission tomography (PET) scanner using the isotope 18-FDG provides amazingly accurate images of cancer size and location anywhere in the body, giving the patient knowledge of whether or not their treatment is working. Is the cancer mass decreasing or increasing in response to treatment? The PET scan will answer this question. To assess cancer treatment, a PET scan three months after starting a cocktail of repurposed anti-cancer drugs indicates success or failure. Treatment protocols can be tailored "on the fly" based on real-time PET scan imaging. Blood tests following serial cancer markers are also useful.

Sharing Stories, Protocols, and Information on Message Boards

The second technological advance is the invention of message groups on the Internet, where large numbers of patients, thousands perhaps, share information about their repurposed drug protocols—their successes as well as failures. This is historic and remarkable, considering that medical information is protected by privacy laws and considered confidential at the doctor's office. Desperate cancer patients may feel they are out of time and have nothing to lose. They seek out others with similar stories on message boards and in groups, hoping for a good outcome with repurposed drugs and supplements.

High-Throughput Drug Screening

The third technological advance has to do with the molecular and cell biology of cancer, also known as "in vitro" cancer cell culture and "in vivo" xenograft animal research, which have elucidated metabolic pathways in cancer cells. These pathways can be targeted by repurposed drugs and botanicals. One such advance is the implementation of automated drug screening. A large drug library of thousands of drugs can be screened for the most effective cancer-killing drug. For example, if basic laboratory studies identify a metabolic pathway in cancer cells that can be selectively targeted while normal cells are left unharmed, then high-throughput screening can be used to find the best drug suited for this purpose.

Basic Science Research Thirty Years Ahead of Clinical Practice

New tools for delving into cellular metabolic pathways have propelled preclinical laboratory cancer research thirty years ahead of actual clinical practice on the oncology wards. *Think about it: Instead of waiting thirty years, what if we could put this new research to work immediately using repurposed drugs. Would we then achieve remissions and cures?*

The answer is affirmative.

The Chemotherapy Concession

Although amazing breakthroughs have been made in non-chemotherapy oncology drugs, such as checkpoint inhibitors and tyrosine kinase inhibitors, oncologists are still limited to chemotherapy and a short list of FDA-approved oncology drugs. The so-called chemotherapy concession, a form of lucrative kickback to oncologists for using chemotherapy, has kept these drugs in the forefront of oncology far too long, artificially extending their life span.

The financial stakes are too high to change the paradigm.

Out of Time

New drugs in the pipeline are slow to arrive at the clinic. Clinical trials required for FDA approval are expensive and laborious. Old off-patent drugs in common use, such as repurposed anti-cancer drugs, may never be properly studied in clinical trials simply because no drug company in its right mind would outlay the huge sums needed for clinical trials, without the profits guaranteed by a patent. But today's desperate cancer patient does not have the luxury of time and cannot wait years for clinical trials that may never be done. These are the brave souls with nothing to lose, sharing stories on Internet message boards and Internet groups about the repurposed drug protocols they are using.

Chemotherapy Disappointment

With the exception of testicular cancer and some lymphoma cell types, chemotherapy remains a disappointment. Granted, chemotherapy can temporarily decrease tumor size and induce a temporary remission. However, the price is cumulative cytotoxicity to normal tissues such as bone marrow, brain, and heart and adverse effects of nausea, vomiting, anorexia, weight loss, hair loss, bone marrow toxicity, neurotoxicity ("chemo brain") and cardiotoxicity. Invariably, the cancers return months to years after completing chemotherapy, when they may be even more aggressive and resistant to further chemotherapy treatment.

The Cancer Stem Cell and Cancer Recurrence

The cancer stem cell (CSC) is the major cause of tumor recurrence after completing chemotherapy. The CSC is resistant to chemotherapy, dormant, and hiding in the recesses of the body waiting for a future opportunity to repopulate. Your oncologist may very well have attended one or more national CSC meetings, sitting in a large hall, listening to speakers drone on about this topic. Even so, the CSC is ignored by oncologists on the hospital wards. They are oblivious to the problem. We will discuss the CSC and treatment solutions in the coming pages.

In 2013, Dr. Claire Pecqueur et al. discussed the CSC problem, suggesting that a reversal of cancer cell metabolism with an agent like dichloroacetate (DCA) could be effective:

> The successful elimination of a cancer requires an anti-cancer therapy that will affect both differentiated cancer cells and CSCs.... At present, conventional therapy that includes radio-, chemo-, and immunotherapy kills rapidly proliferating and differentiated cells. These treatments may cause the tumor to shrink but will not prevent tumor recurrence. Thus, a combination of treatments targeting both rapidly proliferating cancer cells and quiescent or slow-proliferating CSCs would be ideal. Therefore, it is essential to identify specific markers that distinguish between tumorigenic and nontumorigenic stem cells ... a reversal of tumor metabolism [with DCA dichloroacetate] to "normal" might impair tumor growth of cancer cells, causing tumor regression, and differentiation/sensitization to cell death of CSCs, impairing the recurrence of the tumor. (2)

Theories of Cancer

In the coming chapters, we will discuss the theory of cancer as a metabolic disease, as well as the old idea that cancer is a form of parasite that steals nutrition from its host. Supporting this hypothesis is the fact that a number of antiparasitic drugs have been repurposed as anti-cancer drugs. Another old idea is that cancer shares many similarities with the placenta cell called the trophoblast. Like the trophoblast, cancer cells create their own blood supply, using the same molecular circuitry.

Finding the Combination to Open the Lock

Another way to understand cancer is to use the analogy of a combination lock. The walk-in safe at your bank has a combination lock. Unless all the numbers are lined up and the tumblers are in the correct position, the door of the safe will not open. In the same way, if we could discover the combination, we could "crack" cancer and find a cure.

In the case of cancer, the tumblers are the correct combination of cellular pathways targeted by repurposed drugs and supplements. Don't forget the new targeted Food and Drug Administration (FDA) approved oncology drugs. These pathway drugs, like rituximab, ibrutinib, venetoclax, lenalidomide, and chimeric antigen T cell (CAR T) all have a place in our anti-cancer armamentarium.

Can Targeted Therapies with Repurposed Drugs Actually Work?

The next logical question is: Can it really be true that a few repurposed drugs targeting metabolic pathways in cancer can induce complete long-term remissions and even cure?

The answer to this question is an emphatic "yes." Lest you have doubts, allow me point out that this book is heavily referenced to the medical literature. It takes about 20 to 30 years for mainstream medicine to adopt and accept new information from the medical literature. This book gives you information and tools 20 to 30 years ahead of its time.

Since I am not an oncologist, you might ask the obvious question: "What gives me the ability and authority to write a book about cancer? Isn't that reserved for the oncologist?"

Although not an oncologist, I do have credentials as a board-certified diagnostic radiologist. I have spent a 30-year career in the hospital studying cancer on medical images, CAT scans, PET Scans, Ultrasound, X-Rays, Nuclear Imaging, SPECT, etc. I retired from medical imaging and have been seeing patients in a small office setting for the past 15 years. During this time, three of my family members were stricken with cancer, motivating me to research, gain an understanding, and write about cancer. This is the genesis of *Cracking Cancer Toolkit*.

Physician Colleagues with Cancer in Family

Over the years, while working in the hospital setting, many of my physician colleagues shared with me their frustration with mainstream oncology's harsh treatments, adverse side effects, and poor outcomes. Because I had a reputation for being interested in "alternative medicine," they wanted my advice about a family member stricken with cancer. At the time, I could do little to help them. This is another motivation for this book—to enable others, physicians and non-medical people alike, to "get up to speed" rapidly in this field. Picking up the molecular biology jargon and trying to read medical research is like reading a foreign language; it's time consuming and difficult even if you happen to have an MD or a few PhDs in biological science. This learning process took me four years. When a cancer diagnosis strikes a family member, trust me, you don't have four years to study the medical literature. It is my hope *Cracking Cancer Toolkit* will give you a head start, save you valuable time, allow you to rapidly come up to speed, and illuminate the way to a favorable outcome.

Inspirations for this Book

- *Ben Williams—Surviving Glioblastoma:* Ben Williams was a psychology professor at the University of San Diego when he was diagnosed with terminal brain cancer (glioblastoma), a uniformly fatal incurable disease. This was before the Internet and PubMed, so Mr. Williams accessed the University medical library in person, spent hours on research, and devised his own cocktail of repurposed drugs. Many were purchased over the counter by driving across the border to Mexico.

In combination with chemotherapy, brain surgery, and his repurposed drug cocktail, he survived and is alive today. This is noteworthy because, if you ask any neurologist or neurosurgeon, they will tell you that all glioblastoma patients succumb to their disease. There are no survivors. Ben Williams is indeed the rare exception. How he did it is documented in his book, *Surviving "Terminal" Cancer: Clinical Trials, Drug Cocktails and Other Treatments Your Oncologist Won't Tell You About* (Fairview Press, 2002).

- *Joe Tippens's Fenbendazole Story:* Joe Tippens was diagnosed with non-small-cell lung cancer with extensive metastatic disease and sent home to hospice with a projected three months to live. An old friend, a veterinarian, suggested he take a dog de-wormer drug called Fenbendazole. Three months after starting the drug, his PET scan, done at MD Anderson Cancer Center in Houston was completely clear of cancer. I had the pleasure of meeting and briefly chatting with Joe at the Annie Appleseed meeting February 2020. Joe Tippens has a large Facebook group where thousands of cancer patients share stories.

- *Jane McLelland—Starving Cancer*: Jane McLelland is a physiotherapist who survived multiple cancers by devising her own treatment program using a cocktail of repurposed drugs. Jane's Facebook Group has thousands of members sharing their personal stories. Her book, *How to Starve Cancer: Without Starving Yourself,* is rec-

ommended. I have read it many times, and it has inspired and assisted me in writing *Cracking Cancer Toolkit*. I had the pleasure of meeting Jane at her booth at the Annie Appleseed Cancer Meeting in West Palm Beach, Florida, in February 2020, where she spoke about her experiences and gave me an autographed copy of her book. It was a thrill to meet her. Jane is a true pioneer and leader in the field of repurposed drugs for cancer treatment. Here is a quote from *How to Starve Cancer: Without Starving Yourself (Agenor, 2018)*:

Years from now, when the oncology practices finally change, as they must, I feel sure we'll look back in sadness at how many patients died and suffered needlessly. We'll be amazed that the medical profession persisted so long with cruel and destructive treatments.

The Politics of Cancer

A brief note about the politics of cancer. Many of the repurposed drugs and supplements mentioned in this book are still available in the United States. However, this may change. Inside the U.S., the FDA and other government agencies working hand in glove with the drug industry are in the process of banning or may have already banned many of the anti-cancer drugs and supplements discussed here. The reason for this is to protect the profits of the chemotherapy drug industry. The cancer patients and health care practitioners may be forced to seek supplies and expertise outside the U.S., in Canada or Mexico, where they are readily available.

Practical Considerations for Repurposed Drugs

Regarding the use of repurposed drugs and supplements, it is recommended that the patient seek the care of a knowledgeable physician familiar with the approach in this book, monitor for adverse side effects, and perform blood labs, such as liver function tests, blood counts, cancer markers, and other parameters. The following questions should be asked for each agent:

- **Drug Therapeutic Blood Levels— Pharmacokinetics:** *Are we able to reach therapeutic blood levels using standard dosages of the drug or supplement?* In other words, when reading the research literature, can the effective in vitro drug concentration be achieved in humans with an oral tablet or capsule? For example, although the botanical supplement feverfew (parthenolide), commonly used for migraine headaches, shows striking in vitro anti-cancer activity, in a 2004 study by Dr. E. A. Curry, there was no detectable feverfew found in the plasma after a 4 mg dose. (1) A commonly available feverfew extract 500 mg capsule contains 2.5 mg of parthenolides. What is the correct dosage? This type of dosage issue is not a problem for FDA-approved drugs at the corner drugstore that have undergone extensive pharmacokinetic studies showing therapeutic blood levels.

- **Adverse Effects—Drug Toxicity:** *Is the drug too toxic for human use?* What are the adverse effects of the drug or supplement, and do they outweigh the potential benefit? Obviously, those agents with no or minimal adverse effects are preferred.

- **Drug Efficacy in Human Use:** Once anti-cancer activity is demonstrated by in vitro and in vivo animal xenografts, does this translate into efficacy for human use? Many drugs show efficacy in the lab, then fail human clinical trials. Do we have case reports and human clinical trials showing efficacy?

- **Cancer Stem Cell Activity:** Is the drug active against CSCs?

- **Interactions with Other Drugs:** How does the drug interact with other drugs and with the CYP450 enzyme system?

Many of the repurposed drugs, such as itraconazole and cimetidine, interact with the CYP450 enzyme system in the liver, which metabolizes drugs. This means plasma levels of concurrent drugs will be increased, possibly dangerously. Monitoring this type of drug interaction is essential when multiple drugs are used in combination.

How to Read This Book

Before starting the book, you may wish to first read the Final Words (Chapter 42) at the end, and the Glossary and the Quick Reference Guide to give an overview before actually starting the book in earnest. Also, you may wish to skip around in the book to make connections and links between ideas and concepts. There is a large amount of information in this book, and I have found it useful to re-read the book a number of times. An index would be enormously useful. However I decided not to include an index in the paperback version because the searchable kindle version serves this purpose better than any index I could ever do. I suggest obtaining the both the paperback and kindle version (serving as a searchable index).

An added advantage of the kindle version is easier access to the original reference articles. References for each chapter are numbered and listed at the end of each chapter. Open a second window with Google Scholar, and then cut and paste the reference into Google Scholar to find the original publication. We use a lot of molecular and cell biology jargon that may not be familiar to you, so this terminology is explained as we go along. The Glossary is intended to help with this as well.

References for Chapter 1: Introduction

1) Curry, Eardie A., et al. "Phase I dose escalation trial of feverfew with standardized doses of parthenolide in patients with cancer." Investigational new drugs 22.3 (2004): 299-305.

2) Pecqueur, Claire, et al. "Targeting metabolism to induce cell death in cancer cells and cancer stem cells." International journal of cell biology 2013 (2013).

3) Grössmann, Nicole, and Claudia Wild. "Between January 2009 and April 2016, 134 novel anticancer therapies were approved: what is the level of knowledge concerning the clinical benefit at the time of approval?." ESMO open 1.6 (2016): esmoopen-2016.

Chapter 2

Conventional Oncology: Success or Failure?

CANCER IS THE SECOND LEADING cause of death in the United States after heart disease, with about 600,000 deaths in 2017 according to the Centers for Disease Control and Prevention (CDC). Current cancer mortality rates in 2019 remain at roughly the same level as the year 1930, in spite of the decline since 1990 attributed to reduction in cigarette smoking. (1).

Does this sound like we are winning the "war" against cancer? Here is what Dr. Ian Haines wrote in *Lancet* (2014), taking exception to this battlefield analogy:

> The misplaced battlefield analogy has led to 40 years of toxic and overly aggressive chemotherapy in incurable solid cancers for which no studies have shown that maximum tolerated doses of chemotherapy achieve longer survival or better quality of life than do minimum effective doses. This approach has led to inappropriate and toxic therapies for many patients.... (2)

Chemotherapy: Does It Work?

One of the hallmarks of cancer is rapid cell proliferation. The cancer cells replicate at a faster rate than normal cells, thus forming uncontrolled nodules and masses that can spread throughout the body; this is known as metastatic disease. Chemotherapy uses toxic drugs to target rapid proliferation and preferentially kill the cancer cells.

Problems with Chemotherapy

However, there are a number of problems with the chemotherapy approach. The rapidly dividing cancer cells will promptly die-off. This can lead to "tumor lysis syndrome," in which this massive die-off releases toxins into the circulation. If the dying tumor mass is located in a vascular structure such as the renal parenchyma, this could lead to life-threatening bleeding—a dangerous state of affairs requiring hospitalization.

The second problem is that organs and tissues contain normal cells that are rapidly replicating, and these are therefore also targeted along with the cancer cells. Notably, this includes the gut lining, accounting for the nausea and vomiting commonly seen after chemotherapy. The bone marrow that makes our blood cells is also rapidly replicating and therefore sensitive to chemotherapy-induced bone marrow suppression or even bone marrow failure in extreme cases; this explains adverse effects like anemia (low blood count) and neutropenia (low white blood cells). Moreover, depending on the chemotherapy agent, there may be cardiotoxicity (Adriamycin) or nephrotoxicity.

Febrile Neutropenia and Septic Shock after Chemotherapy

In fact, many deaths from chemotherapy are caused by bone marrow suppression with very low white count, which renders the patient immunosuppressed and susceptible to rampant infection. Combine the bone marrow suppression with gastrointestinal (GI) toxicity, and things can get even worse. Denudation of the inner lining of the GI tract from chemotherapy causes "leaky gut." Gram-negative bacteria normally residing in the gut lumen (also called friendly bacteria) can now leak into the bloodstream. The outer coat of gram-negative bacteria, called lipopolysaccharide (LPS) is one of the most dangerous and toxic substances known to man, causing gram-negative septicemia and shock. Normally, white blood cells in the patient's immune system rush to the rescue and neutralize this bacterial invasion of the bloodstream. Unfortunately, after high-dose chemotherapy, the patient may have zero or almost no white blood cells (neutrophils) on the complete blood count (CBC) test. This condition is invariably fatal, causing death from septic shock unless the patient is promptly admitted to the intensive care unit for intravenous (IV) antibiotics and supportive care. (3)

Enter the "Neupogen" Shot

Lucky for the chemotherapy patient, the drug industry developed filgrastim, human granulocyte colony-stimulating factor (G-CSF) , produced by recombinant DNA technology, which was FDA-approved in 1991. The human gene for this G-CSF protein is inserted into E. coli bacteria, which multiply in large vats, mass producing the G-CSF protein. Amgen Inc.'s brand name for filgrastim is Neupogen®. These injections are pricey but do the trick. White counts go up promptly, saving the patient from the unpleasant experience of febrile neutropenia and septic shock.

One might then ask the obvious question: Since filgrastim (G-CSF) is a growth factor for white blood cells, can filgrastim injections stimulate the growth of cancers of the white cells such as leukemia and lymphoma? The FDA package insert says this remains a question that has not yet been adequately answered by clinical studies. However, the cancer patient has no choice in the matter. Either die from febrile neutropenia and septic shock or take your chances with the shot, stimulating cancer growth. Dr. Belinda Yeo et al. (2018) raise this question:

> Over the past 10–15 years it has become increasingly apparent, in preclinical tumour growth and metastasis models, that **G-CSF can support tumour progression** by mobilization of tumour-associated neutrophils which consequently promote tumour dissemination and metastasis. With the increasing use of G-CSF in the clinic, it is pertinent to ask if there is any evidence of a similar promotion of tumour progression in patients…. Limited data indicate **that high serum G-CSF levels in patients are associated with poorer prognosis** [emphasis added]. (37)

Note: All bold face text within quotes wherever appearing in this book is emphasis added by me.

Others have studied G-CSF in various cancer cell lines finding G-CSF stimulates neurogenesis (nerve growth) into the cancer mass and promotes tumor progression, proliferation, migration, invasion and immunosuppression. This is not a good thing. (38–41)

The Unfortunate Story of Procrit

Another common adverse effect of chemotherapy is chronic anemia or low blood cell count, caused by bone marrow suppression. In order to restore the blood count in these patients, the drug industry invented a biotech drug, a form of recombinant erythropoietin, the human hormone that stimulates red blood cell production. This drug, marketed as both Procrit and Epogen, was FDA-approved in 1989 for anemia in chronic renal failure patients and in 1993 for chronic anemia from chemotherapy. Procrit and other recombinant erythropoietin drugs were used for many years. Unfortunately, only later was it found that the drugs stimulate not only the red cells but also cancer growth as well, causing cancer recurrence and shortened survival. Since patient outcomes were being adversely affected, erythropoietin drugs fell into disfavor and are rarely used on the oncology wards, with old-fashioned blood transfusion being the obvious alternative. Will this story be repeated for the filgrastim drugs that stimulate white cells? We await further studies and hope for an answer with the passage of time.

False Hope: Bone Marrow Transplantation for Breast Cancer

Oncologists who believe in chemotherapy also believe that more chemotherapy must be even better. If only we could use more chemotherapy at higher doses!! Perhaps this belief has been encouraged by financial incentives. As *New York Times* health care reporter Reed Abelson noted (Jan 26, 2003):

Among cancer doctors, it is called **the chemotherapy concession**. At a time when overall spending on prescription drugs is soaring, cancer specialists are pocketing hundreds of millions of dollars each year by selling drugs to patients—a practice that almost no other doctors follow. (4)

Whatever the motivation for using ever higher doses of chemotherapy in the belief that more is better, the limiting factor is, again, bone marrow toxicity. Higher dosage chemotherapy completely destroys the bone marrow compartment, leading to early death unless the bone marrow is restored, usually with a procedure called autologous bone marrow transplant. In this procedure, the patient's own bone marrow progenitor (stem) cells are harvested before chemo treatment and then returned to the patient afterwards. This restores the bone marrow.

Incredible as it sounds, this was commonly done in the 1980s on many breast cancer patients. While many women stricken with advanced illness clamored for this "lifesaving" procedure, their health insurance companies balked at paying for an experimental and unproven $400,000 dollar treatment. After a couple of decades harming thousands of severely ill women with an unproven procedure, medical studies eventually showed the procedure had no merit, causing it to be discredited and abandoned, as described by Dr. Edward Stadtmauer in 2008 in *J Clin Oncology*. (5)

This report [Crump M, et al, J ClinOncol, 26:37-43, 2008]... led us to definitively conclude that a high-dose of alkylating agents with autologous stem-cell transplantation, when given in the setting of responding metastatic breast cancer, **does not lead to improved overall survival.** [Emphasis added] (5)

Although it has been discredited and abandoned for breast cancer and other solid malignancies, autologous and allogeneic bone marrow transplantation is still commonly done for hematologic cancers such as leukemia and lymphoma. While there are anecdotal reports of dramatic long-term remissions or "cures," there are also many patients with poor outcomes who succumb to the adverse toxic effects of such a harsh treatment. These adverse outcomes are related to rampant infection associated with prolonged use of immunosuppressive drugs; engraftment failure, leaving the patient with no functioning bone marrow; and the dreaded graft-versus-host disease, a form of auto-immune disease in which allogeneic bone marrow graft attacks the recipient's body as foreign tissue. Autologous transplant (the patient's own cells preserved and re-infused after treatment) safely avoids the risk of graft-versus-host disease and avoids risk of infection from prolonged immunosuppression; it is considered safer than using bone marrow from a donor. In the allogeneic transplant (cells from a donor) there may be a "graft versus tumor" immune response, which justifies its use in some cases of hematologic malignancy. Will bone marrow transplant for hematologic malignancy be vindicated or discredited by future studies? We will have to wait and see.

Chemotherapy's Low Survival Rate

In the 1970s, chemotherapy was regarded as "curative" for testicular cancer and lymphoma. Expectations of similar chemotherapy outcomes extended to other cancers were never realized. In a 2004 *Clinical Oncology* article, Drs. Graeme Morgan et al. reported that chemotherapy contributed only 2.1% to the 5-year survival rate in adult cancers:

> The overall contribution of curative and adjuvant cytotoxic chemotherapy to 5-year survival in adults was estimated to be **2.1%** in the USA… In view of the minimal impact of cytotoxic chemotherapy on 5-year survival, and the lack of major progress over the last 20 years, it follows that **the main role of cytotoxic chemotherapy is in palliation…**. Despite the early claims of chemotherapy as the panacea for curing all cancers, the impact of cytotoxic chemotherapy is limited to small subgroups of patients and mostly occurs in the less common malignancies. (6)

Checkpoint Inhibitors, the Most Important Advance

If we admit the old chemotherapy paradigm is ripe for revolution, have the newer targeted oncology drugs such as Checkpoint Inhibitor immunotherapy drugs fared better? Admitted, the Checkpoint Inhibitor drugs are an important advance in conventional oncology, however, they have a low response rate.

Expressing enthusiasm, Dr. Antoni Ribas and Jedd Wolchok, writing in 2018 about the new checkpoint inhibitor drugs that target PD-1:

> The underlying biology and durable response rates in patients with multiple

types of cancer indicate that therapeutic blockade of the PD-1 pathway (programmed death) is arguably **one of the most important advances in the history of cancer treatment. (36)**

However, low response rates are disappointing as described by Dr. Pramod Darvin in 2018 who writes:

> Mainstream initiation of immune checkpoint therapy to treat cancers is obstructed by the low response rate and immune-related adverse events in some cancer patients. (42)

New Oncology Drugs' Survival Benefit Is Less than Three Months

Unfortunately, according Dr. Peter Wise in *BMJ* (2016) the newer drugs are no better than chemotherapy. He states:

> Despite considerable investment and innovation, chemotherapy drugs have had little effect on survival in adults with metastatic cancer.... **Newer drugs did no better:** 48 new regimens approved by the US Food and Drug Administration between 2002 and 2014 conferred a **median 2.1 month overall survival benefit.** (7)

According to Drs. Nicole Grössmann and Claudia Wild (2016), the majority of the new drugs provide a dismal 2-to-3 month increase in survival:

> Between January 2009 and April 2016, 134 novel anti-cancer therapies were approved... the survival benefit of the approved indications is **less than 3 months in the majority of approved therapies.** (8)

Progress in Chronic Lymphocytic Leukemia

One of the cancers that the "new drugs" are considered to have the greatest progress with is chronic lymphocytic leukemia (CLL). According to Dr. Gregory Masters et al. (2015) in *J. Clinical Oncology*, the addition of the immunotherapy drugs obinutuzumab and ofatumumab, in combination with the chemotherapy drug chlorambucil delay disease progression for a year. (9) Once the disease relapses or becomes chemo-resistant, the disease may then respond to ibrutinib and idelalisib. Ibrutinib is Bruton's tyrosine kinase inhibitor, a targeted pathway drug that inhibits the B-cell receptor and has revolutionized lymphoma treatment. Idelalisib is a phosphoinositide 3-kinase inhibitor (PI-3K), a major upregulated pathway in cancer cells. However, remissions are only temporary, with all cases eventually relapsing upon development of a mutated, drug-resistant cell type.

It's the Cancer Stem Cells, Stupid

Chemotherapy is disappointing because of cancer relapse after completing treatment. The cancer is not totally eradicated and comes back. Relapse is caused by cancer stem cells (CSCs), which are quiescent, not actively replicating, and resistant to chemotherapy drugs. After completing a course of chemotherapy, the tumor bulk may be eradicated, with a negative PET scan. However, hidden from view are the residual microscopic CSCs hiding in their niche, latent, and biding their time until activation is triggered, causing regrowth and relapse of cancer. When the cancer returns, the cell type may become more aggressive and resistant to further chemotherapy.

In 2019, Dr. Fang-Yu Du et al. studied new drugs that target CSCs and determined that chemotherapy cannot kill them:

> Generally, conventional chemotherapy can only inhibit tumor growth and lead to drug resistance, **but cannot kill CSCs [Cancer Stem Cells].** (10)

Testicular cancer is the only exception to this statement by Dr. Du's group—the one cell type in which chemotherapy does in fact kill the CSCs.

Successful Elimination of Cancer

Although oncologists may have just returned from a medical meeting discussing the CSC problem, they go about their daily routine on the oncology ward oblivious to this message. In 2013, Dr. Claire Pecqueur et al. discussed the need for a cancer treatment targeting both the tumor bulk and the CSCs:

> The successful elimination of a cancer requires an anti-cancer therapy that will affect both differentiated cancer cells and CSCs.... At present, conventional therapy that includes radio-, chemo-, and immunotherapy kills rapidly proliferating and differentiated cells. These treatments may cause the tumor to shrink **but will not prevent tumor recurrence.** Thus, a combination of treatments targeting both rapidly proliferating cancer cells and quiescent or slow-proliferating CSCs would be ideal. (11)

Testicular Cancer Cured with Chemotherapy

Unlike most other cancers, testicular cancer can be "cured" by chemotherapy. Why is this the case? The answer is that all cancers consist of two populations of cells. The cells making up the bulk of the tumor mass (tumor bulk cells) are actively replicating and sensitive to chemotherapy, while the CSCs (or progenitor cells) are dormant and not sensitive to chemotherapy. This is reversed for testicular cancer which has CSCs which are more sensitive to chemotherapy than the tumor bulk. This is explained by Dr. Timothy Pierpont et al. using a mouse testicular cancer xenograft study in *Cell Reports* (2017).

> Treatment of tumor-bearing mice with genotoxic chemotherapy not only prolonged survival and reduced tumor size, but selectively eliminated the OCT4-positive **CSCs.** We conclude that the chemo-sensitivity of TGCTs [testicular germ cancer cells] derives from the sensitivity of their cancer stem cells to DNA-damaging chemotherapy. (12–13)

Chemotherapy Activates Cancer Aggressivity

Another problem with chemotherapy is that the drug makes cancer more aggressive by activating massive inflammation in the body. Chemotherapy activates the inflammatory master controller called nuclear factor kappa B (NF-kB), which produces the inflammatory cytokine IL-6. Measure serum IL-6 after a course of chemotherapy and you will find its levels are massively elevated. According to Dr. Yu Rou Puar et al., this massively increased inflammation produced by chemotherapy is responsible for transforming the cancer cell type into a monster. (14):

Inflammation induced by chemotherapy:

1) Stimulates more rapid cancer growth (proliferation).

2) More resistance to apoptosis (programmed cell death).

3) More invasive and metastatic behavior of the cancer.

4) Stimulates angiogenesis (new blood vessel formation).

5) Creates a chemo-resistant cancer cell type. (14)

In *Nature* (2019), Dr. Ioanna Keklikoglou et al. studied breast cancer xenografts in mice, showing that chemotherapy has pro-metastatic effects:

Here we show that two classes of cytotoxic drugs…. taxanes and anthracyclines, elicit tumour-derived extracellular vesicles [EVs] with enhanced pro-metastatic capacity (15)

Chemotherapy Impairs Host Anti-Cancer Immune Response

Another adverse effect of chemotherapy on the host immune system is that it allows the tumor cells to escape immune detection and eradication. Dr. Jin Peng et al. in *Cancer Research* (2015) wrote that

chemotherapy induces local immune-suppression in ovarian cancer through NF-kB–mediated PD-L1 upregulation. [PD-L1 is Programmed Death Ligand] (16)

The Paradigm Shift in Oncology: Non-Chemo Targeted Pathway Approach

Even within the ranks of mainstream oncology, there is clamor for revolutionary change in the old chemotherapy paradigm. This sentiment was expressed by Drs. Daphne Day and Lillian Siu in 2016. They assert that the existing framework for cancer drug development is inefficient and unsustainable. Instead, Drs. Day and Siu contend that we should be using new technology, "systematic high-throughput methods" for screening libraries of drugs for their anti-cancer efficacy. They urge clinical trials that understand tumor biology and can find effective new drug combinations and useful biomarkers (lab tests):

It is apparent that the existing framework of oncological drug development… is inefficient and ultimately unsustainable. Systematic high-throughput methods…. can be utilized to explore novel therapeutic targets and identify synergistic or additive drug combinations. Clinical trial designs should be informed by comprehensive understanding of tumor biology and pharmacology…. and investigate new drug combinations…. co-development of biomarkers must be prioritized to refine and optimize patient selection. (17)

The Big Lie about Finding the Cure for Cancer

One of my favorite movies is the 1992 film *Medicine Man,* starring Sean Connery and Lorraine Bracco. Connery plays the role of a biologist doing cancer research in the Amazon rainforest who discovers a cure for cancer in a rare flowing plant. The flower extract is tested on an Amazonian tribal child suffering from cancer who miraculously recovers. Unfortunately, the message of the movie is based on the "big lie" that the "cure for cancer" is some rare, elusive flowering plant hidden deep in the rainforest. The reality is that 3,000 plant species worldwide have been identified as having anti-cancer activity. (18–19) If you look outside your window at your neighbor's garden or even the distant landscape, chances are that some of the greenery has anti-cancer activity, possibly providing the basis for the next generation of cancer drugs. (20–21)

The Repurposed Drug Revolution

A repurposed drug is an old drug that the FDA originally approved for a specific purpose, now used "off-label" for something else. Drugs repurposed for use against cancer include antifungal, antiparasitic, and antibacterial drugs; platelet inhibitors; COX-2 inhibitors; antihistamines; cardiac drugs; and the anti-diabetic drug metformin. Of the thousands of old drugs on the shelf at your local pharmacy, FDA-approved and ready to dispense, Dr. Pan Pantziarka et al. identified 268 such drugs repurposed as anti-cancer drugs. (22–23) In the pages to follow, we will discuss a few of these that seem most promising. I apologize in advance for skipping over or slighting any of the list of 268 repurposed drugs not mentioned. (24–25)

Expanding the Cancer Therapy Toolbox with Drug Repurposing

The need to incorporate repurposed drugs into cancer therapy is recognized by many experts in cancer research. Drs. Andresen Vibeke and Bjørn T. Gjertsen (2017) write:

> Cancer therapy needs a larger therapy toolbox and effective repurposing may be one important tool that increases the number of therapy responders in cancer. (26)

Repurposing Drugs for Prostate Cancer Treatment

In 2018, Dr. Beste Turanli et al. summarized a proposed list of repurposed drugs for prostate cancer treatment (27). This list includes:

- Dexamethasone—steroidal, anti-inflammatory
- Aspirin (ASA)—COX-1 and COX-2 inhibitor
- Diclofenac NSAID—COX-2 inhibitor
- Celecoxib NSAID—COX-2 inhibitor
- Minocycline, doxycycline, tetracycline—Antibiotic, anti-inflammatory
- Niclosamide—antiparasitic, potent Wnt/β-catenin inhibitor
- Itraconazole—antifungal; reversed drug resistance by inhibiting P-glycoprotein, Hedgehog, and Wnt/β-catenin pathways; inhibits angiogenesis
- Digoxin—cardiology drug used for congestive heart failure
- Valproic acid—HDAC inhibitor used for seizure disorder
- Statins—HMG-CoA reductase inhibitors; inhibit mevalonate pathway; used for reducing cholesterol

- Mifepristone—progesterone-receptor blocking drug (PR), used as an abortion drug
- Disulfiram—treatment of alcohol addiction
- Metformin—popular anti-diabetic drug.

Repurposed Drugs for Pancreatic Cancer

In 2019, Dr. Matthias Ilmer provided an updated list of repurposed drugs for pancreatic cancer, including (28):

- Hydroxychloroquine—antimalarial autophagy inhibitor
- Disulfiram—(Antabuse) for alcohol addiction
- Itraconazole—antifungal
- Propranolol—beta blocker
- Vitamin D3

In 2019, Drs. Mrugank Parmar and Shital Panchal suggested the following list of repurposed drugs using a pharmaco-vigilance approach. (29)

- Propranolol—beta blocker
- Metformin—anti-diabetic
- Pioglitazone
- Dabigatran

These and others will be discussed in the pages to follow (30–33).

Care Oncology METRICS Study

In 2017, Care Oncology Clinic (COC) in London launched an observational study—the first of its kind—of a combination of repurposed oral anti-cancer drugs in 207 cancer patients. The primary study completion date is May 2023 (Clinical Trial Identifier: NCT02201381) (34).

Two hundred and seven cancer patients will receive the following drugs:

- Atorvastatin (statin drug) 80mg/day.
- Metformin 1000–2000 mg/day
- Doxycycline 100mg/day
- Mebendazole 100mg/day

METRICS and the COC Protocol for Cancer Doubles Survival in Glioblastoma

In 2019, Dr. Samir Gupt Agarwal et al. of COC proposed their protocol for cancer, which involves use of the four of the repurposed drugs mentioned above: metformin, atorvastatin, mebendazole, and doxycycline. Preliminary data was presented in 2019 for 95 glioblastoma patients in their clinical trial (METRICS study NCT02201381). The preliminary data showed the COC protocol nearly doubled the survival time of glioblastoma patients from 14 to 28 months and doubled the number of patients surviving to the 2-year mark. (34)

List of Repurposed Drugs in Clinical Trials

In 2019, Dr. A. Luciano et al. reported a list of drugs repurposed for colorectal cancer treatment currently in clinical trials. This list includes: aspirin, celecoxib, doxycycline, etodolac, indomethacin, mebendazole, metformin, niclosamide, propranolol, simvastatin, and valproate. (35)

Preventing Cancer with Selenium, Iodine, Vitamin D3, and Di-Indole Methane

How can we reduce the incidence of cancer in the population? Deficiencies in blood levels of selenium, iodine and vitamin D3 are associated with increased cancer risk. Therefore, we routinely test for selenium, iodine and vitamin D3 levels and supplement if found low. Di-Indole Methane (DIM), derived from cruciferous vegetables such as broccoli, is a breast cancer preventive, exerting beneficial effects on estrogen metabolism, and is given routinely to all females. This is our basic in-office cancer prevention program. (43-47)

Change Is Coming: The Paradigm Shift

The wheels of progress in medicine turn slowly. Institutional change may not happen anytime soon. However, in spite of heavy resistance by mainstream oncology, the paradigm is shifting. No one could have predicted it. Yet the revolution in cancer treatment is happening with a grassroots movement of people using repurposed drugs to target metabolic pathways in both bulk tumor and CSCs. As is true for many modern revolutions, the Internet is the catalyst, providing a platform for people to share stories and advice. This is an historic revolution in the history of medicine. Will you join ranks and be part of the revolution?

References for Chapter 2: Conventional Oncology Success or Failure?

1) Siegel, Rebecca L., Kimberly D. Miller, and Ahmedin Jemal. "Cancer statistics, 2019." CA: a cancer journal for clinicians 69.1 (2019): 7-34.

2) Haines, Ian. "The war on cancer: time for a new terminology." Lancet 383.1883 (2014): 60907-7.

3) Cupp, Julia, et al. "Analysis of factors associated with in-hospital mortality in lung cancer chemotherapy patients with neutropenia." Clinical lung cancer 19.2 (2018): e163-e169

4) Drug Sales Bring Huge Profits, And Scrutiny, to Cancer Doctors, By Reed Abelson New York times Jan. 26, 2003

5) Stadtmauer, Edward A. "A dramatic story of hope and reality." Journal of Clinical Oncology 26.1 (2008): 11-12.

6) Morgan, Graeme, Robyn Ward, and Michael Barton. "The contribution of cytotoxic chemotherapy to 5-year survival in adult malignancies." Clinical oncology 16.8 (2004): 549-560.

7) Wise, Peter H. "Cancer drugs, survival, and ethics." BMJ 355 (2016): i5792.

8) Grössmann, Nicole, and Claudia Wild. "Between January 2009 and April 2016, 134 novel anticancer therapies were approved: what is the level of knowledge concerning the clinical benefit at the time of approval?." ESMO open 1.6 (2016): esmoopen-2016.

9) Masters, Gregory A., et al. "Clinical cancer advances 2015: annual report on progress against cancer from the American Society of Clinical Oncology." Journal of Clinical Oncology 33.7 (2015): 786-809.

10) Du, Fang-Yu, et al. "Targeting cancer stem cells in drug discovery: Current state and future perspectives." World journal of stem cells 11.7 (2019): 398.

11) Pecqueur, Claire, et al. "Targeting metabolism to induce cell death in cancer cells and cancer stem cells." International journal of cell biology 2013 (2013).

12) Pierpont, Timothy M., et al. "Chemotherapy-induced depletion of OCT4-positive cancer stem cells in a mouse model of malignant testicular cancer." Cell reports 21.7 (2017): 1896-1909.

13) Pierpont, Timothy Michael. "A Novel Mouse Model To Elucidate The Origins And Therapeutic Sensitivity Of Testicular Germ Cell Tumors." (2017).

14) Puar, Yu Rou, et al. "Evidence for the involvement of the master transcription factor NF-κB in cancer initiation and progression." Biomedicines 6.3 (2018): 82.

15) Keklikoglou, Ioanna, et al. "Chemotherapy elicits pro-metastatic extracellular vesicles in breast cancer models." Nature cell biology 21.2 (2019): 190.

16) Peng, Jin, et al. "Chemotherapy induces programmed cell death-ligand 1 overexpression via the nuclear factor-κB to foster an immunosuppressive tumor microenvironment in ovarian cancer." Cancer research 75.23 (2015): 5034-5045.

17) Day, Daphne, and Lillian L. Siu. "Approaches to modernize the combination drug development paradigm." Genome medicine 8.1 (2016): 115.

18) Solowey, Elisha, et al. "Evaluating medicinal plants for anticancer activity." The Scientific World Journal 2014 (2014).

19) Seca, Ana ML, and Diana CGA Pinto. "Plant secondary metabolites as anticancer agents: successes in clinical trials and therapeutic application." International journal of molecular sciences 19.1 (2018): 263.

20) Greenwell, M., and P. K. S. M. Rahman. "Medicinal plants: their use in anticancer treatment." International journal of pharmaceutical sciences and research 6.10 (2015): 4103.

21) Poonam, Sharma, and Majee Chandana. "A review on anticancer natural drugs." International Journal of PharmTech Research 8.7 (2015): 131-141.

22) Pantziarka, Pan, et al. "Repurposing non-cancer drugs in oncology—how many drugs are out there?." bioRxiv (2017): 197434.

23) Pantziarka, Pan, et al. "ReDO_DB: the repurposing drugs in oncology database." ecancermedicalscience 12 (2018).

24) Pantziarka, Pan, et al. "Repurposing drugs in your medicine cabinet: untapped opportunities for cancer therapy?" Future Oncol 11.2 (2015): 182.

25) Antoszczak, Michał, et al. "Old wine in new bottles: Drug repurposing in oncology." European journal of pharmacology 866 (2020): 172784.

26) Andresen, Vibeke, and Bjørn T. Gjertsen. "Drug repurposing for the treatment of acute myeloid leukemia." Frontiers in medicine 4 (2017): 211.

27) Turanli, Beste, et al. "Drug repositioning for effective prostate cancer treatment." Frontiers in Physiology 9 (2018).

28) Ilmer, Matthias, et al. "Repurposed drugs in pancreatic ductal adenocarcinoma: An update." The Cancer Journal 25.2 (2019): 134-138.

29) Parmar, Mrugank, and Shital Panchal. "Drug Repostioning of Non-Cancer Drugs for Cancer Treatment Through Pharmacovigilance Approach - Repurposing Drugs in Oncology." Asian J Pharm Clin Res 12.2 (2019): 310-314.

30) Nowak-Sliwinska, Patrycja, Leonardo Scapozza, and Ariel Ruiz i Altaba. "Drug repurposing in oncology: Compounds, pathways, phenotypes and computational approaches for colorectal cancer." Biochimica et Biophysica Acta (BBA)-Reviews on Cancer (2019).

31) Wuerth, Roberto, et al. "Drug-repositioning opportunities for cancer therapy: novel molecular targets for known compounds." Drug discovery today 21.1 (2016): 190-199.

32) Crispino, Sergio, et al. "Repurposing non-cancer drugs for Breast Cancer? An emerging opportunity." European Journal of Cancer 92 (2018): S93-S94.

33) Ozsvári, Béla, Rebecca Lamb, and Michael P. Lisanti. "Repurposing of FDA-approved drugs against cancer—Focus on metastasis." Aging 8.4 (2016): 567.

34) Agrawal, Samir Gupt, et al. "A new method for ethical and efficient evidence generation for off-label medication use in oncology (A case study in Glioblastoma)." Frontiers in Pharmacology 10 (2019): 681.

35) Luciano, A., F. Malizia, and M. M. Menacho. "Modern Strategies in Cancer Study: Drug Repositioning in Colorectal Cancer Treatment." (2019).

36) Ribas, Antoni, and Jedd D. Wolchok. "Cancer immunotherapy using checkpoint blockade." Science 359.6382 (2018): 1350-1355.

37) Yeo, Belinda, et al. "The dark side of granulocyte-colony stimulating factor: a supportive therapy with potential to promote tumour progression."

Clinical & experimental metastasis 35.4 (2018): 255-267.

38) Dobrenis, Kostantin, et al. "Granulocyte colony-stimulating factor off-target effect on nerve outgrowth promotes prostate cancer development." International journal of cancer 136.4 (2015): 982-988.

39) Wang, Juntao, et al. "Granulocyte-colony stimulating factor promotes proliferation, migration and invasion in glioma cells." Cancer biology & therapy 13.6 (2012): 389-400.

40) Kast, Richard E., et al. "Glioblastoma-synthesized G-CSF and GM-CSF contribute to growth and immunosuppression: Potential therapeutic benefit from dapsone, fenofibrate, and ribavirin." Tumor Biology 39.5 (2017).

41) Zhang, Xinghua, et al. "Upregulation of microRNA-125b by G-CSF promotes metastasis in colorectal cancer." Oncotarget 8.31 (2017): 50642.

42) Darvin, Pramod, et al. "Immune checkpoint inhibitors: recent progress and potential biomarkers." Experimental & molecular medicine 50.12 (2018): 1-11.

43) Gandin, Valentina, et al. "Organic selenium compounds as potential chemotherapeutic agents for improved cancer treatment." Free Radical Biology and Medicine 127 (2018): 80-97.

44) Grant, William B. "A review of the evidence supporting the vitamin D-cancer prevention hypothesis in 2017." Anticancer research 38.2 (2018): 1121-1136.

45) Kargar, Saeed, et al. "Urinary Iodine Concentrations in Cancer Patients." Asian Pacific journal of cancer prevention: APJCP 18.3 (2017): 819.

46) Rappaport, Jay. "Changes in dietary iodine explains increasing incidence of breast cancer with distant involvement in young women." Journal of Cancer 8.2 (2017): 174.

47) Thomson, Cynthia A., Emily Ho, and Meghan B. Strom. "Chemopreventive properties of 3, 3'-diindolylmethane in breast cancer: evidence from experimental and human studies." Nutrition reviews 74.7 (2016): 432-443.

Chapter 3

The Ten Hallmarks of Cancer

IN ORDER TO BETTER UNDERSTAND how to target metabolic pathways in cancer cells, let's examine their characteristics and the ways they are different from normal cells. Perhaps the two most seminal articles on this topic come from Drs. Douglas Hanahan and Robert A. Weinberg, entitled "The Ten Hallmarks Cancer," published in *Cell* in 2000, and revised in 2011 (1–2). For those less technically oriented, I recommend the *Scientific American* series by molecular biologist Dr. Buddhini Samarasinghe, which covers the topic nicely. (3)

Here are the ten hallmarks of cancer according to Drs. Hanahan and Weinberg:

1) Self-sufficiency in growth signals—proliferative growth signals are made by the cancer cells themselves or from hijacked surrounding stromal cells.

2) Insensitivity to anti-growth signals.

3) Evasion of apoptosis (programmed cell death). This includes upregulation of the BCL-2 apoptotic protein, attachment of HKII to the voltage-dependent anion channels (VDAC), mutation of the P53 gene, etc.

4) Replicative immortality—i.e., no Hayflick Limit. The Hayflick Limit, or Hayflick phenomenon, named after its discoverer Leonard Hayflick, is the number of times a normal human cell population will divide before cell division stops. The cancer cell replicates indefinitely.

5) Induction of angiogenesis, also called tumor vascularity.

6) Invasion and metastasis, the cancer spreads throughout the body.

7) Genome instability, the cancer cells have many mutations that keep changing.

8) Upregulation of inflammation with activation of inflammatory pathways (NF-kB, COX-2, 5-LOX etc.)

9) Reprograming of energy metabolism—Relocation of hexokinase 2 (HK2) to the VDAC located on the Mitochondrial Outer Membrane (MOM), upregulation of pyruvate dehydrogenase kinase (PDK); inhibition of pyruvate dehydrogenase complex (PDC); inhibition of the mitochondrial oxidative phosphorylation (OXPHOS) system; stimulation of GLYCOLYSIS (the Warburg effect).

10) Evasion of destruction by the host immune system, cancer cells disable the host immune system, also called immune suppression.

Modification of Hanahan and Weinberg's Ten Hallmarks for Cracking Cancer Toolkit

For the purposes of the *Cracking Cancer Toolkit*, we will modify, simplify, and re-prioritize these ten hallmarks of cancer. At the top of our list is my new concept, which I call the "three pillars of cancer cell metabolism." Using "metabolic plasticity", the cancer cell switches among these three pillars in order to maintain survival.

To achieve what's known as "synthetic lethality," we must block all three at the same time.

The three pillars of cancer cell metabolism are:

1) OXPHOS—Oxidative phosphorylation in the mitochondria.

2) GLYCOLYSIS—Metabolism of glucose in the cytoplasm (Warburg Effect).

3) Autophagy—Cells literally "eat themselves" by engulfing and digesting organelles.

4) The Fourth Pillar, the Immune System, is of equal importance to the first three. Restoring host anti-cancer immunity is discussed in later chapters.

Note: In this book, we will use the term GLYCOLYSIS in capital letters to denote aerobic glycolysis, also called the Warburg Effect, a characteristic of cancer cells. This is different from anaerobic glycolysis which occurs in normal cells, for example hypoxic skeletal muscle cells will use anaerobic glycolysis.

These next five pathways are considered important targets for *Cracking Cancer Toolkit*

1) HK2 attached to VDAC. (Hexokinase II is the first enzymatic step in GLYCOLYSIS)

2) Cancer stem cells and Wnt, Hedgehog, and Notch pathways.

3) Tumor evasion of the immune system.

4) Inflammatory Pathways

5) The tumor micro-environment. Recruitment of stromal cells provides growth factors and nutrients to the tumor.

We will discuss these "three pillars of cancer cell metabolism" and five additional pathways throughout the book.

Weinberg's Ten Hallmarks of Cancer: A Closer Look

Let's look at Drs. Hanahan and Weinberg's ten hallmarks of cancer in greater detail:

1. Self-Sufficiency in Growth Signals

Growth Signaling factors such as PDGF (platelet-derived growth factor), VEGF (vascular endothelial growth factor), EGF (epidermal growth factor), OGF (opiate derived growth factor) and Estrogen bind to cell membrane receptors which then activate the MAPk/Erk signaling pathway, which "turns on" genetic expression for cell growth and proliferation. Normally, adult cells stop growing, and spend most of the time in a quiescent phase doing their specialized jobs as "worker bees" in the hierarchy of the organism. In order to leave the dormant state, start growing and replicating, the cell requires growth factors which overcome a critical checkpoint, which would normally prevent uncontrolled growth. However, the cancer cell has bypassed this checkpoint by either generating its own growth factors, or eliminating the need for them, usually by mutating the Ras protein into "the permanent on signal."

2. Insensitivity to Anti-Growth Signals

Normally, anti-growth signaling proteins outside the cancer cell tell it to behave and stop replicating. These are the anti-growth signals. Cancer cells are no longer responsive to cell-signaling proteins which normally provide checkpoints in the cell cycle. Thus, cancer cells become insensitive to anti-growth signals and divide uncontrollably.

3. Evading Apoptosis

Apoptosis is the cell-signaling pathway leading to programmed cell death (PCD). For the purpose of our discussion, evading apoptosis is perhaps one of the most important of the ten hallmarks of cancer. Apoptosis is a normal part of the cell cycle, and a mechanism for destroying unwanted or damaged cells, such as cancer cells, in the body.

Do you remember those old spy movies? Just before being sent off on a new mission, the secret agent was handed a cyanide pill in case of capture. Committing suicide was preferable to inevitable torture and disclosure of secret information to the enemy. Well, all of our cells have a similar "suicide pill," ready when the time comes. If activated, molecular programs "hard wired" inside the cell trigger an irreversible cascade, culminating in organized cell death.

We are no strangers to apoptosis. Ten million of our own cells commit apoptosis (suicide) every day. They have become damaged and dysfunctional, so they are instructed to undergo apoptosis. These lost cells require replacement cells to take their place (4–6).

The cancer cell, however, evades apoptosis by placing Hexokinase II at the VDAC pore on the outer mitochondrial membrane, preventing apoptosis.

Apoptosis is enormously important in biol

ogy, embryology, health and medicine. The 2002 Nobel Prize for Physiology or Medicine was awarded to Drs. Sydney Brenner, H. Robert Horvitz, and John E. Sulston for their work on apoptosis (33).

Embryology Relies on Apoptosis

Embryologic development relies on apoptosis to remove unwanted cells in order to form appendages, organs, and tissue layers. An example is the transformation of a tadpole into a frog. The tadpole's tail is removed by apoptosis. Another example is the webbing between the fingers of a human embryo; again, these webbing cells are removed by apoptosis to form well-defined fingers. In disease states, there may be disruption in the cellular machinery or signaling pathways that control apoptosis. Excessive apoptosis may cause neurodegenerative disease. Not enough apoptosis may cause cancer. (4–6)

Apoptosis vs. Necrosis

Apoptosis is characterized by cell shrinkage and preservation of the cell membrane, which keeps cell contents nice and neat as the cell goes through organized dissolution and digestion. This must be distinguished from cell necrosis, a more brutal form of cell death caused by toxic injury associated with chemotherapy treatment. Necrotic cells typically show cytoplasmic swelling and rupture of the cell membrane, with release of cellular debris into the surrounding tissues, which evokes an inflammatory response. A quote from Bruce Alberts in his book, *Molecular Biology of the Cell* explains this difference.

Cells that die as a result of acute injury typically swell and burst. They spill their contents all over their neighbors—a process called cell necrosis—causing a potentially damaging inflammatory response. By contrast, a cell that undergoes apoptosis dies neatly, without damaging its neighbors. The cell shrinks and condenses. The cytoskeleton collapses, the nuclear envelope disassembles, and the nuclear DNA breaks up into fragments. Most importantly, the cell surface is altered, displaying properties that cause the dying cell to be rapidly phagocytosed [ingested by phagocytes], either by a neighboring cell or by a macrophage, before any leakage of its contents occurs. This not only avoids the damaging consequences of cell necrosis but also allows the organic components of the dead cell to be recycled by the cell that ingests it. (7)

The Mitochondria Control Apoptosis

There are many pathways leading to apoptotic cell death, and most of them converge on the mitochondria, little oval organelles involved in energy production. Signaling proteins (such as Bax) attach to the mitochondrial membrane, which then releases cytochrome C, which binds to a protein called apaf-1, which in turn induces formation of the apoptosome, a seven-spoke wheel protein that activates the caspase cascade, an irreversible event leading to cell death.

The P53 Gene—"Guardian of the Genome"

Our DNA may be damaged by environmental chemicals, irradiation, or even by oxidation generated by normal cellular energy production. The P53 Gene, dubbed "guardian of the genome," detects this DNA damage in the nucleus. In the event of DNA damage, the cell cycle is arrested to initiate DNA repair. If the damage exceeds our capacity for repair, then apoptosis is triggered by the P53 gene with the death-signal protein Bax, which tells the mitochondria to release cytochrome c and activate the caspase cascade. A common method used by the cancer cell to evade apoptosis is to harbor a mutation in the P53 gene, rendering it non-functional. Roughly half of all cancers harbor such a mutation.

The Biology of Cancer: What Causes Cancer?

If you ask your local doctor, "What causes cancer?" more than likely they may tell you "We just don't know." This is not entirely correct. We do know. Even the American Cancer society admits that carcinogenic chemicals in the environment cause cancer.

Try this experiment: Go to your local university and ask a cancer researcher the following question: "How do you give cancer to your experimental mice?" The cancer researcher will typically reply: "We give the mice carcinogenic chemicals." These cancer-causing chemicals cause oxidative damage to the nuclear and mitochondrial DNA. Of course, our cells are prepared for this and will quickly repair the oxidative damage with the seleno-protein repair system. However, our DNA repair mechanisms can be overwhelmed, leading to transformation of the normal cell to a cancer cell.

4. Replicative Immortality

Normal cells have a well-defined life cycle, starting out as a primitive stem cell, they differentiate into their predestined specialized cell type (liver cell, muscle cell, nerve cell, light receptor cell, red blood cell, etc.) Once differentiated, these mature cells have a limited life span, replicating about fifty to sixty times, governed by the Hayflick Limit, named after Leonard Hayflick, who discovered it.

During the life span of a cell, as a result of the aging process, cell damage accumulates and causes loss of function. This aging process is caused by oxidative damage to cell organelles, a normal adverse effect of mitochondrial energy production. Once the cell becomes dysfunctional, internal mechanisms signal it is time for PCD by apoptosis and autophagy, two cell mechanisms we will discuss in more detail below. This end of life event for the cell is called "cell senescence."

The Cell Time Clock: The Telomere

The time clock that controls the Hayflick Limit is located at the end of each chromosome. Called the telomere, this region shortens slightly every time cell division takes place. Like a candle burning down, when the telomere eventually becomes too short, it signals the cell to enter senescence and ultimately apoptotic cell death.

The Hayflick Limit Does Not Apply to Cancer!

For cancer cells, the Hayflick Limit does not apply, as cancer cells are immortal and will replicate indefinitely. Cancer cells have escaped the final instruction of PCD. The cancer cell laughs at "cell senescence," proliferates uncontrollably, and is seemingly immune to normal control. How do cancer cells avoid the telomere-shortening mechanism that limits the total number of cell replications, the Hayflick Limit? Cancer cells have the ability to re-grow their telomeres by making an enzyme called telomerase. They are free from control and can replicate indefinitely. However, the price of immortality is continuous accumulation of genetic damage, which is visible upon microscopic examination of the cancer cell.

5. Inducing Angiogenesis

A growing cancer mass has a voracious appetite for nutrition, mostly in the form of massive amounts of glucose. These nutrients can only be supplied by blood flow; therefore, cancers need new blood vessels to provide nourishment. Growth factors such as VEGF signal the vascular tree to grow new blood vessels, a process called angiogenesis. In normal organisms, angiogenesis is a carefully controlled physiologic event found in wound healing, embryogenesis, ischemia and inflammation. However, angiogenesis induced by tumors is uncontrolled, resulting in tangle of disorderly vessels responsible for the "tumor blush" visible on contrast-enhanced imaging with CAT or MRI scans, a telltale sign of a growing malignancy.

6. Tissue Invasion and Metastases

A growing lump detected somewhere in our body is bad enough. Even worse, cancer cells have the perfidious ability to spread elsewhere and grow satellite masses in distant locations throughout the body. This is called metastatic disease, a poor prognostic indicator, and the major cause of cancer-related mortality. The production of proteolytic enzymes called matrix metalloproteases, which dissolve the extracellular matrix, allows the cancer cells to become locally invasive. This frightful ability of the cancer cell to invade is a feature shared by the trophoblast cell of the placenta, and is the basis for the trophoblast theory of cancer, originally proposed in 1906 by the Scottish embryologist John Beard. For over 100 years, the theory was largely ignored by the scientific community until recent advances in molecular biology have indeed confirmed that cancer cells share many of the molecular pathways and circuits of the trophoblast. (8) For more on this, see chapter 25, on the trophoblastic theory of cancer.

7. Genome Instability and Mutation

Polyploidy and Aneuploidy

Normal human cells have 46 chromosomes, while cancer cells have more. This unusual increased number of chromosomes in cancer cells is called *polyploidy* or *aneuploidy*. (9)

The increased number of chromosomes is caused by a defect in the machinery of cell division. The increased amount of nuclear material (chromatin) may be visible on histologic examination using light or electron microscopy.

Cancer cells have lost the ability to repair damaged DNA and are genetically unstable. In addition to the frequent mutations, cancer cells may have deletions of genetic material and loss or duplication of whole chromosomes, etc. Now that we have tools that allow us to sequence cancer genomes, we have discovered that while they are all vastly different, nearly all cancer genomes have loss of DNA repair mechanisms, accumulating more and more genetic damage and instability over time. (10)

The breast cancer (BRCA) gene mutation, which confers increased risk of breast and ovarian cancer, involves the inability to repair damaged DNA, thought to be related to deficient seleno-protein repair mechanisms, since selenium supplementation reverses the defect. (11)

8. Upregulated Inflammation

The successful cancer hijacks our immune system by activating nuclear factor kappa B (NF-kB), the inflammatory master controller that causes massive elevations in inflammatory cytokines such as IL-6. Thus, the well-known inflammatory response that creates a "wound that won't heal." For example, the ulcerated breast mass looks like a superficial open wound. However, unlike a typical wound, which eventually seals over and heals, the cancer mass continues to grow and ulcerate.

9. Reprogramming of Energy Metabolism

The Warburg effect describes the way in which cancer-cell energy production shifts from normal oxidative respiration (OXPHOS) to GLYCOLYSIS, a more primitive state, similar to a fermenting yeast cell in which glucose is converted to energy with lactic acid as a byproduct. (12)

Normal mammalian cells use oxygen to produce energy through oxidative phosphorylation (OXPHOS), which takes place in the mitochondrial electron transport chain. Energy production reverts to GLYCOLYSIS under conditions of oxygen deprivation (hypoxia). In cancer cells, however, mitochondrial energy production is locked into the GLYCOLYSIS pathway, even in the presence of plentiful oxygen, a state called *aerobic fermentation* or *aerobic glycolysis*. In this book, we refer to this simply as GLYCOLYSIS, in capital letters to denote the Warburg Effect.

Cancer as a Metabolic Disease— the Warburg Effect

By the way, our friend the trophoblast cell also utilizes GLYCOLYSIS, just like cancer cells. (13) Some experts regard the reprogramming of energy metabolism as the most significant of the cancer hallmarks, providing a more unified understanding of cancer biology and subsequent treatment strategies.

In *Cancer Cell* (2008), Drs. Guido Kroemer and Jacques Pouyssegur write, "Tumor cell metabolism is cancer's Achilles' heel."(14)

This topic could very well fill an entire book. In fact, that book has already been published and is entitled *Cancer as a Metabolic Disease: On the Origin, Management, and Prevention of Cancer*, by Thomas Seyfried (2012), professor of biology at Boston College. I was fortunate to be in the audience for Dr. Seyfried's presentation at the 2013 American College for the Advancement of Medicine (ACAM) medical meeting at the Diplomat Hotel in Hollywood. According to Dr. Seyfried, cancer is not a "somatic genetic disease"; rather, it is a perturbation of mitochondrial energy metabolism. (15) Another book, perhaps more accessible to the layman, is *Tripping Over the Truth: The Metabolic Theory of Cancer*, by Travis Christofferson. (16)

As mentioned above, under conditions of oxygen deprivation (hypoxia), normal cells will shift into an alternate form of energy production, called anaerobic glycolysis, which preferentially utilizes glucose in the cytoplasm, resulting in production of the byproduct lactic acid. This tissue buildup of lactic acid is called *lactic acidosis,* which causes the muscle pain of long distance marathon runners. Even in the presence of oxygen, cancer cells preferentially utilize GLYCOLYSIS in the cytoplasm. The Warburg Effect in cancer cells, also called "aerobic glycolysis", requires massive amounts of glucose to meet nutrient demands of the proliferating cancer mass. The exception of course, is the CSC, which is dormant, has slowed its metabolic rate, has arrested cell replication, and uses very little glucose. For the purpose of this book, GLYCOLYSIS (in capital letters) refers to the Warburg Effect in cancer cells.

Mitochondria—Are They Defective or Not?

Followers of Otto Warburg, who believe in the metabolic basis of cancer, consider the disease to originate in the mitochondria, which reside in the cytoplasm of cancer cells. It was predicted that the mitochondria in cancer cells would be defective or absent, and indeed, this was found to be the case, as demonstrated by electron microscopy. In contradiction, cancer cells grown in culture (in vitro) appear to have intact, fairly normal appearing mitochondria. Nonetheless, even though they may appear morphologically normal, the mitochondria of cancer cells have been reprogrammed to serve as "biosynthetic organelles" whose main job is to grow the tumor biomass involved in consuming massive amounts of glucose and other nutrients to sustain rapid growth and proliferation. (12–15)

PET-Scanning– High Glucose Uptake by Cancer Cells

The avid uptake of glucose by the cancer cell is the basis for modern cancer imaging at the hospital. Positron emission tomography (PET scanning) with the flouro-deoxy-glucose (F-18-FDG) tracer "lights up" cancer masses, and serves as an excellent way to visualize cancer deposits anywhere in the body. The pitfall of the PET scan is that the CSC is dormant, quiescent, and not actively metabolizing glucose, rendering it invisible on the PET scan. (17)

Insulin-Induced Hypoglycemia

Avid glucose uptake and utilization by cancer cells might suggest a possible cancer therapy. Starve the cancer of its main nutrient, glucose, by reducing blood sugar levels. This can be done with dietary modifications that reduce blood sugar, such as ketogenic and low-carbohydrate diets. This can also be done with insulin, a hormone produced by the pancreas to control blood sugar. Injection of insulin causes blood sugar levels to plummet.

Insulin Shock Therapy

An old medical practice from the 1950s, now considered obsolete, was the psychiatric treatment for depression called insulin shock therapy, which induced a hypoglycemic coma, a form of "shock therapy." The patient is given intravenous insulin under controlled circumstances causing profound hypoglycemia, a drastic reduction in blood glucose levels and a temporary insulin-coma. Doctors observed that in some patients undergoing this treatment who also harbored malignancies, the cancers would go into remission. In 1962, two such reports of cancer remission from insulin shock therapy appeared in the psychiatric literature. The doctors speculated that the treatment induced low blood sugar, which starved the cancer mass, causing metabolic catastrophe and cancer cell death. (18–19)

Insulin-Potentiated Chemotherapy

The cancer cells have a voracious appetite for glucose and can be "starved" by insulin-induced hypoglycemia. This became the basis for a cancer treatment called IPT (insulin-potentiated therapy) involving the intravenous administration of insulin combined with low-dose chemotherapy. The cancer cell membranes contain microscopic pores that open in response to insulin, allowing rapid influx of either glucose or drug into the cancer cell. This maneuver "tricks" the cancer cell into taking up the chemotherapy drug instead of glucose, making the chemotherapy more effective at a lower dose. The concurrent use of insulin allows the reduction in chemotherapy dosage while achieving the same anti-cancer effect, achieving a reduction in toxicity of the chemotherapy treatment. (20–23)

The "Greek Test"—Research Genetics Cancer Center (RGCC) Group

The selection of chemotherapy agent can be critical, and in order to increase the odds of success, IPT is usually combined with some form of chemotherapy sensitivity testing. One such test is called the "Greek Test," from the RGCC, established in 2004 by Dr. Ioannis Papasotiriou. The Greek Test uses a patient blood sample to isolate circulating tumor cells, which are then grown in culture. The next step is isolation and extraction of the messenger RNA from the circulating tumor cells, which can then identify upregulated cancer cell pathways targeted for treatment. In addition, the isolated circulating tumor cells are tested against a battery of drugs and supplements for anti-cancer activity, providing a useful sensitivity chart that indicates which drugs are effective and which drugs are not effective for this particular cancer cell type. (24–30)

Dr. Panagiotis Apostolou et al. write (2017):

> The RNA was used as template for micro-array experiments in the Human MI ReadyArray platform, while a universal reference RNA was used as reference… the data was then used to determine upregulated metabolic pathways, and sensitivities to various treatments with natural substances and drugs. (24)

10. Tumor Immune Evasion

Normally, our immune system serves as a cancer surveillance mechanism: The cancer cell dies by apoptosis and our macrophages then gobble up the dead cells. The successful cancer hijacks our immune system, suppressing our innate immunity from cancer.

Restoring our immune system's ability to kill cancer cells is an important part of any cancer treatment program. Until recently, conventional oncology completely ignored this important aspect of cancer treatment. However, this is changing with the introduction of immunother-

apies in the form of checkpoint inhibitors and CAR T cell therapies. The successful anti-cancer program includes restoration of the host immune system's anti-cancer functions.

Many of the drugs discussed in this book modify the immune response. A few examples are: cimetidine (Tagamet®); dichloroacetate (DCA), propranolol, and mifepristone (RU-486). See chapters 26-30 for in-depth discussion of restoring host anti-cancer immunity. See the Quick Reference Guide for a more complete list of these agents.

Tumor Microenvironment

Now that we have concluded the ten hallmarks of cancer, let's look at a few more important aspects of cancer that deserve to be included on the list. The tumor micro-environment (TME) must be mentioned. Cancer tumors hijack normal stromal cells in the surrounding tissues, such as cancer-associated fibroblasts (CAFs), to secrete growth factors and provide nutrients to the growing cancer mass. Two microenvironment agents discussed in this book, for example, are pyrvinium and sulfasalazine.

In 2003, Drs. Peter Gout et al. studied the effect of an old rheumatology drug, sulfasalazine (Azulfidine®), on the tumor microenvironment of lymphoma. In order to survive, lymphoma cells need cysteine from the cells of their microenvironment. Sulfasalazine blocks cysteine transport from the micro-environment into the cancer cell. Dr. Gout et al. propose that the anti-cancer effect of sulfasalazine:

> involves inhibition of cysteine secretion by tumor-associated somatic cells (macro-

phages, dendritic cells), leading to cysteine starvation of the tumor cells and apoptosis. (31)

Metabolic Plasticity of Cancer Stem Cells

The reason for relapse after chemotherapy is the dormant CSC. Although ignored by conventional oncology, eradicating the CSC is the key to a successful anti-cancer program. Recent studies reveal that CSCs display heterogeneity and metabolic plasticity, meaning they shift their metabolic pathways, as well as their nutrient sources, depending on the micro-environment, shifting back and forth from OXPHOS to GLYCOLYSIS. Dr. Géraldine Gentric et al. (2017) write:

> Glucose utilization and carbon sources in tumors are much more heterogeneous than initially thought. Indeed, new studies emerged and revealed a dual capacity of tumor cells for Glycolytic and oxidative phosphorylation (OXPHOS) metabolism. (32)

The third metabolic pathway is "protective autophagy," which allows the stressed cancer cell to survive against the most toxic chemotherapy regimen. Autophagy inhibitors are discussed in later chapters 31-35.

Conclusion

Cracking Cancer Toolkit proposes a new approach to addressing all three pillars of cancer-cell metabolism, OXPHOS, GLYCOLYSIS, and Autophagy. The metabolic plasticity of the cancer cell requires the use of a combination of two or more anti-cancer agents to block all three pathways, thereby achieving "synthetic lethality."

References for Chapter 3: The Ten Hallmarks of Cancer

1) Hanahan, Douglas, and Robert A. Weinberg. "The hallmarks of cancer." cell 100.1 (2000): 57-70.

2) Hanahan, Douglas, and Robert A. Weinberg. "Hallmarks of cancer: the next generation." cell 144.5 (2011): 646-674.

3) Samarasinghe, Buddhini. The Hallmarks of Cancer 9: Reprogramming Energy Metabolism. October 8th, 2014. Scientific American Guest Blog.

4) Kerr, John FR, Andrew H. Wyllie, and Alastair R. Currie. "Apoptosis: a basic biological phenomenon with wide ranging implications in tissue kinetics." British journal of cancer 26.4 (1972): 239.

5) Fadeel, B., and S. Orrenius. "Apoptosis: a basic biological phenomenon with wide-ranging implications in human disease." Journal of internal medicine 258.6 (2005): 479-517.

6) Elmore, Susan. "Apoptosis: a review of programmed cell death." Toxicologic pathology 35.4 (2007): 495-516.

7) Alberts, Bruce, et al. "Molecular Biology of the Cell 4th edn (New York: Garland Science)." Ann Bot 91 (2002): 401.

8) Ferretti, C., et al. "Molecular circuits shared by placental and cancer cells, and their implications in the proliferative, invasive and migratory capacities of trophoblasts." Human reproduction update 13.2 (2007): 121-141.

9) Duesberg, Peter, and David Rasnick. "Aneuploidy, the somatic mutation that makes cancer a species of its own." Cell motility and the cytoskeleton 47.2 (2000): 81-107.

10) Shen, Zhiyuan. "Genomic instability and cancer: an introduction." Journal of molecular cell biology 3.1 (2011): 1-3.

11) Kowalska E.,et al.(2005) Increased rates of chromosome breakage in BRCA1 carriers are normalized by oral selenium supplementation. Cancer Epidemiol. Biomarkers Prev., 14, 1302–1306.

12) Ward, Patrick S., and Craig B. Thompson. "Metabolic reprogramming: a cancer hallmark even Warburg did not anticipate." Cancer cell 21.3 (2012): 297-308.

13) Bax, Bridget E., and David L. Bloxam. "Energy metabolism and glycolysis in human placental trophoblast cells during differentiation." Biochimica et Biophysica Acta (BBA)-Bioenergetics 1319.2-3 (1997): 283-292.

14) Kroemer, Guido, and Jacques Pouyssegur. "Tumor cell metabolism: cancer's Achilles' heel." Cancer cell 13.6 (2008): 472-482.

15) Seyfried, Thomas N., et al. "Cancer as a metabolic disease: implications for novel therapeutics." Carcinogenesis 35.3 (2013): 515-527.

16) Christofferson, Travis. Tripping Over the Truth: How the Metabolic Theory of Cancer is Overturning One of Medicine's Most Entrenched Paradigms. Chelsea Green Publishing, 2017.

17) Rigo, Pierre, et al. "Oncological applications of positron emission tomography with fluorine-18 fluorodeoxyglucose." European journal of nuclear medicine 23.12 (1996): 1641-1674.

18) Koroljow, S. Two cases of malignant tumors with metastases apparently treated successfully with hypoglycemic coma. Psychiatric Quarterly 1962; 36(1):261-270.

19) Neufeld, O. Insulin therapy in terminal cancer: a preliminary report. J Amer Geriatric Soc 1962; 10(3):274-6.

20) Agrawal, Siddarth, et al. "Insulin-induced enhancement of MCF-7 breast cancer cell response to 5-fluorouracil and cyclophosphamide." Tumor Biology 39.6 (2017).

21) Agrawal, Siddarth, et al. "Insulin enhancement of the antitumor activity of chemotherapeutic agents in colorectal cancer is linked with downregulating PIK3CA and GRB2." Scientific reports 9.1 (2019): 1-14.

22) Geeraert, Luc, and CAM-Cancer Consortium. "Insulin potentiation therapy." (2011).

23) Ayre, S. G., DP Garcia y Bellon, and D. P. Garcia Jr. "Insulin, chemotherapy, and the mechanisms of malignancy: the design and the demise of cancer." Medical hypotheses 55.4 (2000): 330-334.

24) Apostolou, Panagiotis, et al. "P-280 The molecular profile of colon cancer cells." Annals of Oncology 28. suppl 3 (2017).

25) Guadagni, Stefano, et al. "Precision oncotherapy based on liquid biopsies in multidisciplinary treatment of unresectable recurrent rectal cancer: a retrospective cohort study." Journal of Cancer Research and Clinical Oncology 146.1 (2020): 205-219.

26) deleted

27) Papasotiriou, Ioannis, et al. "Detection of circulating tumor cells in patients with breast, prostate, pancreatic, colon and melanoma cancer: A blinded comparative study using healthy donors." Journal of Cancer Therapy 6.07 (2015): 543.

28) Toloudi, Maria, et al. "Comparison of the growth curves of cancer cells and cancer stem cells." Current stem cell research & therapy 9.2 (2014): 112-116.

29) Toloudi, Maria, et al. "A possible clinical benefit of the identification and characterization of colon cancer stem cells." Asian Pacific Journal of Tropical Disease 5.1 (2015): 22-27.

30) Ntanovasilis, Dimitrios-Athanasios, Panagiotis Apostolou, and Ioannis Papasotiriou. "Flow Cytometric Detection of Circulating Tumor Cells in Breast Cancer Patients: A Blinded Study." Journal of Cancer Therapy 10.08 (2019): 708.

31) Gout, Peter W., Chris R. Simms, and May C. Robertson. "In vitro studies on the lymphoma growth-inhibitory activity of sulfasalazine." Anticancer drugs 14.1 (2003): 21-29.

32) Gentric, Géraldine, Virginie Mieulet, and Fatima Mechta-Grigoriou. "Heterogeneity in cancer metabolism: new concepts in an old field." Antioxidants & redox signaling 26.9 (2017): 462-485.

33) Lendahl, U., and S. Orrenius. "Sydney Brenner, Robert Horvitz and John Sulston. Winners of the 2002 Nobel Prize in medicine or physiology. Genetic regulation of organ development and programmed cell death." Lakartidningen 99.41 (2002): 4026.

Chapter 4

Cancer as a Metabolic Disease

THE OBVIOUS FLAW IN CANCER treatment is non-selectivity. Chemotherapy targets *all* rapidly replicating cells in both the cancer and the patient. Because certain normal tissues of the body, such as the bone marrow and the GI tract, also undergo rapid cell replication, they are sensitive to the toxic effects of chemotherapy. This unwanted toxicity to the GI tract, bone marrow, brain, and heart accounts for most of the adverse side effects of chemotherapy, including nausea, vomiting, loss of appetite, weight loss, hair loss, bone marrow suppression with anemia, cardiotoxicity, "chemo brain," and chronic fatigue.

Another criticism of the so-called "chemotherapy paradigm" relates to the ten hallmarks of cancer cells, which were explored in the previous chapter. Chemotherapy targets only one of these ten hallmarks, rapid cell proliferation, and ignores the others. Rather than ignore them, this book will prioritize and utilize all the "Hallmarks of Cancer" to selectively target cancer stem cells.

Finding a Selective Cancer Treatment and Leaving Normal Cells Unharmed

The optimal cancer treatment is selective in that it will kill the cancer while leaving the rest of the patient unharmed. Can we find such a selective cancer treatment? What if we could identify subtle differences in the metabolism of cancer cells that will allow us to target them in a more selective way, thus sparing normal cells?

An analogy can be found in antibiotics, which kill invading bacteria without harming the body, or in antiparasitic drugs, which kill parasites without harming us. Are there such selective anti-cancer treatments? The answer is yes: Repurposed drugs can be used to selectively target metabolic pathways in cancer cells.

Cancer as a Metabolic Disease

One difference between metabolism in cancer cells and normal cells, the Warburg effect, describes how a metabolic switch called aerobic glycolysis is turned on in the cancer cell. In 2014, Dr. Thomas Seyfried came to an important realization, that all the hallmarks of cancer described by Weinberg and Hanahan in the previous chapter are "downstream" to this primary metabolic disturbance in the mitochondria. In *Carcinogenesis* (2014), Seyfried writes:

> Emerging evidence indicates that cancer is primarily a metabolic disease involving disturbances in energy production through respiration and fermentation. The genomic instability observed in tumor cells and all other recognized hallmarks of cancer are considered downstream epiphenomena of the initial disturbance of cellular energy metabolism. The disturbances in tumor cell energy metabolism can be linked to abnor-

malities in the structure and function of the mitochondria. (1)

Electron microscope studies of cancer cells indeed show abnormalities in the mitochondria. (2) The cancer cell's mitochondria have undergone "metabolic reprogramming" and exhibit a key difference that can be exploited to devise a more selective cancer treatment. (3–4)

Metabolic Reprogramming of the Cancer Cell

Mammalian cells have two metabolic pathways. The first is oxidative phosphorylation (OXPHOS), which is aerobic, and takes place in the mitochondria. The second is glycolysis, also called non-oxidative or anaerobic, which takes place in the cytoplasm. Since the mitochondrial oxidative pathway is the more efficient one, under normal circumstances with abundant oxygen, this pathway is preferred. Under conditions of hypoxia (low oxygen), however, normal cells will use the anaerobic pathways (glycolytic), producing lactic acid as a byproduct. Unlike normal cells, cancer cells have *preferentially* switched their metabolism from oxidative (OXPHOS) to non-oxidative (GLYCOLYSIS), consuming vast amounts of glucose and producing lactic acid.

3-Bromopyruvate (3BP) and Hexokinase 2 (HK2)

In 2009, Drs. Y. H. Ko and J. L. Pederson uncovered an important key to the metabolic reprogramming of the mitochondria of cancer cells. In cancer cells, an embryonic form of HK, called HK2, which is not usually present in nor-

mal cells, is attached to the outer membrane pores of the mitochondria, called the voltage-dependent anion channel (VDAC). HK2 is the first enzyme in the metabolism of glucose, and its aberrant location on the mitochondria outer membrane (MOM) allows for the massive utilization of glucose to feed the rapidly growing tumor mass.

Separating HK2 from the VDAC

What if we could somehow separate the HK2 enzyme from the VDAC? Would this help? Yes, it would be very helpful, because this would trigger apoptosis in the cancer cell while sparing normal cells. (5–6) This is exactly what we are looking for.

Drs. Shoshan-Barmatz and M. Golan (2012) write about mitochondrial HK binding to voltage dependent anion channel 1 (VDAC1) as a rational therapeutic target:

> The upregulation of HK expression in tumor cells and its binding to VDAC provide both a metabolic benefit and apoptosis-suppressive capacity that offers the cell a growth advantage and increases its resistance to chemotherapy. **VDAC has also been recognized as a key protein in mitochondria-mediated apoptosis** since it is the proposed target for the pro- and anti-apoptotic Bcl-2-family of proteins, as well as due to its function in the release of apoptotic proteins located in the inter-membrane space. These and other functions point to **VDAC1 as being a rational target** for the development of a new generation of therapeutics. (7)

Note: See the Glossary for more information on HK2, VDAC and BCL-2.

Deletion of HK2 is Therapeutic

Dr. K. C. Patra et al. (2013) concluded that HK2 is required for cancer cell maintenance and blocking HK2 is therapeutic in mouse xenograft models of cancer:

> Hexokinase 2 is required for tumor initiation and maintenance and its systemic deletion is therapeutic in mouse models of cancer. (8–9)

Discovery of 3BP by Dr. Ko

Drs. Y. H. Ko and Pederson discovered a small molecule called 3-bromo-pyruvate (3BP) that throws a "monkey wrench" into the metabolic machinery of the cancer cell and induces apoptosis via separation of Hexokinase 2 from the outer mitochondrial membrane. 3BP is a small nontoxic molecule that induces apoptosis in cancer cells while sparing normal cells, thus providing the most promising cancer treatment in years. Sadly, in-fighting over patent rights by the key players has delayed drug development and commercialization. 3BP as a commercial product for cancer treatment may never come to fruition. (5-6)(10–12)

Natural Compounds that Disassociate HK2 from VDAC

Thankfully, there are many other drugs and natural substances that separate the HK2 from the VDAC, selectively inducing apoptosis in cancer cells while sparing normal cells. Many of these have already been commercialized and are available at the local drugstore and health food store. We will mention a few here, discussed more fully in chapters 10-12 on natural substances and repurposed drugs as anti-cancer stem cell agents.

Resveratrol and Pterostilbenes

Resveratrol from grapes and its derivative pterostilbene have been extensively studied and demonstrate striking anti-cancer activity; they may indirectly inhibit HK2. Dr. Dora Moon et al. (2013) studied in vitro breast cancer cells showing that pterostilbene induces apoptosis via the mitochondrial pathway in breast cancer cell lines. (13)

In 2014, Dr. Hsiao Pei-Ching et al., using acute myeloid leukemia cells, found pterostilbene induced apoptosis in cancer cells via mitochondrial pathways (with activation of the caspase system). (14)

A 2015 study by Julie A. Alosi et al. on pterostilbene in breast cancer showed similar findings with apoptosis induced by mitochondrial pathways. (15)

A 2012 study by Yanshang Wang et al. showed pterostilbene induces apoptosis and cell-cycle arrest in breast cancer cells. (16)

Pterostilbene is a dimethylated analog of resveratrol. In 2013, Dr. Dong Hoon Suh et al. wrote that although there is no evidence of direct inhibition of HK2 activity by resveratrol (pterostilbene), there is evidence of inhibition of the PI3K/AKT/mTOR pathway, which indirectly inhibits HK2, and inhibition of HIF-1 (hypoxia-inducible factor):

> There is no evidence suggesting that resveratrol directly inhibits the enhanced activity of HK2 in tumor cells. However, growing evidence supports indirect HK2

inhibition by resveratrol through the inhibitory effect of resveratrol on the PI3K/AKT/mTOR pathway in many types of cancer cells. Resveratrol-induced HK2 inhibition also seems to be mediated through the inhibition of hypoxia-inducible factor-1α (HIF-1α), a transcription factor that reprograms cancer cell metabolism. (17)

Note: See the glossary for more on HIF and the PI3K/AKT/mTOR pathway, a major cancer pathway. See chapter 16 for more on pterostilbene.

Methyl Jasmonate

Methyl jasmonate has been extensively studied and found to disassociate HK2 from the VDAC at the outer mitochondria membrane, thus inducing apoptosis in cancer cells. The net effect is inhibition of GLYCOLYSIS (the Warburg Effect) in the cancer cell. Methyl jasmonate is ubiquitous in the plant world and found in the jasmine flower. It is used extensively by the fragrance industry for perfumes and is available as jasmine tea. Unfortunately, no commercially marketed anti-cancer drug version of methyl jasmonate has been developed by the drug industry as yet. (18–23)

Chinese Skullcap, Baicalin, Oroxylin A

Chinese Skullcap (also called Oroxylin A and Baicalin) is extracted from a medicinal plant called Scutellaria baicalensis Georgi. Researchers found that Chinese Skullcap inhibits GLYCOLYSIS and induces disassociation of HK2 from the mitochondria in human breast carcinoma cell lines, thus inducing apoptosis. Chinese Skullcap blocked the translocation of the anti-apoptotic protein Bcl-2 to the mitochondria, keeping the VDAC pores open, allowing apoptosis to take place. (24–25)

Dr. Xin-Eng Huang studied oroxylin A (Chinese Skullcap) in a hepatoma cell model showing apoptosis through the mitochondrial pathway in human hepatoma HepG2 cells with activation of mitochondrial permeability transition pores (VDAC). (26)

Chinese skullcap was also effective as an anti-cancer agent in lung cancer, acute myeloid leukemia (AML), and glioblastoma cell models. (27–33) Baicalin (Chinese skullcap root) penetrates into the CNS, according to Stephen Harrod Buhner, and baicalin is concentrated in the brain, striatum, thalamus, and hippocampus. (34)

Curcumin

Curcumin was studied by Dr. Ke Wang et al. in an animal model of colorectal cancer, showing that curcumin inhibits aerobic glycolysis (Warburg Effect) and induces mitochondrial-mediated apoptosis. Curcumin downregulates HK2 and disassociates HK2 from the mitochondria. The mechanism was different from 3 BP in that "the phosphorylation of mitochondrial HK2 through AKT was responsible for the curcumin-induced dissociation of HK2." (35)

In 2015, Dr. Tewari found that curcumin attaches to the VDAC, causing the pore to close, and that "curcumin-induced apoptosis is possibly associated with VDAC-closure." (36) Curcumin is available as a spice at the grocery store and is sold as capsules at the health food store.

Aspirin and the VDAC

In 2017, Dr. Debanjan Tewari et al. studied the effect of aspirin on the VDAC in cervical cancer cells, finding aspirin disassociated HK2 from the VDAC.

> Aspirin dissociated bound Hexokinase 2 (HK II) from mitochondria. Further, aspirin promoted the closure of recombinant human VDAC1, reconstituted in planar lipid bilayer. Taken together, these results imply that VDAC1 serves as a novel target for aspirin. Modulation of VDAC1 is possibly associated with the cell death and anti-cancer effects of aspirin. (37)

In 2018, Dr. Doaa Ali Abdelmonsif et al. studied the combination of aspirin and metformin in hepatocellular cancer (HepG2) cells in vitro, finding synergy with the combination:

> The Metformin/aspirin combined treatment had a synergistic effect on cell cycle arrest... and apoptosis... Additionally, metformin/aspirin combined treatment enhanced membrane localization of β-catenin expression in HepG2 cells.... (38)

The β-catenin protein is the key signal for the Wnt pathway involved in CSC (cancer stem cell) maintenance. Nuclear localization of beta-catenin promotes aggressive behavior with invasion and metastatic spread of tumor cells. Cell-membrane localization is just the opposite, denoting a more benign behavior of the tumor cell. See the Glossary for more on Beta-Catenin and the Wnt Pathway.

Cannabidiol Binds to VDAC

In 2013, Dr. Rimmerman studied microglial (brain) cells treated with cannabidiol (CBD), the non-psychoactive component of cannabis, finding that CBD binds to VDAC and inhibits its function, possibly accounting for immunosuppressive and anti-cancer effects. (39) For more on this, see chapter 19, on cannabis.

Quercetin Glycolysis Inhibitor

Quercetin (QUE) is a well-known bioflavonoid present in onions, capers, and many other foods having anti-oxidant, anti-inflammatory, antiplatelet, antihistamine, and antiviral properties, and is widely used for metabolic and inflammatory disorders. (40–41)

In 2019, Dr. Honguan Wu et al. studied the anti-cancer effects of the bioflavonoid QUE on hepatocellular carcinoma cell lines in vitro, showing glycolysis inhibition by reducing Hexokinase 2 and inhibition of the Akt-mTOR pathway. (42)

In 2018, Dr. Lijun Jia et al. studied the anti-cancer effects of QUE in a breast cancer model using in vitro and in vivo xenografts. Dr. Jia found that QUE blocked cancer-cell GLYCOLYSIS, inhibited glucose uptake, decreased lactic acid, and decreased glycolysis-related proteins such as pyruvate kinase, glucose transporter1 (GLUT1), and lactate dehydrogenase A (LDHA). As expected, inhibition of mTOR resulted in autophagy induction in this model. Dr. Jia's group writes:

> Quercetin suppressed the progression of breast cancer by inhibiting cell mobility and glycolysis through Akt-mTOR pathway mediated autophagy induction and may provide a potential therapeutic target for breast cancer treatment. (43)

In 2019, Drs. Marjorie Reyes-Farias and Catalina Carrasco-Pozo summarized the anti-cancer effect of QUE as a glycolysis inhibitor:

Effects of (Quercetin) are predominantly anti-carcinogenic by targeting glycolysis.... By interfering in PI3K/Akt/mTOR pathways, QUE exerts its metabolic effect on cancer, inhibiting key enzymes of glycolysis and glucose uptake. (44)

Note: The mTOR pathway controls autophagy, and inhibition of the mTOR pathway triggers "protective autophagy."

Targeting Multiple Metabolic Pathways with Repurposed Drugs

Targeting a single metabolic pathway is usually ineffective as an anti-cancer strategy because cancer compensates by switching to alternate metabolic pathways. If cancer cells are using OXPHOS, inhibition of OXPHOS causes a switch to GLYCOLYSIS. If cancer cells are using GLYCOLYSIS, inhibition of GLYCOLYSIS causes a switch to OXPHOS. If both are inhibited, then the cell may enter a dormant mode called "protective autophagy", under the control of mTOR. This ability to switch among three metabolic pathways is called "metabolic plasticity."

Goal of Cracking Cancer Toolkit

The goal of *Cracking Cancer Toolkit* is to use repurposed drugs and supplements to target all three pillars of cancer-cell metabolism—OXPHOS, GLYCOLYSIS and Autophagy, to induce metabolic catastrophe and restore apoptosis to the cancer cell. At the same time, we will also target five other important pathways:

Inflammation, cell replication, HK2-VDAC, immune restoration, and the micro-environment. The goal is to produce a more robust anti-cancer effect, achieving "synthetic lethality" with curative intent.

Conclusion

As we have seen, all ten hallmarks of cancer are "downstream" from the metabolic derangements in the mitochondria of cancer cells. In the following chapters, we will examine a number of repurposed drugs and natural substances targeting all "three pillars of metabolism"—OXPHOS, GLYCOLYSIS, and autophagy—in the cancer cell, to achieve synthetic lethality.

References for Chapter 4: Cancer as a Metabolic Disease

1) Seyfried, Thomas N., et al. "Cancer as a metabolic disease: implications for novel therapeutics." Carcinogenesis 35.3 (2013): 515-527.

2) Arismendi-Morillo, Gabriel. "Electron microscopy morphology of the mitochondrial network in human cancer." The international journal of biochemistry & cell biology 41.10 (2009): 2062-2068.

3) Ward, Patrick S., and Craig B. Thompson. "Metabolic reprogramming: a cancer hallmark even Warburg did not anticipate." Cancer cell 21.3 (2012): 297-308.

4) Kroemer, Guido, and Jacques Pouyssegur. "Tumor cell metabolism: cancer's Achilles' heel." Cancer cell 13.6 (2008): 472-482.

5) Mathupala, Saroj P., Young H. Ko, and Peter L. Pedersen. "Hexokinase-2 bound to mitochondria: cancer's stygian link to the "Warburg Effect" and a pivotal target for effective therapy." Seminars in cancer biology. Vol. 19. No. 1. Academic Press, 2009.

6) Mathupala, Saroj P., Young H. Ko, and Peter L. Pedersen. "The pivotal roles of mitochondria in

cancer: Warburg and beyond and encouraging prospects for effective therapies." Biochimica et Biophysica Acta (BBA)-Bioenergetics 1797.6-7 (2010): 1225-1230.

(7) Shoshan-Barmatz, V., and M. Golan. "Mitochondrial VDAC1: function in cell life and death and a target for cancer therapy." Current medicinal chemistry 19.5 (2012): 714-735.

8) Patra K.C., Hay N. Hexokinase 2 as oncotarget. Oncotarget. 2013;4:1862–1863.

9) Patra K.C., Wang Q., Bhaskar P.T., Miller L., Wang Z., Wheaton W. Hexokinase 2 is required for tumor initiation and maintenance and its systemic deletion is therapeutic in mouse models of cancer. Cancer Cell. 2013;24:213–228.

10) Moss, Ralph. "War on cancer: 3BP and the metabolic approach to cancer: a visit with Peter Pedersen and Young Hee Ko." Townsend Letter › June 1, 2013.

11) Xian, Shu-Lin, et al. "Inhibitory effects of 3-bromopyruvate on human gastric cancer implant tumors in nude mice." Asian Pacific J. Cancer Prev 15 (2014): 3175-3178.

12) Chen, Zhao, et al. "Role of mitochondria-associated hexokinase II in cancer cell death induced by 3-bromopyruvate." Biochimica et Biophysica Acta (BBA)-Bioenergetics 1787.5 (2009): 553-560.

13) Moon, Dora, et al. "Pterostilbene induces mitochondrially derived apoptosis in breast cancer cells in vitro." Journal of Surgical Research 180.2 (2013): 208-215.

14) Hsiao, Pei-Ching, et al. "Pterostilbene simultaneously induced G0/G1-phase arrest and MAPK-mediated mitochondrial-derived apoptosis in human acute myeloid leukemia cell lines." PLoS One 9.8 (2014): e105342.

15) Alosi, Julie A., et al. "Pterostilbene inhibits breast cancer in vitro through mitochondrial depolarization and induction of caspase-dependent apoptosis." Journal of Surgical Research 161.2 (2010): 195-201.

16) Wang, Yanshang, et al. "Pterostilbene simultaneously induces apoptosis, cell cycle arrest and cyto-protective autophagy in breast cancer cells." American journal of translational research 4, no. 1 (2012): 44.

17) Suh, Dong Hoon, et al. "Cancer-specific therapeutic potential of resveratrol: metabolic approach against hallmarks of cancer." Functional Foods in Health and Disease 3.8 (2013): 332-343.

18) Cesari, Italo Mario, et al. "Methyl jasmonate: putative mechanisms of action on cancer cells cycle, metabolism, and apoptosis." International journal of cell biology 2014 (2014).

19) Goldin, N., et al. "Methyl jasmonate binds to and detaches mitochondria-bound hexokinase." Oncogene 27.34 (2008): 4636-4643.

20) Galluzzi, L., et al. "Disruption of the hexokinase–VDAC complex for tumor therapy." Oncogene 27.34 (2008): 4633-4635.

21) Krasnov, George S., et al. "Targeting VDAC-bound hexokinase II: a promising approach for concomitant anti-cancer therapy." Expert opinion on therapeutic targets 17.10 (2013): 1221-1233.

22) Li, Jingjing, et al. "Methyl jasmonate leads to necrosis and apoptosis in hepatocellular carcinoma cells via inhibition of glycolysis and represses tumor growth in mice." Oncotarget 8.28 (2017): 45965.

23) Sucu, Bilgesu Onur, et al. "Synthesis of novel methyl jasmonate derivatives and evaluation of their biological activity in various cancer cell lines." Bioorganic chemistry 91 (2019): 103146.

24) Wei, L., et al. "Oroxylin A induces dissociation of hexokinase II from the mitochondria and inhibits glycolysis by SIRT3-mediated deacetylation of cyclophilin D in breast carcinoma." Cell death & disease 4.4 (2013): e601.

25) Qiao, Chen, et al. "UCP2-related mitochondrial pathway participates in oroxylin A-induced apoptosis in human colon cancer cells." Journal of cellular physiology (2014).

26) Huang, Xin-Eng, et al. "MPTP related mitochondrial pathway in oroxylin A induced-apoptosis in HepG2 cancer cells." Int J Clin Exp Pathol 9.11 (2016): 11139-11148

27) Wei, Libin, et al. "Oroxylin A sensitizes non-small cell lung cancer cells to anoikis via glucose-deprivation-like mechanisms: c-Src and hexokinase II." Biochimica et Biophysica Acta (BBA)-General Subjects 1830.6 (2013): 3835-3845.

28) Hui, Hui, et al. "Oroxylin A has therapeutic potential in acute myelogenous leukemia by dual effects targeting PPARγ and RXRα." International journal of cancer 134.5 (2014): 1195-1206.

29) Gao, Ying, et al. "Anticancer properties of baicalein: a review." Medicinal Chemistry Research 25.8 (2016): 1515-1523.

30) Chen, Haijun, et al. "Exploring therapeutic potentials of baicalin and its aglycone baicalein for hematological malignancies." Cancer letters 354.1 (2014): 5-11.

31) Chen YJ, Wu CS, Shieh JJ, Wu JH, Chen HY, Chung TW, Chen YK, Lin CC (2013c) Baicalein triggers mitochondria-mediated apoptosis and enhances the antileukemic effect of vincristine in childhood acute lymphoblastic leukemia CCRF-CEM cells. Evid Based Complementary Altern Med 2013:124747

32) Fong, Yui Kau, et al. "In vitro and in situ evaluation of herb–drug interactions during intestinal metabolism and absorption of baicalein." Journal of ethnopharmacology 141.2 (2012): 742-753.

33) Li, Min, et al. "Safety, tolerability, and pharmacokinetics of a single ascending dose of baicalein chewable tablets in healthy subjects." Journal of ethnopharmacology 156 (2014): 210-215.

34) Buhner, Stephen Harrod. Herbal Antivirals: Natural Remedies for Emerging & Resistant Viral Infections. Storey Publishing, 2013.

35) Wang, Ke, et al. "Curcumin inhibits aerobic glycolysis and induces mitochondrial-mediated apoptosis through hexokinase II in human colorectal cancer cells in vitro." Anti-cancer drugs 26.1 (2015): 15-24.

36) Tewari, Debanjan, et al. "Modulation of the mitochondrial voltage dependent anion channel (VDAC) by curcumin." Biochimica et Biophysica Acta (BBA)-Biomembranes 1848.1 (2015): 151-158.

37) Tewari, Debanjan, et al. "Aspirin induces cell death by directly modulating mitochondrial voltage-dependent anion channel (VDAC)." Scientific reports 7.1 (2017): 1-9.

38) Abdelmonsif, Doaa Ali, et al. "Targeting AMPK, mTOR and β-catenin by combined metformin and aspirin therapy in HCC: an appraisal in Egyptian HCC patients." Molecular diagnosis & therapy 22.1 (2018): 115-127.

39) Rimmerman, N., et al. "Direct modulation of the outer mitochondrial membrane channel, voltage-dependent anion channel 1 (VDAC1) by cannabidiol: a novel mechanism for cannabinoid-induced cell death." Cell death & disease 4.12 (2013): e949-e949.

40) David, Alexander Victor Anand, Radhakrishnan Arulmoli, and Subramani Parasuraman. "Overviews of biological importance of quercetin: A bioactive flavonoid." Pharmacognosy reviews 10.20 (2016): 84.

41) Shah, Palak Mayur, Vishnu V. Priya, and R. Gayathri. "Quercetin-a flavonoid: a systematic review." Journal of Pharmaceutical Sciences and Research 8.8 (2016): 878.

42) Wu, Hongyan, et al. "Quercetin inhibits the proliferation of glycolysis-addicted HCC cells by reducing hexokinase 2 and Akt-mTOR pathway." Molecules 24.10 (2019): 1993

43) Jia, Lijun, et al. "Quercetin suppresses the mobility of breast cancer by suppressing glycolysis through Akt-mTOR pathway mediated autophagy induction." Life sciences 208 (2018): 123-130.

44) Reyes-Farias, Marjorie, and Catalina Carrasco-Pozo. "The anti-cancer effect of quercetin: Molecular implications in cancer metabolism." International journal of molecular sciences 20.13 (2019): 3177.

Chapter 5

Dichloroacetate (DCA): Breakthrough Anti-Cancer Agent

MARY, A LONG-TIME PATIENT OF mine, called to ask for advice about her husband, Jim, a 63-year-old who had been quite healthy for many years. Jim recently noticed some back pain, and his primary care doctor ordered a CAT scan, which showed a large lung mass and destructive lesions in the spine. Biopsies confirmed the lung mass was indeed cancer, with metastatic spread to the thoracic vertebral bodies. Jim was referred to the local oncologist, who started radiation and chemotherapy. After the first week of chemotherapy, Jim was miserable from its adverse effects, with nausea, vomiting, and loss of appetite. He felt so bad, he declined any further chemotherapy treatment. Mary asked if I had any suggestions.

Integrative Oncology Clinics in Canada

I had just returned from Seattle, where I had attended an integrative cancer meeting organized by Paul Anderson, ND, director of the Seattle clinic Advanced Medical Specialties. Dr. Anderson, author of *Out of the Box Cancer,* pioneered the use of the orphan drug* dichloroacetate (DCA), which shares synergy with a vitamin supplement called poly-MVA. (1–4)

One of the Truly Big Advances

Dr. Anderson declares:

The combined use of DCA and Poly-MVA has been one of the truly big advances in integrative cancer therapies in the past 20 years. (1)

Whenever I hear the phrase, "truly big advances," it really garners my attention.

Adding Solomon's Seal

Dr. Neil McKinney, ND, author of *Naturopathic Oncology*, was a keynote speaker at the meeting. (5) Dr. McKinney is director of Vital Victoria, an integrative cancer clinic in Victoria, British Columbia. His program includes DCA and R-ALA in a nebulized version available from York Downs Compounding Pharmacy in Toronto. An additional supplement is Dr McKinney's Mito-SAP which contains Carnitine, Quercetin, R-Alpha-Lipoic acid, Grape seed extract, Thiamine and Coenzyme Q10. During his talk, Dr. McKinney made the observation that patient outcomes using the DCA/R-ALA combination improved dramatically with the addition of a botanical extract, Solomon's seal. See chapter 18 on Solomon's seal. Dr. McKinney announced his retirement in October 2020 while writing this book. The clinic remains open under the direction of his colleagues. (6–8)

---

* An orphan drug is a needed drug that a pharmaceutical company might not normally develop without government support, due to a lack of financial incentive

Medicor Clinic, Toronto—Dr. Akbar Khan

Another Canadian integrative cancer doctor not attending the meeting, but prominently mentioned was Dr. Akbar Khan, director of the Medicor Clinic in Toronto. Dr. Khan was a keynote speaker at the October 2018 International College of Integrative Medicine (ICIM) cancer meeting in Minneapolis and has published many case reports detailing his extensive experience with DCA as a cancer treatment. (9–12)

For people like Jim who decline conventional treatment because of adverse effects, all three clinics are good options, offering integrative oncology with DCA , given with supportive vitamins, thiamine (benfotiamine) and R-alpha lipoic acid, which can be taken individually or in a combination called Poly-MVA. These vitamins are necessary to avoid neuropathy induced by DCA. We will discuss this in more detail later. First, a little background on targeting cancer cell metabolism.

Metabolic Reprogramming of the Cancer Cell—The Warburg Effect

Cancer cell biology reveals that cancer is a metabolic disease. In other words, cancer cells have a fundamental metabolic derangement, named the Warburg effect. Targeting the metabolic pathways of the cancer cell while leaving normal cells unharmed provides a safer and more effective treatment, and avoids the toxic effects of chemotherapy.

Warburg Effect—Aerobic Glycolysis

Normal cells have two quite different energy pathways, oxidative and non-oxidative. The oxidative (aerobic) pathway uses oxygen in the mitochondria and the non-oxidative (anaerobic) pathway metabolizes glucose in the cytoplasm. Normal cells prefer the more efficient, oxidative pathway. However, the cancer cell has "switched off" the oxidative pathway in the mitochondria and instead prefers the non-oxidative pathway in the cytoplasm, called GLYCOLYSIS. The cancer cells shift their energy production to the cytoplasm, a form of "fermentation" also called "aerobic glycolysis" (Warburg effect). According to Dr. Thomas McFate et al. in 2008:

> High lactate generation and low glucose oxidation, despite normal oxygen conditions, are commonly seen in cancer cells and tumors.... Historically known as the Warburg Effect ... High lactate accumulation, despite adequate oxygen availability, is a metabolic pattern commonly associated with malignant transformation of the uncontrolled dividing cell. This metabolic phenotype, termed **aerobic glycolysis and historically known as the Warburg Effect**, is characterized by high glycolytic rates and reduced mitochondrial oxidation. (13)

Drs. Gopinath Sutendra and Evangelos D. Michelakis (2013) write:

> The unique metabolism of most solid tumors.... all result in a switch in metabolism from mitochondria-based glucose oxidation (OXPHOS) to cytoplasm-based Glycolysis even under normoxia [normal oxygen levels], also known as the Warburg Effect. (14)

Reprogramming the Metabolic Switch with DCA

One might then ask the next logical question: What is the exact mechanism by which cancer cells turn off the mitochondrial oxidative pathway, and how can we switch it back on? Many years after Warburg's discovery, molecular biology clarified the metabolic reprogramming of the cancer cell. The key is an enzyme called pyruvate dehydrogenase complex (PDC), which sits at the control point for entry of pyruvate into the mitochondria. Pyruvate is derived from glucose and the main fuel for the mitochondria. Cancer cells turn off PDC by upregulating pyruvate dehydrogenase kinase (PDK). Inhibition of PDC in the cancer cell is the key step in metabolic reprogramming. According to Dr. Peter Stacpoole (2017):

> The mitochondrial pyruvate dehydrogenase complex [PDC] irreversibly decarboxylates pyruvate to acetyl coenzyme A, thereby linking glycolysis to the tricarboxylic acid cycle [oxidative in the mitochondria] and defining a critical step in cellular bioenergetics ... Inhibition of PDC activity by pyruvate dehydrogenase kinase [PDK]–mediated phosphorylation has been associated with the pathobiology of many disorders of metabolic integration, including cancer. Consequently, the PDC/PDK axis has long been a therapeutic target. (15)

The Achilles heel of the cancer cell is the PDC/PDK axis. If we could somehow inhibit PDK, this would reverse the metabolic reprogramming of the cancer cell and unlock the cancer cell from a state of apoptosis resistance. (14–16)

Note: Apoptosis is programmed cell death. See the Glossary.

Drs. Sutendra and Michelakis (2013) write:

> The unique metabolism of most solid tumors integrates many molecular and genetic proximal signals, which all result in a switch in metabolism from mitochondria-based glucose oxidation [GO] to cytoplasm-based glycolysis even under normoxia, also known as the Warburg Effect.... Therefore, by reversing this mitochondrial remodeling, it is possible to "unlock" these cells from a state of apoptosis resistance, selectively inducing cancer cell death. (14)

DCA Glycolysis Inhibitor

The glycolysis inhibitor DCA (dichloroacetate) inhibits PDK and is exactly what we are looking for. DCA is an "orphan drug," meaning it is an old, off-patent drug originally used for rare genetic mitochondrial diseases causing lactic acidosis. (17–18) Since DCA is off-patent and not profitable, drug companies are unlikely to fund large-scale clinical trials looking at efficacy for cancer patients. Even so, a number of cancer based clinical trials have been completed or are underway.

DCA Inhibits PDK

Remember the Warburg effect? Cancer cells have deranged metabolism that has been switched from OXPHOS in mitochondria to GLYCOLYSIS in the cytoplasm. The inhibition of PDK by DCA results in a "vastly diminished GLYCOLYSIS " in the cancer cell. By inhibiting PDK, DCA is a "glycolysis inhibitor," "forcing cancer cells to use OXPHOS in the mitochondria as the main ATP generator." Dr. Martin Villalba et al. (2014) write:

> One enzyme implicated in tumor metabolic remodeling and whose expression is regulated by oncogenic transcription factors is pyruvate dehydrogenase kinase 1 [PDK1], which is inhibited by dichloroacetate [DCA]. PDK1 inhibition leads to pyruvate dehydrogenase [PDH] activation and forces cells to use mitochondria as the main ATP generator. As a result, **glycolysis is vastly diminished.** (16)

Production of Lactic Acid and Acidity in the Microenvironment

A byproduct of the Warburg Effect is the production of excess lactic acid, which exits the cancer cells and creates an acidic microenvironment, playing a role in tumor immune evasion. DCA restores anti-cancer host immunity in the microenvironment by inhibiting acidic lactate production. (20) Dr. Toshimitsu Ohashi (2013) says in the *International Journal of Cancer*: "Dichloroacetate improves immune dysfunction caused by tumor-secreted lactic acid and increases anti-tumor immunoreactivity." (24–26)

DCA Synergy with Anti-VEGF Antibody (Avastin)

In 2013, Dr. Krishan Kumar et al. used an in vivo glioblastoma xenograft model to study drug resistance to the anti-angiogenic drug bevacizumab, an anti-VEGF antibody (VEGF=vascular endothelial growth factor). The two drugs, bevacizumab and DCA used together "dramatically blocked tumor growth" compared to either drug alone, making it a potent anti-cancer strategy. (27)

DCA Induces Protective Autophagy

In 2014, Dr. G. Lin et al. studied DCA in a colorectal and prostate cancer xenograft model in vivo, expecting to find cancer cells dying from apoptosis. They did not find the expected apoptosis of cancer cells. Instead, they found increased expression of autophagy after DCA treatment, both in vitro and in vivo.

The induction of "protective autophagy" by cancer cells is a well-known response to stress or anti-cancer drug treatment. This can be overcome by adding an autophagy inhibitor drug, such as propranolol. (DCA synergy with the autophagy inhibitor propranolol is discussed below.) In addition, Dr. Lin's group found that DCA treatment increased reactive oxygen species (ROS), inhibited mTOR pathway signaling, and reduced lactate production. (28) Similar induction of "protective autophagy" occurred in cancer cells after DCA treatment in esophageal cancer and colon cancer in vitro. (29–30)

DCA Modulates Embryonic Stem Cell Pluripotency

Embryonic stem cells share many similarities with cancer cells. They both have a glycolytic profile and use similar signaling pathways. Researchers study mouse embryonic stem cells (mESC) to shed light on cancer cell biology. Both tissue hypoxia and mitochondrial inhibition are needed for embryonic stem cell (ESC) pluripotency, and pyruvate dehydrogenase kinase (PDK) is upregulated in mESC to maintain a glycolytic phenotype.

DCA Reduces Hypoxia-Inducible (HIF–1) Factor

In 2015, Dr. Ana Sofia Rodrigues et al. studied the effect of DCA on mESC pluripotency and stem cell metabolism. In the presence of DCA, embryonic stem cells began to differentiate and become more mature. Dr. Rodrigues's group found that DCA inhibits PDK, resulting in downstream reduction in hypoxia-inducible factor HIF-1, HIF-2, p53, and HK2, disrupting the glycolytic profile. They write:

> We can conclude that DCA promotes pluripotency loss and a shift in metabolism ... It is tempting to propose that if PDHK [PDK] is inhibited.... cells will adapt their metabolic regulatory circuitry in order to have a more active PDH. This adaptation will result in lower levels of Hif-1α, Hif-2α, p53, HK2, PDHK1 and PKM1/2, ultimately leading to **more active mitochondria, and disrupting the glycolytic metabolic profile** necessary to maintain pluripotency. (31)

Note: PDHK and PDK are the same. HIF-1, HIF-2 and HIF-3 are isoforms of a transcription factor called HIF (hypoxia inducible factor) which has multiple target genes controlling response to hypoxia (low oxygen). In cancer cells, HIFs regulate angiogenesis, glucose metabolism, cell growth, and metastatic behavior. Reduction in HIF is a valid anti-cancer strategy.

DCA Inhibits Angiogenesis and HIF-1

The HIF target genes are frequently upregulated in cancer, responsible for angiogenesis, the formation of new vessels in the micro-environment which feed the growing tumor mass.

In 2013, Dr. G. Sutendra et al. used animal xenografts of non-small-cell lung cancer and breast cancer to study DCA inhibition of HIF-1 and angiogenesis. They observed that DCA increases pyruvate dehydrogenase (PDH) activity, inhibiting GLYCOLYSIS, which inhibited cancer cell proliferation and induced apoptosis. In addition, DCA treatment suppressed new tumor vessel formation (angiogenesis), and also inhibited HIF1α. They write:

> Effective inhibition of HIF1α is shown by a decrease in the expression of several HIF1α regulated gene products as well as **inhibition of angiogenesis** in vitro in matrigel assays.... DCA increases pyruvate dehydrogenase activity ... pro-apoptotic and antiproliferative effects and suppresses angiogenesis as well, normalizing the pseudo-hypoxic signals that lead to normoxic HIF1α activation in solid tumors. (32)

Thiamine and R-Alpha Lipoic Acid Analogous to DCA

In 2014, Dr. Bradley Hanberry et al. studied high-dose thiamine in pancreatic cancer and neuroblastoma cell lines in vitro, finding that the mechanism of reduction in proliferation was similar to that of DCA:

> Thiamine exhibited a lower IC50 value in both cell lines compared to DCA. Both thiamine and DCA reduced the extent of PDH phosphorylation [PDH inactivation], reduced glucose consumption, lactate production, and mitochondrial membrane potential. High-dose thiamine and DCA did not increase ROS but increased caspase-3 activity [apoptosis].... Our findings suggest that **high-dose thiamine reduces cancer cell proliferation by a mechanism similar to that described for dichloroacetate.** (33)

Both thiamine and alpha lipoic acid are

co-factors for the PDC complex, standing at the entry point for pyruvate into the mitochondrial electron transport chain. Both thiamine and alpha lipoic acid are routinely recommended along with DCA, either separately or all together in a liquid supplement called Poly-MVA, prominently mentioned by Dr. Paul Anderson in his (2018) book, *Outside the Box Cancer Therapies*.(1) Poly-MVA is a liquid polymer containing palladium, thiamine, and alpha lipoic acid. The addition of the rare earth metal, palladium, serving as electron donor, provides added synergy.

Translocation of Hexokinase II (HK2) from Cytoplasm to Mitochondria: HK2 Binds to and Inhibits VDAC

Another prominent feature of metabolic reprogramming of the cancer cell involves the HK enzyme, the first step in GLYCOLYSIS in the cytoplasm. Cancer cells have switched to an embryonic form of hexokinase called HK2, which then trans-locates from the cytoplasm to the outer mitochondrial membrane, where it attaches to the voltage-dependent anion channel (VDAC). The VDAC is a pore-like opening in the outer membrane involved in shuttling nutrients and signaling molecules in and out of the mitochondria. (20–23)

HK2 is not present in normal cells (with the exception of skeletal muscle, heart, and adipose tissue). This is an important difference between cancer cells and normal cells that can be targeted. Dr. Gopinath Sutendra et al. (2013) write:

> The resultant concomitant upregulation of

glycolysis is associated with a translocation of hexokinase 2 from the cytoplasm to the mitochondrial membranes, where it has been shown to bind and further inhibit VDAC ... (14)

Hexokinase normally resides in the cytoplasm and is the enzyme for the first step in glycolysis in normal cells. However, in cancer cells, HK has been replaced by HK2, translocated to the mitochondrial outer membrane, where it gains access to energy in the form of adenosine triphosphate (ATP) from the mitochondria and blocks mitochondrial apoptosis, effectively "immortalizing" the cancer cell. Dr. Saroj Mathupala et al. (2009) write:

> Significantly, HK-2 is the major bound hexokinase isoform expressed in cancers that exhibit a "Warburg Effect." This includes most cancers that metastasize and kill their human host. By stationing itself on the outer mitochondrial membrane, **HK-2 also helps immortalize cancer cells**, escapes product inhibition and gains preferential access to newly synthesized ATP for phosphorylating glucose. (20)

DCA does not specifically bind to or detach HK2 from the VDAC, so additional agents that act on HK2 and VDAC would be synergistic.

Other Agents That Target Mitochondria
Itraconazole and Fenofibrate Separate HK2 from VDAC

The attachment of HK2 to the VDAC on the outer mitochondrial membrane creates a state of apoptosis resistance and shunts ATP out of the mitochondria to the cytoplasm to support GLYCOLYSIS. (20)

It then follows logically that repurposed

drugs and natural substances that separate HK2 from the VDAC are effective "anti-cancer" drugs. (34–38)

Among many on the list, two such commonly available repurposed drugs are fenofibrate, a lipid-lowering drug, and itraconazole, an antifungal. I am highlighting these two drugs because they are widely available, have a long track record of safety, and are well tolerated for long-term use.

Dr. Jan Chia-Ing et al. write that fenofibrate is more potent than 3- bromopyruvate in disrupting HK2 from VDAC:

> Fenofibrate disrupted the interaction of Hexokinase 2 and VDAC more potently than 3-BrPA [3-Bromo-Pyruvate] in both SAS and OECM1 [cancer] cells. (39)

Note: SAS=human high-grade malignant oral cancer cell line; OECM1= low-grade malignant oral cancer cell line.

See chapters 36 and 37 on itraconazole and fenofibrate as anti-cancer drugs for in-depth information about each drug.

Itraconazole Targets the VDAC on Outer Mitochondrial Membrane

In 2015, Dr. Sarah Head et al. used a fluorescent probe to identify the VDAC as the molecular target of itraconazole. Dr. Head's group found that itraconazole is 1,000 times more effective than metformin in activating adenosine monophosphate-activated protein kinase (AMPK). They write:

> In the present study, we used a photoaffinity labeling approach using a biologically active itraconazole photoaffinity probe

in live cells to identify the OMM [Outer Mitochondrial Membrane] channel VDAC1 as a molecular target of itraconazole ... the concentrations of metformin required to activate AMPK in HUVEC are at least **1,000 times higher** than those required of itraconazole [in the range of low millimoles], suggesting that itraconazole might be significantly more effective than metformin at inhibiting angiogenesis in patients..... Itraconazole is pharmacologically distinct from other azole antifungal agents in that it is the only inhibitor in this class that has been shown to inhibit both the hedgehog signaling pathway and angiogenesis. (40)

In *Blood* (2016), Dr. Juan J. Gu et al. studied chemotherapy resistant NHL (Non-Hodgkin's Lymphoma) cell lines in vitro and found that itraconazole disrupts HK2 from the mitochondria and enhances the efficacy of chemotherapy agents.

> The disruption of HK2 from mitochondria following itraconazole exposure may contribute to lower the mitochondrial membrane potential and enhance the chemotherapeutic efficacy. (41)

For more on itraconazole as an anti-cancer drug, see chapter 36. (42–46)

3 Bromopyruvate Disassociates HK2 from VDAC

3 bromopyruvate (3BP) is a pyruvate analog, a small molecule with anti-cancer activity studied by Drs. Ko and Pederson. (47)

In 2009, Dr. Zhao Chen et al. found that 3BP:

> directly triggered the dissociation of HK2 from mitochondria, leading to a specific

release of apoptosis-inducing factor [AIF] from the mitochondria to cytosol and eventual cell death. (48)

Disputes over patent rights may prevent the 3BP drug from ever coming to practical use in the clinic.

Lithium Detaches HK2 from Mitochondria

Lithium is available at the vitamin store as 5 mg lithium orotate capsules and at the corner drugstore as prescription 300 mg lithium carbonate tablets, used to treat bipolar disorder. Dr. J. Penso and R. Beitner write (2003) that lithium detaches Hexokinase 2 from the mitochondria and inhibits melanoma cancer cells. (49)

Note: checking serum lithium levels is prudent when using lithium carbonate, as high levels can approach toxicity. This is not required for lithium orotate, however.

Clotrimazole

Another small molecule, clotrimazole, is an antifungal drug known to detach hexokinase from the outer mitochondrial membrane. Drs. Penso and Beitner (1998) write that clotrimazole induces a dose-dependent detachment of hexokinase from the mitochondria of B16 melanoma cells. (50)

Dr. S. Kadavakollu et al. wrote an excellent review in *Medicinal Chemistry* (2014) of all the in vitro, animal xenograft, and clinical studies of clotrimazole as an anti-cancer drug. Their review summarizes efforts to enhance the anti-cancer activity of clotrimazole by forming a complex with rare earth metals such as palladium:

The nitrogen atom present in the imidazole ring of clotrimazole facilitates coordination with transition metal ions such as Pt, as well as Ru, Pd, Cu, Co, Zn and Ni. Ravera et al. synthesized Pt(II) complexes containing bis(clotrimazole) ligands, which were shown to effectively inhibit the growth of MCF-7, SKBR-3, HT-29, and B16/BL6 cell lines. (51)

With the above in mind, one might speculate synergy of clotrimazole (and perhaps other azoles) with poly-MVA (MVA=minerals, vitamins, amino acids), which contains palladium in a liquid polymer with alpha lipoic acid and thiamine. Unfortunately, we have yet to see development of a commercially available clotrizamole anti-cancer pruduct.

Methyl Jasmonate Detaches HK2 from Mitochondria

Methyl jasmonate is a "stress hormone" found in the jasmine plant. The oil is widely available, used in cosmetics, perfumes, and aromatherapy. The methyl jasmonate molecule has been extensively studied in vitro and xenograft animal models, showing excellent results, with separation of HK2 from the mitochondrial membrane and induction of cancer cell death with virtually no toxic effects on normal cells. Unfortunately, we have yet to see any effort to develop a marketable drug or practical anti-cancer application from the natural substance methyl jasmonate. (52–63)

Chrysin Targets HK2 and Inhibits Complex II and V

One might speculate regarding a possible synergy of DCA with chrysin, which has been shown to target HK2 and inhibit complexes II and V of the electron transport chain (ETC). (64–65)

Resveratrol, Pterostilbene, and VDAC

In 2019, Dr. Mengyuan Tian showed that resveratrol and pterostilbene phosphorylated the VDAC and reduced interaction with HK2. In vitro cancer cell studies show resveratrol "phosphorylated VDAC1 and showed increased affinity to Bax, whereas interaction with hexokinase 2 (HK2) was reduced....."(66)

One might therefore expect synergy of pterostilbene with DCA.

Synergy of DCA with Metformin and other Electron Transport Chain Agents

Another way to amplify the effect or create synergy with DCA is to use another agent that causes defects in the mitochondrial electron transport chain (ETC). DCA increases the electron flux through the ETC. So if we can throw a "monkey wrench" into the ETC machinery by inhibiting complex I of the ETC, then this will amplify the anti-cancer effect of DCA.

Dr. Luke Stockwin et al. (2010) write:

Sodium dichloroacetate [DCA] selectively targets cells with defects in the mitochondrial ETC. (67)

Metformin, a popular anti-diabetic drug used by millions, inhibits complex I of the ETC.

Indeed, numerous studies show anti-cancer synergy of metformin with DCA. The metformin makes cancer cells more sensitive to DCA treatment. (68–78)

Dr. Thomas Seyfried writes (2015):

Our data indicate that **metformin enhancement of DCA cytotoxicity is dependent on complex I inhibition.** Particularly, that complex I inhibition cooperates with DCA-induction of glucose oxidation [OXPHOS] to enhance cytotoxic oxidative stress in VM-M3 GBM (glioblastoma) cells. (68)

In *Oncotarget* (2015), Dr. Vitalba Ruggieri et al., working with DCA and oral squamous carcinoma cells, came to the same conclusion:

The therapeutic efficacy of DCA may depend on the specific metabolic profile adopted by the cancer cells with those exhibiting a deficient mitochondrial oxidative phosphorylation resulting in more sensitivity to the drug treatment. (79)

DCA Synergy with Antibiotics Doxycycline and Clarithromycin

Another way to induce defects in the electron transport chain in mitochondria is with the common antibiotics doxycycline and clarithromycin, which inhibit bacterial (and therefore mitochondrial) ribosomal protein production, thus impairing the production of protein components of the ETC. (80–89)

Targeting Mitochondria to Eradicate Cancer Stem Cells

An added bonus when targeting cancer-cell mitochondria is the eradication of CSCs, which depend on OXPHOS. Dr. Federica Sotgia et al.

studied repurposing the following commonly used antibiotics for targeting mitochondria in CSCs: (82)

- Doxycycline
- Azithromycin (clarithromycin)
- Pyrvinium pamoate (salt)
- Atovaquone
- Bedaquiline

They write (2018):

Doxycycline and Azithromycin are known to inhibit mitochondrial protein translation as an off-target side effect. They are used clinically as antibiotics to inhibit bacterial protein synthesis. Similarly, Pyrvinium pamoate and Atovaquone are known to inhibit OXPHOS (related to mitochondrial complex II/III), as a side effect. Bedaquiline was originally designed to inhibit the bacterial ATP synthase, which is analogous to mitochondrial complex V. (82)

Similar to the way metformin sensitizes cancer cells to DCA, one might speculate that long-term use of one or a combination of these antibiotics would interrupt mitochondrial function (inhibiting OXPHOS), shunt metabolism toward GLYCOLYSIS, and sensitize the cancer cells to DCA treatment.

See chapter 9 on doxycycline and vitamin C anti-cancer synergy and chapter 35 on clarithromycin anti-cancer antibiotic.

DCA May Be a Cancer Stem Cell Agent!!

In their excellent review in *Oxidative Medicine and Cellular Longevity* (2019), Drs. Tiziani Tataranni and Claudia Piccoli suggests that DCA may have anti-cancer properties against CSCs:

Interestingly, **DCA could significantly affect cancer stem cell fraction and contribute to cancer eradication**.... DCA treatment seems to improve the efficacy of chemotherapy, and is a radiation sensitizer. DCA synergizes with many other drugs and natural substances.... the possible sensitivity of CSC [cancer stem cell] fraction to DCA has been hypothesized and tested in different cancer models (19)

DCA and Pancreatic Cancer Stem Cells

Drs. Tataranni and Piccoli (2018) studied DCA in pancreatic cancer cell lines in vitro and in vivo using a xenograft mouse model and found downregulation of CSC markers and inhibition of spheroid formation and viability, concluding:

The novelty that DCA might affect the cancer stem cell compartment is therapeutically relevant. (90)

DCA and Hepatocellular Cancer Stem Cells

A 2015 study by Dr. Kyoungsub Song et al. nicely demonstrates anti-cancer stem cell activity of DCA in a highly glycolytic (CD133+) hepatocellular CSC line. Treatment with DCA-decreased stem cell markers, spheroid formation, and overall proliferation and restored sensitivity to sorafenib, a kinase inhibitor that was FDA-approved in 2007 for hepatocellular carcinoma. (91)

DCA from Glioblastoma Stem Cells

Glioblastoma cells and their stem cells are highly glycolytic and a good target for the glycolysis inhibitor DCA, which easily crosses the blood-brain barrier (BBB). In 2010, Dr. E. D. Michelakis et al. studied the effect of DCA on glioblastoma cells (GBM) freshly isolated from 49 patients. In addition, 5 patients with GBM were treated with oral DCA over 15 months, together with the oral methylator temozolomide, with promising results. Both glioblastoma bulk tumor cells as well as (CD 133+) stem cells showed an excellent response to the DCA. They conclude:

> DCA treatment was associated in some GBM patients with prolonged radiologic stabilization or tumor regression and, in general, displayed an overall good safety profile. This early, first-in-human report provides a rationale for extended studies with this generic small molecule in patients with GBM. (92)

In 2012, Dr. Marie Morfouace et al. found that DCA in combination with etoposide or radiation potentiated apoptosis in glioblastoma CSCs in vitro and reduced proliferation in vivo, via a Bax pathway. Bax is a pro-apoptotic protein and member of the BCL-2 family. (93)

DCA for Breast Cancer Stem Cells

In 2014, Dr. Weiguo Feng et al. studied the anti-CSC effects of DCA in a breast cancer model, finding that the CSCs (called TICs, for tumor-initiating cells) have a "pro-glycolytic phenotype" with fewer, less active mitochondria. Dr. Feng found that breast CSCs rely on GLYCOLYSIS and are eliminated in vitro and in vivo by metabolic reprogramming with a glycolysis inhibitor, such as DCA. Dr. Feng's group concludes:

Transcriptome profiling using RNA-Seq revealed TICs [tumor-initiating cells, cancer stem cells] under-express genes involved in mitochondrial biology and mitochondrial oxidative phosphorylation and metabolic analyses revealed TICs preferentially perform glycolysis over oxidative phosphorylation compared to NTCs [non-tumor-initiating cells]. Mechanistic analyses demonstrated that decreased expression and activity of pyruvate dehydrogenase [PDH], a key regulator of oxidative phosphorylation, play a critical role in promoting the pro-glycolytic phenotype of TICs. Metabolic reprogramming [with DCA] via forced activation of PDH preferentially eliminates TICs both in vitro and in vivo. (94)

Note: Transcriptome profiling using RNA-Seq (RNA Sequencing) is a laboratory technique using next-generation gene sequencing of the messenger RNA (mRNA) output of a cancer cell culture in-vitro. Knowing the mRNA output is key to understanding the oncogenes and metabolic derangements in the cancer cells, as well as response to various drug treatments.

Metformin Synergy with Venetoclax

In 2016, Dr. Juliana Velez et al. found that metformin used in combination with DCA, synergizes with venetoclax, a new oncology drug approved for use in lymphomas known to express high levels of the BCL-2 protein that inhibits apoptosis. Venetoclax is commonly given in combination with ibrutinib, a B-cell receptor blocker, for B-cell lymphoma and chronic lymphocytic leukemia (CLL). Thus, the combination of metformin, DCA, ibrutinib, and venetoclax would be expected to show synergy and high efficacy in treatment of B-cell lymphoma. We await future studies for confirmation. (95)

Synergy Combination of DCA and Fenbendazole

The anti-cancer activity of the antiparasitic drug fenbendazole (FZ) was found to be "**strongly synergistic**" with DCA. FZ increased P53 protein, which translocated to the mitochondria, resulting in a mitochondrial cell-death pathway. FZ inhibited glucose uptake, reduced lactate levels, and reduced HK2 activity. Dr. Nilambra Dogera et al. write (2018) :

> We evaluated the effect of FZ in combination with the microtubule targeting drug taxol, glycolytic inhibitor 2 deoxyglucose [2DG] and dichloroacetate [DCA] - a pyruvate dehydrogenase kinase inhibitor which acts by shifting the metabolism towards glucose oxidation over glycolysis.**.... there was a strong synergism by FZ and DCA.** (96)

Synergy Combination of DCA and Omaprazole (PPI Drug)

The combination of DCA with metformin provides inhibition of two of our three pillars of cancer cell metabolism. What if we addressed the third pillar, autophagy, by adding an autophagy inhibitor drug? Would this provide synergy? The answer is yes. In 2012, Dr. Tatsuaki Ishiguro et al. studied human fibrosarcoma cells in vitro, finding the combination of DCA with the autophagy inhibitor, omeprazole (OMP) highly synergistic. Omaprazole is a widely available PPI proton pump inhibitor commonly used over-the-counter as anti-acid drug. OMP inhibits the acid pump called V-ATPase in lysosomes, rendering them non-functional, thereby inhibiting autophagy. Dr. Tatsuaki Ishiguro writes:

> Cotreatment with DCA and OMP exhibits a synergistic antiproliferative effect on malignant tumors... Since OMP and DCA may be administered orally and have been used clinically for several years without major side effects, we believe that this combination therapy could be readily translated to treat malignant tumors. (97)

Note: See Chapter 33 on PPI drugs as autophagy inhibitors for more on this topic.

Synergy of DCA with Propranolol

The beta blocker propranolol has been repurposed as an excellent anti-cancer drug. (98)

In 2018, Dr. Christopher Lucido et al. studied propranolol combined with DCA in head-and-neck squamous cell cancer (HNSCC) in vitro and in vivo, finding propranolol heightened glycolytic activity, promoting a state of glucose dependence in the cancer cells. The authors hypothesized that combining propranolol with the glycolysis inhibitor DCA, would be a highly effective combination, with no evidence of toxicity:

> Propranolol synergizes with the glycolytic inhibitor dichloroacetate [DCA] to dramatically attenuate tumor cell metabolism and mTOR signaling.... significantly delays tumor growth in vivo with no evidence of toxicity. Additionally, the combination of propranolol and DCA enhances the effects of and sensitizes resistant cells to chemo-radiation. (99)

See chapter 6 on propranolol for more information.

DCA Alone Induces Protective Autophagy

As is typical for most effective anti-cancer agents, including GLYCOLYSIS and OXPHOS inhibitors, DCA induces protective autophagy by inhibiting mTOR. A number of studies show DCA activates protective autophagy.

In 2013, Dr. F. Gong et al. studied the effect of DCA on a colon cancer cell line, finding induction of protective autophagy. Firstly, the reversal of metabolism from GLYCOLYSIS to OXPHOS increased damaging ROS. Secondly, DCA treatment suppressed the Akt-mTOR pathway, which directly activates protective autophagy. (149) These findings were updated by Dr. Gigin Lin in 2014 in colorectal and prostate cancer xenografts, again showing DCA induces protective autophagy. (150)

In 2017, Dr. HongYu Jia et al. studied the effect of DCA on an esophageal cancer cell line, again finding suppression of Akt-mTOR pathway with induction of protective autophagy, thus confirming Dr. Gong's 2013 results. The inhibition of DCA-induced autophagy serves to increase apoptosis and cancer cell sensitivity to combined treatment with low concentrations of DCA and 5-FU (5 flouro-uracil chemotherapy). Dr. Jia suggested combined use of DCA with autophagy inhibitors as an effective strategy. Dr. Jia and colleagues write:

> Autophagy inhibition by Atg5 siRNA or 3-MA treatment significantly improved DCA-induced apoptosis and drug sensitivity in TE-1 [esophageal cancer] cells. These

results suggest that autophagy plays a protective role in tumor cells in response to DCA treatment. Hence, low-concentration DCA treatment in conjunction with autophagy inhibitors may exert anti-tumor activity. (151)

Note: Atg5 siRNA (short interfering RNA) inhibits Atg5 (autophagy-related gene) expression. The Atg5 gene controls autophagy. 3-MA (3-Methyladenine) inhibits phosphatidylinositol 3-kinase (PI3K), inhibiting autophagy. Both are laboratory agents used for autophagy inhibition in cancer cell models, and not approved for human use. For more on autophagy inhibitors see chapters 31-35.

DCA Combined with Chemotherapy Inhibits Autophagy

As we have seen, DCA alone induces protective autophagy. However, this effect is reversed when DCA is used in combination with chemotherapy. In this scenario, the DCA now inhibits the protective autophagy induced by the chemotherapy agent. In 2017, Dr. Minghao Wang et al. studied the effect of DCA in combination with Doxorubicin (DOX) in a breast cancer cell model, finding DCA significantly inhibits the autophagy induced by DOX, markedly enhancing cancer cell death in vitro and in vivo with prolongation of mouse survival time. Dr. Wang's group writes:

> DCA inhibit[s] doxorubicin-inducing autophagy and provide[s] a novel strategy for improving the anti-cancer efficacy of chemotherapy. (152)

In 2018, Dr. Xiao Lu et al. studied the effect of DCA in combination with the chemotherapy agent paclitaxel, finding DCA inhibits autophagy, with marked enhancement of apoptosis in a lung cancer mouse xenograft model. They write:

> Our results suggest that DCA can inhibit cell autophagy induced by chemotherapeutics, providing a new avenue for cancer chemotherapy sensitization. (153)

Curcumin and Other Drugs Synergy with DCA

In 2018, Dr. Ping-Chuan Kan et al. suggested that coupling curcumin with DCA "significantly enhances" anti-cancer potential, allowing for reduction in DCA dosage. (100)

Anti-cancer effects of DCA synergizes with many other drugs and natural substances including:

- Fenbendazole ("exhibits strong synergy") (96)
- Omeprazole (PPI) (97)
- Propranolol (99)
- Curcumin (100)
- Metformin (72–74)(101–103)
- Celecoxib (Celebrex COX-2 Inhibitor) (104)
- Phenylbutyrate (105)
- Sulindac NSAID (106–107)
- Bevacizumab Avastin (Anti-VEGF antibody) (27)
- Sorafinib, (approved hepatocellular carcinoma)(108–109)
- Salinomycin (125)

Anti-Cancer Effects of DCA on Various Cancers:

- Non-Hodgkin's lymphoma (110–111)
- Colorectal cancer cells (112)(125)
- Endometrial cancer cells (113)
- Breast cancer (114)
- Glioblastoma (115–116)
- Multiple myeloma (117–118) (improves sensitivity to bortezomib)
- B-cell leukemia (119)
- T cell lymphoma (120)
- Gastric cancer (121)
- Ovarian cancer (72)
- Lung cancer (73)(123–124)(126)
- Oral squamous cell cancer (74)(79)
- Esophageal squamous (29)
- Pancreatic cancer (90)
- Neuroblastoma (122)
- NHL lymphoma (110–111)
- T cell lymphoma (120)
- Hepatocellular carcinoma (91)(108–109)
- Enhances effects of chemotherapy (126–133)
- Enhances effects of radiation (134–135)

DCA Has Immunomodulatory Activity toward T1 Function

As an added bonus, DCA has benefits for the host immune system, restoring cancer immune surveillance. Dr. Badr writes in *Oncotarget* (2014):

> DCA has immunomodulatory activity, mainly via activation of the IL-12–IFN-gamma pathway and is able to modulate cytokines toward T-helper 1 lymphocyte function. (136)

Note: T-Helper-1 (TH1) lymphocytes carry out

cell-mediated immunity, while TH2 cells provide humoral immunity with antibody production. TH1 function is important for host anti-cancer immunity. IL-12 (Interleukin 12) is a pro-inflammatory cytokine which shifts T cell differentiation to TH1 cell mediated immunity, enhancing NK cell function and anti-tumor immunity. One might speculate that DCA's immune enhancing effects could be useful as an adjunct to CAR-T therapy, providing a beneficial TH1 shift similar to that of ibrutinub when combined with CAR-T therapy as discussed by Dr. Jim Qin (2020). (154)

DCA has been studied in ALS (amyotrophic lateral sclerosis) and chronic fatigue syndrome. (137–138)

Case Report "Durable Complete Remission" of NHL with DCA

Dr. Stephen Strum (2012) et al. report on a 52-year-old male (TM) who had a 6 year history of B-Cell Lymphoma, now presenting with recurrent disease causing drenching night sweats and PET scan showing extensive abdominal and cervical lymphadenopathy. The patient's B-cell lymphoma recurrence was treated with conventional chemotherapy (rituximab-CHOP, R-CHOP), achieving complete remission of short duration, which lasted about seven months, at which time the patient again relapsed with symptoms of weight loss, night sweats, and a new PET scan showing hypermetabolic foci (recurrent lymphadenopathy). At this time, the patient declined any further chemotherapy and instead started taking DCA on his own. Dr. Strum and colleagues write:

> His [the patient TM] "DCA protocol" consisted of: DCA 1,000 mg per day in one daily dose. The DCA was mixed with 10 ounces of Mountain Dew™ containing 55 mg of

caffeine. TM also used vitamin B1 at 500 mg/d [through 12/10/08], alpha lipoic acid 600 mg bid, green tea [Jarrow™] 500 mg bid containing 74 mg of EGCG and 35 mg of caffeine per 500 mg. (111)

Within two weeks on the DCA regimen, the patient reported significant improvement in symptoms and disappearance of palpable neck nodes; a follow-up PET scan four months later showed resolution of all abnormalities seen on the previous study. The patient remained in "durable complete remission" with a negative PET scan over the next four years of follow-up. (110–111)

Adverse Side Effects of DCA

Neurotoxicity is a well-known reversible adverse side effect of dichloroacetate, with a peripheral neuropathy with tingling and numbness in the extremities as the most common symptoms. (139–144)

DCA-Induced Hand Tremor Reversed with Decreased Dose

Hand tremor is a neurotoxic adverse side effect of DCA. In 2018, Dr. Frank Comhaire reported improvement in hand tremor upon decreasing the DCA dosage. (138)

Avoiding Neurotoxicity with Supplements

Neurotoxicity can be avoided by supplementing with thiamine (benfotiamine) and R-alpha lipoic acid, and reducing dosage of the DCA. Poly-MVA, a liquid polymer containing palladium, thiamine and alpha lipoic acid, is also useful for reducing the incidence of neuropathy, reversible upon stopping the DCA. According to Drs. Tataranni and Piccoli (2019), DCA-induced neuropathy is more common with the oral administration and can be avoided with IV (intravenous) DCA and (inhaled) nebulized administration. (19)

Fatal Outcome Combining DCA and Artesunate

In 2016, Dr. Martin Uhl et al. published a case report of fatal outcome using the combination of DCA and Artesunate in a Glioblastoma patient who experienced both fatal liver failure and bone marrow toxicity after combined use of DCA and Artesunate. Therefore, it would be prudent to use extreme caution or avoid this combination. The two agents have different mechanisms of action. DCA is a glycolysis inhibitor, shifting metabolism back to mitochondrial OXPHOS, which creates increased reactive oxygen species (ROS). Artesunate also creates ROS by reacting with Iron in lysosomes. This case highlights the importance of using a knowledgeable physician who can monitor adverse side effects and serial blood labs such as liver function tests (LFTs) during treatment for early detection of adverse events. For more on this, see chapter 21 on artesunate. (142)

Long-Term DCA—Prostate and Epididymis Toxicity

Long term DCA studies in mice show testicular, prostate and epididymis toxicity which may result in decreased testosterone levels and impaired fertility with reduction in sperm production. Monitoring testosterone levels is advised when using DCA in males. One study suggests ingesting palm date fruit extract to prevent DCA induced testicular toxicity. (143-147)

Conclusion

DCA is an excellent GLYCOLYSIS inhibitor that creates lethal synergy in combination with OXPHOS inhibitors such as metformin and propranolol. Metformin targets complex I of the ETC while propranolol inhibits ATPase, thus both inhibit mitochondrial OXPHOS. There is strong in vitro synergy of DCA with fenbendazole, a veterinary antiparasitic drug made popular by Joe Tippens.

Concurrent use of thiamine and alpha lipoic acid or Poly-MVA with DCA is necessary to avoid DCA's adverse effect of neuropathy. For now, the combination of DCA and artesunate is to be avoided, until it can be studied further.

An added bonus of DCA is that it targets CSCs, especially in combination with OXPHOS inhibitors, such as metformin, doxycycline, propranolol, etc.

DCA restores host anti-cancer immunity by decreasing acidic lactate in the micro-environment, and by increasing IL-12 and "modulating cytokines toward T-helper 1 (TH1) lymphocyte function."

Similar to many other potent anti-cancer drugs, DCA inhibits mTOR, which triggers "protective autophagy." The DCA/Propranolol combination is appealing because propranolol, in addition to being an OXPHOS inhibitor, is also an autophagy inhibitor. Thus, the DCA/Propranolol combination targets all "three pillars of cancer metabolism". Similar to many other glycolysis inhibitors that stimulate OXPHOS and mitochondrial electron flux, DCA will increase ROS, which is damaging to the cancer cell. Additional agents that downregulate ROS defenses by decreasing intracellular glutathione, such as sulforaphane and sulfasalazine, will augment DCA's ROS damage to the cancer cell.

Note: Sulfasalazine is discussed later its own chapter 11, and may also be associated with testicular toxicity. (148)

Suggested add-ons: Frankincense (boswellia) and Solomon's seal. See respective chapters 17 and 18 on each of these essential oils.

Overwhelming evidence has accumulated over the years supporting a paradigm shift in cancer treatment using targeted drugs such as DCA, metformin, doxycycline, and propranolol to inhibit metabolic pathways in cancer cells. In spite of its promise, DCA is not routinely used and is not available on the oncology wards of U.S. hospitals. When it will become available is anyone's guess. Until then, DCA treatment will be restricted to the integrative oncology practitioner, outside of conventional oncology.

References for Chapter 5: DCA Dichloroacetate

1) Stengler, Mark and Anderson Paul. Outside the Box Cancer Therapies: Alternative Therapies that Treat and Prevent Cancer. Hay House, Inc, 2018.

2) Metabolic Therapies in Advanced "Salvage" Cancer Cases by Dr. Paul S. Anderson, NMD Townsend Letter Aug /Sept 2018

3) Rationale for and Protocol for the use of combined Dichloroacetate (DCA) and Lipoic Acid Mineral Complex (LAMC) in advanced Cancer Patients as developed by Paul S. Anderson for patients treated at Anderson Medical Specialty Associates and in the Bastyr University Clinical Research Center (BCRC)

4) Poly-MVA as an integrative approach to the treatment of cancer: evidence-based through case reports. Sheri Lieberman Aug 2008 Townsend letter.

5) Neil McKinney Naturopathic Oncology. Creative Guy Publishing; Third edition edition (January 6, 2016)

6) Wang, Shu-ya, et al. "Polygonatum cyrtonema lectin, a potential antineoplastic drug targeting programmed cell death pathways." Biochemical and biophysical research communications 406.4 (2011): 497-500.

7) Ouyang, Liang, et al. "Polygonatum odoratum lectin induces apoptosis and autophagy via targeting EGFR-mediated Ras-Raf-MEK-ERK pathway in human MCF-7 breast cancer cells." Phytomedicine 21.12 (2014): 1658-1665.

8) Liu, Tao, et al. "Role of reactive oxygen species-mediated MAPK and NF-κB activation in polygonatum cyrtonema lectin-induced apoptosis and autophagy in human lung adenocarcinoma A549 cells." The Journal of Biochemistry 160.6 (2016): 315-324.

9) Khan, Akbar, et al. "A novel form of dichloroacetate therapy for patients with advanced cancer: a report of 3 cases." Alternative Therapies in Health & Medicine 20 (2014).

10) Khan, Akbar, Douglas Andrews, and Anneke C. Blackburn. "Long-term stabilization of stage 4 colon cancer using sodium dichloroacetate therapy." World journal of clinical cases 4.10 (2016): 336.

11) Khan, Akbar, et al. "Long-term stabilization of metastatic melanoma with sodium dichloroacetate." World journal of clinical oncology 8.4 (2017): 371.

12) Khan, Akbar, et al. "Long-term stabilization of metastatic melanoma with sodium dichloroacetate." World journal of clinical oncology 8.4 (2017): 371.

13) McFate, Thomas, et al. "Pyruvate dehydrogenase complex activity controls metabolic and malignant phenotype in cancer cells." Journal of Biological Chemistry 283.33 (2008): 22700-22708.

14) Sutendra, Gopinath, and Evangelos D. Michelakis. "Pyruvate dehydrogenase kinase as a novel therapeutic target in oncology." Frontiers in oncology 3 (2013): 38.

15) Stacpoole, Peter W. "Therapeutic targeting of the pyruvate dehydrogenase complex/pyruvate dehydrogenase kinase (PDC/PDK) axis in cancer." JNCI: Journal of the National Cancer Institute 109.11 (2017).

16) Villalba, Martin, et al. "Chemical metabolic inhibitors for the treatment of blood-borne cancers." Anti-Cancer Agents in Medicinal Chemistry (Formerly Current Medicinal Chemistry-Anti-Cancer Agents) 14.2 (2014): 223-232.

17) Stacpoole, Peter W., et al. "Treatment of congenital lactic acidosis with dichloroacetate." Archives of disease in childhood 77.6 (1997): 535-541.

18) Stacpoole, Peter W., et al. "Role of dichloroacetate in the treatment of genetic mitochondrial diseases." Advanced drug delivery reviews 60.13-14 (2008): 1478-1487.

19) Tataranni, Tiziana, and Claudia Piccoli. "Dichloroacetate (DCA) and Cancer: An Overview towards Clinical Applications." Oxidative Medicine and Cellular Longevity 2019 (2019).

20) Mathupala, Saroj P., Young H. Ko, and Peter L. Pedersen. "Hexokinase-2 bound to mitochondria: cancer's stygian link to the "Warburg Effect" and a pivotal target for effective therapy." Seminars in cancer biology. Vol. 19. No. 1. Academic Press, 2009.

21) Bustamante E, Morris HP, Pedersen PL. Energy metabolism of tumor cells. Requirement for a form of hexokinase with a propensity for mitochondrial binding. J Biol Chem 1981; 256 (16):8699–704].

22) Ko YH, Smith BL, Wang Y, Pomper MG, Rini DA, Torbenson MS, et al. Advanced cancers: eradication in all cases using 3-bromopyruvate therapy to deplete ATP. Biochem Biophys Res Commun 2004; 324(1):269–75]

23) Chen, Zhao, et al. "Role of mitochondria-associated hexokinase II in cancer cell death induced by 3-bromopyruvate." Biochimica et Biophysica Acta (BBA)-Bioenergetics 1787.5 (2009): 553-560.

24) Ohashi, Toshimitsu, et al. "Dichloroacetate improves immune dysfunction caused by tumor-secreted lactic acid and increases antitumor immunoreactivity." International journal of cancer 133.5 (2013): 1107-1118.

25) Santos, Nuno, et al. "Lactate as a Regulator of Cancer Inflammation and Immunity." Immunometabolism 1.2 (2019).

26) Kim, Jaehong. "Regulation of immune cell functions by metabolic reprogramming." Journal of immunology research 2018 (2018).

27) Kumar, Krishan, et al. "Dichloroacetate reverses the hypoxic adaptation to bevacizumab and enhances its antitumor effects in mouse xenografts." Journal of molecular medicine 91.6 (2013): 749-758.

28) Lin, G., et al. "Dichloroacetate induces autophagy in colorectal cancer cells and tumours." British journal of cancer 111.2 (2014): 375-385.

29) Jia, Hong-Yu, et al. "Dichloroacetate induces protective autophagy in esophageal squamous carcinoma cells." Oncology letters 14.3 (2017): 2765-2770.

30) Gong, F., et al. "Dichloroacetate induces protective autophagy in LoVo cells: involvement of cathepsin D/thioredoxin-like protein 1 and Akt-mTOR-mediated signaling." Cell death & disease 4.11 (2013): e913-e913.

31) Rodrigues, Ana Sofia, et al. "Dichloroacetate, the pyruvate dehydrogenase complex and the modulation of mESC pluripotency." PloS one 10.7 (2015): e0131663.

32) Sutendra, G., et al. "Mitochondrial activation by inhibition of PDKII suppresses HIF1a signaling and angiogenesis in cancer." Oncogene 32.13 (2013): 1638.

33) Hanberry, Bradley S., Ryan Berger, and Jason A. Zastre. "High-dose vitamin B1 reduces proliferation in cancer cell lines analogous to dichloroacetate." Cancer chemotherapy and pharmacology 73.3 (2014): 585-594.

34) Krasnov, George S., et al. "Targeting VDAC-bound hexokinase II: a promising approach for concomitant anti-cancer therapy." Expert opinion on therapeutic targets 17.10 (2013): 1221-1233.

35) Shoshan-Barmatz, Varda, et al. "Voltage-dependent anion channel 1 as an emerging drug target for novel anti-cancer therapeutics." Frontiers in oncology 7 (2017): 154.

36) Camara, Amadou KS, et al. "Mitochondrial VDAC1: a key gatekeeper as potential therapeutic target." Frontiers in physiology 8 (2017): 460.

37) Magrì, Andrea, Simona Reina, and Vito De Pinto. "VDAC1 as pharmacological target in cancer and neurodegeneration: focus on its role in apoptosis." Frontiers in chemistry 6 (2018): 108.

38) Huang, Li, et al. "A new fungal diterpene induces VDAC1-dependent apoptosis in Bax/Bak-deficient cells." Journal of Biological Chemistry 290.39 (2015): 23563-23578.

39) Jan, Chia-Ing, et al. "Fenofibrate suppresses oral tumorigenesis via reprogramming metabolic processes: potential drug repurposing for oral cancer." International journal of biological sciences 12.7 (2016): 786.

40) Head, Sarah A., et al. "Antifungal drug itraconazole targets VDAC1 to modulate the AMPK/mTOR signaling axis in endothelial cells." Proceedings of the National Academy of Sciences 112.52 (2015): E7276-E7285.

41) Gu, Juan J., et al. "Itraconazole, an Oral Antifungal Drug, Is Active in Chemotherapy Resistant B-Cell Non-Hodgkin Lymphoma and Enhances the Anti-Tumor Activity of Chemotherapy Agents." Blood. (2016): 5138-5138.

42) Pantziarka, Pan, et al. "Repurposing Drugs in Oncology (ReDO)—itraconazole as an anti-cancer agent." ecancermedicalscience 9 (2015).

43) Tsubamoto, Hiroshi, et al. "Repurposing itraconazole as an anticancer agent." Oncology Letters 14.2 (2017): 1240-1246.

44) Head, Sarah A., et al. "Simultaneous Targeting of NPC1 and VDAC1 by Itraconazole Leads to Synergistic Inhibition of mTOR Signaling and Angiogenesis." ACS chemical biology 12.1 (2016): 174-182.

45) Ueda, Tomoko, et al. "Itraconazole modulates hedgehog, WNT/β-catenin, as well as Akt Signalling, and inhibits proliferation of cervical Cancer cells." Anticancer research 37.7 (2017): 3521-3526.

46) Pounds R, Leonard S, Dawson C, Kehoe S. Repurposing itraconazole for the treatment of cancer. Oncology Letters. 2017;14(3):2587-2597.

47) Ko YH, Smith BL, Wang Y, Pomper MG, Rini DA, Torbenson MS, et al. Advanced cancers: eradication in all cases using 3-bromopyruvate therapy to deplete ATP. Biochem Biophys Res Commun 2004;324(1):269–75]

48) Chen, Zhao, et al. "Role of mitochondria-associated hexokinase II in cancer cell death induced by 3-bromopyruvate." Biochimica et Biophysica Acta (BBA)-Bioenergetics 1787.5 (2009): 553-560.

49) Penso J1, Beitner R. Lithium detaches hexokinase from mitochondria and inhibits proliferation of B16 melanoma cells.Mol Genet Metab. 2003 Jan;78(1):74-8.

50) Penso, Julia, and Rivka Beitner. "Clotrimazole and bifonazole detach hexokinase from mitochondria of melanoma cells." European journal of pharmacology 342.1 (1998): 113-117.

51) Kadavakollu, S., et al. "Clotrimazole as a cancer drug: a short review." Medicinal chemistry 4.11 (2014): 722.

52) Goldin N1, Arzoine L, Heyfets A, Israelson A, Zaslavsky Z, Bravman T, Bronner V, Notcovich A, Shoshan-Barmatz V, Flescher E. Methyl jasmonate binds to and detaches mitochondria-bound hexokinase. Oncogene. 2008 Aug 7;27(34):4636-43

53) Fingrut O1, Reischer D, Rotem R, Goldin N, Altboum I, Zan-Bar I, Flescher E. Jasmonates induce nonapoptotic death in high-resistance mutant p53-expressing B-lymphoma cells. Br J Pharmacol. 2005 Nov;146(6):800-8.

54) Sucu, Bilgesu Onur, et al. "Synthesis of novel methyl jasmonate derivatives and evaluation of their biological activity in various cancer cell lines." Bioorganic chemistry 91 (2019): 103146.

55) Li, Jingjing, et al. "Methyl jasmonate leads to necrosis and apoptosis in hepatocellular carcinoma cells via inhibition of glycolysis and represses tumor growth in mice." Oncotarget 8.28 (2017): 45965.

56) Wang, Yao, et al. "EZH2 inhibition promotes methyl jasmonate-induced apoptosis of human colorectal cancer through the Wnt/β-catenin pathway." Oncology letters 16.1 (2018): 1231-1236.

57) Yehia, Rania, et al. "Anti-tumor efficacy of an integrated methyl dihydrojasmonate transdermal microemulsion system targeting breast cancer cells:

in vitro and in vivo studies." Colloids and Surfaces B: Biointerfaces 155 (2017): 512-521.

58) Zhang, Mutian, et al. "Methyl jasmonate induces apoptosis and pro-apoptotic autophagy via the ROS pathway in human non-small cell lung cancer." American journal of cancer research 6.2 (2016): 187.

59) Cesari, Italo Mario, et al. "Methyl jasmonate: putative mechanisms of action on cancer cells cycle, metabolism, and apoptosis." International journal of cell biology 2014 (2014).

60) Tong, Qiang-Song, et al. "Methyl jasmonate downregulates expression of proliferating cell nuclear antigen and induces apoptosis in human neuroblastoma cell lines." Anti-Cancer Drugs 19.6 (2008): 573-581.

61) Fingrut, O., and E. Flescher. "Plant stress hormones suppress the proliferation and induce apoptosis in human cancer cells." Leukemia 16.4 (2002): 608.

62) Kim JH, Lee SY, Oh, SY, Han SI, Park HG, Yoo M, Kang HS. Methyl jasmonate induces apoptosis through induction of Bax/Bcl-XS and activation of caspase-3 via ROS production in A549 cells. Oncol Rep 2004; 12:1233-8;

63) Rotem R, Heyfets A, Fingrut O, Blickstein D, Shaklai M, Flescher E. Jasmonates: novel anticancer agents acting directly and selectively on human cancer cell mitochondria. Canc Res 2005; 65:1981-993;

64) Xu, Dong, et al. "Chrysin inhibited tumor glycolysis and induced apoptosis in hepatocellular carcinoma by targeting hexokinase-2." Journal of Experimental & Clinical Cancer Research 36.1 (2017): 44.

65) Salimi, Ahmad, et al. "Chrysin as an anti-cancer agent exerts selective toxicity by directly inhibiting mitochondrial complex II and V in CLL B-lymphocytes." Cancer investigation 35.3 (2017): 174-186.

66) Tian, Mengyuan, et al. "Resveratrol protects cardiomyocytes against anoxia/reoxygenation via dephosphorylation of VDAC1 by Akt-GSK3 β pathway." European journal of pharmacology 843 (2019): 80-87.

67) Stockwin, Luke H., et al. "Sodium dichloroacetate selectively targets cells with defects in the mitochondrial ETC." International journal of cancer 127.11 (2010): 2510-2519.

68) Seyfried, Thomas N. "Cancer as a mitochondrial metabolic disease." Frontiers in cell and developmental biology 3 (2015): 43.

69) Ward, Nathan Patrick. "Therapeutic Modulation of Cancer Metabolism with Dichloroacetate and Metformin." (2017).

70) Ward, Nathan P., et al. "Complex I inhibition augments dichloroacetate cytotoxicity through enhancing oxidative stress in VM-M3 glioblastoma cells." PloS one 12.6 (2017): e0180061.

71) Florio, Rosalba, et al. "Effects of dichloroacetate as single agent or in combination with GW6471 and metformin in paraganglioma cells." Scientific reports 8.1 (2018): 13610.

72) Li, Bo, et al. "Dichloroacetate and metformin synergistically suppress the growth of ovarian cancer cells." Oncotarget 7.37 (2016): 59458.

73) Kolesnik, D. L., et al. "Time-dependent cytotoxicity of dichloroacetate and metformin against Lewis lung carcinoma." Experimental oncology 41.1 (2019): 14-19.

74) Inanc, Seniz, et al. "Metformin and Dichloroacetate Combination Exert A Synergistic Effect On Cell Viability Of Oral Squamous Cell Carcinoma." ENT Updates 9.2 (2019): 68-73.

75) Vial, Guillaume, Dominique Detaille, and Bruno Guigas. "Role of Mitochondria in the Mechanism (s) of Action of Metformin." Frontiers in endocrinology 10 (2019): 294.

76) Voltan, Rebecca, et al. "Metformin combined with sodium dichloroacetate promotes B leukemic cell death by suppressing anti-apoptotic protein Mcl-1." Oncotarget 7.14 (2016): 18965.

77) Choi, Yong Won, and In Kyoung Lim. "Sensitization of metformin-cytotoxicity by dichloroacetate via reprogramming glucose metabolism in cancer cells." Cancer letters 346.2 (2014): 300-308.

78) Haugrud, Allison B., et al. "Dichloroacetate enhances apoptotic cell death via oxidative damage and attenuates lactate production in metformin-treated breast cancer cells." Breast cancer research and treatment 147.3 (2014): 539-550.

79) Ruggieri, Vitalba, et al. "Dichloroacetate, a selective mitochondria-targeting drug for oral squamous

cell carcinoma: a metabolic perspective of treatment." Oncotarget 6.2 (2015): 1217.

80) Woodhead, Jeffrey L., et al. "Analyzing the Mechanisms Behind Macrolide Antibiotic-Induced Liver Injury Using Quantitative Systems Toxicology Modeling." Pharmaceutical research 36.3 (2019): 48.

81) Fiorillo, Marco, et al. "Repurposing atovaquone: targeting mitochondrial complex III and OXPHOS to eradicate cancer stem cells." Oncotarget 7.23 (2016): 34084.

82) Sotgia, Federica, et al. "A mitochondrial based oncology platform for targeting cancer stem cells (CSCs): MITO-ONC-RX." Cell Cycle 17.17 (2018): 2091-2100.

83) Srivastava, Indresh K., Hagai Rottenberg, and Akhil B. Vaidya. "Atovaquone, a broad spectrum antiparasitic drug, collapses mitochondrial membrane potential in a malarial parasite." Journal of Biological Chemistry 272.7 (1997): 3961-3966.

84) Tan, Qian, et al. "Induction of mitochondrial dysfunction and oxidative damage by antibiotic drug doxycycline enhances the responsiveness of glioblastoma to chemotherapy." Medical science monitor: international medical journal of experimental and clinical research 23 (2017): 4117.

87) Zhao, Yan, et al. "Doxycycline inhibits proliferation and induces apoptosis of both human papillomavirus positive and negative cervical cancer cell lines." Canadian journal of physiology and pharmacology 94.5 (2016): 526-533.

88) Ahler, Ethan, et al. "Doxycycline alters metabolism and proliferation of human cell lines." PloS one 8.5 (2013): e64561.

89) Lleonart, Matilde E., et al. "Mitochondrial dysfunction and potential anticancer therapy." Medicinal Research Reviews 37.6 (2017): 1275-1298.

90) Tataranni, Tiziana, et al. "Dichloroacetate Affects Mitochondrial Function and Stemness-Associated Properties in Pancreatic Cancer Cell Lines." Cells 8.5 (2019): 478.

91) Song, Kyoungsub, et al. "Active glycolytic metabolism in CD133 (+) hepatocellular cancer stem cells: regulation by MIR-122." Oncotarget 6.38 (2015): 40822.

92) Michelakis, E. D., et al. "Metabolic modulation of glioblastoma with dichloroacetate." Science translational medicine 2.31 (2010): 31ra34-31ra34.

93) Morfouace, Marie, et al. "Comparison of spheroids formed by rat glioma stem cells and neural stem cells reveals differences in glucose metabolism and promising therapeutic applications." Journal of Biological Chemistry 287.40 (2012): 33664-33674.

94) Feng, Weiguo, et al. "Targeting unique metabolic properties of breast tumor initiating cells." Stem cells 32.7 (2014): 1734-1745.

95) Velez, Juliana, et al. "Biguanides sensitize leukemia cells to ABT-737-induced apoptosis by inhibiting mitochondrial electron transport." Oncotarget 7.32 (2016): 51435.

96) Dogra, Nilambra, Ashok Kumar, and Tapas Mukhopadhyay. "Fenbendazole acts as a moderate microtubule destabilizing agent and causes cancer cell death by modulating multiple cellular pathways." Scientific reports 8.1 (2018): 1-15.

97) Ishiguro, Tatsuaki, et al. "Cotreatment with dichloroacetate and omeprazole exhibits a synergistic antiproliferative effect on malignant tumors." Oncology letters 3.3 (2012): 726-728.

98) Pantziarka, Pan, et al. "Repurposing Drugs in Oncology (ReDO)—Propranolol as an anti-cancer agent." ecancermedicalscience 10 (2016).

99) Lucido, Christopher T., W. Keith Miskimins, and Paola D. Vermeer. "Propranolol Promotes Glucose Dependence and Synergizes with Dichloroacetate for Anti-Cancer Activity in HNSCC." Cancers 10.12 (2018).

100) Kan, Ping-Chuan, et al. "Coupling dichloroacetate treatment with curcumin significantly enhances anticancer potential." Anticancer research 38.11 (2018): 6253-6261.

101) Kolesnik, D. L., et al. "Metformin enhances antitumor action of sodium dichloroacetate against glioma C6." Experimental oncology 41.2 (2019): 123-129.

102) Kolesnik, D. L., et al. "Time-dependent cytotoxicity of dichloroacetate and metformin against Lewis lung carcinoma." Experimental oncology 41.1 (2019): 14-19.

103) Inanc, Seniz, et al. "Metformin And Dichloroacetate Combination Exert A Synergistic Effect On Cell Viability Of Oral Squamous Cell Carcinoma." ENT Updates 9.2 (2019): 68-73.

104) Li, Bo, et al. "Inhibition of COX2 enhances the chemosensitivity of dichloroacetate in cervical cancer cells." Oncotarget 8.31 (2017): 51748.

105) Ferriero, Rosa, et al. "Differential inhibition of PDKs by phenylbutyrate and enhancement of pyruvate dehydrogenase complex activity by combination with dichloroacetate." Journal of Inherited Metabolic Disease 38.5 (2015): 895.

106) Aono, Yuichi, et al. "Sulindac sulfone inhibits the mTORC1 pathway in colon cancer cells by directly targeting voltage-dependent anion channel 1 and 2." Biochemical and biophysical research communications 505.4 (2018): 1203-1210.

107) Ayyanathan, Kasirajan, et al. "Combination of sulindac and dichloroacetate kills cancer cells via oxidative damage." PloS one 7.7 (2012): e39949.

108) SUN, Liangbo, et al. "Dichloroacetate enhances sorafenib's inhibitory effect on proliferation of hepatocellular carcinoma cells by activating ROS-JNK pathway."

109) Shen, Y. C., et al. "Activating oxidative phosphorylation by a pyruvate dehydrogenase kinase inhibitor overcomes sorafenib resistance of hepatocellular carcinoma." British journal of cancer 108.1 (2013): 72-81.

110) Strum, Dana F. "Non-Hodgkin's lymphoma reversal with dichloroacetate." Journal of oncology 2010 (2010).

111) Strum, Stephen B., et al. "Case report: Sodium dichloroacetate (DCA) inhibition of the "Warburg Effect" in a human cancer patient: complete response in non-Hodgkin's lymphoma after disease progression with rituximab-CHOP." Journal of bioenergetics and biomembranes 45.3 (2013): 307-315.

112) Madhok, B. M., et al. "Dichloroacetate induces apoptosis and cell-cycle arrest in colorectal cancer cells." British journal of cancer 102.12 (2010): 1746.

113) Wong, Jason YY, et al. "Dichloroacetate induces apoptosis in endometrial cancer cells." Gynecologic oncology 109.3 (2008): 394-402.

114) Sun, Ramon C., et al. "Reversal of the glycolytic phenotype by dichloroacetate inhibits metastatic breast cancer cell growth in vitro and in vivo." Breast cancer research and treatment 120.1 (2010): 253-260.

115) Garnier, Delphine, et al. "Glioblastoma stem-like cells, metabolic strategy to kill a challenging target." Frontiers in oncology 9 (2019).

116) Pecqueur, Claire, et al. "Targeting metabolism to induce cell death in cancer cells and cancer stem cells." International journal of cell biology 2013 (2013).

117) Tian, Dandan. "Repurposing Dichloroacetate for the Treatment of Multiple Myeloma." (2018).

118) Sanchez, W. Y., et al. "Dichloroacetate inhibits aerobic glycolysis in multiple myeloma cells and increases sensitivity to bortezomib." British journal of cancer 108.8 (2013): 1624-1633.

119) Voltan, Rebecca, et al. "Metformin combined with sodium dichloroacetate promotes B leukemic cell death by suppressing anti-apoptotic protein Mcl-1." Oncotarget 7.14 (2016): 18965.

120) Kumar, Ajay, Shiva Kant, and Sukh Mahendra Singh. "Novel molecular mechanisms of antitumor action of dichloroacetate against T cell lymphoma: Implication of altered glucose metabolism, pH homeostasis and cell survival regulation." Chemico-biological interactions 199.1 (2012): 29-37.

121) Xuan, Yi, et al. "Dichloroacetate attenuates hypoxia-induced resistance to 5-fluorouracil in gastric cancer through the regulation of glucose metabolism." Experimental cell research 321.2 (2014): 219-230.

122) Vella, Serena, et al. "Dichloroacetate inhibits neuroblastoma growth by specifically acting against malignant undifferentiated cells." International journal of cancer 130.7 (2012): 1484-1493.

123) Otterson, G. A., et al. "Effect of dichloroacetate in combination with chemotherapy on human lung cancer cells." Journal of Clinical Oncology 26.15_suppl (2008): 14637-14637.

124) Lu, Xiao, et al. "Dichloroacetate enhances the antitumor efficacy of chemotherapeutic agents via inhibiting autophagy in non-small-cell lung cancer." Cancer management and research 10 (2018): 1231.

125) Skeberdytė, Aistė, et al. "Dichloroacetate and salinomycin exert a synergistic cytotoxic effect in colorectal cancer cell lines." Scientific reports 8.1 (2018): 1-13.

126) Garon, Edward B., et al. "Dichloroacetate should be considered with platinum-based chemotherapy in hypoxic tumors rather than as a single agent in advanced non-small cell lung cancer." Journal of cancer research and clinical oncology 140.3 (2014): 443-452.

127) Fiebiger, Wolfgang, et al. "In vitro cytotoxicity of novel platinum-based drugs and dichloroacetate against lung carcinoid cell lines." Clinical and Translational Oncology 13.1 (2011): 43-49.

128) Olszewski, Ulrike, et al. "In vitro cytotoxicity of combinations of dichloroacetate with anticancer platinum compounds." Clinical pharmacology: advances and applications 2 (2010): 177.

129) Tong, Jingtao, et al. "Synergistic antitumor effect of dichloroacetate in combination with 5-fluorouracil in colorectal cancer." BioMed Research International 2011 (2011).

130) Xie, Jing, et al. "Dichloroacetate shifts the metabolism from glycolysis to glucose oxidation and exhibits synergistic growth inhibition with cisplatin in HeLa cells." International journal of oncology 38.2 (2011): 409-417.

131) Wang, Minghao, et al. "Sensitization of breast cancer cells to paclitaxel by dichloroacetate through inhibiting autophagy." Biochemical and biophysical research communications 489.2 (2017): 103-108.

132) Dai, Yunhai, et al. "Dichloroacetate enhances adriamycin-induced hepatoma cell toxicity in vitro and in vivo by increasing reactive oxygen species levels." PLoS One 9.4 (2014).

133) LazarÃn, Ana Luisa Rivera, and Alejandro Zugasti Cruz. "Synergistic cytotoxic effect of sodium dichloroacetate combined with chemotherapeutic drugs on B16F10 murine melanoma cell line." (2019).

134) Cao, Wengang, et al. "Dichloroacetate (DCA) sensitizes both wild-type and over expressing Bcl-2 prostate cancer cells in vitro to radiation." The Prostate 68.11 (2008): 1223-1231.

135) Allen, Kah Tan, et al. "Dichloroacetate alters Warburg metabolism, inhibits cell growth, and increases the X-ray sensitivity of human A549 and H1299 NSC lung cancer cells." Free Radical Biology and Medicine 89 (2015): 263-273.

136) Badr, Mujtaba M., et al. "Dichloroacetate modulates cytokines toward T helper 1 function via induction of the interleukin-12–interferon-gamma pathway." OncoTargets and therapy 7 (2014): 193.

137) Martínez-Palma, Laura, et al. "Mitochondrial Modulation by Dichloroacetate Reduces Toxicity of Aberrant Glial Cells and Gliosis in the SOD1G93A Rat Model of Amyotrophic Lateral Sclerosis." Neurotherapeutics 16.1 (2019): 203-215.

138) Comhaire, Frank. "Treating patients suffering from myalgic encephalopathy/chronic fatigue syndrome (ME/CFS) with sodium dichloroacetate: An open-label, proof-of-principle pilot trial." Medical hypotheses 114 (2018): 45-48.

139) Brandsma, Dieta, et al. "Severe encephalopathy and polyneuropathy induced by dichloroacetate." Journal of neurology 257.12 (2010): 2099-2100.Severe encephalopathy and polyneuropathy induced by dichloroacetate Brandsma J neurology 2010

140) Stacpoole, Peter W., et al. "Dichloroacetate-induced peripheral neuropathy." International review of neurobiology 145 (2019): 211-238.

141) Djordjević, Mladen, and Ivan Petković. "Dichloroacetate-Induced Neuropathy in High Grade Follicular Lymphoma Patient." Acta Medica Medianae 58.1 (2019): 102-105

142) Uhl, Martin, Stefan Schwab, and Thomas Efferth. "Fatal liver and bone marrow toxicity by combination treatment of dichloroacetate and artesunate in a glioblastoma multiforme patient: case report and review of the literature." Frontiers in oncology 6 (2016): 204.

143) Sen, R., et al. "Long-Term Administration of DCA Induces Epididymus Toxixity in Male Albino Rats." Advances in Pharmacology and Toxicology 17.1 (2016): 21.

144) Sen, R., et al. "A Toxicological Study of Dichloroacetate Acid (DCA) on the Prostate Gland of Male Albino Rats." Advances in Pharmacology & Toxicology 16.3 (2015).

145) El Arem, Amira, et al. "Dichloroacetic acid-induced testicular toxicity in male rats and the protective

effect of date fruit extract." BMC Pharmacology and Toxicology 18.1 (2017): 17.

146) Toth, G. P., et al. "Adverse male reproductive effects following subchronic exposure of rats to sodium dichloroacetate." Fundamental and Applied Toxicology 19.1 (1992): 57-63.

147) Linder, Ralph E., et al. "Spermatotoxicity of dichloroacetic acid." Reproductive Toxicology 11.5 (1997): 681-688.

148) Hoyt, J. A., L. F. Fisher, and D. K. Swisher. "Short-term male reproductive toxicity study with sulfasalazine in the rat." Reproductive Toxicology 9.3 (1995): 315-326.

149) Gong, F., et al. "Dichloroacetate induces protective autophagy in LoVo cells: involvement of cathepsin D/thioredoxin-like protein 1 and Akt-mTOR-mediated signaling." Cell death & disease 4.11 (2013): e913-e913.

150) Lin, G., et al. "Dichloroacetate induces autophagy in colorectal cancer cells and tumours." British journal of cancer 111.2 (2014): 375-385.

151) Jia, HongYu, et al. "Dichloroacetate induces protective autophagy in esophageal squamous carcinoma cells." Oncology letters 14.3 (2017): 2765-2770.

152) Wang, Minghao, et al. "Sensitization of breast cancer cells to paclitaxel by dichloroacetate through inhibiting autophagy." Biochemical and biophysical research communications 489.2 (2017): 103-108.

153) Lu, Xiao, et al. "Dichloroacetate enhances the antitumor efficacy of chemotherapeutic agents via inhibiting autophagy in non-small-cell lung cancer." Cancer management and research 10 (2018): 1231.

154) Qin, Jim S., et al. "Antitumor potency of an anti-CD19 chimeric antigen receptor T-cell therapy, lisocabtagene maraleucel in combination with ibrutinib or acalabrutinib." Journal of Immunotherapy (Hagerstown, Md.: 1997) 43.4 (2020): 107.

Chapter 6

Propranolol Beta Blocker Anti-Cancer Drug

JIM IS A 54-YEAR-OLD ACCOUNTANT who lives alone in a small apartment in an overcrowded part of a big city. He takes the subway every day to a small cubicle on the 46th floor, the location of his high-pressure job. Needless to say, the daily stresses are sometimes overwhelming, mostly because Jim's boss is a bully who berates him on a daily basis for insignificant things. Eventually, Jim got sick and stayed in bed for a week, refusing to go to work. A friend found him and took Jim to the emergency room, where the doctor ordered lab tests and a CAT scan, which showed Jim had pancreatic cancer with metastatic spread to the liver. Jim's parents were shocked and upset and wanted to know if Jim's stressful lifestyle had caused the cancer.

According to Dr. Corona Kim-Fuchs et al. (2014), the answer is yes: "Chronic stress accelerates pancreatic cancer growth and invasion."[1] Chronic stress activates the sympathetic nervous system, which secretes catecholamines, which feed cancer growth. *(1–5)*

Note: Catecholamines are epinephrine, and norepinephrine.

More to the point, in 2010, Dr. A. Yuan et al. write:

> Accumulating data indicate that the psychological stress caused by chronic stressors is a major risk factor for cancer occurrence, growth, and metastasis. (2)

The molecular mechanism has been elucidated. Stress causes the body to secrete "stress hormones" called catecholamines, which attach to receptors on the cancer cells, stimulating growth, proliferation, and invasion. (3)

Dr. Steven Cole et al. (2015) write that in vivo animal models of stress show accelerated cancer growth, preventable with an old beta-blocker drug (propranolol):

> Experimental analyses with in vivo animal models have now shown that behavioral stress can accelerate the progression of breast, prostate, and ovarian carcinomas, neuroblastomas, malignant melanomas, pancreatic carcinoma, and some haematopoietic cancers such as leukaemia. In many of these experimental models, the biological effects of stress could be efficiently blocked by βeta-adrenergic antagonists and mimicked by pharmacologic βeta-agonists. (4)

Chronic Stress Is a Bad Thing

Chronic stress is undoubtedly a bad thing because of the release of massive adrenal hormones called catecholamines. This is extremely deleterious to our immune system, increases susceptibility to viral infection, and delays wound healing. Chronic stress has been implicated in cardiovascular disease, osteoporosis, arthritis, type 2 diabetes, gastric ulcer, as well as cancer (6–7)

Can Chronic Stress Cause Cancer?

This leads us to the main question of this chapter: Can chronic stress cause cancer? Let's examine three animal models of chronic stress using lymphoma, ovarian, and breast cancer xenografts in a mouse model of restraint stress to answer this question.

Lymphoma in Animal Model of Chronic Stress

The animal model of chronic stress involves restraining mice in narrow plastic tubes for a few hours every day. To make matters worse, the restrained mouse may be immersed in cold water, with only the nose above water for breathing. As you can imagine, this really aggravates the mouse's discomfort and panic.

In 2012, Dr. Donald Lamkin et al. used a lymphoblastic leukemia model in mice undergoing restraint stress to answer the question, "Does chronic stress cause cancer?" Dr. Lamkin's 2012 study, published in *Brain Behavior*, showed that mice suffering from restraint stress had accelerated progression of lymphoma compared to controls. (8)

Effect of Beta Blockers on Stress

The effect of stress was abrogated by giving the mice propranolol, which blocks the activation of the sympathetic nervous system. The propranolol-treated mice actually showed regression of cancer compared to controls. Thus, proving that beta-adrenergic stimulation drives cancer growth, and by blocking the effect of chronic stress with a beta blocker drug, we can slow the progression of cancer. Stressed mice had increased cancer growth compared to controls. Beta-blocker-propranolol-treated mice had actual regression of cancer compared to controls. (8)

Chronic Stress Promotes Ovarian Cancer

Similarly, in 2006, Dr. Premal Thaker et al. showed that chronic stress promotes growth and angiogenesis (new blood vessels) in a mouse model of ovarian cancer. Stressed mice had higher levels of stress hormones called catecholamines due to upregulation of the beta-adrenergic and cyclic AMP-kinase (cAMP-K) pathways. Stressed mice had larger tumors and more metastatic spread of ovarian cancer in a mouse xenograft model. Tumors in the stressed mice had increased tumor vessel formation (neo-vascularity) and increased vascular endothelial growth factor (VEGF). (9)

Thirty-Fold Increase in Metastatic Lesions

Similarly, in 2010, Dr. Erica Sloan et al. studied the effect of stress-induced neuroendocrine activation in a mouse model of breast cancer using in vivo bioluminescence imaging to track metastatic spread of disease. This study revealed that stress-increased beta-adrenergic signaling, which increased macrophage infiltration into the tumor, induced a pro-metastatic gene expression and induced a **30-fold increase** in distant metastatic lesions. This effect was blocked by treating the animals with the beta blocker propranolol. Dr. Sloan et al. conclude:

These findings identify activation of the

sympathetic nervous system as a novel neural regulator of breast cancer metastasis and suggest new strategies for antimetastatic therapies that target the βeta-adrenergic induction of pro-metastatic gene expression in primary breast cancers. (10)

Neurogenesis—New Nerve Growth into Tumors

Others have observed ingrowth of nerves from the autonomic nervous system into the tumor mass that enhances beta-adrenergic signaling. In addition, cancer stem cells (CSCs) are capable of generating neurons (sympathetic and parasympathetic) in the micro-environment involved in maintaining the cancer mass. (11–14)

Neupogen Stimulates Neurogenesis

Granulocyte colony-stimulating factor (G-CSF), marketed as Neupogen, is routinely used in cancer patients after chemotherapy to increase the white blood cell count, thus avoiding febrile neutropenia. G-CSF stimulates the bone marrow to make white blood cells. However, G-CSF also stimulates cancer neurogenesis in the micro-environment, promoting cancer development. One might therefore speculate about the cancer-promoting properties of G-CSF treatments. One might also speculate that concurrent use of a beta blocker drug such as propranolol would be beneficial in blocking the nerve growth stimulation from G-CSF. (15)

Stress and Beta-Adrenergic Stimulation

Chronic stress stimulates the adrenal medulla to secrete massive amounts of catecholamines, epinephrine, and norepinephrine. These stress hormones stimulate the beta-adrenergic receptors in the nervous system, inducing the fight-or-flight reaction. (16) Beta-adrenergic receptors are overexpressed in many cancers, playing a key role in invasion and metastatic behavior. (17) In addition, beta-adrenergic signaling plays a role in the tumor micro-environment, inducing immuno-suppression, and enhancing tumor immune evasion by impairing host anti-tumor immunity. (16–18)

Propranolol Anti-Cancer Effects

Preclinical studies show blocking beta-adrenergic receptors with propranolol reduces cancer-cell proliferation and migration (i.e., metastatic disease). In vivo studies show decreased cancer proliferation, decreased metastatic behavior, and improved survival. Propranolol synergizes with conventional chemotherapy with augmented anti-cancer efficacy.

According to Dr. Alexa Montoya et al. (2019), retrospective studies using propranolol (beta-adrenergic antagonists) in breast cancer patients showed reduced tumor proliferation, decreased mortality, decreased metastases, longer survival, and reduced cancer recurrence. Most significantly, propranolol downregulates hexokinase 2 and inhibits glucose metabolism. Propranolol has anti-angiogenic effects, as well. (19–20)

Adrenal Masses on CAT Scan

Circulating tumor cells may migrate to the adrenal glands, seeking the adrenal medulla for its high concentration of catecholamines, thus producing large bilateral adrenal masses on CAT scan imaging. In such cases, adrenal insufficiency or adrenal failure may require urgent treatment with adrenal hormone replacement with hydrocortisone (Cortef®). (21–25)

The González Method

In addition to the use of beta blocker drugs like propranolol, the sympathetic nervous system can be downregulated by dietary intervention, a method used by Nicholas González, MD, in his cancer treatment protocol based on the work of Drs. William Donald Kelley and Max Gerson. ** (26–28)

Repurposing Propranolol as an Anti-Cancer Drug

In 2016, Dr. Pan Pantziarka et al. reviewed the nonselective beta blocker propranolol as a repurposed anti-cancer drug. Propanolol anti-cancer activities include:

- Abrogates norepinephrine-induced increased migratory activity in breast cancer cells (blocks metastatic spread).
- Exerts an anti-angiogenic effect by downregulating VEGF in cancers and infantile hemangiomas. (29)

The Most Striking Discovery to Date

According to Drs. Frank Entschladen et al. (2016):

To date, the by far **most striking discovery** in the context of drug repurposing in oncology is the antimetastatic function of beta blockers. (30)

Propranolol Beta Blocker

Propranolol, like its cousin carvedilol, is a nonselective beta blocker, used safely for decades by cardiologists to treat hypertension, slow the heart rate, and reduce anxiety. Originally approved for medical use in 1964, propranolol (Inderal®) and other beta blockers are useful for slowing the heart in hyperthyroidism and for relieving tachycardia related to performance anxiety (stage fright). About 18 million people take beta blockers annually. Over many years, physicians have observed beta blocker use associated with reduced mortality from cancer and reduced rate of metastatic disease. (31–33)

Propranolol for Breast Cancer Patients

In 2013, Dr. Edoardo Botteri et al. identified 800 post-menopausal women who underwent surgery to remove a triple-negative breast cancer (negative for hormone receptors). Of the 800, 74 women were coincidentally on beta blockers.

Beta blocker (BB) intake was associated with a significantly decreased risk of recurrence, metastasis, and death from breast cancer.

The hazard ratio (HR) for women on beta blockers was 0.32 for metastases and 0.42 for death from breast cancer, compared to controls

---

** Dr. Gonzalez died unexpectedly on July 21, 2015, at the age of 67. His wife and medical colleague, Dr. Linda Issacs, continues their work in New York City.

---

not on beta blockers. This is remarkable. (34)

In 2011, Dr. Amal Melhem-Bertrandt et al. found improved relapse-free survival in the cohort of women using beta blocker drugs. (HR = 0.32) (35)

In 2015, Dr. Kurtis Childers et al. did a meta-analysis, finding risk of death from breast cancer reduced in half:

> Breast cancer death results were contained in 4 studies, which also suggested a significant reduction in risk (HR, 0.50; 95% CI, 0.32–0.80). (36)

In 2011, Dr. Thomas Barron et al. analyzed women with breast cancer in Ireland over a 5-year period from 2001 to 2006. Compared to matched controls, women taking propranolol had less locally invasive or metastatic cancers at diagnosis, with marked reduction in metastases (OR, 0.20; 95% CI, 0.04 to 0.88) and striking reduction in breast cancer mortality (HR, 0.19; 95% CI, 0.06 to 0.60). Propranolol has been suggested as an adjunct to breast cancer treatment. Additional studies describe beta blockers conferring similar reduction in cancer mortality in prostate cancer, melanoma, colon, ovarian, prostate, non-small-cell lung, and hepatocellular, multiple myeloma. (37)

Evaluation of Cancer Markers after Propranolol

In 2019, Dr. Alexa Montoya et al. studied late-stage breast cancer in a 44-year-old female with a 6.5 cm. invasive lobular breast cancer. After initial biopsy, the patient was treated with propranolol, 80 mg per day for 25 days and then underwent definitive radical mastectomy. The histology on microscopic slides of both biopsy sample and mastectomy sample were compared. The use of propranolol decreased the Ki-67 proliferation marker, the BCL-2 anti-apoptosis protein, and increased pro-apoptosis p53 expression on the surgical specimen histology slides. (19)

Hexokinase 2, the Achilles Heel of the Cancer Cell

An embryonic form of hexokinase called HK2 is present in cancer cells and is usually absent in normal cells, the exception being skeletal muscle, heart, and adipose tissue. (20) In cancer cells, the HK2 is translocated to the voltage dependent anion channel (VDAC) on the mitochondrial membrane. In normal cells, the hexokinase enzyme is found in the cytoplasm.

In 1995, Dr. H. Osawa et al. studied the regulation of the HK2 gene, finding that the beta receptor agonist isoproterenol, cyclic AMP (cAMP) and insulin all selectively increase HK2 gene transcription, increased HK2 protein production, and increased glucose phosphorylation and utilization. Beta-adrenergic stimulation turns on the genetic machinery to produce more HK2 and increases the glucose utilization in the cancer cell. (20)

Therefore, blocking this machinery with a beta blocker (propranolol) would seem logical.

Propranolol Reduces Hexokinase 2 in Brown Adipose Tissue

Abundant amounts of HK2 are present in brown adipose tissue under the control of the sympathetic nervous system. Brown adipose tissue is involved in thermal regulation of the body, and beta blockers reduce brown adipose activity 30% below control group on routine PET Scans. (38) Patients are routinely given propranolol 20 mg one hour before their PET scan to prevent false positive 18-FDG isotope uptake in the brown adipose tissue. (39)

Propranolol Reduces HK2 and PET Uptake in Breast Cancer

In 2014, Dr. Fei Kang et al. studied breast cancer using in vitro and in vivo mouse xenografts. Their studies showed that beta-adrenergic receptors were overexpressed in breast cancer cell lines. Propranolol significantly decreased HK2 protein levels through post-transcription mechanisms. In vivo studies using propranolol in this animal model of breast cancer showed reduced expression of HK2. In addition, PET scans of the propranolol-treated mice showed reduced 18-FDG uptake in tumor and brown adipose tissue. Dr. Kang et al. suggested the use of propranolol in humans might reduce true-positive PET scan uptake in small or low-uptake lesions, concluding:

> The expression of HK-2 was regulated by the activation of ADRB2 [Adrenergic Receptor Beta2] in 4T1 [mouse] breast cancer cells primarily at the post-transcriptional level. Additionally, propranolol prevented glucose metabolism and 18F-FDG PET imaging of 4T1 breast cancer tumors. (40)

Synergy of Propranolol with Metformin in Breast Cancer Model

In *Oncotarget* (2017), Dr. Maria Rico et al. studied the combination of metformin and propranolol in a breast cancer cell model, finding reduction in cancer progression, metastasis, and reduced migratory and invasive behavior of the cancer cells. The combination of metformin and propranolol showed a "strong inhibition of mitochondrial bioenergetics" and "drastically activated glycolysis...abolished mitochondrial respiratory activity...with a noticeable increase in glycolysis." The metabolic pathway of the cancer cell was skewed away from mitochondrial OXPHOS and toward GLYCOLYSIS. Dr. Rico et al. theorize that this metabolic derangement starved the cancer cells of glucose, causing cell death:

> By enhancing glycolysis to an extraordinarily high rate, the combination probably leads to glucose deprivation in the tumor cell micro-environment... ultimately produce synthetic lethality, as glucose levels decrease. (41)

Metformin is more fully discussed in Chapter 14.

Synergy of Propranolol with DCA in HNSCC

In *Cancers* (2018), Dr. Christopher Lucido et al., using head-and-neck squamous cell cancer (HNSCC) studied in vivo mouse xenografts with the combination of propranolol and dichloroacetate (DCA) and found significant delay in tumor growth with no toxicity and improved sensitivity to chemotherapy and radiation. Dr. Lucido observed that propranolol alone inhibited mitochondrial metabolism (with decreased oxygen consumption) and heightened glycolytic activity, promoting a state of glucose dependence; he hypothesized that adding a glycolytic inhibitor such as DCA could be a "highly effective therapeutic combination" and the logical next step. Dr. Lucido's group report no toxicity to the animals studied with this combination. The effect was selective for tumor cells, as normal epithelial cells were unaffected. They write:

> The rational combination of propranolol and dichloroacetate [DCA], a clinically available glycolytic inhibitor, dramatically attenuates tumor cell metabolism and mTOR signaling, inhibits proliferation and colony formation, and induces apoptosis. (42)

Note: The combination of DCA with Propranolol looks promising because it targets all three major pillars of cancer cell metabolism, OXPHOS, GLYCOLYSIS and Autophagy. DCA is more fully discussed in Chapter 5.

Glucose Starvation and Anti-Cancer Diets

Glucose starvation in combination with propranolol showed augmented cancer cell inhibition. The fasting-mimicking diet has received attention for reducing serum glucose levels, starving the cancer of glucose and may prove useful for the cancer patient. (43–47)

Starve the Cancer Cell of Glucose

Another way to starve the cancer cell of glucose is to use a glycolysis inhibitor such as dichloroacetate (DCA). By inactivating pyruvate dehydrogenase kinase (PDK), the inhibitor of pyruvate dehydrogenase (PDH), DCA frees PDH to convert pyruvate to acetyl-CoA which feeds mitochondrial oxidative energy production (OXPHOS). The net effect is to shunt energy metabolism away from GLYCOLYSIS in the cytoplasm and back to the mitochondria as OXPHOS, which inhibits mTOR signaling. Dr. Lucido et al. write that mTOR is the "master regulatory pathway controlling cellular metabolism and growth, and is critical in the progression of both of these tumor models."(42)

In vivo mouse xenograft studies showed that this combination (propranolol and DCA), led to a 50% reduction in tumor volume (HNSCC) without toxicity or weight loss. Dr. Lucido et al. conclude:

> As FDA-approved drugs, propranolol and DCA have the potential for rapid translation from the bench to the clinical oncology setting…. Perhaps most importantly, both drugs are generally well tolerated, suggesting the potential for therapeutic benefit without significantly increasing treatment-associated morbidity. (42)

Propranolol Is an OXPHOS Inhibitor

In 1985, Dr. Yau-Huei Wei et al. elucidated the mechanism of propranolol as a mitochondrial OXPHOS inhibitor. Propranolol has no effect on elements of the electron transport chain (ETC). Rather, it impairs mitochondrial respiration and oxidative phosphorylation by inhibiting ATPase, the enzyme responsible for ATP (Adenosine-Triphosphate) energy production in mitochondria. (48–49)

Propranolol Autophagy Inhibitor!!! Prostate Cancer in Vivo

Similar to the Lucido study above, combining propranolol with a glycolysis inhibitor, 2DG (2-deoxyglucose), was found quite effective in a prostate cancer model in 2018 by Dr. Laura Brohée et al. who observed that this combination led to a massive accumulation of autophagosomes indicating inhibition of autophagy in the prostate cancer cells. Dr. Brohée's group write:

> The propranolol + 2DG treatment efficiently prevents prostate cancer cell proliferation, induces cell apoptosis, alters mitochondrial morphology, inhibits mitochondrial bioenergetics and aggravates ER [endoplasmic reticulum] stress in vitro and also suppresses tumor growth in vivo..... The blockage by propranolol of the autophagy flux induced by 2-DG resulted in a strong accumulation of LC3-II and p62 and in a massive accumulation of autophagic vesicles.... Propranolol is also an inhibitor of the PAP [phosphatidate phosphatase] activity of lipins, which probably explains why it inhibits autophagy flux. (50)

Note: PAP is a major regulator of lipid metabolism and controls the autophagy process. Both PAP and Lipin-1 have emerged as good targets for anti-cancer treatment. (51–57)

One might speculate that DCA could serve the same purpose as glycolysis Inhibitor, replacing the 2-DG in the above study.

Propranolol Is a Chloroquine-Like Autophagy Inhibitor

Propranolol was identified as an autophagy inhibitor by Dr. Yuan Li et al. in 2016, with high thru-put screening, suggesting propranolol may be a "chloroquine-like autophagy inhibitor." (58)

The fact that propranolol is both an OXPHOS Inhibitor as well as an autophagy inhibitor is fortuitous, because as we will see in later chapters, cancer cells respond to OXPHOS inhibition by stimulating "protective autophagy" as a survival mechanism. Inhibiting this "protective autophagy" will push the cancer cells "over the apoptotic cliff," with induction of programmed cell death.

Blocking All Three Metabolic Pathways

Propranolol's dual role of OXPHOS inhibitor and autophagy inhibitor promotes this drug as a major player in our anti-cancer toolkit. Combining propranolol with the glycolysis inhibitor DCA effectively blocks all three major metabolic pathways in the cancer cell—OXPHOS, GLYCOLYSIS, and Autophagy.

Other autophagy inhibitors discussed in this book are: mefloquine, chloroquine, hydroxychloroquine, pyrvinium, niclosamide-(late-stage autophagy), clarithromycin, thymoquinone, loratadine and PPI drugs. See chapters 31-35 for more on autophagy inhibitors.

Beta Blockers in Ovarian Cancer and Lung Cancer

A 2013 study by Dr. Guolin Gao et al. used chronic stress to promote progression of a mouse model of ovarian cancer. (59) Similarly, in 2011, Dr. A. V. Amikishieva et al. found stress enhanced the metastatic spread in a mouse model of Lewis lung cancer. (60)

In a 2015 human clinical study of ovarian cancer patients led by Dr. Jack Watkins, users of nonselective beta blockers had more than double the overall survival time when compared to non-users (90 months vs. 38.2 months P<0.001). (32)

Population Study Beta Blockers Reduce Cancer

In 2015, Dr. Pig Ying Chang et al. reviewed a database of 24,238 patients over a 12-year follow-up. Dr. Chang's group report:

> Patients with propranolol treatment exhibited significantly lower risks of cancers in head and neck (HR: 0.58), esophagus (HR: 0.35), stomach (HR: 0.54), colon (HR: 0.68), and prostate cancers (HR: 0.52). [HR= Hazard Ratio]. (33)

Propranolol Effective for Cancer Cell Types

- Neuroblastoma (beta blockers improve the efficacy of chemotherapy in neuroblastoma) (61–63)

- Angiosarcoma –(propranolol has been approved for treatment of soft tissue sarcoma by the European Medicines Agency (64–68)

- Breast cancer (69–73)(83)

- Melanoma (74–75)

- Lung cancer (76–77)

- Multiple myeloma (78–79)

- Cervical cancer (80)

- Canine osteosarcoma (81)

- Leukemia (82)

- Hepatocellular carcinoma (84)

- Infantile hemangioma (85–89)

- Ovarian cancer (90–91)(9)(32)

- Prostate cancer (92)(12)(50)

- Pancreatic cancer (93–95)(1)

- Bone sarcoma (63)

Propranolol in Breast Cancer Epidemiology Study

In 2010, Dr. Desmond Powe et al. reviewed the medical records of 466 women with operable breast cancer with more than 10 years follow-up. Women on beta blockers (propranolol) had a 57% reduction in metastatic disease and recurrence, and a 71% reduction in mortality compared to controls not on propranolol. Dr. Powe writes:

> We performed an epidemiological study of breast cancer patients with long-term clinical follow-up [>10 years] and showed that patients receiving antihypertensive beta-blocker drugs [propranolol] significantly benefit by a **57% reduction** in distant metastasis formation and a **71% reduced risk** of dying from breast cancer compared to control patients..... (71–72)

In 2019, Dr. A. Spini et al. reviewed the preclinical and clinical evidence for use of beta blockers (propranolol) for TNBC, finding 616 published studies, including 62 preclinical (in vitro and in vivo). The clinical studies included four retrospective observational cohort studies showing TNBC patients using beta blockers (propranolol) had a 65% reduction in mortality, and a 68% reduction in metastatic disease. Dr. Spini and colleagues write:

> The in vitro studies showed a high expression of Beta-2 adrenoreceptors in TNBC cell lines. Propranolol (and carvedilol) significantly decreased proliferation, migration and invasion of TNBC cells.... In vivo studies reported a reduction of metastasis, angiogenesis and tumor growth in animals exposed to propranolol. (73)

Immunotherapy with Beta Blockade—Propranolol

Tumor immune suppression, tumor growth stimulation, and metastasis are all supported and enhanced by beta-adrenergic signaling from the sympathetic nervous system. Beta blockade with Propranolol is beneficial. In 2019, Drs. Wei Wang and Xuefang Cao reviewed beta-adrenergic signaling in cancer, writing:

> Beta-adrenergic receptors expressed on immune cells engage with neurotransmitters released by the sympathetic nervous system and mediate immunosuppression in the tumor micro-environment by recruiting tumor-associated macrophages and dampening cytotoxic T and NK cells ... Therefore, blockade of the beta-adrenergic signaling [with propranolol] implies a promising strategy to improve current immunotherapy. (96)

Not only does beta-adrenergic signaling stimulate tumor cell growth and angiogenesis, it also suppresses anti-tumor immunity.

Immunosuppressive Effect of Beta-Adrenergic Signaling

In 2017, Dr. Michael Nissen et al. studied beta-adrenergic signaling in a mouse model of lymphoma, finding that chronic beta-adrenergic signaling enhanced tumor immune evasion by inhibiting CD8+ T cell response.

> Chronic ßAR [Beta-Adrenergic Receptor] signaling has an immunosuppressive effect on CD8+ T cells, which decreases the efficacy of CD8+ T cell-targeting immunotherapies. (97)

In 2019, Dr. Clara Daher et al. studied the blockade of adrenergic receptors in a mouse model of anti-cancer vaccine-based immunotherapy, finding Beta Blockage (Propranolol) restored activation of anti-tumor CD8+ T Cells:

> β-AR [Beta-Adrenergic Receptor] signaling suppresses the initial priming phase of anti-tumor CD8+ T cell responses, providing a rationale to use clinically available β-blockers [propranolol] in patients to improve cancer immunotherapies. (98)

Others studies are in agreement. (99-100)

Adverse Effects of Propranolol

In general, propranolol is well-tolerated. However, it can be associated with adverse effects related to slowing the heart rate (bradycardia), reduction in blood pressure, and reduction in blood sugar. (101–102)

Mitochondrial Toxins

Both statin drugs and propranolol decrease cellular ATP levels and are regarded as mitochondrial toxins. Concurrent use of propranolol and statin drug may aggravate statin-induced myopathy, so caution is advised when combining propranolol with a statin drug. In my opinion, this combination should be avoided unless the patient is closely monitored for muscle pain and symptoms of myopathy related to mitochondrial toxicity. (103–106)

Conclusion

In the field of repurposed anti-cancer drugs, propranolol is **"the most striking discovery to date."** Activities include: reduced tumor proliferation, decreased mortality, decreased metastases, longer survival, and reduced cancer recurrence. Propranolol has anti-angiogenic effects, reduces HK2 protein levels, activates GLYCOLYSIS, and inhibits mitochondrial OXPHOS. Propranolol is an autophagy inhibitor, and may replace chloroquine in this role. With regard to immunotherapy, propranolol restores anti-tumor immune function. The combination of DCA and propranolol is appealing because it effectively blocks all three major metabolic pathways in the cancer cell—OXPHOS, GLYCOLYSIS, and Autophagy. This combination looks promising as a safe, potent, synergistic anti-cancer cocktail. We await further in vivo animal studies and human clinical trials to evaluate efficacy and potential toxicity. (107–108)

References Chapter 6: Propranolol Anti-Cancer Drug

1) Kim-Fuchs, Corina, et al. "Chronic stress accelerates pancreatic cancer growth and invasion: a critical role for beta-adrenergic signaling in the pancreatic microenvironment." Brain, behavior, and immunity 40 (2014): 40-47.

2) Yuan, Aihua, et al. "Psychological aspect of cancer: From stressor to cancer progression (Review)." Experimental and therapeutic medicine 1.1 (2010): 13-18.

3) Jin Shin, Kyeong, et al. "Molecular mechanisms underlying psychological stress and cancer." Current pharmaceutical design 22.16 (2016): 2389-2402.

4) Cole, Steven W., et al. "Sympathetic nervous system regulation of the tumour microenvironment." Nature Reviews Cancer 15.9 (2015): 563-572.

5) Krizanova, O., Petr Babula, and K. Pacak. "Stress, catecholaminergic system and cancer." Stress 19.4 (2016): 419-428.

6) Glaser, Ronald, and Janice K. Kiecolt-Glaser. "Stress-induced immune dysfunction: implications for health." Nature Reviews Immunology 5.3 (2005): 243-251.

7) Reiche, Edna Maria Vissoci, Sandra Odebrecht Vargas Nunes, and Helena Kaminami Morimoto. "Stress, depression, the immune system, and cancer." The lancet oncology 5.10 (2004): 617-625.

8) Lamkin, Donald M., et al. "Chronic stress enhances progression of acute lymphoblastic leukemia via ß-adrenergic signaling." Brain, behavior, and immunity 26.4 (2012): 635-641.

9) Thaker, Premal H., et al. "Chronic stress promotes tumor growth and angiogenesis in a mouse model of ovarian carcinoma." Nature medicine 12.8 (2006): 939.

10) Sloan, Erica K., et al. "The sympathetic nervous system induces a metastatic switch in primary breast cancer." Cancer research 70.18 (2010): 7042-7052.

11) Magnon, Claire. "Role of the autonomic nervous system in tumorigenesis and metastasis." Molecular & cellular oncology 2.2 (2015): e975643.

12) Magnon, Claire, et al. "Autonomic nerve development contributes to prostate cancer progression." Science 341.6142 (2013).

13) Pundavela, Jay, et al. "Nerve fibers infiltrate the tumor microenvironment and are associated with nerve growth factor production and lymph node

invasion in breast cancer." Molecular oncology 9.8 (2015): 1626-1635.

14) Lu, Ran, et al. "Neurons generated from carcinoma stem cells support cancer progression." Signal transduction and targeted therapy 2.1 (2017): 1-10.

15) Dobrenis, Kostantin, et al. "Granulocyte colony-stimulating factor off-target effect on nerve outgrowth promotes prostate cancer development." International journal of cancer 136.4 (2015): 982-988.

16) Eng, Jason W-L., et al. "A nervous tumor microenvironment: the impact of adrenergic stress on cancer cells, immunosuppression, and immunotherapeutic response." Cancer Immunology, Immunotherapy 63.11 (2014): 1115-1128.

17) Rains, Steven L., Clarissa N. Amaya, and Brad A. Bryan. "Beta-adrenergic receptors are expressed across diverse cancers." Oncoscience 4.7-8 (2017): 95.

18) Nissen, Michael D., Erica K. Sloan, and Stephen R. Mattarollo. "β-adrenergic signaling impairs antitumor CD8+ T-cell responses to B-cell lymphoma immunotherapy." Cancer immunology research 6.1 (2018): 98-109.

19) Montoya, Alexa, et al. "The beta adrenergic receptor antagonist propranolol alters mitogenic and apoptotic signaling in late stage breast cancer." Biomedical Journal 42.3 (2019): 155.

20) Osawa, H., et al. "Regulation of hexokinase II gene transcription and glucose phosphorylation by catecholamines, cyclic AMP, and insulin." Diabetes 44.12 (1995): 1426.

21) Hassan, Muhammad, et al. "Gastric diffuse large B-cell lymphoma with bilateral adrenal metastasis." BMJ Case Reports CP 12.7 (2019).

22) Wakabayashi, Mutsumi, et al. "Diffuse large B-cell lymphoma solely involving bilateral adrenal glands and stomach: report of an extremely rare case with review of the literature." International journal of clinical and experimental pathology 7.11 (2014): 8190.

23) Nishiuchi, Takamasa, et al. "A case of non-Hodgkin's lymphoma primary arising in both adrenal glands associated with adrenal failure." Endocrine 35.1 (2009): 34-37.

24) Karimi, Fariba. "Primary adrenal lymphoma presenting with adrenal failure: a case report and review of the literature." International journal of endocrinology and metabolism 15.4 (2017).

25) de Sousa Lages, Adriana, et al. "Diffuse large B-cell lymphoma of the adrenal gland: a rare cause of primary adrenal insufficiency." Case Reports 2016 (2016).

26) Gonzalez, Nicholas J. Nutrition and the Autonomic Nervous System: The Scientific Foundations of the Gonzalez Protocol. New Spring Press, 2017.

27) Gonzalez, Nicholas James, and Linda Lee Isaacs. "Evaluation of pancreatic proteolytic enzyme treatment of adenocarcinoma of the pancreas, with nutrition and detoxification support." Nutrition and cancer 33.2 (1999): 117-124.

28) Gonzalez, Nicholas J., and Linda L. Isaacs. "The Gonzalez therapy and cancer: A collection of case reports." Alternative therapies in health and medicine 13.1 (2007): 46.

29) Pantziarka, Pan, et al. "Propranolol and breast cancer—A work in progress." ecancermedicalscience 12 (2018).

30) Entschladen, Frank, Dane A. Thyssen, and David W. Drell. "Re-Use of Established Drugs for Anti-Metastatic Indications." Cells 5.1 (2016): 2.

31) Nagaraja, Archana S., et al. "ß-blockers: a new role in cancer chemotherapy?" Expert opinion on investigational drugs 22.11 (2013): 1359-1363.

32) Watkins, Jack L., et al. "Clinical impact of selective and nonselective beta-blockers on survival in patients with ovarian cancer." Cancer 121.19 (2015): 3444-3451.

33) Chang, Ping-Ying, et al. "Propranolol reduces Cancer risk: a population-based cohort study." Medicine 94.27 (2015).

34) Botteri, Edoardo, et al. "Therapeutic effect of β-blockers in triple-negative breast cancer postmenopausal women." Breast cancer research and treatment 140.3 (2013): 567-575.

35) Melhem-Bertrandt, Amal, et al. "Beta-blocker use is associated with improved relapse-free survival in patients with triple-negative breast cancer." Journal of clinical oncology 29.19 (2011): 2645.

36) Childers, W. Kurtis, Christopher S. Hollenbeak, and Pramil Cheriyath. "β-blockers reduce breast cancer recurrence and breast cancer death: a meta-analysis." Clinical breast cancer 15.6 (2015): 426-431.

37) Barron, Thomas I., et al. "Beta blockers and breast cancer mortality: a population-based study." J Clin Oncol 29.19 (2011): 2635-2644.

38) Hao, Ruirui, et al. "Brown adipose tissue: distribution and influencing factors on FDG PET/CT scan." Journal of Pediatric Endocrinology and Metabolism 25.3-4 (2012): 233-237.

39) Surasi, Devaki Shilpa, et al. "18F-FDG PET and PET/CT patient preparation: a review of the literature." Journal of nuclear medicine technology 42.1 (2014): 5-13.

40) Kang, Fei, et al. "Propranolol inhibits glucose metabolism and 18F-FDG uptake of breast cancer through posttranscriptional downregulation of hexokinase-2." Journal of Nuclear Medicine 55.3 (2014): 439-445.

41) Rico, María, et al. "Metformin and propranolol combination prevents cancer progression and metastasis in different breast cancer models." Oncotarget 8.2 (2017): 2874.

42) Lucido, Christopher T., W. Keith Miskimins, and Paola D. Vermeer. "Propranolol Promotes Glucose Dependence and Synergizes with Dichloroacetate for Anti-Cancer Activity in HNSCC." Cancers 10.12 (2018).

43) Brandhorst, Sebastian, et al. "Periodic fasting mimicking diet delays cancer development and progression." (2016): 4313-4313.

44) Di Biase, Stefano, et al. "Fasting-mimicking diet reduces HO-1 to promote T cell-mediated tumor cytotoxicity." Cancer cell 30.1 (2016): 136-146.

45) Nencioni, Alessio, et al. "Fasting and cancer: molecular mechanisms and clinical application." Nature Reviews Cancer 18.11 (2018): 707.

46) Wei, Min, et al. "Fasting-mimicking diet and markers/risk factors for aging, diabetes, cancer, and cardiovascular disease." Science translational medicine 9.377 (2017): eaai8700.

47) de Braud, Filippo, et al. "Abstract B022: Metabolic and immunologic effects of the fasting mimicking diet in cancer patients." (2018): B022-B022.

48) Wei, Yau-Huei, et al. "Inhibition of the mitochondrial Mg2+-ATPase by propranolol." Biochemical pharmacology 34.7 (1985): 911-917.

49) Almotrefi, Abdulrahman A., and Nduna Dzimiri. "Effects of β-adrenoceptor blockers on mitochondrial ATPase activity in guinea pig heart preparations." European journal of pharmacology 215.2-3 (1992): 231-236.

50) Brohée, Laura, et al. "Propranolol sensitizes prostate cancer cells to glucose metabolism inhibition and prevents cancer progression." Scientific reports 8.1 (2018): 7050.

51) Pascual, Florencia, and George M. Carman. "Phosphatidate phosphatase, a key regulator of lipid homeostasis." *Biochimica et Biophysica Acta (BBA)-Molecular and Cell Biology of Lipids* 1831.3 (2013): 514-522.

52) Zhang, Peixiang, M. Anthony Verity, and Karen Reue. "Lipin-1 regulates autophagy clearance and intersects with statin drug effects in skeletal muscle." Cell metabolism 20.2 (2014): 267-279.

53) Dall'Armi, Claudia, Kelly A. Devereaux, and Gilbert Di Paolo. "The role of lipids in the control of autophagy." Current Biology 23.1 (2013): R33-R45.

54) Brohée, Laura. Lipin-1 regulates cancer cell phenotype and is a potential target to amplify the effect of metabolic inhibitors. Diss. Université de Liège, Liège, Belgique, 2017.

55) Brohée, Laura, et al. "Lipin-1 regulates cancer cell phenotype and is a potential target to potentiate rapamycin treatment." Oncotarget 6.13 (2015): 11264.

56) Fan, Xueyu, et al. "Lipin-1 determines lung cancer cell survival and chemotherapy sensitivity by regulation of endoplasmic reticulum homeostasis and autophagy." Cancer medicine 7.6 (2018): 2541-2554.

57) Shaughnessy, Ronan, et al. "Epidermal growth factor receptor endocytic traffic perturbation by phosphatidate phosphohydrolase (PAP) inhibition: new strategy against cancer." The FEBS journal 281.9 (2014): 2172-2189.

58) Li, Yuan, et al. "A cell-based quantitative high-throughput image screening identified novel autophagy modulators." Pharmacological research 110 (2016): 35-49.

59) Gao, Guolan, et al. "Chronic stress promoted the growth of ovarian carcinoma via increasing serum levels of norepinephrine and interleukin-10 and altering nm23 and NDRG1 expression in tumor tissues in nude mice." Bioscience trends 7.1 (2013): 56-63.

60) Amikishieva, A. V., et al. "Depressive-like psychoemotional state versus acute stresses enhances Lewis lung carcinoma metastasis in C57BL/6J mice." Experimental oncology (2011).

61) Pasquier, E., et al. "Reply: Comment on 'Beta-blockers increase response to chemotherapy via direct anti-tumour and anti-angiogenic mechanisms in neuroblastoma'–β-blockers are potent anti-angiogenic and chemo-sensitising agents, rather than cytotoxic drugs." British journal of cancer 109.7 (2013): 2024-2025.

62) Pasquier, E., et al. "β-blockers increase response to chemotherapy via direct antitumour and anti-angiogenic mechanisms in neuroblastoma." British journal of cancer 108.12 (2013): 2485.

63) Wolter, Jennifer K., et al. "Anti-tumor activity of the beta-adrenergic receptor antagonist propranolol in neuroblastoma." Oncotarget 5.1 (2014): 161.

64) Banavali, Shripad, Eddy Pasquier, and Nicolas Andre. "Targeted therapy with propranolol and metronomic chemotherapy combination: sustained complete response of a relapsing metastatic angiosarcoma." Ecancermedicalscience 9 (2015).

65) Pasquier, Eddy, et al. "Effective management of advanced angiosarcoma by the synergistic combination of propranolol and vinblastine-based metronomic chemotherapy: a bench to bedside study." EBioMedicine 6 (2016): 87-95.

67) Daguzé, Justine, et al. "Visceral metastatic angiosarcoma treated effectively with oral cyclophosphamide combined with propranolol." JAAD case reports 2.6 (2016): 497-499.

68) Chow, William, et al. "Growth attenuation of cutaneous angiosarcoma with propranolol-mediated β-blockade." JAMA dermatology 151.11 (2015): 1226-1229.

69) Hiller, Jonathan G., et al. "Pre-operative β-blockade with propranolol reduces biomarkers of metastasis in breast cancer: a Phase II randomized trial." Clinical Cancer Research (2019).

70) Pasquier, Eddy, et al. "Propranolol potentiates the anti-angiogenic effects and anti-tumor efficacy of chemotherapy agents: implication in breast cancer treatment." Oncotarget 2.10 (2011): 797.

71) Powe, Desmond G., et al. "Beta-blocker drug therapy reduces secondary cancer formation in breast cancer and improves cancer specific survival." Oncotarget 1.7 (2010): 628.

72) Powe, D. G., et al. "Alpha-and beta-adrenergic receptor (AR) protein expression is associated with poor clinical outcome in breast cancer: an immunohistochemical study." Breast cancer research and treatment 130.2 (2011): 457-463

73) Spini, A., et al. "Abstract P3-14-08: Preclinical and clinical evidence about the use of betablockers for the treatment of triple negative breast cancer: A systematic review." (2019): P3-14.

74) Calvani, Maura, et al. "ß3-Adrenoceptor as a potential immuno-suppressor agent in melanoma." British journal of pharmacology 176.14 (2019): 2509-2524.

75) De Giorgi, Vincenzo, et al. "Propranolol for off-label treatment of patients with melanoma: results from a cohort study." JAMA oncology 4.2 (2018): e172908-e172908.

76) Xia, Yun, et al. "Catecholamines contribute to the neovascularization of lung cancer via tumor-associated macrophages." Brain, behavior, and immunity (2019).

77) Huang, Qi, et al. "The role of adrenergic receptors in lung cancer." American journal of cancer research 8.11 (2018): 2227.

78) Hwa, Yi L., et al. "Beta-blockers improve survival outcomes in patients with multiple myeloma: a retrospective evaluation." American journal of hematology 92.1 (2017): 50-55.

79) Kozanoglu, Ilknur, et al. "New indication for therapeutic potential of an old well-known drug

(propranolol) for multiple myeloma." Journal of cancer research and clinical oncology 139.2 (2013): 327-335.

80) Gong, Liuyun, et al. "Propranolol selectively inhibits cervical cancer cell growth by suppressing the cGMP/PKG pathway." Biomedicine & Pharmacotherapy 111 (2019): 1243-1248.

81) Duckett, Megan M., et al. "The adrenergic receptor antagonists propranolol and carvedilol decrease bone sarcoma cell viability and sustained carvedilol reduces clonogenic survival and increases radiosensitivity in canine osteosarcoma cells." Veterinary and comparative oncology (2019).

82) Gaeini, Amirhossein, and Fatemeh Hajighasemi. "Sensitivity of human leukemic cells to carvedilol." Journal of Basic and Clinical Pathophysiology 7.1 (2019): 37-42.

83) Dezong, Gao, et al. "Carvedilol suppresses migration and invasion of malignant breast cells by inactivating Src involving cAMP/PKA and PKCδ signaling pathway." Journal of cancer research and therapeutics 10.4 (2014): 991.

84) Suna, N., et al. "Effect of Propranolol Treatment on the Incidence of Hepatocellular Carcinoma in Patients Waiting for Liver Transplant With Cirrhosis: A Retrospective, Surveillance Study in a Tertiary Center." Experimental and clinical transplantation. (2019).

85) Prasad, Arun, et al. "Individualized dosing of oral propranolol for treatment of infantile hemangioma: a prospective study." Pan African Medical Journal 32.155 (2019).

86) Tsai, Mu-Chieh, Hsi-Che Liu, and Chun-Yan Yeung. "Efficacy of infantile hepatic hemangioma with propranolol treatment: A case report." Medicine 98.4 (2019).

87) Grech, Jamie Alexander, et al. "Necrosis of infantile haemangioma with propranolol therapy." Archives of disease in childhood (2019): e316478.

88) Wu, Wenli, et al. "Therapeutic efficacy of propranolol for infantile hemangiomas." Oral surgery, oral medicine, oral pathology and oral radiology (2019).

89) Pan, Wei-Kang, et al. "Propranolol induces regression of hemangioma cells via the down-regulation of the PI3K/Akt/eNOS/VEGF pathway." Pediatric blood & cancer 62.8 (2015): 1414-1420.

90) Jang, Hye-In, et al. "Perioperative administration of propranolol to women undergoing ovarian cancer surgery: A pilot study." Obstetrics & gynecology science 60.2 (2017): 170-177.

91) Diaz, E. S., B. Y. Karlan, and A. J. Li. "Impact of beta blockers on epithelial ovarian cancer survival." Gynecologic oncology 127.2 (2012): 375.

92) Lu, Saihua, et al. "Propranolol Inhibits Androgen Deprivation-induced Neuroendocrine Differentiation of Prostate Cancer." Pharmacology 15.8 (2019): 986-993.

93) Partecke, Lars Ivo, et al. "Chronic stress increases experimental pancreatic cancer growth, reduces survival and can be antagonised by beta-adrenergic receptor blockade." Pancreatology 16.3 (2016): 423-433.

94) Ilmer, Matthias, et al. "Repurposed drugs in pancreatic ductal adenocarcinoma: An update." The Cancer Journal 25.2 (2019): 134-138.

95) Blair, Alex, et al. "345—Non-Selective β-Adrenergic Blockade Impacts Pancreatic Cancer Tumor Biology, Decreases Perineural Invasion and Improves Patient Survival." Gastroenterology 156.6 (2019): S-1394.

96) Wang, Wei, and Xuefang Cao. "Beta-adrenergic signaling in tumor immunology and immunotherapy." Critical Reviews™ in Immunology 39.2 (2019).

97) Nissen, Michael D., Erica K. Sloan, and Stephen R. Mattarollo. "Beta-adrenergic signaling impairs anti-tumor CD8+ T cell responses to B cell lymphoma immunotherapy." Cancer Immunology Research (2017): canimm-0401.

98) Daher, Clara, et al. "Blockade of ß-adrenergic receptors improves CD8+ T-cell priming and cancer vaccine efficacy." Cancer immunology research 7.11 (2019): 1849-1863.

99) Armaiz-Pena, Guillermo N., Claudia B. Colon-Echevarria, and Rocio Lamboy-Caraballo. "Neuroendocrine regulation of tumor-associated immune cells." Frontiers in oncology 9 (2019): 1077

100) Kurozumi, Sasagu, et al. "ß 2-Adrenergic receptor expression is associated with biomarkers of tumor immunity and predicts poor prognosis in estrogen receptor-negative breast cancer." Breast cancer research and treatment 177.3 (2019): 603-610.

101) Linde, Klaus, and Karin Rossnagel. "Propranolol for migraine prophylaxis." Cochrane Database of Systematic Reviews 2 (2004).

102) Miller, Richard A. "Propranolol and impotence." Annals of internal medicine 85.5 (1976): 682-683.

103) Setoguchi, Soko, et al. "Propranolol and the risk of hospitalized myopathy: Translating chemical genomics findings into population-level hypotheses." American heart journal 159.3 (2010): 428-433.

104) Zhang, Peixiang, M. Anthony Verity, and Karen Reue. "Lipin-1 regulates autophagy clearance and intersects with statin drug effects in skeletal muscle." Cell metabolism 20.2 (2014): 267-279.

105) Wagner, Bridget K., et al. "Large-scale chemical dissection of mitochondrial function." Nature biotechnology 26.3 (2008): 343-351.

106) Bouitbir, Jamal, et al. "Statins trigger mitochondrial reactive oxygen species-induced apoptosis in glycolytic skeletal muscle." Antioxidants & redox signaling 24.2 (2016): 84-98.

107) Hondermarck, Hubert, and Phillip Jobling. "The sympathetic nervous system drives tumor angiogenesis." Trends in cancer 4.2 (2018): 93-94.

108) Phadke, Sneha, and Gerald Clamon. "Beta Blockade as Adjunctive Breast Cancer Therapy: A Review." Critical reviews in oncology/hematology (2019).

Chapter 7

Alpha Lipoic Acid, Low-Dose Naltrexone, and Melatonin

In 1977, I was just finishing medical school. That same year, Dr. Burton Berkson was saving his first patient from an agonizing death from hepatic necrosis after he had eaten the poison mushroom Amanita verna, "the destroying angel." Dr. Berkson, who had earned his Ph.D. in mycology at Rutgers, recalled an article about alpha lipoic acid (ALA; also known as thioctic acid) as an antidote for mushroom poisoning. (1) Realizing the drug could save his patent's life, he placed a call to Fred Bartter, an old friend at the National Institutes of Health (NIH) and asked for a prompt overnight air shipment of ALA to his hospital. Upon infusing the drug into the dying patient, much to the disbelief of his superiors, the patient miraculously recovered and is still alive today. (2)

Drs. Berkson and Fred Bartter later collaborated in the treatment of 79 similar patients, all dying of hepatic failure. Seventy-five of the 79 patients survived with the intravenous ALA treatment, a remarkable accomplishment. Bartter and Berkson filed for a new drug application (NDA) with the Food and Drug Administration, and for the next 23 years Dr. Berkson was deemed "FDA principal investigator" for ALA. (3)

A New Discovery: ALA Effective for Cancer

After finishing his training, Dr. Berkson embarked on his medical career treating liver disease with ALA at his clinic in Las Cruces, New Mexico. There he observed something unexpected in liver disease patients who also had cancer. Pancreatic and hepatic cancer patients went into remission after IV alpha lipoic acid treatment. (4) The alpha lipoic acid had a beneficial side effect, selectively killing cancer cells while leaving normal cells unharmed.

Molecular Mechanism of Alpha Lipoic Acid Effect on Cancer Cells

The exact molecular mechanism for this remarkable cell-killing effect was elucidated in a series of studies by Drs. Paul Bingham, Bastian Dörsam, Perrine Kafara, Lioubov G. Korotchkina, Uwe Wenzel, and Benedikt Feuerecker. (7–12)

In 2019, Dr. Ivana Damnjanovic studied alpha lipoic acid (ALA) in a human colon cancer cell line, finding inhibition of the anti-apoptotic protein BCL-2 and activation of the pro-apoptotic BAX protein. This finding suggests that ALA is a BH3 mimetic similar to the new FDA-approved drug, venetoclax (ABT-199), a selective BCL-2 inhibitor. (7)

Note: BH3 mimetics inhibit BCL-2, the main anti-apoptotic protein that immortalizes the cancer cell. Inhibition of BCL-2 allows the cancer cell to undergo programmed cell death (apoptosis).

Pyruvate Dehydrogenase Complex

ALA is the key enzyme and regulator of the pyruvate dehydrogenase complex (PDC), the primary gateway for carbon fuel into the tricarboxylic acid cycle (TCA), which drives the oxygen-dependent mitochondrial electron transport chain (ETC). Lipoic acid plays a key role in the PDC cycle, which converts pyruvate to acetyl Co-A. Thiamine-pyro-phosphate (TPP) is an important co-factor in the reaction. Another needed co-factor is carnitine, which shuttles the acetyl-CoA into the mitochondria. (9–13)

Note: The nutritional supplement POLY-MVA, developed by Merrill Garnett, contains both alpha lipoic acid and thiamine, the two co-factors mentioned above, as well as the rare earth metal, palladium.

PDK Upregulation, a Central Element of Cancer Cell Metabolism

The upregulation of PDK and downregulation of PDC is the central element in cancer cell metabolism. First, the cancer cell's metabolism is upregulated, with increased uptake of both glucose and glutamine. Second, the cancer cell metabolism is redirected away from mitochondrial OXPHOS to GLYCOLYSIS in the cytoplasm (the Warburg Effect), providing increased anabolic substrates for the nucleotide and amino acid synthesis needed for rapid cell proliferation.

Third, PDK is upregulated in cancer cells, thus inhibiting PDC. This in turn downregulates carbon flow through the pyruvate dehydrogenase (PDH) pathway. **Note**: PDH is the first component of PDC. This upregulation of PDK and downregulation of PDC—the central element in cancer cell metabolism—shunts metabolism away from mitochondrial OXPHOS toward GLYCOLYSIS in the cytoplasm. (9–13)

Lipoic Acid Increases PDC Activity

According to Drs. Lioubov Korotchkina et al:

An inhibitory effect of lipoic acid on PDKs would result in... increased PDC pyruvate dehydrogenase complex (PDC) activity. This finding provides a possible mechanism for a glucose (and lactate) lowering effect of R-lipoic acid in diabetic subjects. (10)

Dr. U. Wenzel et al. studied the effect of ALA on colon cancer cells, finding:

ALA was able to increase Oxygen generation inside mitochondria. Increased mitochondrial O2 production was preceded by an increased influx of lactate or pyruvate into mitochondria, and resulted in the downregulation of the anti-apoptotic protein BCL-2.... In contrast to HT-29 [colon cancer] cells, no apoptosis was observed in non-transformed human colonocytes [normal cells] in response to ALA. (11)

ALA Compared to DCA Dichloroacetic Acid: Both ALA and DCA are Glycolysis Inhibitors

In 2012, Dr. Benedikt Feuerecker et al. studied the effect of ALA compared to dichloroacetate (DCA) on neuroblastoma and breast cancer cells in vitro; in addition, in vivo animal xenograft studies were done with breast cancer cells

---

treated with ALA. Dr. Feuerecker's group found ALA to be more effective than DCA in reducing cancer cell viability/proliferation at low concentrations (2.5 to 10 milliMolar), reducing the 18-FDG (18-flouro-deoxy-glucose) uptake in the cancer cells, suggesting a shift from GLYCOLYSIS to mitochondrial OXPHOS, which requires less glucose. However, compared to ALA, the DCA required much higher doses (25–30 milliMoles/L) to reduce 18-FDG uptake.

The effect of ALA on cancer cells involves:

- Reduced cancer cell viability/proliferation.

- Reduced uptake of radio-labeled glucose (18F-FDG).

- Reduced lactate production.

- Increased apoptosis in all investigated cancer cell lines, demonstrated by dose-dependent increase in caspase-3 **Note:** caspase-3 is the executioner protein involved in triggering apoptosis. (12)

See chapter 5 on DCA for more on this topic.

Aerobic GLYCOLYSIS Versus OXPHOS

Aerobic glycolysis (the Warburg Effect) preferentially used by cancer cells is inefficient, producing only two molecules of adenosine triphosphate (ATP) per molecule of glucose. In comparison, mitochondrial OXPHOS (oxidation of glucose to CO_2 and H_2O) produces more than 32 molecules of ATP per molecule of glucose. Although aerobic glycolysis is inefficient, it shunts much needed carbon into building materials for rapid cell replication. Normal cells use the PDC to direct pyruvate into the more efficient mitochondrial electron transport chain, producing large amounts of energy per carbon atom. Operating this electron transport chain produces damaging oxidative byproducts called reactive oxygen species (ROS). This is no problem for the normal cell, which has anti-oxidant protection. The cancer cell, on the other hand, has little protection from this oxidative onslaught, making it susceptible to oxidative therapies, such as ALA. (13)

Note: in this book, we refer to aerobic glycolysis (the Warburg Effect) with the word, GLYCOLYSIS in capital letters.

Oxidative Therapies

Other oxidative therapies include hyperbaric oxygen and ozone therapy, which are useful as adjunctive treatments for cancer patients. (114–118)

Shunting Carbon into the Mitochondrial Electron Transport

As mentioned above, the central metabolic feature of the cancer cell is the inhibition of the PDC, which blocks entry of carbon into the ETC. If we could find some way to force the cancer cell to use the mitochondrial ETC, this would overwhelm the mitochondria, which would then "burn up" and trigger apoptosis, i.e., programmed cell death. This is exactly what alpha lipoic acid does at the molecular level.

PDC Gateway for Carbon Flux into Mitochondria

The PDC and PDK enzyme are the primary gateway for carbon metabolism. The alpha lipoic acid inhibits PDK, which upregulates the

PDC. This forces the cancer cell to use the mitochondrial electron transport chain, an intolerable state inducing mitochondrial apoptosis of the cancer cell.

High-Dose ALA Causes Adverse Effects on Mitochondria

In 2014, Dr. Michael Vigil et al. studied high-dose ALA in monkeys. Transmission electron microscope images in control (normal) animals showed mitochondria with intact membranes and cristae ultrastructure. However high-dose ALA treatment resulted in disrupted ultrastructure of mitochondria, caused by excess ROS and lipid peroxidation.

Although these effects are seen with excess amounts of alpha lipoic acid in a monkey model, similar effects occur in cancer cells that cannot tolerate the increased electron flux through the mitochondrial respiratory chain, resulting in lipid peroxidation and oxidative damage to the ultrastructure of the membranes and cristae, triggering release of cytochrome C and caspase-induced mitochondrial apoptosis. (14)

Low-Dose Naltrexone (LDN)

FDA-approved in 1984, naltrexone is an opiate blocker developed as part of Ronald Reagan's "war on drugs" as a treatment for drug addiction. The chemical structure is similar to the opiate receptor blocker Narcan, a drug commonly used by paramedics to wake up drug-overdose victims and by anesthesiologists to wake up patients after surgery. Naltrexone comes as a 50 milligram tablet, and LDN comes as a 4.5 mg. compounded capsule. LDN, usu-ally taken at night before sleep, shows remarkable benefits for auto-immune disease, cancer, chronic fatigue/fibromyalgia, and chronic pain syndromes. LDN blocks the opiate growth factor receptor (OGFr) implicated in breast and pancreatic cancer proliferation. (15)

In 2013, Dr. Ian Zagon et al. studied OGFr in triple-negative breast cancer in vitro, finding opiate growth factor (OGF) inhibited cancer proliferation.

> OGF treatment inhibited TNBC [breast cancer] cells in a dosage related, receptor mediated, and reversible manner. OGF was the specific endogenous opioid to inhibit cell proliferation, and this was mediated by p21 cyclin dependent inhibitory kinase pathways, and required protein and RNA synthesis. OGFr was the specific receptor involved … OGF is an endogenously produced pentapeptide that inhibits cell replication by interacting with OGFr and upregulating cyclin-dependent inhibitory kinase pathways thus reducing DNA synthesis. (16)

Similarly, Dr. Zagon also studied OGF in pancreatic and ovarian cancer. (17–18)

In 2019, Dr. Ruizhe Wang et al. reviewed this topic and concluded that naltrexone could bind to the opiate receptor and serve in place of OGF (also called met-enkephalin, an endogenous opioid), thereby inhibiting cancer proliferation. OGF and naltrexone at suitable dosage range could inhibit tumor growth through binding to opioid receptors. (19)

In 2020, Dr. Alshimaa Aboalsoud et al. studied the anti-cancer effects of LDN in a mouse xenograft study using Ehrlich's carcinoma, with and without the chemotherapy agent 5 flouro-uracil (5FU). These mouse xenograft studies confirmed the earlier 2013 study by Dr. Ian Zagon et al., using LDN instead of OGF:

> All drug-treated groups showed reduction in tumor weight and volume…. LDN led to significant increase in OGFr [Opiate Growth Factor Receptor] both in solo and in combination with 5FU. Serum IFN-γ [interferon gamma] is significantly increased by LDN but decreased by 5-FU. Also, LDN and 5FU increased immune-histochemical staining of p21 [cyclin-dependent kinase inhibitor] while decreased immunostaining of Bcl2 [anti-apoptosis protein]. In animals treated with a combination of LDN and 5FU a maximal downregulation of the anti-apoptotic mediator BCL2 was observed. (20)

Note: Interferon (IFN)-γ is a cytokine involved in anti-tumor immunity, increased by DCA, LDN and Cimetidine.

Combining LDN with Aged Garlic in Mouse Fibrosarcoma

In 2013, Dr. Soheil Ebrahimpour et al. found the combination of LDN and aged garlic to be synergistic in a mouse xenograft model of fibrosarcoma, resulting in improved immune response and longer survival times. (21)

Long-Term Remission in Carcinoma of Tongue with LDN

In 2014, Dr. Akbar Khan reported a case of LDN-induced long-term remission of carcinoma of the tongue. Note that Met-enkephalin is another name for OGF.

Dr. Khan writes:

> Low Dose Naltrexone [LDN] in the range of 3–4.5 mg per day has been shown to…

[induce] brief opiate receptor blockade with resulting upregulation of endogenous opiate production. Through the work of Bihari and Zagon, it has been determined that the level of the endogenous opiate methionine-enkephalin [OGF] is increased by LDN. Met-enkephalin [OGF] is involved in regulating cell proliferation and can inhibit cancer cell growth in multiple cell lines. **Increased met-enkephalin [OGF] levels created by LDN thus have the potential to inhibit cancer growth in humans.**(22)

Combination of ALA and LDN: Case Report of Metastatic Pancreatic Cancer

In 2009, Dr. Burton Berkson reported a series of remarkable cancer remissions using the combination of ALA and LDN in pancreatic cancer and B-cell lymphoma. (23–25)

A 46-year-old male sought medical attention for abdominal pain, which was biopsy-proven to be pancreatic cancer metastatic to the liver. The patient was then treated with conventional chemotherapy (gemcitabine and carboplatin), which caused leukopenia and thrombocytopenia. The patient tolerated the chemotherapy poorly, seeking a second opinion from a different oncologist who advised "any further treatment would ultimately be fruitless." (24)

The patient sought medical care with Dr. Berkson, who started treatment with intravenous ALA, 300 to 600 mg twice a week, and LDN 4.5 mg at bedtime. Supplements given were: oral ALA (600 mg/d), selenium (200 mcg twice daily), and silymarin (300 mg, four times a day). There was also dietary and lifestyle modification. This treatment program resulted in comparatively "stable disease for more than a 3-year period." (24)

Case Report B-Cell Lymphoma Remission

A 61-year-old male with progressive follicular lymphoma who declined conventional chemotherapy sought medical care at Dr. Berkson's clinic. The patient was treated solely with nine intravenous (IV) ALA treatments and was continued on oral LDN 4.5 mg nightly. Six months later, the enlarged lymph nodes had resolved, and the patient remained in remission for another year, after which he was lost to follow-up. (25)

Considering the above studies and reports, LDN is a promising addition to any integrative oncology protocol. The opposite approach, the use of narcotics and opiate drugs, should be regarded as stimulatory to cancer proliferation and to be avoided as discussed by Dr. Frances Lennon (2012). (26)

Cancer Cell Types Studied with ALA

ALA anti-cancer effects have been studied in:

- Bladder cancer (5)
- Colorectal cancer (6–7)(54)
- Non-small-cell lung cancer (8)
- Ovarian cancer (41)
- Breast cancer (42–49)
- Lung cancer (50–53)
- Hepatoma (55–56)
- Gastric cancer (57)
- Leukemia (58)
- Ehrlich ascites carcinoma (119)

Treating Diabetic Neuropathy with ALA

ALA is well known for its benefits in diabetes and diabetic neuropathy patients. They recommend taking ALA 30 minutes before meals to improve absorption. Treatment of diabetics with 300 to 1200 mg ALA daily for six months produced a decrease in hemoglobin- A1C (HgbA1c) and fasting blood sugar. In diabetic neuropathy patients, intravenous ALA, 600 mg daily for three weeks, provided significant improvement, with reduction in neuropathy symptoms of pain, numbness, and burning compared to placebo. (59–61)

ALA Effective for Ovarian Cancer

In 2015, Dr. Perrine Kafara et al. studied the anti-cancer effects of ALA on two ovarian cancer cell lines showing induction of ROS, suppression of growth, and downregulation of anti-apoptotic proteins. Dr. Kafara and colleagues write:

ALA [Alpha Lipoic Acid] suppressed growth proliferation and induced apoptosis in both ovarian [cancer] cell lines. Moreover, ALA provoked a **downregulation of two anti-apoptotic proteins, Mcl-1 and Bcl-xL** protein and a strong induction of the BH3-only protein Bim. Furthermore, ALA induced **ROS generation.** (41)

Synergy of ALA with IV Vitamin C

The anti-cancer effect of alpha lipoic acid is synergistic with high-dose Intravenous vitamin C (20–75 grams) serving as a pro-oxidant in the mitochondria. (27–28)

In 2001, Dr. J. J. Casciari et al. wrote that ALA synergistically enhances vitamin C anti-cancer toxicity:

Lipoic acid synergistically enhanced ascorbate cytotoxicity, reducing the 2-day LC50 [lethal concentration 50%] in hollow fibre tumors from 34 mM to 4 mM. Lipoic acid, unlike ascorbate, was equally effective against proliferating and non-proliferating cells. Ascorbate levels in human blood plasma were measured during and after intravenous ascorbate infusions. Infusions of 60 g produced peak plasma concentrations exceeding 20 mM, with an area under the curve [24 h] of 76 mM h. Thus, tumoricidal concentrations may be achievable in vivo. Ascorbate efficacy was enhanced in an additive fashion by vitamin K3. (28)

The ALA is commonly given as a 600 mg IV bolus following the IV vitamin C infusion, useful in diabetic peripheral neuropathy. (59–61) See chapter 8 on IV Vitamin C as cancer chemotherapy.

Addition of Hydroxy Citrate Improves Effect of ALA

ATP citrate lyase (also called ATP-citric synthase) is frequently upregulated in cancer. ATP citrate lyase is a central enzyme involved in glucose metabolism and lipid biogenesis and a useful anti-cancer target. In 2010, Dr. Schwartz studied the combination of ALA and hydroxycitrate (a known inhibitor of ATP Citrate Lyase) in vitro and in vivo mouse xenografts, finding an augmented anti-cancer effect. Other ATP citrate lyase inhibitors are under development, such as dehydrocurvularin, an irreversible inhibitor. (31–36)

Benfotiamine (Thiamine) and Carnitine

Both thiamine and carnitine are co-factors for PDC delivery of carbon to the TCA and mitochondrial electron transport chain. Thus, similar to ALA, they are activators of the PDH complex. Adding these vitamins synergizes and augments the ALA anti-cancer effect because they increase PDC activity, driving carbon flux into the mitochondrial ETC, causing apoptosis of the cancer cell. For example, benfotiamine has in vivo anti-cancer activity. (37–38)

Thiamine for Breast Cancer

In 2018, Dr. Xiaowen Liu studied the effect of thiamine on breast cancer cells in vitro, finding an anti-cancer mechanism similar to ALA:

The treatment of MCF7 breast cancer cells with 1–2 microgram/mL of thiamine for 24 hours significantly reduced their proliferation. This reduction is associated with **a reduction in glycolysis and activation of the PDH complex in breast cancer cells.** (39)

In 2014, Dr. Bradley Hanberry, using two cancer cell lines, pancreatic cancer and neuroblastoma, found that high-dose thiamine reduced cancer cell proliferation. The mechanism was analogous to dichloroactetate (DCA), as both are glycolysis inhibitors. (40)

ALA Synergy with Melatonin

Melatonin is another glycolysis inhibitor, discovered over 60 years ago. Melatonin is a sleep hormone produced by the pineal gland. Analogous to ALA, thiamine, and DCA, melatonin switches cancer cells from GLYCOLYSIS in the cytosol to OXPHOS in the mitochondria. Melatonin selectively causes apoptosis in cancer cells by downregulating the Warburg Effect, while sparing normal cells. Melatonin taken as a supplement or produced nightly during darkness enters cancer cells via glucose transporters. Similar to bacteria, mitochondria also contain high concentrations of melatonin obtained by their own synthesis from acetyl-CoA.

Circadian Rhythm and Melatonin

Melatonin levels rise at night during darkness and fall during daylight. In mouse breast cancer xenograft and in human breast cancer studies, high nighttime circulating melatonin switches the breast cancer cells from GLYCOLYSIS to OXPHOS. Dr. Russel Reiter et al. speculate this is done by inhibition of PDK, the same target as DCA. In this way, the anti-cancer mechanism of melatonin is similar to that of DCA. Dr. Reiter also predicts that mitochondria in cancer cells lose their ability to synthesize melatonin, a function maintained in normal cells. The mechanism by which cancer cells shut down melatonin production is yet to be determined. Dr. Reiter's group notes:

> Melatonin is in high concentration in the mitochondria of normal cells, where it is synthesized, but absent or in lower levels in cancer cell mitochondria where it is not synthesized ... melatonin restricts the initiation, progression and metastasis of tumors ... limiting growth factor uptake, improving immune surveillance, reducing oxidative/nitrosative stress, controlling angiogenesis, synchronizing circadian rhythms ... (62)

Dr. Reiter et al. (2014) further state:

> Melatonin behaves as a "smart killer," i.e., modulating anti-apoptotic processes in normal cells, and triggering pro-apoptotic signals in cancer cells... indeed, melatonin induces apoptosis in several types of tumors: colon cancer cells, hepatocarcinoma, glioma and neuroblastoma, Ehrlich ascites carcinoma cells, lymphoma, leukemia cells, etc. (62–64)

Melatonin Effect Similar to DCA, Thiamine, and ALA

In 2016, Dr. Nicola Pacini and Fabio Borziani wrote a brilliant review of melatonin's anti-cancer effects, which includes a decoupling effect, and stimulation of ETC respiratory complexes I, II, and IV and a marked effect on complex III, all similar to the effects of DCA, ALA and Thiamine:

> Mitochondria of neoplastic cells actually have a strong decoupling of the oxidative phosphorylation.... the production of ROS is extremely harmful for the mitochondrial structures... the paradoxical action of MLT [melatonin], able to induce cellular death in cancer cells and cytoprotection in models of neurodegeneration is quite appropriate. Melatonin stimulates the activity of respiratory complexes I, II, and IV, and has a marked effect on complex III, thus being able to achieve a strong perturbation of the electron transport chain in neoplastic cells, also preventing the braking action of BCL-2 and overstimulating an already metastable cellular system, characterized by a high electron flow through the electron transport chain, high oxygen consumption, UCP [Uncoupling Proteins]-mediated uncoupling and high sensitivity to ROS...

substances that, also at the end of respiratory complexes, force the cellular respiration, such as **dichloroacetate, thiamine or R-lipoic acid,** induce ROS-mediated cell death in neoplastic cells and neuroprotection in many neurodegenerative diseases. (66)

In 2018, Dr. Yi Wang et al. reviewed the use of melatonin for cancer patients, saying melatonin exerts such positive effects as:

improving tumor remission rate and overall survival rate, while reducing the incidence of chemotherapy side effects. (67)

Melatonin Accumulates in Cancer Cells

In 2018, Dr. Gaia Favero et al. wrote that melatonin accumulates in cancer cells, inhibiting proliferation and inducing cell cycle arrest. Melatonin prevents EMT (epithelial to mesenchymal transition), is involved in cytoskeletal reorganization, modulates the cell matrix, inhibits angiogenesis, has antimetastatic properties, and induces apoptosis in cancer cells only while sparing normal cells. Melatonin works in synergy with chemotherapy and radiation therapy while reducing their toxicity. (68–71)

Melatonin Is a Cancer Stem Cell Agent

Cancer stem cells are highly resistant to chemotherapy, and residual CSCs will then repopulate the tumor mass after chemotherapy, causing cancer relapse with a more invasive metastatic cell type. EMT allows for this invasive, metastatic behavior. The primitive, embryonic Wnt pathway activated by Beta-Catenin is key for the CSCs.

In 2016, Dr. Naiane do Nascimento Goncalves et al. studied melatonin in breast CSCs in human and canine lines, finding melatonin effective for EMT markers and reducing invasive properties. Melatonin inhibits EMT by degrading Beta-Catenin via activation of GSK3-Beta. This prevents the Beta-Catenin from translocating to the nucleus, and complexing with TCF/LEF to induce transcription of Wnt target genes. Melatonin promotes apoptosis and inhibits invasiveness of CSCs, effective at the 1 millimolar concentration. (72–78) Melatonin has synergy with ATRA (all-trans retinoic acid, a vitamin A analog) and berberine. (79–80) Melatonin has synergy with most chemotherapies and oncology drugs, while reducing the toxicity of chemotherapy. (81–84)

Embryonic Cancer Stem Cells (P19): Synergy of DCA and Melatonin

The embryonic CSC is a useful model for studying the efficacy of anti-cancer agents.

In 2015, Dr. Rute Loureiro et al. studied the effect of melatonin on highly glycolytic embryonal carcinoma stem cells (ESC), finding synergy with dichloroacetate, DCA. (97) The stem cells can be induced to undergo differentiation by growing in a glucose-free galactose medium. This environment causes the stem cells to switch metabolism from GLYCOLYSIS to mitochondrial OXPHOS. Dr. Loureiro's group write:

P19 CSCs [Embryonic Cancer Stem Cells] are highly glycolytic and their differentiation is characterized by a more oxidative metabolism…. In fact, when forcing mitochondrial metabolism by growing P19 cells in galactose [glucose-free], glutamine/

pyruvate-containing medium (Gal-CSCs), cells increase their mitochondrial activity, reduce proliferation and pluripotency and, spontaneously differentiate. In addition, when P19 Gal-CSCs are treated with retinoic acid [vitamin A], the resultant cells (Gal-dCCs) show the highest degree of mitochondrial development and function. (97)

These cells are sensitive to melatonin.

The Gal-dCCs (differentiated cancer cells grown in galactose and treated with vitamin A) are the cell group with the largest degree of cell differentiation and upregulated mitochondrial function (OXPHOS). These are susceptible to inhibition with melatonin, which has a pro-oxidant effect, inducing S-phase arrest, altered mitochondrial membrane potential, decreased oxygen consumption, and reduced BCL-2 protein with induction of cell death.

While the cancer cells relying on OXPHOS were sensitive to melatonin, the highly glycolytic CSCs "were less susceptible to melatonin anti-tumoral effects." (97)

However, these highly resistant glycolytic stem cells could be re-sensitized to the anti-cancer effects of melatonin by co-treating them with dichloroacetate (DCA), which forced them to shift mitochondrial metabolism to OXPHOS. Dr. Tiziana Tataranni et al. (2019) write:

> DCA treatment of ESCs [embryonic stem cells] promotes loss of pluripotency and **shifts towards a more active oxidative metabolism**, accompanied by **a significant decrease in HIF1a and p53 expression**. (98)

> Surprisingly, when we combined 1 mM melatonin and 10 mM dichloroacetate,

cytotoxicity in the highly resistant [glycolytic] Glu-CSCs was observed. These results are of great importance considering that to our knowledge, this is the only treatment showing an efficient and viable effect against [highly glycolytic] P19 Glu-CSCs. Furthermore, the synergistic capability of this treatment combination was observed in P19 cells with the most active mitochondrial metabolism. (97)

Our hypothesis ascribes an anti-tumor effect for melatonin only in differentiated cancer cells with an active oxidative metabolism, triggering a type of mitochondrial-mediated cell death which is likely to be characterized by an arrest at S-phase, reduction of the mitochondrial ETC, generation of reactive oxygen species, BCL-2 downregulation and AIF release. Thus, the treatment with melatonin and the stimulation of mitochondrial metabolism [i.e., with DCA] constitute promising strategies against resistant CSCs. (97)

Drs. Mu-Tai Liu and Russel Reiter write in 2018:

> Combination therapy with melatonin and the activation of mitochondrial metabolism **[with DCA]** represents promising strategies reducing cancer stem cell resistance. (100)

Important!! The combined use of melatonin and DCA appears to be a valid anti-CSC strategy.

Melatonin Is Chemo- and Radioprotective

A number of studies reveal protective effects of melatonin and ALA against toxic effects of radiation therapy and chemotherapy (101–105)

Anti-Cancer Effects of Melatonin Considered Hugely Exciting

In 2019, Dr. Shahrokh Iravani et al. studied the role of melatonin in colorectal cancer finding **anti-cancer effects of melatonin hugely exciting and a "possible cure"**, writing:

> Overall, the anti-cancer activity of melatonin, combined with its actions via multiple signaling pathways, is considered **hugely exciting** to use this drug as a possible treatment strategy to **cure cancer.** Apart from its anti-cancer potential, this drug has shown to induce modulation of chemotherapy toxicity and improving its therapeutic efficacy. (94)

Melatonin has antiproliferative, anti-angiogenic, pro-apoptotic and immunomodulatory effects on many cancer types including:

- Hodgkin's lymphoma (85)
- Hematologic neoplasms, B Cell Lymphoma (86–88)
- Breast cancer (89)
- Ovarian cancer (90–92)
- Colorectal, (93–95)
- Gastric (121)
- Osteosarcoma (122)
- Prostate (123)

Melatonin also has the beneficial effect of boosting the host immune system. (96)

Since both ALA and melatonin are glycolysis inhibitors and increase electron flux through the mitochondrial electron transport chain, one might speculate synergistic anti-cancer effects. However, we await further studies to confirm this hypothesis.

ALA for Diabetic Neuropathy and Autonomic Neuropathy

A large number of studies show that IV or oral ALA is beneficial in diabetic peripheral neuropathy (106–107) and autonomic neuropathy (29–30) (59–61)

ALA and PQQ

Pyrroloquinoline-quinine (PQQ) is a newly discovered vitamin co-factor which has "exceptionally high redox recycling ability," making it useful as an anti-neurodegenerative and anti-cancer agent. (108) According to Drs. H. S. Misra et al. (2012), "PQQ stimulates mitochondrial complex 1 activity in vitro."(109)

In 2010, Dr. Bhavani Shankar et al. studied the effect of PQQ on leukemia cells, finding:

> PQQ induced apoptosis in human promonocytic leukemia U937 cells, accompanied by depletion of the major cellular anti-oxidant glutathione and increase in intracellular reactive oxygen species (ROS). (110)

In a 2014 *Journal of Cancer* report, Dr. Zhihui Min et al. remark that

> PQQ could induce apoptosis in human promonocytic leukemia U937 and lymphoma EL-4 cells. The underlying mechanism might be relevant to the increase of intracellular reactive oxygen species (ROS) and depletion of glutathione. (111)

PQQ is also neuroprotective and synergizes with lithium in this role. (112–113)

These findings suggest PQQ would work in synergy with alpha lipoic acid to increase electron flux through the mitochondrial electron transport chain, thus increasing ROS, depleting glutathione, and causing mitochondrial apoptosis in the cancer cell. However, we await further studies for confirmation of this hypothesis.

Dichloroacetate and Alpha Lipoic Acid Combination

Dr. Paul Anderson's book, *Out of the Box Cancer Treatments,* discusses the combination of DCA and Poly-MVA as an important tool in the anti-cancer armamentarium. (114) Poly-MVA is a proprietary palladium, alpha lipoic acid, thiamine complex developed by Merrill Garnett. The metabolic effect of DCA is similar to that of alpha lipoic acid, as they are both GLYCOLYSIS inhibitors. Both drive the PDC reaction forward, feeding electrons (from pyruvate) into the mitochondrial ETC. Thus, both agents block GLYCOLYSIS and drive electron flux through the mitochondria, which is intolerable to cancer cells.

Conclusion

The experience of Dr. Berkson with alpha lipoic acid as an anti-cancer agent is intriguing, with case reports of cancer remission. The combination of LDN and melatonin provides additional synergy. ALA is a remarkably safe and effective anti-cancer agent, serving as a cornerstone for any cancer prevention or treatment program. Regarding melatonin, in the words of Dr. Shahrokh Iravani (2019): "[it is] **hugely exciting** to use this drug [melatonin] **as a possible treatment strategy to cure cancer**." The added synergy of melatonin when combined with DCA is remarkable, a highly effective anti-cancer strategy deserving prominence in our *Cracking Cancer Toolkit.*

References for Chapter 7: Alpha Lipoic Acid and LDN

1) Becker, Charles E., et al. "Diagnosis and treatment of Amanita phalloides-type mushroom poisoning: use of thioctic acid." Western Journal of Medicine 125.2 (1976): 100.

2) Berkson, Burton M. "Alpha-lipoic acid (thioctic acid): my experience with this outstanding therapeutic agent." Journal of Orthomolecular Medicine 13.1 (1998): 44-48.

3) Berkson, Burton M. "Alpha lipoic acid and liver disease." Townsend Letter for Doctors and Patients 293 (2007): 80.

4) Berkson, Burton M., Daniel M. Rubin, and Arthur J. Berkson. "Revisiting the ALA/N (α-Lipoic Acid/Low-Dose Naltrexone) protocol for people with metastatic and nonmetastatic pancreatic cancer: a report of 3 new cases." Integrative cancer therapies 8.4 (2009): 416-422.

5) Yamasaki, Masao, et al. "α-Lipoic acid suppresses migration and invasion via downregulation of cell surface β1-integrin expression in bladder cancer cells." Journal of clinical biochemistry and nutrition (2013): 13-57.

6) Dörsam, Bastian, et al. "Lipoic acid induces p53-independent cell death in colorectal cancer cells and potentiates the cytotoxicity of 5-fluorouracil." Archives of toxicology 89.10 (2015): 1829-1846.

7) Damnjanovic, Ivana, et al. "Possible molecular mechanisms and pathways involved in BH3 mimetic activity of alpha-lipoic acid on human colon cancer cell line." Farmacia (2019).

8) Michikoshi, Hiromitsu, et al. "α-Lipoic acid-induced inhibition of proliferation and met phosphorylation in human non-small cell lung cancer cells." Cancer letters 335.2 (2013): 472-478.

9) Bingham, Paul M., Shawn D. Stuart, and Zuzana Zachar. "Lipoic acid and lipoic acid analogs in cancer

metabolism and chemotherapy." Expert review of clinical pharmacology 7.6 (2014): 837-846.

10) Korotchkina, Lioubov G., Sukhdeep Sidhu, and Mulchand S. Patel. "R-lipoic acid inhibits mammalian pyruvate dehydrogenase kinase." Free radical research 38.10 (2004): 1083-1092.

11) Wenzel, U., A. Nickel, and H. Daniel. "Alpha-lipoic acid induces apoptosis in human colon cancer cells by increasing mitochondrial respiration with a concomitant O2 generation." Apoptosis 10.2 (2005): 359-368.

12) Feuerecker, Benedikt, et al. "Lipoic acid inhibits cell proliferation of tumor cells in vitro and in vivo." Cancer biology & therapy 13.14 (2012): 1425-1435.

13) Bingham, Paul M., Zuzana Zachar, and R. A. Canuto. "The pyruvate dehydrogenase complex in cancer: implications for the transformed state and cancer chemotherapy." Dehydrogenases. Intech, 2012.

14) Vigil, Michael, Burton M. Berkson, and Ana Patricia Garcia. "Adverse effects of high doses of intravenous alpha lipoic acid on liver mitochondria." Global Advances in Health and Medicine 3.1 (2014): 25-27.

15) Li, Zijian, et al. "Low-dose naltrexone (LDN): A promising treatment in immune-related diseases and cancer therapy." International immunopharmacology 61 (2018): 178-184.

16) Zagon, Ian S., Nancy K. Porterfield, and Patricia J. McLaughlin. "Opioid growth factor–opioid growth factor receptor axis inhibits proliferation of triple negative breast cancer." Experimental Biology and Medicine 238.6 (2013): 589-599.

17) Zagon, Ian S., and Patricia J. McLaughlin. "Opioid growth factor and the treatment of human pancreatic cancer: a review." World Journal of Gastroenterology: WJG 20.9 (2014): 2218.

18) Zagon, Ian S., Renee Donahue, and Patricia J. McLaughlin. "Targeting the opioid growth factor: opioid growth factor receptor axis for treatment of human ovarian cancer." Experimental Biology and Medicine 238.5 (2013): 579-587.

19) Wang, Ruizhe, Yi Zhang, and Fengping Shan. "Interaction of opioid growth factor (OGF) and opioid antagonist and their significance in cancer therapy." International immunopharmacology 75 (2019): 105785.

20) Aboalsoud, Alshimaa, et al. "The effect of low-dose naltrexone on solid Ehrlich carcinoma in mice: The role of OGFr, BCL2, and immune response." International Immunopharmacology 78 (2020): 106068.

21) Ebrahimpour, Soheil, et al. "Synergistic effect of aged garlic extract and naltrexone on improving immune responses to experimentally induced fibrosarcoma tumor in BALB/c mice." Pharmacognosy research 5.3 (2013): 189.

22) Khan, Akbar. "Long-Term Remission of Adenoid Cystic Tongue Carcinoma with Low Dose Naltrexone and Vitamin D3–A Case Report." Oral Health Dent Manag 13.3 (2014): 721-724.

23) Berkson, Burton M., Daniel M. Rubin, and Arthur J. Berkson. "Revisiting the ALA/N (α-Lipoic Acid/Low-Dose Naltrexone) protocol for people with metastatic and nonmetastatic pancreatic cancer: a report of 3 new cases." Integrative cancer therapies 8.4 (2009): 416-422.

24) Berkson, Burton M., Daniel M. Rubin, and Arthur J. Berkson. "The long-term survival of a patient with pancreatic cancer with metastases to the liver after treatment with the intravenous α-lipoic acid/low-dose naltrexone protocol." Integrative cancer therapies 5.1 (2006): 83-89.

25) Berkson, Burton M., Daniel M. Rubin, and Arthur J. Berkson. "Reversal of signs and symptoms of a B-cell lymphoma in a patient using only low-dose naltrexone." Integrative cancer therapies 6.3 (2007): 293-296.

26) Lennon, Frances E., Jonathan Moss, and Patrick A. Singleton. "The-Opioid Receptor in Cancer Progression." Anesthesiology 116.4 (2012): 940-5.

27) Ngo, Bryan, et al. "Targeting cancer vulnerabilities with high-dose vitamin C." Nature Reviews Cancer 19.5 (2019): 271-282.

28) Casciari, J. J., Riordan et al. "Cytotoxicity of ascorbate, lipoic acid, and other antioxidants in hollow fibre in vitro tumours." British journal of cancer 84.11 (2001): 1544. 88)

29) Ziegler, Dan, and F. Arnold Gries. "Alpha-lipoic acid in the treatment of diabetic peripheral and cardiac autonomic neuropathy"Diabetes 46.Supplement 2 (1997): S62-S66.

30) Ziegler, Dan, et al. "Treatment of symptomatic diabetic polyneuropathy with the antioxidant alpha-lipoic acid: a 7-month multicenter randomized controlled trial (ALADIN III Study). ALADIN III Study Group. Alpha-Lipoic Acid in Diabetic Neuropathy." Diabetes care 22.8 (1999): 1296-1301.

31) Icard, Philippe, et al. "ATP citrate lyase: a central metabolic enzyme in cancer." Cancer Letters (2019).

32) Devi Khwairakpam, Amrita, et al. "ATP citrate lyase (ACLY): a promising target for cancer prevention and treatment." Current drug targets 16.2 (2015): 156-163.

33) Schwartz, Laurent, et al. "A combination of alpha lipoic acid and calcium hydroxycitrate is efficient against mouse cancer models: preliminary results." Oncology reports 23.5 (2010): 1407-1416.

34) Granchi, Carlotta. "ATP citrate lyase (ACLY) inhibitors: an anti-cancer strategy at the crossroads of glucose and lipid metabolism." European journal of medicinal chemistry 157 (2018): 1276-1291.

35) Zu, Xu-Yu, et al. "ATP citrate lyase inhibitors as novel cancer therapeutic agents." Recent patents on anti-cancer drug discovery 7.2 (2012): 154-167.

36) Deng, Zhangshuang, et al. "Dehydrocurvularin is a potent antineoplastic agent irreversibly blocking ATP-citrate lyase: evidence from chemoproteomics." Chemical Communications 55.29 (2019): 4194-4197.

37) J Nutr. 2005 Jun; 135(6):1510-4. Increased carnitine-dependent fatty acid uptake into mitochondria of human colon cancer cells induces apoptosis. Wenzel U1, Nickel A, Daniel H.

38) Jonus, Hunter C., et al. "Thiamine mimetics sulbutiamine and benfotiamine as a nutraceutical approach to anticancer therapy." Biomedicine & Pharmacotherapy 121 (2020): 109648.

39) Liu, Xiaowen, et al. "The effects of thiamine on breast cancer cells." Molecules 23.6 (2018): 1464.

40) Hanberry, Bradley S., Ryan Berger, and Jason A. Zastre. "High-dose vitamin B1 reduces proliferation in cancer cell lines analogous to dichloroacetate." Cancer chemotherapy and pharmacology 73.3 (2014): 585-594.

41) Kafara, Perrine, et al. "Lipoic acid decreases Mcl-1, Bcl-x L and up regulates Bim on ovarian carcinoma cells leading to cell death." Journal of ovarian research 8.1 (2015): 1.

42) Tripathy, Joytirmay, et al. "α-Lipoic acid inhibits the migration and invasion of breast cancer cells through inhibition of TGFβ signaling." Life sciences 207 (2018): 15-22.

43) Na, Mi Hee, Eun Young Seo, and Woo Kyoung Kim. "Effects of α-lipoic acid on cell proliferation and apoptosis in MDA-MB-231 human breast cells." Nutrition research and practice 3.4 (2009): 265-271.

44) Kuban-Jankowska, Alicja, Magdalena Gorska-Ponikowska, and Michal Wozniak. "Lipoic acid decreases the viability of breast cancer cells and activity of PTP1B and SHP2." Anticancer research 37.6 (2017): 2893-2898.

45) Nur, Gökhan, Mustafa Nazıroğlu, and Haci Ahmet Deveci. "Synergic prooxidant, apoptotic and TRPV1 channel activator effects of alpha-lipoic acid and cisplatin in MCF-7 breast cancer cells." Journal of Receptors and Signal Transduction 37.6 (2017): 569-577.

46) Li, B. J., et al. "Effect of lipoic acid combined with paclitaxel on breast cancer cells." Genet Mol Res 14 (2015): 17934-17940.

48) Dozio E, Ruscica M, Passafaro L, et al. The natural antioxidant alpha-lipoic acid induces p27(Kip1)-dependent cell cycle arrest and apoptosis in MCF-7 human breast cancer cells. Eur J Pharmacol. 2010 Sep 1;641(1):29-34

49) Lee HS, Na MH, Kim WK. alpha-Lipoic acid reduces matrix metalloproteinase activity in MDA-MB-231 human breast cancer cells. Nutr Res. 2010 Jun;30(6):403-9

50) Phiboonchaiyanan, Preeyaporn Plaimee, and Pithi Chanvorachote. "Suppression of a cancer stem-like phenotype mediated by alpha-lipoic acid in human lung cancer cells through down-regulation of β-catenin and Oct-4." Cellular Oncology 40.5 (2017): 497-510.

51) Puchsaka, Punyawee, Chatchai Chaotham, and Pithi Chanvorachote. "α-Lipoic acid sensitizes lung cancer cells to chemotherapeutic agents and anoikis via integrin β1/β3 downregulation." International journal of oncology 49.4 (2016): 1445-1456.

52) Yang, Lan, et al. "α-Lipoic acid inhibits human lung cancer cell proliferation through Grb2-mediated

EGFR downregulation." Biochemical and biophysical research communications 494.1-2 (2017): 325-331.

53) Choi SY, Yu JH, Kim H. Mechanism of alpha-lipoic acid-induced apoptosis of lung cancer cells. Ann N Y Acad Sci. 2009 Aug;1171:149-55. Choi alpha lipoic acid induced apoptosis lung cancer Ann N Y Acad Sci 2009

54) Neitzel, Carina, et al. "Lipoic Acid Synergizes with Antineoplastic Drugs in Colorectal Cancer by Targeting p53 for Proteasomal Degradation." Cells 8.8 (2019): 794.

55) Ikuta, Naoko, et al. "Time course effect of R-alpha-lipoic acid on cellular metabolomics in cultured hepatoma cells." Journal of medicinal food 20.3 (2017): 211-222.

56) Shi DY, Liu HL, Stern JS, Yu PZ, Liu SL. Alpha-lipoic acid induces apoptosis in hepatoma cells via the PTEN/Akt pathway. FEBS Lett. 2008 May 28;582(12):1667-71.

57) Yang, Yu, et al. "The Antioxidant Alpha-Lipoic Acid Inhibits Proliferation and Invasion of Human Gastric Cancer Cells via Suppression of STAT3-Mediated MUC4 Gene Expression." Oxidative Medicine and Cellular Longevity 2019 (2019).

58) Selvakumar E, Hsieh TC. Regulation of cell cycle transition and induction of apoptosis in HL-60 leukemia cells by lipoic acid: role in cancer prevention and therapy. J Hematol Oncol. 2008;1:4.

59) Gomes MB and Negrato CA. Alpha-lipoic acid as a pleiotropic compound with potential therapeutic use in diabetes and other chronic diseases. DiabetolMetabSyndr. 2014 Jul; 6:80.

60) Han, T., et al. "A systematic review and meta-analysis of α-lipoic acid in the treatment of diabetic peripheral neuropathy." European journal of endocrinology/European Federation of Endocrine Societies 167.4 (2012): 465.

61) Tankova, Tsvetalina, D. Koev, and L. Dakovska. "Alpha-lipoic acid in the treatment of autonomic diabetic neuropathy (controlled, randomized, open-label study)." Romanian Journal of Internal Medicine. 42.2 (2003): 457-464.

62) Reiter, Russel J., et al. "Inhibition of mitochondrial pyruvate dehydrogenase kinase: a proposed mechanism by which melatonin causes cancer cells to overcome cytosolic glycolysis, reduce tumor biomass and reverse insensitivity to chemotherapy." Melatonin Research 2.3 (2019): 105-119.

63) Reiter, Russel J., et al. "Melatonin, a full service anti-cancer agent: inhibition of initiation, progression and metastasis." International journal of molecular sciences 18.4 (2017): 843.

64) Reiter, Russel J., Dun Xian Tan, and Annia Galano. "Melatonin: exceeding expectations." Physiology 29.5 (2014): 325-333.

65) Liu, Mu-Tai, and Russel J. Reiter. "The Impact of Melatonin and Ionizing Radiation on Autophagy in Cancer Cells." EC Emergency Medicine and Critical Care 4.2 (2020): 01-16.

66) Pacini, Nicola, and Fabio Borziani. "Oncostatic-Cytoprotective Effect of Melatonin and Other Bioactive Molecules: A Common Target in Mitochondrial Respiration." International journal of molecular sciences 17.3 (2016): 341.

67) Wang, Yi, et al. "Therapeutic strategies of melatonin in cancer patients: a systematic review and meta-analysis." OncoTargets and therapy 11 (2018): 7895.

68) Favero, Gaia, et al. "Promising antineoplastic actions of melatonin." Frontiers in pharmacology 9 (2018): 1086.

69) Najafi, Masoud, et al. "Adjuvant chemotherapy with melatonin for targeting human cancers: A review." Journal of cellular physiology 234.3 (2019): 2356-2372.

70) Li, Ya, et al. "Melatonin for the prevention and treatment of cancer." Oncotarget 8.24 (2017): 39896.

71) Cardinali, D., et al. "Melatonin-Induced Oncostasis, Mechanisms and Clinical Relevance." J Integr Oncol S 1 (2016): 2.

72) do Nascimento Goncalves, Naiane, et al. "Effect of melatonin in epithelial mesenchymal transition markers and invasive properties of breast cancer stem cells of canine and human cell lines." PloS one 11.3 (2016).

73) Zhou, Bin, et al. "Targeting miR-193a-AML1-ETO-β-catenin axis by melatonin suppresses the self-renewal of leukaemia stem cells in leukaemia with t (8; 21) translocation." Journal of cellular and molecular medicine 23.8 (2019): 5246-5258.

74) Yang, Yi-Chen, et al. "Melatonin reduces lung cancer stemness through inhibiting of PLC, ERK, p38, β-catenin, and Twist pathways." Environmental toxicology 34.2 (2019): 203-209.

75) Serrano, Consuelo, et al. "Melatonin decreases in vitro viability and migration of spheres derived from CF41. Mg canine mammary carcinoma cells." BMC veterinary research 15.1 (2019): 390.

76) Akbarzadeh M, et al. (2017) The potential therapeutic effect of melatonin on human ovarian cancer by inhibition of invasion and migration of cancer stem cells. Sci, Rep, 7 (1):17062.

77) Lee, Jun Hee, et al. "Melatonin and 5-fluorouracil co-suppress colon cancer stem cells by regulating cellular prion protein-Oct4 axis." Journal of pineal research 65.4 (2018): e12519.

78) Hao, Jiaojiao, et al. "Melatonin synergizes BRAF-targeting agent vemurafenib in melanoma treatment by inhibiting iNOS/hTERT signaling and cancer-stem cell traits." Journal of Experimental & Clinical Cancer Research 38.1 (2019): 48.

79) Margheri M, et al. (2012) Combined effects of melatonin and all-trans retinoic acid and somatostatin on breast cancer cell proliferation and death: molecular basis for the anticancer effect of these molecules.

80) Lu, Jian-Jun, et al. "Melatonin inhibits AP-2β/hTERT, NF-κB/COX-2 and Akt/ERK and activates caspase/Cyto C signaling to enhance the antitumor activity of berberine in lung cancer cells." Oncotarget 7.3 (2016): 2985.

81) Gao, Yue, et al. "Melatonin synergizes the chemotherapeutic effect of 5-fluorouracil in colon cancer by suppressing PI 3K/AKT and NF-κB/iNOS signaling pathways." Journal of pineal research 62.2 (2017): e12380.

82) Lin, Shibo, et al. "Melatonin promotes sorafenib-induced apoptosis through synergistic activation of JNK/c-jun pathway in human hepatocellular carcinoma." Journal of pineal research 62.3 (2017): e12398.

83) Plaimee, P., et al. "Melatonin potentiates cisplatin-induced apoptosis and cell cycle arrest in human lung adenocarcinoma cells." Cell proliferation 48.1 (2015): 67-77.

84) Öz, Eser, et al. "Prevention of doxorubicin-induced cardiotoxicity by melatonin." Molecular and cellular biochemistry 282.1-2 (2006): 31-37.

85) Yan, Gege, et al. "Melatonin triggers autophagic cell death by regulating RORC in Hodgkin lymphoma." Biomedicine & Pharmacotherapy 123 (2020): 109811.

86) Li, Tian, et al. "Melatonin: does it have utility in the treatment of haematological neoplasms?." British journal of pharmacology 175.16 (2018): 3251-3262.

87) Trubiani, Oriana, et al. "Melatonin provokes cell death in human B-lymphoma cells by mitochondrial-dependent apoptotic pathway activation." Journal of pineal research 39.4 (2005): 425-431.

88) Shafabakhsh, Rana, Hamed Mirzaei, and Zatollah Asemi. "Melatonin: A promising agent targeting leukemia." Journal of cellular biochemistry (2019).

89) Amin, Negin, et al. "Melatonin is an appropriate candidate for breast cancer treatment: Based on known molecular mechanisms." Journal of cellular biochemistry 120.8 (2019): 12208-12215.

90) Zare, Hadis, et al. "Melatonin is a potential inhibitor of ovarian cancer: molecular aspects." Journal of ovarian research 12.1 (2019): 26.

91) Chuffa, Luiz Gustavo de Almeida, Russel J. Reiter, and Luiz Antonio Lupi. "Melatonin as a promising agent to treat ovarian cancer: molecular mechanisms." Carcinogenesis 38.10 (2017): 945-952.

92) Shen, Ching-Ju, et al. "Melatonin suppresses the growth of ovarian cancer cell lines (OVCAR-429 and PA-1) and potentiates the effect of G1 arrest by targeting CDKs." International journal of molecular sciences 17.2 (2016): 176.

93) Gil-Martín, Emilio, et al. "The emergence of melatonin in oncology: Focus on colorectal cancer." Medicinal Research Reviews 39.6 (2019): 2239-2285.

94) Iravani, Shahrokh, et al. "The Role of Melatonin in Colorectal Cancer." Journal of Gastrointestinal Cancer (2019): 1-6.

95) Xin, Zhenlong, et al. "Melatonin as a treatment for gastrointestinal cancer: a review." Journal of pineal research 58.4 (2015): 375-387.

96) Mortezaee, Keywan, et al. "Boosting immune system against cancer by melatonin: A mechanistic viewpoint." Life sciences (2019): 116960.

97) Loureiro, Rute, et al. "Melatonin antiproliferative effects require active mitochondrial function in embryonal carcinoma cells." Oncotarget 6.19 (2015): 17081.

98) Tataranni, Tiziana, and Claudia Piccoli. "Dichloroacetate (DCA) and Cancer: An Overview towards Clinical Applications." Oxidative Medicine and Cellular Longevity 2019 (2019).

99) deleted

100) Liu, Mu-Tai, and Russel J. Reiter. "The Impact of Melatonin and Carbon Ion Irradiation on Mitochondria of Cancer Cells." SCIAEON J Radiol (2018)

101) Uttenthal, Lars Otto. "Melatonin for Preventing and Treating Radiation Vaginitis and Proctitis." U.S. Patent Application No. 15/553,562.

102) Amini, Peyman, et al. "Mechanisms for radioprotection by melatonin; can it be used as a radiation countermeasure?." Current molecular pharmacology 12.1 (2019): 2-11.

103) Adikwu, Elias, Nelson Clement Ebinyo, and Bonsome Bokolo. "Melatonin and alpha lipoic acid attenuate methotrexate/cisplatin-induced kidney toxicity in albino rats." Journal of Nephropharmacology 9.2 (2020).

104) Tuncer, Seckin, et al. "Comparative effects of alpha lipoic acid and melatonin on cisplatin-induced neurotoxicity." International Journal of Neuroscience 120.10 (2010): 655-663.

105) Hussein, Samy Ali, M. Omnia, and A. M. Fayed. "Protective effects of alpha-lipoic acid and melatonin against cadmium-induced oxidative stress in erythrocytes of rats." J. Pharmacol. Toxicol 9 (2014): 1-24.

106) Ziegler, D., et al. "Treatment of symptomatic diabetic polyneuropathy with the antioxidant α-lipoic acid: a meta-analysis." Diabetic Medicine 21.2 (2004): 114-121.

107) Han, T., et al. "A systematic review and meta-analysis of α-lipoic acid in the treatment of diabetic peripheral neuropathy." European journal of endocrinology/ European Federation of Endocrine Societies 167.4 (2012): 465.

108) Rucker, Robert, Winyoo Chowanadisai, and Masahiko Nakano. Potential physiological importance of pyrroloquinoline quinone " Alternative Medicine Review 14.3 (2009): 268.

109) Misra, H. S., Y. S. Rajpurohit, and N. P. Khairnar. "Pyrroloquinoline-quinone and its versatile roles in biological processes." Journal of biosciences 37.2 (2012): 313.

110) Shankar, Bhavani S., et al. "Role of glutathione in augmenting the anticancer activity of pyrroloquinoline quinone (PQQ)." Redox Report 15.4 (2010): 146-154.

111) Min, Zhihui, et al. "Pyrroloquinoline Quinone Induces Cancer Cell Apoptosis via Mitochondrial-Dependent Pathway and Down-Regulating Cellular Bcl-2 Protein Expression." Journal of Cancer 5.7 (2014): 609-624.

112) Kuo, Yung-Ting, et al. "Pyrroloquinoline Quinone Resists Denervation-Induced Skeletal Muscle Atrophy by Activating PGC-1α and Integrating Mitochondrial Electron Transport Chain Complexes." PloS one 10.12 (2015): e0143600.

113) Zhao, Lei, et al. "Beneficial synergistic effects of microdose lithium with pyrroloquinoline quinone in an Alzheimer's disease mouse model." Neurobiology of aging 35.12 (2014): 2736-2745.

114) Stengler, Mark. Outside the Box Cancer Therapies: Alternative Therapies that Treat and Prevent Cancer. Hay House, Inc, 2018.

115) Luongo, Margherita, et al. "Possible therapeutic effects of ozone mixture on hypoxia in tumor development." Anticancer research 37.2 (2017): 425-435.

116) Sweet, Frederick, et al. "Ozone selectively inhibits growth of human cancer cells." Science 209.4459 (1980): 931-933.

117) Bocci, Velio, Alessandra Larini, and Vanna Micheli. "Restoration of normoxia by ozone therapy may control neoplastic growth: a review and a working hypothesis." Journal of Alternative & Complementary Medicine 11.2 (2005): 257-265.

118) Moen, Ingrid, and Linda EB Stuhr. "Hyperbaric oxygen therapy and cancer—a review." Targeted oncology 7.4 (2012): 233-242.

119) Al Abdan, M. "Alfa-lipoic acid controls tumor growth and modulates hepatic redox state in Ehrlich-ascites-carcinoma-bearing mice." The Scientific World Journal 2012 (2012). Ehrlich tumor is an experimental model for breast cancer.

120) deleted

121) Song, Jun, et al. "Melatonin induces the apoptosis and inhibits the proliferation of human gastric cancer cells via blockade of the AKT/MDM2 pathway." Oncology reports 39.4 (2018): 1975-1983.

122) T.Liu, Lifeng, Ying Xu, and Russel J. Reiter. "Melatonin inhibits the proliferation of human osteosarcoma cell line MG-63." Bone 55.2 (2013): 432-438.: 1483-1496.

123) Paroni, Rita, et al. "Antitumour activity of melatonin in a mouse model of human prostate cancer: relationship with hypoxia signalling." Journal of pineal research 57.1 (2014): 43-52.

Chapter 8

Intravenous Vitamin C as Cancer Chemotherapy

SUSAN IS A NEW PATIENT interested in hormone replacement for relief of menopausal symptoms. During our first visit, she mentioned that her OB/GYN doctor has been following her for a "pelvic mass" that was noted on a sonogram she had taken six months earlier for fullness and discomfort in her lower abdomen. Before doing anything else, we sent Susan for a follow-up sonogram. Sure enough, the mass had increased in size over the last 6 months, highly characteristic for a growing cancer mass. So, Susan was sent back to her OB/GYN for laparoscopic surgery. This revealed that Susan indeed had ovarian cancer, which had already spread to the peritoneal cavity. The surgeon then did a complete hysterectomy and debulked the peritoneal metastatic deposits. Susan recovered quickly from surgery and was then scheduled for chemotherapy with an oncologist.

Sister Recommends IV Vitamin C for Susan

Susan's sister told her about Intravenous (IV) vitamin C (ascorbate) for cancer patients. So, Susan called one of my colleagues in Boca Raton, who offers this treatment. However, when she mentioned it to her oncologist, he practically hit the ceiling. He was very opposed to it, saying the IV vitamin C would reduce the effectiveness of the chemotherapy.

IV Vitamin C Makes Ovarian Cancer More Chemo Sensitive and Reduces Adverse Effects of Chemo

Susan's oncologist is quite wrong about this. This question has been studied over the last 20 years, revealing that, in fact, the opposite is true. High-dose intravenous (IV) vitamin C actually synergizes and augments conventional chemotherapy, making the chemotherapy more effective. In 1996, Dr. Christian Kubacher et al. reported that vitamin C improves the antineoplastic activity of doxorubicin, cisplatin, and paclitaxel in breast cancer cells in vitro. (1)

This is also true for ovarian cancer chemotherapy. A study by Dr. Jeanne Drisko et al. in the 2003 *Journal of the American College of Nutrition* and a more recent study by Dr. Yan Ma et al. (2014) in *Science Translational Medicine* are to this point. (2–3) They state that "high-dose parenteral ascorbate enhanced chemo-sensitivity of ovarian cancer and reduced toxicity of chemotherapy."(2–3)

Vitamin C—the Safest and Most Valuable Substance

After reviewing the medical literature on high-dose IV vitamin C for cancer patients, Drs. Michael J González and Hugh D. Riordan state (2005): "AA Ascorbic Acid (vitamin C) is one of the safest and most valuable substances available to the physician for treating cancer."(45)

Overwhelming Evidence for IV Vitamin C

In this chapter, we pull together a huge volume of published studies on high-dose intravenous (IV) vitamin C for the cancer patient showing overwhelming evidence that not only is this safe and effective along with conventional chemotherapy, IV Vitamin C may also be regarded as an effective stand-alone chemotherapy agent, killing cancer cells through a well-described pro-oxidative mechanism.

Lymphomas Are Sensitive

Lymphoma cells are especially sensitive to IV vitamin C at low serum concentrations (LD50 of 0.5 mmol/L). (4–5) Downregulating the dual anti-oxidant system with auranofin, which inhibits the thioredoxin reductase system, and a second agent such as celecoxib, which attenuates glutathione levels, potentiates the cytotoxic effects of vitamin C. (6–8)

Sulforaphane, derived from broccoli, may also be useful for downregulating the glutathione anti-oxidant system, rendering the cancer cell more vulnerable to the pro-oxidant effect of IV vitamin C. (9)

Iron-Containing Multiple Myeloma is Sensitive to Vitamin C

In 2017, Dr. Jiliang Xia et al. studied IV vitamin C for multiple myeloma in vitro and in vivo, showing its efficacy at pharmacologic doses due to formation of ROS and depletion of glutathione. Dr. Jiliang Xia et al. write that multiple myeloma cells contain high amounts of iron, targeted by the vitamin-C-producing reactive oxygen species (ROS):

We show that pharmacologically-dosed ascorbic acid (PAA), in the presence of iron, leads to the formation of highly reactive oxygen species [ROS] resulting in cell death. PAA selectively kills CD138+ MM [Multiple Myeloma] tumor cells.... PAA alone or in combination with melphalan inhibits tumor formation in MM xenograft mice. This study shows PAA efficacy on primary cancer cells and cell lines in vitro and in vivo. (82)

Vitamin C Mechanism of Action

The mechanism by which high-dose vitamin C kills cancer cells selectively while leaving normal cells unharmed has been extensively studied. Notice that the chemical structure of vitamin C is similar to that of glucose. Indeed, in non-primate mammals, glucose is converted to vitamin C by three enzymes in the liver. The final enzyme gulano lactone oxidase (GLO) has a mutated gene in primates, explaining why primates (including humans) cannot make their own vitamin C and must acquire it through dietary intake.

Vitamin C is avidly taken up into the cancer cell by glucose transporters (GLUT1) and serves as a pro-oxidant, with production of hydrogen peroxide, an oxidant that is toxic to cancer cells since they have reduced levels of the catalase enzyme needed for degradation of hydrogen peroxide. Extracellular spaces and normal cells, however, contain plenty of catalase enzymes, which promptly degrade the hydrogen peroxide, explaining why normal cells are unharmed. (10–11)(85–92)

Vitamin C Targets Cancer Stem Cells

The bulk of a cancer mass consists of rapidly replicating cancer cells. However, lurking in the mass are a smaller number of CSCs that are dormant, not actively replicating, and are therefore immune to the cell-killing effects of chemotherapy. This explains why chemotherapy treatments may induce a brief remission with a "clean" PET scan. The cancer mass is debulked by the cell-killing effects of the chemotherapy, leaving a few CSCs behind to repopulate the cancer mass later on. Cancer relapse is inevitable after an interval of time, depending on the proliferation rate of the cell type. This is why the cancers re-grow and are not cured. Unlike conventional chemotherapy, which is unable to kill CSCs, combination therapy with IV vitamin C attacks the CSCs and may result in a complete cure with no further relapse, as discussed in 2020 by Dr. N. J. Satheesh et al. (81)

Vitamin C Depletes Glutathione, Inhibits GLYCOLYSIS, and Targets Cancer Stem Cells

In 2017, Dr. Bonuccelli et al. studied the effect of vitamin C (ascorbate) on breast cancer cell cultures and stated that ascorbate depletes the glutathione pool, inhibits GLYCOLYSIS, and targets CSCs:

> Vitamin C has two mechanisms of action. First, it is a potent pro-oxidant, that actively depletes the reduced glutathione pool, leading to cellular oxidative stress and apoptosis in cancer cells. Moreover, it also behaves as an inhibitor of glycolysis, by targeting the activity of GAPDH, a key glycolytic enzyme... Here, we show that

Vitamin C can also be used to target the CSC Cancer Stem Cell population, as it is an inhibitor of energy metabolism that feeds into the mitochondrial TCA cycle [TriCarboxylic Acid Cycle] and OXPHOS.... A breast cancer based clinical study has already shown that the use of Vitamin C, concurrent with or within 6 months of chemotherapy, significantly reduces both tumor recurrence and patient mortality. (12)

Cancer Cells Have Large Amounts of Iron—Artemisinin

In addition to lacking catalase, cancer cells contain larger amounts of iron, which react with the peroxide to produce damaging ROS. (13–15) The iron reaction with oxygen results in a form of apoptosis, or cell death, called ferroptosis, and is augmented by concurrent use of artemisinin, which contains an endoperoxide bridge that delivers additional oxidative therapy to the cancer cells. (16) The intravenous (IV) version of artemisinin is artesunate, widely available and recommended by the World Health Organization (WHO) for first-line treatment of severe malaria. See chapter 21, on artemisinin, which explains why it is such a highly effective anti-cancer agent.

Hyperbaric Oxygen or Ozone Sauna

Concomitant use of hyperbaric oxygen or ozone sauna therapy augments the pro-oxidative effect of IV vitamin C. (17–18)

Alpha Lipoic Acid Augments Cancer-Killing Effect of Vitamin C

As mentioned in chapter 7, on alpha lipoic acid (ALA), the addition of R-ALA to the IV vitamin C augments the cancer-cell-killing effect at lower serum concentrations of vitamin C. ALA increases the electron flux through the mitochondria of the cancer cell, an intolerable state of affairs that triggers mitochondrial-induced apoptosis of the cancer cell. (19–20)

In 2001, Drs. J. J. Casciari and N. H. Riordan studied the combination of high-dose IV vitamin C with ALA. They write:

> Lipoic acid synergistically enhanced ascorbate cytotoxicity, reducing the 2-day LC 50 (Lethal Concentration 50%) in hollow fibre tumours from 34 mM to 4 mM [millimolar]. Lipoic acid, unlike ascorbate, was equally effective against proliferating and non-proliferating cells. Ascorbate levels in human blood plasma were measured during and after intravenous ascorbate infusions. Infusions of 60 g produced peak plasma concentrations exceeding 20 mM with an area under the curve (24 h) of 76 mM h. Thus, tumoricidal concentrations may be achievable in vivo. (19)

The R-ALA (for injection) is usually given in a chaser bag to follow the IV vitamin C infusion. In 2004, Drs. Dan Zeigler and F. Arnold Gries reported that daily IV infusions of 600 mg ALA for three weeks is safe. (21–22)

Dr. Neil McKinney, an integrative oncologist from Victoria, British Colombia, recommends use of the R-lipoic acid isomer rather than the more commonly available racemic mixture for best results. (23)

Menadione Vitamin K3, Ubiquinol, PQQ

Other agents similar to R-Alpha Lipoic Acid, which increase electron flux through the mitochondrial electron transport chain, include vitamin K3, CoQ10, pyrroloquinoline quino (PQQ), etc. As expected, these all synergize and augment the cancer-cell-killing effects of IV vitamin C. These are all vitamins, so they can be safely added to the IV vitamin C program. (24–30)

In 2019, Dr. X. Ren et al. studied the combination of ascorbate and menadione (vitamin K3) in a ratio of (100:1), finding inhibition of cell replication, as well as apoptosis from elevated ROS causing oxidation of lipids (lipid peroxidation):

> We found that VC/VK3 [vitamin C and vitamin K3] inhibited glutathione peroxidase activity and led to an elevated level of lipid peroxidation, which triggered apoptosis-inducing factor [AIF] mediated cell death pathway. Therefore, the combination not only induced replicative stress by inhibiting RNR [ribonucleotide reductase], but also oxidative stress by targeting anti-oxidant systems and triggered AIF-mediated cancer cell death. (93)

Simultaneous Autophagy and Apoptosis

Anti-cancer effects of the quinones, vitamin K2 and K3, have been extensively studied over the years, finding vitamin K simultaneously induces both apoptosis and autophagy in various cancer cell types. (94–107)

Synergy of IV Vitamin C/Vitamin K with Chemotherapy Drugs

In 2018, Dr. Donika Inanova et al. studied the combination of IV vitamin C with vitamin K3 in a lymphocytic leukemia cell line treated with 15 different anti-cancer drugs (chemotherapies), finding the combination of vitamin C/K3 allowed a lower dose of the chemotherapy drug while minimizing its adverse effects:

> The combined treatment with anti-cancer drug and vitamin C&K3 can be considered as a new therapeutic approach—to sensitize cancer cells **and to achieve a lower effective dose** of the drug, **minimizing the harmful side effects of conventional chemotherapy.** (107)

Synergy Combination IV Vitamin C with Auranofin

Auranofin is a gold-containing rheumatology drug used for many years for arthritis patients. It has been repurposed as an anti-cancer drug. Auranofin inhibits the thioredoxin reductase system, which increases ROS in the cancer cells. (6–7) The combination of IV ascorbate (vitamin C) and auranofin was found to be "strongly" synergistic in vitro for malignant B cells (lymphoma) and in a mouse xenograft breast cancer model as reported by Drs. Agnieszka Graczyk et al. (2019) and Dr. Elie Hatem et al. (2018). (31–32)

Chinese Skullcap and Oroxylin A

The botanical Chinese skullcap, which contains oroxylin A, acts as a glycolysis inhibitor in cancer cells and is recommended as a safe treatment for the cancer patent. Researchers found that oroxylin A binds to hexokinase 2 (HK2), attached to mitochondria in human breast carcinoma cell lines, inhibiting GLYCOLYSIS (utilization of glucose) and thus inducing apoptosis (cell death). Chinese skullcap is effective as an anti-cancer agent in lung cancer, acute myeloid (AML) leukemia, and glioblastoma cell models. The scientific name for Chinese skullcap is Scutellaria baicalensis Georgi. Chinese skullcap is discussed in chapter 10, Natural Substances Targeting Cancer Stem Cells.

Doxycycline and High-Dose IV Vitamin C—A Lethal Combination for Cancer Stem Cells

The common antibiotic doxycycline works by blocking bacterial ribosomal protein production. Combining doxycycline with IV vitamin C is a lethal combination for eradication of CSCs.

Mammalian mitochondria share many similarities with bacterial life forms. Based on this similarity, Dr. Lynn Margulis invented the "endo-symbiotic theory," the idea that billions of years ago, mitochondria evolved through the symbiotic incorporation of bacteria into eukaryotic single-celled organisms. Symbiotic relationship means they are assisting and helping each other rather than competing with each other. If mitochondria are thus related to bacteria, then many of the routine antibiotics that target bacteria can be expected to also target mitochondrial functions in cancer cells, with the added bonus of targeting CSCs.

This has been found to be the case by Michael Lisanti's group in an elegant 2015 study entitled "Antibiotics that target mitochondria effectively eradicate CSCs, across multiple tumor types: Treating cancer like an infectious disease," published in *Oncotarget* 6.7 (2015): 4569–4584. This explains the ability of doxycycline to induce clinical remission and in some cases "cure" for patients with periorbital and gastric MALT lymphomas. (33–34) In 2015, Dr. Lisanti's group published a study using an in vitro breast cancer cell model showing that doxycycline and high-dose IV Vitamin C induced "synthetic lethality," leading to eradication of CSCs. (35)(81)

Intravenous Vitamin C for Septic Shock

Cancer patients are frequently found to be vitamin C deficient (36), as are critically ill patients in the ICU. Forty-four critically ill patients in the ICU studied by Dr. Anitra Carr et al. in 2017 were found to be vitamin C deficient, suffering from scurvy. (37–38) Until 2016, septic shock was considered incurable, with a high mortality rate of 50 percent. However, in *Chest* (2016), Dr. Paul Marik et al. reported that IV vitamin C, hydrocortisone, and thiamine can be "curative" for septic shock patients in the ICU, dramatically improving outcomes. (39)

Safety of High-Dose IV Vitamin C

In 2014, Dr. Hiroshi Kawada et al. evaluated the safety of IV vitamin C in a phase one clinical trial of three patients with B-cell lymphoma given 75 grams of ascorbate intravenously. Serum ascorbate levels exceeded 15 mMoles/L with no adverse effects. (11).

In 2017, Dr. Junwen Ou et al. reported a second clinical trial in thirty-five lung cancer patients given high-dose IV vitamin C three times a week for 4 weeks who likewise showed no adverse effects. Ascorbate serum levels were recorded in the range of 15–20 mMoles/L range. (40).

Adverse Effects, Drug Interactions

The use of vitamin K will reverse the blood thinning effect of warfarin, a vitamin K antagonist. Therefore, caution is advised when using vitamin K and warfarin together.

Conclusion

It is quite obvious that high-dose intravenous vitamin C is an extremely safe and beneficial therapy for cancer patients and electively kills cancer cells while leaving normal cells unharmed. In fact, it should be offered routinely on all hospital oncology wards as an adjunct to the chemotherapy infusions. The fact that mainstream oncology has rejected and ignored this inexpensive, safe, and effective therapy is simply astounding. You can change things by giving your doctor a copy of this book.

References Chapter 8: Vitamin C as Chemotherapy

1) Kurbacher, Christian M., et al. "Ascorbic acid (vitamin C) improves the antineoplastic activity of doxorubicin, cisplatin, and paclitaxel in human breast carcinoma cells in vitro." Cancer letters 103.2 (1996): 183-189.

2) Drisko, Jeanne A., Julia Chapman, and Verda J. Hunter. "The use of antioxidants with first-line chemotherapy in two cases of ovarian cancer." Journal of the American College of Nutrition 22.2 (2003): 118-123.

3) Ma, Yan, et al. "High-dose parenteral ascorbate enhanced chemosensitivity of ovarian cancer and reduced toxicity of chemotherapy." Science translational medicine 6.222 (2014): 222ra18-222ra18.

4) Graczyk-Jarzynka, Agnieszka, et al. "New insights into redox homeostasis as a therapeutic target in B-cell malignancies." Current opinion in hematology 24.4 (2017): 393.

5) Chen, Qi, et al. "Pharmacologic ascorbic acid concentrations selectively kill cancer cells: action as a pro-drug to deliver hydrogen peroxide to tissues." Proceedings of the national academy of sciences of the United States of America 102.38 (2005): 13604-13609.

6) Cancer Res. 2010 Nov 15; 70(22):9505-14. Loss of thioredoxin reductase 1 renders tumors highly susceptible to pharmacologic glutathione deprivation. Mandal PK1, Schneider M, Kölle P, Kuhlencordt P, Förster H, Beck H, Bornkamm GW, Conrad M.

7) Kiebala, Michelle, et al. "Dual targeting of the thioredoxin and glutathione antioxidant systems in malignant B cells: a novel synergistic therapeutic approach." Experimental hematology 43.2 (2015): 89-99.

8) Bernard, M. P., et al. "Targeting cyclooxygenase-2 in hematological malignancies: rationale and promise." Current pharmaceutical design 14.21 (2008): 2051-2060.–

9) Clarke, John D., Roderick H. Dashwood, and Emily Ho. "Multi-targeted prevention of cancer by sulforaphane." Cancer letters 269.2 (2008): 291-304.

10) Doskey, Claire M., et al. "Tumor cells have decreased ability to metabolize H2O2: Implications for pharmacological ascorbate in cancer therapy." Redox Biology 10 (2016): 274-284.

11) Kawada, Hiroshi, et al. "Phase I Clinical Trial of Intravenous L-ascorbic Acid Following Salvage Chemotherapy for Relapsed B-cell non-Hodgkin's Lymphoma." The Tokai journal of experimental and clinical medicine 39.3 (2014): 111-115.

12) Bonuccelli G, De Francesco EM, de Boer R, Tanowitz HB, Lisanti MP. NADH autofluorescence, a new metabolic biomarker for cancer stem cells: Identification of Vitamin C and CAPE as natural products targeting "stemness." Oncotarget. 2017;8(13):20667-20678.

13) Schoenfeld, Joshua D., et al. "O2*–and H2O2–mediated disruption of Fe metabolism causes the differential susceptibility of NSCLC and GBM cancer cells to pharmacological ascorbate." Cancer cell 31.4 (2017): 487-500.

14) Toyokuni, Shinya, et al. "Iron and thiol redox signaling in cancer: an exquisite balance to escape ferroptosis." Free Radical Biology and Medicine (2017).

15) McCarty, Mark Frederick, and Francisco Contreras. "Increasing superoxide production and the labile iron pool in tumor cells may sensitize them to extracellular ascorbate." Frontiers in oncology 4 (2014).

16) Gerhardt, Thomas, et al. "Effects of antioxidants and pro-oxidants on cytotoxicity of dihydroartemisinin to Molt-4 human leukemia cells." Anticancer research 35.4 (2015): 1867-1871.

17) Increasing the Effectiveness of Intravenous Vitamin C as an Anticancer Agent. Journal of Orthomolecular Medicine Volume 32, Number 1, 2017. JOM Archives, Volume 30, Number 1, 2015

18) DeBlasi, Janine M., et al. "Anti-Cancer Effects of Ascorbic Acid and Hyperbaric Oxygen Therapy in vitro." The FASEB Journal 31.1_supplement (2017): 879-4.

19) Casciari, J. J., Riordan et al. "Cytotoxicity of ascorbate, lipoic acid, and other antioxidants in hollow fibre in vitro tumours." British journal of cancer 84.11 (2001): 1544. 88)

20) US Patent: Treatment of cancer using lipoic acid in combination with ascorbic acid. Hugh Riordan Clinic. US 6448287 B1

21) Ziegler, Dan, and F. Arnold Gries. "Alpha-lipoic acid in the treatment of diabetic peripheral and cardiac autonomic neuropathy"Diabetes 46.Supplement 2 (1997): S62-S66.

22) Ziegler, D., et al. "Treatment of symptomatic diabetic polyneuropathy with the antioxidant α-lipoic acid: a meta-analysis." Diabetic Medicine 21.2 (2004): 114-121.

23) McKinney, Neil. Naturopathic Oncology: An Encyclopedic Guide for Patients & Physicians. Liaison Press, 2012.

24) Verrax, Julien, et al. "Redox-active quinones and ascorbate: an innovative cancer therapy that exploits

the vulnerability of cancer cells to oxidative stress." Anti-Cancer Agents in Medicinal Chemistry (Formerly Current Medicinal Chemistry-Anti-Cancer Agents) 11.2 (2011): 213-221.

25) Tareen, Basir, et al. "A 12 week, open label, phase I/IIa study using apatone for the treatment of prostate cancer patients who have failed standard therapy." Int J Med Sci 5.2 (2008): 62-67.

26) Patent: Ascorbate, vitamin K3 and hydroxytolans in the treatment of cancer US 8680142 B2

27) Gilloteaux, Jacques, et al. "Synergistic antitumor cytotoxic actions of ascorbate and menadione on human prostate (DU145) cancer cells in vitro: nucleus and other injuries preceding cell death by autoschizis." Ultrastructural pathology 38.2 (2014): 116-140.

28) Lamson, Davis W., et al. "The vitamin C: vitamin K3 system-enhancers and inhibitors of the anticancer effect." Altern Med Rev 15.4 (2010): 345-351.

29) Bonilla-Porras, Angelica R., Marlene Jimenez-Del-Rio, and Carlos Velez-Pardo. "Vitamin K3 and vitamin C alone or in combination induced apoptosis in leukemia cells by a similar oxidative stress signalling mechanism." Cancer cell international 11.1 (2011): 19.

30) Gonzalez, Michael J., and Jorge R. Miranda-Massari. New insights on vitamin C and cancer. Springer New York, 2014. New Insights vitamin C and Cancer Gonzalez Michael Springer 2014.

31) Graczyk-Jarzynka, Agnieszka, et al. "Inhibition of thioredoxin-dependent H2O2 removal sensitizes malignant B-cells to pharmacological ascorbate." Redox biology 21 (2019): 101062.

32) Hatem, Elie, et al. "Auranofin/vitamin C: a novel drug combination targeting triple-negative breast Cancer." JNCI: Journal of the National Cancer Institute 111.6 (2018): 597-608.

33) Han, Jae Joon, et al. "Long-term outcomes of first-line treatment with doxycycline in patients with previously untreated ocular adnexal marginal zone B cell lymphoma." Annals of hematology 94.4 (2015): 575-581.

34) Raderer, Markus, et al. "Antibiotic treatment as sole management of Helicobacter pylori-negative gastric MALT lymphoma: a single center experience with prolonged follow-up." Annals of hematology 94.6 (2015): 969-973.

35) Ernestina Marianna De Francesco, Gloria Bonuccelli, Marcello Maggiolini, Federica Sotgia, Michael P. Lisanti. Vitamin C and Doxycycline: A synthetic lethal combination therapy targeting metabolic flexibility in cancer stem cells (CSCs). Oncotarget, 2015;

36) Mayland, Catriona R., Michael I. Bennett, and Keith Allan. "Vitamin C deficiency in cancer patients." Palliative medicine 19.1 (2005): 17-20.

37) Carr, Anitra C., et al. "Hypovitaminosis C and vitamin C deficiency in critically ill patients despite recommended enteral and parenteral intakes." Critical Care 21 (2017).

38) Marik, Paul E., and Michael H. Hooper. "Doctor—your septic patients have scurvy!." (2018): 23.

39) Marik, Paul E., et al. "Hydrocortisone, Vitamin C and Thiamine for the Treatment of Severe Sepsis and Septic Shock: A Retrospective Before-After Study." CHEST Journal (2016).

40) Ou, Junwen, et al. "The safety and pharmacokinetics of high dose intravenous ascorbic acid synergy with modulated electrohyperthermia in Chinese patients with stage III-IV non-small cell lung cancer." European Journal of Pharmaceutical Sciences 109 (2017): 412-418.

41) Mastrangelo, Domenico, et al. "Cytotoxic effects of high concentrations of sodium ascorbate on human myeloid cell lines." Annals of hematology 94.11 (2015): 1807-1816.

42) Goodman, Annekathryn. "Vitamin C and cancer." AIMS Medical Science 3.1 (2016): 41-51.

43) Seo, Min-Seok, Ja-Kyung Kim, and Jae-Yong Shim. "High-dose vitamin C promotes regression of multiple pulmonary metastases originating from hepatocellular carcinoma." Yonsei medical journal 56.5 (2015): 1449-1452.

44) Mastrangelo, D. "The Cure from Nature: The Extraordinary Anticancer Properties of Ascorbate (Vitamin C)." J Integr Oncol 5 (2016): 157.

45) González, Michael J., et al. "Orthomolecular oncology review: ascorbic acid and cancer 25 years later." Integrative cancer therapies 4.1 (2005): 32-44.

46) Levine, Mark, Sebastian J. Padayatty, and Michael Graham Espey. "Vitamin C: a concentration-function approach yields pharmacology and therapeutic discoveries." Advances in Nutrition: An International Review Journal 2.2 (2011): 78-88.

47) Frömberg, Anja, et al. "Ascorbate exerts anti-proliferative effects through cell cycle inhibition and sensitizes tumor cells towards cytostatic drugs." Cancer chemotherapy and pharmacology 67.5 (2011): 1157-1166.

48) Du, Juan, et al. "Mechanisms of ascorbate-induced cytotoxicity in pancreatic cancer." Clinical Cancer Research 16.2 (2010): 509-520.

49) Verrax, Julien, and Pedro Buc Calderon. "Pharmacologic concentrations of ascorbate are achieved by parenteral administration and exhibit antitumoral effects." Free Radical Biology and Medicine 47.1 (2009): 32-40.

50) Riordan, N. H., H. D. Riordan, and R. E. Hunninghake. "Intravenous ascorbate as a chemotherapeutic and biologic response modifying agent." Bio-communications Research Institute (1997).

51) Mlkirova, Nina, and Ronald Hunninghake. "Effect of high dose vitamin C on Epstein-Barr viral infection." Medical Science Monitor 20 (2014): 725-732.

52) Chen, Qi, et al. "Pharmacologic doses of ascorbate act as a prooxidant and decrease growth of aggressive tumor xenografts in mice." Proceedings of the National Academy of Sciences 105.32 (2008): 11105-11109.

53) Chen, Qi, et al. "Ascorbate in pharmacologic concentrations selectively generates ascorbate radical and hydrogen peroxide in extracellular fluid in vivo." Proceedings of the National Academy of Sciences 104.21 (2007): 8749-8754.

54) Padayatty, Sebastian J., et al. "Intravenously administered vitamin C as cancer therapy: three cases." Canadian Medical Association Journal 174.7 (2006): 937-942.

55) Hoffer, L. J. "Vitamin C: Case History of an Alternative Cancer Therapy." Journal of Orthomolecular Medicine 15.4 (2000): 181-188.

56) Hoffer, L. John, et al. "High-dose intravenous vitamin C combined with cytotoxic chemotherapy in patients with advanced cancer: a phase I-II clinical trial." PloS one 10.4 (2015): e0120228.

57) Olney, Kristen E., et al. "Inhibitors of hydroperoxide metabolism enhance ascorbate-induced cytotoxicity." Free radical research 47.3 (2013): 154-163.

58) Satoshi, et al. "High-dose vitamin C (ascorbic acid) therapy in the treatment of patients with advanced cancer." Anticancer research 29.3 (2009): 809-815.

59) Frei, Balz, and Stephen Lawson. "Vitamin C and cancer revisited." Proceedings of the National Academy of Sciences 105.32 (2008): 11037-11038.

60) Cameron, Ewan, and Linus Pauling. "Supplemental ascorbate in the supportive treatment of cancer: Prolongation of survival times in terminal human cancer." Proceedings of the National Academy of Sciences 73.10 (1976): 3685-3689.

61) Cameron, Ewan, and Linus Pauling. "Supplemental ascorbate in the supportive treatment of cancer: reevaluation of prolongation of survival times in terminal human cancer." Proceedings of the National Academy of Sciences 75.9 (1978): 4538-4542.

62) Riordan, N. H., et al. "Intravenous ascorbate as a tumor cytotoxic chemotherapeutic agent." Medical hypotheses 44.3 (1995): 207-213.

63) Pollard, Harvey B., et al. "Pharmacological ascorbic acid suppresses syngeneic tumor growth and metastases in hormone-refractory prostate cancer." in vivo 24.3 (2010): 249-255.

64) Mata, Ana Maria Oliveira Ferreira da, et al. "Ascorbic acid in the prevention and treatment of cancer." Revista da Associação Médica Brasileira 62.7 (2016): 680-686.

65) Xia, Jiliang, et al. "Multiple myeloma tumor cells are selectively killed by pharmacologically-dosed ascorbic acid." EBioMedicine 18 (2017): 41-49.

66) Yun, Jihye, et al."Vitamin C selectively kills KRAS and BRAF mutant colorectal cancer cells by targeting GAPDH." Science 350.6266 (2015): 1391-1396.

67) Garcia, Keishla M., et al. "Intravenous Vitamin C and Metabolic Correction as Adjuvant Therapy for prostate Cancer: a Case Report." (2016).

68) Gilloteaux, J., et al. "Autoschizis: A Mode of Cell Death of Cancer Cells Induced by a Prooxidant

Treatment In Vitro and In Vivo." Apoptosis and Beyond: The Many Ways Cells Die (2018): 583-694.

69) Bonilla-Porras, Angelica R., Marlene Jimenez-Del-Rio, and Carlos Velez-Pardo. "Vitamin K3 and vitamin C alone or in combination induced apoptosis in leukemia cells by a similar oxidative stress signalling mechanism." Cancer cell international 11.1 (2011): 19.

70) Gonzalez, Michael J., Miguel J. Berdiel, and Amanda V. Cintrón. "High Dose IV Vitamin C and Metastatic Breast Cancer: A Case Report." Journal of Orthomolecular Medicine 32.6 (2017).

71) Huijskens, Mirelle JAJ, et al. "Ascorbic acid serum levels are reduced in patients with hematological malignancies." Results in immunology 6 (2016): 8-10.

72) Ohno, Satoshi, et al. "High-dose vitamin C (ascorbic acid) therapy in the treatment of patients with advanced cancer." Anticancer research 29.3 (2009): 809-815.

73) Levine, Mark, Michael Graham Espey, and Qi Chen. "Losing and finding a way at C: new promise for pharmacologic ascorbate in cancer treatment." Free radical biology & medicine 47.1 (2009): 27.

74) Lee, Min Ho, et al. "Menadione induces G2/M arrest in gastric cancer cells by down-regulation of CDC25C and proteasome mediated degradation of CDK1 and cyclin B1." American Journal of Translational Research 8.12 (2016): 5246.

75) Vissers, Margreet CM, and Andrew B. Das. "Potential Mechanisms of Action for Vitamin C in Cancer: Reviewing the Evidence."

76) Ang, Abel, et al. "Vitamin C and immune cell function in inflammation and cancer." Biochemical Society Transactions 46.5 (2018): 1147-1159.

77) Badu-Boateng, Charles, and Richard J. Naftalin. "Ascorbate and ferritin interactions: Consequences for iron release in vitro and in vivo and implications for inflammation." Free Radical Biology and Medicine 133 (2019): 75-87.

78) Ngo, Bryan, et al. "Targeting cancer vulnerabilities with high-dose vitamin C." Nature Reviews Cancer (2019): 1.

79) Corti, Alessandro, Eugenia Belcastro, and Alfonso Pompella. "Antitumoral effects of pharmacological ascorbate on gastric cancer cells: GLUT1 expression may not tell the whole story." Theranostics 8.21 (2018): 6035.

80) Mikirova, Nina, Joseph Casciari, and Ronald Hunninghake. "Continuous intravenous vitamin C in the cancer treatment: re-evaluation of a Phase I clinical study." Functional Foods in Health and Disease 9.3 (2019): 180-204.

81) Satheesh, Noothan Jyothi, Samson Mathews Samuel, and Dietrich Büsselberg. "Combination Therapy with Vitamin C Could Eradicate Cancer Stem Cells." Biomolecules 10.1 (2020): 79.

82) Xia, Jiliang, et al. "Multiple myeloma tumor cells are selectively killed by pharmacologically-dosed ascorbic acid." EBioMedicine 18 (2017): 41-49.

83) Franqui-Machin, Reinaldo, et al. "Multiple Myeloma Tumor Cells Are Selectively Killed By Pharmacologically-Dosed Ascorbic Acid." Blood 130. Supplement 1 (2017): 5391-5391.

84) Violet, Pierre-Christian, and Mark Levine. "Pharmacologic Ascorbate in Myeloma Treatment: Doses Matter." EBioMedicine 18 (2017): 9-10.

85) Ye, Mingtong, et al. "Oxidized vitamin C (DHA) overcomes resistance to EGFR-targeted therapy of lung cancer through disturbing energy homeostasis." Journal of Cancer 10.3 (2019): 757.

86) Ngo, Bryan, et al. "Targeting cancer vulnerabilities with high-dose vitamin C." Nature Reviews Cancer 19.5 (2019): 271-282.

87) Vissers, Margreet, and Andrew B. Das. "Potential mechanisms of action for vitamin C in cancer: reviewing the evidence." Frontiers in physiology 9 (2018): 809.

88) Carr, Anitra C., and John Cook. "Intravenous vitamin C for cancer therapy–identifying the current gaps in our knowledge." Frontiers in physiology 9 (2018): 1182.

89) Mastrangelo, Domenico, et al. "Mechanisms of anti-cancer effects of ascorbate: Cytotoxic activity and epigenetic modulation." Blood Cells, Molecules, and Diseases 69 (2018): 57-64.

90) Shenoy, Niraj, et al. "Ascorbic acid in cancer treatment: let the phoenix fly." Cancer cell 34.5 (2018): 700-706.

91) Christianto, Victor, and Florentin Smarandache. "On the Efficacy of High-dose Ascorbic Acid as Anticancer Treatment: A Literature Survey." BAOJ Cancer Res Ther 4 (2018): 056.

92) Bakalova, Rumiana, et al. "Vitamin C versus Cancer: Ascorbic Acid Radical and Impairment of Mitochondrial Respiration?" Oxidative Medicine and Cellular Longevity 2020 (2020).

93) Ren, X., et al. "The combination of ascorbate and menadione causes cancer cell death by oxidative stress and replicative stress." Free radical biology & medicine 134 (2019): 350.

94) Dahlberg, Sofia, Jacob Ede, and Ulf Schött. "Vitamin K and cancer." Scandinavian journal of clinical and laboratory investigation 77.8 (2017): 555-567.

95) Dasari, Subramanyam, et al. "Vitamin K2, a menaquinone present in dairy products targets castration-resistant prostate cancer cell-line by activating apoptosis signaling." Food and chemical toxicology 115 (2018): 218-227.

96) Dasari, Subramanyam, et al. "Vitamin K and its analogs: Potential avenues for prostate cancer management." Oncotarget 8.34 (2017): 57782.

97) Kiely, Maeve, et al. "Real-time cell analysis of the inhibitory effect of vitamin K2 on adhesion and proliferation of breast cancer cells." Nutrition Research 35.8 (2015): 736-743.

98) Nakaya, K., et al. Vitamin K2 as a Chemotherapeutic Agent for Treating Ovarian Cancer. INTECH Open Access Publisher, 2012.

99) Yao, Yuting, et al. "Enhanced therapeutic efficacy of vitamin K2 by silencing BCL-2 expression in SMMC-7721 hepatocellular carcinoma cells." Oncology letters 4.1 (2012): 163-167.

100) Tokita, Hiromi, et al. "Vitamin K2-induced antitumor effects via cell-cycle arrest and apoptosis in gastric cancer cell lines." International journal of molecular medicine 17.2 (2006): 235-243.

101) Shibayama-Imazu, Toshiko, et al. "Production of superoxide and dissipation of mitochondrial transmembrane potential by vitamin K2 trigger apoptosis in human ovarian cancer TYK-nu cells." Apoptosis 11.9 (2006): 1535-1543.

102) Li, Lu, et al. "Induction of apoptosis in hepatocellular carcinoma Smmc-7721 cells by vitamin K2 is associated with p53 and independent of the intrinsic apoptotic pathway." Molecular and cellular biochemistry 342.1-2 (2010): 125-131.

103) Takumi, Naofumi, et al. "Dietary vitamin K alleviates the reduction in testosterone production induced by lipopolysaccharide administration in rat testis." Food & function 2.7 (2011): 406-411.

104) Shibayama-Imazu, Toshiko, Toshihiro Aiuchi, and Kazuyasu Nakaya. "Vitamin K2-mediated apoptosis in cancer cells: Role of mitochondrial transmembrane potential." Vitamins & Hormones 78 (2008): 211-226.

105) Kawakita, Hideaki, et al. "Growth inhibitory effects of vitamin K2 on colon cancer cell lines via different types of cell death including autophagy and apoptosis." International journal of molecular medicine 23.6 (2009): 709-716.

106) Yokoyama, Tomohisa, et al. "Vitamin K2 induces autophagy and apoptosis simultaneously in leukemia cells." Autophagy 4.5 (2008): 629-640.

107) Ivanova, Donika, et al. "Vitamin K: redox-modulation, prevention of mitochondrial dysfunction and anticancer effect." Redox biology 16 (2018): 352-358

Chapter 9

Doxycycline/ Vitamin C Anti-Cancer Synergy

It's the Stem Cells, Stupid!

AS MENTIONED PREVIOUSLY, MODERN-DAY ONCOLOGY clings dogmatically to the old chemotherapy paradigm. Admittedly, chemotherapy can "debulk" the tumor mass, inducing a temporary remission for the cancer patient. However, chemotherapy leaves behind the cancer stem cell (CSC), dormant and resistant to chemotherapy, inevitably leading to relapse. The CSCs are a tiny fraction of the tumor mass, estimated to be about 0.001 to 0.01 percent, and live in a dormant, quiescent, drug-resistant state with a low proliferation rate. Cancer stem cells are adaptable to their environment, changing their metabolic pathways as needed to survive. Similar to normal stem cells, CSCs can be identified by characteristic surface markers—CD24, CD133, CD44, CD49, CXCR4 and LGR5—or intracellular markers like aldehyde dehydrogenase (ALDH). The CSCs activated pathways include Wnt, Notch, and Hedgehog signaling. (1)

Hypoxic Cancer Stem Cells

Tumor hypoxia is a common problem that creates a protective niche for CSCs to survive in the face of conventional chemotherapy. This is where doxycycline can be useful. In 2019, Dr. Lisanti's group found that doxycycline targets hypoxic CSCs, halting mitochondrial biogenesis and propagation. The effect was augmented by the taxane chemotherapy drug paclitaxel. (2–3)

Activating the Dormant Cancer Stem Cell

Another feature of CSCs discussed by Dr. Lisanti's group (2018) is their ability to shift from a dormant glycolytic state (usually in a hypoxic environment) to an activated energetic proliferative state with oxidative phenotype (using OXPHOS). (4–5)

These activated or "energetic" CSCs are characterized by increased mitochondrial biogenesis, i.e., increased mitochondrial mass involved in OXPHOS metabolic duties. By inhibiting mitochondrial protein production, doxycycline functions as a "nontoxic inhibitor of mitochondrial biogenesis," thereby targeting CSCs. (6–8)

Doxycycline and Ascorbate— Lethal Synergy

In *Oncotarget* (2017), Dr. Lisanti's group studied the synergy of doxycycline and IV vitamin C for eradication of CSCs. This is a really huge breakthrough in our quest for effective nontoxic cancer treatment. Working with MCF7 breast cancer-cell cultures, the Lisanti Group showed that the combined use of doxycycline and vitamin C was a "lethal metabolic strategy for eradicating cancer stem cells." (9)

Doxycycline is a safe, common antibiotic that has been used for 50 years. I have seen patients come into the office who have been on doxycycline for months or even years for treatment of acne or rosacea. Likewise, vitamin C is about as safe a substance as you can find. A clinical trial safety study on relapsed B-cell lymphoma patients receiving 75 grams of vitamin C intravenously reported no adverse effects. (10)

Reversibility of Metabolic Plasticity

The Lisanti group's understanding of CSC bioenergetics was built on 2013 work using a myeloid leukemia cell line by Dr. Bozhena Jhas et al., who found that inhibition of mitochondrial protein production with a tetracycline antibiotic, tigecycline, over four months eventually created a population of leukemia cells resistant to the antibiotic with a purely GLYCOLYTIC phenotype, abnormally swollen mitochondria, and an irregular cristae structure (these are mitochondrial internal membranes, the site of energy production). Upon removal of the antibiotic, the cells reverted back to an OXPHOS phenotype using mitochondrial oxidative metabolism, revealing the reversibility of metabolic plasticity. (11)

Cancer Stem Cells That Develop Resistance to Doxycycline Become Purely GLYCOLYTIC Phenotype

In an elegant study, Lisanti's group created doxycycline-resistant CSCs by passing them through successively higher doses of doxycycline. Most of the cells were killed by the doxycycline. However, the few surviving cells were then allowed to multiply and repopulate and were again treated with higher doses of dox-

ycycline. This process was repeated until the final cells were indeed immune to the antibiotic. Lisanti's group then did next-generation molecular studies on the doxycycline-resistant (Dox-R) CSCs, showing they had assumed a purely glycolytic phenotype, meaning metabolism had shifted away from the OXPHOS in the mitochondria to GLYCOLYSIS in the cytoplasm. (9)

These DOX-R breast CSCs were in a dormant state, as discussed by Dr. Luke Horton et al. (2016). (12)

The DOX-R CSCs were now sensitive to eradication with metabolic perturbation from high-dose vitamin C, acting as a glycolysis inhibitor by targeting glyceraldehyde 3-phosphate dehydrogenase (GAPDH), the 6th step in glycolysis. Vitamin C also depletes the nicotinamide adenine dinucleotide (NAD) pool. NAD is the primary electron donor in the mitochondrial respiratory electron transport chain (ETC).

High-dose IV vitamin C easily reached serum concentrations for these lethal effects in the clinical setting. A few other drugs and natural substances are also effective, namely berberine (OXPHOS-Complex I ETC inhibitor), chloroquine (autophagy inhibitor), niclosamide (OXPHOS inhibitor) and atovaquone (OXPHOS inhibitor). Dr. Lisanti's group writes:

> Understanding the metabolic basis of Doxycycline-resistance has ultimately helped us to develop a new synthetic lethal strategy, for more effectively targeting CSCs. (9) (13–14)

Doxycycline Plus: The Invention of "Triple Therapy"

The basic concept demonstrated by the work of the Lisanti group is that "triple therapy" with the combination of these three agents:

1) OXPHOS inhibitor (doxycycline, metformin, atavoquone, niclosamide, berberine etc.)

2) GLYCOLYSIS inhibitor (DCA, vitamin C, 2DG 2-De-Oxyglucose)

3) Autophagy inhibitor (propranolol, chloroquine, etc.),

The use of these three agents combined is potent anti-cancer strategy for synthetic lethality and eradication of CSCs. (3) (5) (9)

Metabolic plasticity of the CSC can be overcome using this type of combination approach. A partial approach, omitting one or more of the triple therapy components, is ill advised, leading to relapse with a more aggressive cancer cell type, as you will see below from the metformin study of Dr. Patricia Sancho et al. with pancreatic CSCs.

Triple Combination: Doxycycline, Azithromycin, Ascorbate

There are two ribosomes in mitochondria, a smaller (28s) and a larger (39s) one. The doxycycline targets only smaller ribosome, inhibiting its protein production. Proteins produced by mitochondrial ribosomes are incorporated into complex 1–4 of the election transport chain (ETC). What if we could use a second drug to simultaneously block the larger (39s) ribosome and induce more profound inhibition of protein production? This is exactly what was done in 2019 by the Fiorillo/Lisanti Group by adding azithromycin (commonly known as the Z-pack), a commonly used antibiotic that targets the larger ribosome.

Note: Clarithromycin is in the same drug family and can be used in place of azithromycin.

As expected, there was more complete eradication of CSCs in a breast cancer model with this triple combination at low concentration. Dr. Marco Fiorillo et al. (2020) stated:

> Remarkably, treatment with a combination of Doxycycline (1 μM MicroMolar), Azithromycin (1 μM) plus Vitamin C (250 μM) very potently inhibited CSC [Cancer Stem Cell] propagation by >90%, using the MCF7 ER(+) breast cancer cell line as a model system … showed a complete eradication of CSC propagation. The synergistic effect of these compounds on the breast cancer cell line MCF7 were induced by the inhibition of two key targets, namely the large [39 s] and small mitochondrial ribosomes [28 s] (2)

Note: the authors are referring to eradication of CSC propagation, not eradication of the CSCs themselves.

Berberine, Metformin, and Cancer Stem Cells

Dr. Lisanti's group found the botanical supplement berberine effective against CSCs. Both berberine and metformin are OXPHOS inhibitors, which target CSCs by inhibiting complex one of the mitochondrial ETC.

Pancreatic Cancer Stem Cell Model—Dr. Sancho

In 2015, Dr. Patricia Sancho et al. studied a pancreatic cancer cell model and found metformin to be an effective CSC agent. Dr. Sancho's group found that CSCs are a minor population (0.001 to 0.1%) of the entire cancer. The stem cells had a low proliferation rate, remaining dormant, and a high level of drug resistance to chemotherapy. They displayed stem cell surface markers such as CD44 and CD133 and intracellular marker aldehyde dehydrogenase (ALDH). Signaling pathways for CSCs include Wnt, Notch, and Hedgehog (15).

Shifting Metabolic Pathways

The CSCs were able to adapt to the micro-environment by shifting energy production from OXPHOS to GLYCOLYSIS and back again. Dr. Sancho's group found that the CSCs relied on OXPHOS (oxidative phosphorylation) while (non-stem) cancer cells were highly GLYCOLYTIC. Metformin treatment, which impairs mitochondrial OXPHOS, killed most of the CSCs. However, the few remaining CSCs were resistant to metformin because they had switched their metabolic pathway from OXPHOS to a GLYCOLYTIC phenotype.

As noted above, this conversion to a GLYCOLYTIC phenotype is exactly what Lisanti's group found when treating breast CSCs with doxycycline, producing a GLYCOLYTIC phenotype now vulnerable to the lethal effects of high-dose IV vitamin C, which served as a glycolysis inhibitor. Dr. Sancho et al. were disappointed to find that pancreatic tumors developed resistance to metformin and then progressed to a more aggressive form in cancer xenografts. On the other hand, treatment with menadione (Vitamin K3), which inhibited complex one and increased ROS, was lethal to the cancer xenografts without inducing resistant cell types. (15)

This experience highlights the dangers of CSC treatments that merely induce resistant cancer cell types that are more aggressive and more difficult to treat. Another problem: We do not know when all the CSCs have been eradicated and when it is safe to stop treatment. We cannot rely on a PET Scan for this because the dormant CSCs are not visible on the scan. Blood testing for cancer markers, such as circulating tumor cells (CTC s) may help, but markers may be unreliable because residual CSCs are dormant and not circulating in the blood stream. If treatment is stopped too soon, then resistant CSCs are left behind to induce a relapse after a variable latency period. This is a major problem that awaits further research. Perhaps the answer is to maintain a long-term maintenance program on a nontoxic anti-cancer protocol of repurposed drugs.

Atovaquone-Doxycycline Combination for Stem Cells

Dr. Lisanti's group found doxycycline effective for eradication of CSCs when combined with the OXPHOS inhibitor atovaquone, an antimalarial drug that inhibits complex III of the mitochondrial ETC. Atovaquone's chemical structure is similar to CoQ-10, and competes with it, thereby inhibiting oxidative respiration in the mitochondria of the CSC. Atavaquone is already FDA-approved for malaria and prevention of pneumocystis pneumonia in immunosuppressed patients, and easily reaches effective serum levels with routine dosage of 750 mg BID with food. Atovaquone is commonly prescribed long-term for the immune-suppressed oncology patient for pneumocystis prophylaxis. (13–14)

Ignoring the Cancer Stem Cells— the Failure of Oncology

For rapidly proliferating cancer cell types (high Ki-67), chemotherapy provides a temporary remission or reduction in tumor size. However, CSCs are unaffected by chemotherapy and will induce cancer relapse. The more aggressive, highly proliferative cell types relapse within months, while the more indolent cell types (low Ki-67) take longer and relapse after a few years. Clearly, targeting CSCs is imperative in order to prevent relapse. Unfortunately, current day oncology has failed the cancer patient by ignoring CSCs and has been blindly forging ahead with the old chemotherapy protocols, as if medical science is still in the 1960s, and nothing has changed.

Estrogen and Exemestane—Aromatase Inhibitor for Breast Cancer

Regardless of serum estrogen levels, which may be quite low in post-menopausal women, many tumors use intracrine (local) estrogen production to stimulate cell growth. The tumor cells contain upregulated aromatase enzymes to produce estrogen locally. This local estro-

gen production at the tumor site uses the same mechanism as the ovary, namely, aromatase conversion of testosterone to estrogen. The aromatase enzyme removes one hydrogen atom from testosterone, and behold, we now have an estrogen molecule. In this scenario, aromatase blockers such as exemestane are beneficial as a cancer treatment, as they also prevent local estrogen production at the tumor site.

Exemestane for Lung Cancer and Mesothelioma

Exemestane is a third-generation irreversible aromatase inhibitor and a conventional oncology success story that stands out. In addition to its aromatase blocking activity, exemestane metabolites induce very effective mitochondrial-mediated apoptosis of breast cancer cells. Exemestane also seems effective in lung cancer, which frequently expresses estrogen receptors and has aromatase activity (16–18). Exemestane may synergize with doxycycline in treatment of mesothelioma (19–20).

In Situ Aromatase Activity in Skin Cancers

The skin is a "steroidal organ," meaning the skin can produce and metabolize various hormones very similar to those of breast tissue cells. (21) Dr. Georgios Nikolakis et al. (2016) write:

> The skin is an important extra-gonadal steroidogenic organ, capable of metabolizing various hormones from their precursors, as well as of synthesizing de novo a broad palette of sex steroids and glucocorticoids from cholesterol. (22)

Like their cousin, the breast cancer cell, skin cancer cells will upregulate aromatase activity to stimulate growth via intra-tumoral, in situ, estrogen production (intracrine) independent of serum concentrations, which may be quite low in post-menopausal women. Blocking aromatase activity, which blocks local estrogen production, has been shown to be effective for skin cancers. After all, breast tissue is an appendage of the skin, so estrogen production by the skin via aromatase activity is not as strange as it sounds. (23–24)

In- Situ (Intracrine) Aromatase Activity in Colon Cancer

One does not usually associate estrogen production with colonic epithelium or colon cancer cells. However, Dr. Sato et al. in 2012 found that *"colon carcinoma expresses functional aromatase, and that estrogens are locally synthesized in the tumor tissues."(25)*

Synergy of mTOR Inhibition (Itraconazole) with Exemestane

A number of studies show a synergistic cancer-cell-killing effect when an mTOR inhibitor drug (such as itraconazole), is combined with the aromatase inhibitor, exemestane. (26–29)

Exemestane Synergy with Simvastatin

Statin drugs such as simvastatin have stand-alone anti-cancer activity by activating the intrinsic apoptosis pathway. (30) In vitro studies show statin drugs induce apoptosis in B-cell lymphoma via suppression of the mevalonate pathway. (31)

Using a breast cancer cell line in 2015, Dr. Yuanyuan Shen studied the synergy of combining exemestane with simvastatin (a common statin drug) showing that it:

markedly increased the efficacy, as compared with the single-agent treatment, suggesting that **combination treatment could become a highly effective approach for breast cancer**…. co-administration of exemestane and simvastatin was shown to result in marked inhibition of tumor cell proliferation, significant cell cycle arrest at G0/G1 phase and induction of apoptosis, as compared with that of the control and individual drug-treated cells. (32)

More Drug Combinations

A combination that includes all or some of the following: exemestane, doxycycline, itraconazole, fenofibrate, clarithromycin, simvastatin, metformin, etc. might be suggested for breast cancer patients, along with weekly intravenous high-dose vitamin C. Other aromatase-producing cancer-cell types (colon, lung, skin etc.) might also benefit from such a combination of drugs that block molecular pathways in cancer cells.

Bone Metastasis on Zoledronic Acid

In those with bone metastasis from breast cancer already on Zoledronic acid, the addition of doxycycline to the Zoledronic acid might be synergistic and more effective than each single agent. (33–34)

Exemestane and Anti-Cancer Metabolites

In the drug development for exemestane, researchers may have accidentally stumbled upon a highly effective anti-cancer drug by virtue of the metabolites of exemestane, which seem to have a potent biological effect, inducing *"cell cycle arrest and apoptosis via mitochondrial pathway, involving caspase-8 activation."* Dr. Cristina Amaral et al. (2015) write:

> Our results indicate that metabolites induced, in sensitive breast cancer cells, cell cycle arrest and apoptosis via mitochondrial pathway, involving caspase-8 activation... It was also concluded that.... **the biological effects of [exemestane] metabolites are different from the ones of exemestane,** which suggests that exemestane efficacy in breast cancer treatment may also be dependent on its metabolites. **Note:** caspase 8 activation initiates apoptosis. (35)

Doxycycline—Benefits in Ascites and Pleural Effusions

Back in the day (1976–2005), working as an interventional radiologist, we commonly did a procedure called thoracentesis, removing malignant pleural fluid from breast cancer patients, and then injected doxycycline as a "sclerosing agent" into the pleural space. In 1994, Dr. Wakai discovered that doxycycline (the synthetic form of tetracycline [TCN]) suppresses malignant effusions in a mouse fibrosarcoma model by suppressing tumor growth, writing:

> it appears that TCNs [Doxycycline] injected

into the pleural cavity to manage malignant effusions in man [i.e., humans] exert their activity, at least in part, by suppressing malignant cell growth. (36)

Doxycycline as Stand-alone Anti-Cancer Drug More Effective than Chemotherapy

Studies show that doxycycline may be considered an effective stand-alone anti-cancer therapy. In 2016, Dr. Chen studied 21 cancer cell lines in vitro and 4 kinds of tumor-bearing mouse models in vivo. Dr. Chen found that many of the cancer cell lines were *"very sensitive"* to doxycycline, killing them at low concentrations. IC50 (Inhibitory Concentration 50%) was less than 5 microMolar. Dr. Chen makes the remarkable observation that doxycycline was more effective than the standard chemotherapy drug cyclophosphamide, concluding:

> Doxycycline elicits a remarkable inhibitory effect on cancer cells. In our animal experiments, the inhibitory rates of doxycycline were higher than those of cyclophosphamide. Doxycycline could also improve the survival condition of mice. Therefore, doxycycline is a promising anti-cancer agent because it inhibits cancer cell proliferation, induces fewer toxic and other side effects than other drugs do... (37)

Doxycycline for Lymphoma

In 2015, Drs. David Barbie and Brian Kennedy summarized the preclinical work of Dr. Mary Pulvino et al. on doxycycline for B-cell lymphoma. Doxycycline accumulates in lymphoma cells in high concentrations. Summarizing the work of Pulvino, Drs. Barbie and Kennedy wrote:

Notably, doxycycline was also effective at inhibiting the growth of DLBCL [Diffuse Large B-cell Lymphoma] xenografts at physiologically achievable doses.... (38–39)

Others have written extensively on the use of doxycycline as a potential anti-CSC agent and radiation sensitizer. (40–42)

Doxycycline Synergy with Celecoxib in Colon Cancer

In 2006, Dr. Toshinao Onoda reported that doxycycline induces apoptosis via the mitochondrial pathways in colon cancer cells (in vitro), finding the combination of doxycycline and COX-2 inhibitor (celecoxib) synergistic. (43–44)

Doxycycline for Breast Cancer Stem Cells

Doxycycline preclinical studies have shown favorable results for breast CSCs by inhibiting the cancer stem phenotype epithelial to mesenchymal transition (EMT). In 2016, Dr. Le Zhang et al. studied breast cancer cells in vitro, building on the 2015 work by Dr. Rebecca Lamb's group, finding doxycycline:

> inhibition of the viability and proliferation of breast cancer cells and BCSCs [stem cells], decrease mammosphere forming efficiency, migration and invasion, and EMT [epithelial to mesenchymal transition] of breast cancer cells. Expression of stem cell factors Oct4, Sox2, Nanog and CD44 were also significantly downregulated after doxycycline treatment. (45)

Doxycycline Autophagy Inhibitor

Dr. Zhang further writes that doxycycline treatment of breast cancer cells induced a decrease in LC3B protein marker, indicating inhibition of autophagy. In addition, inhibition of autophagy specifically targets CSCs:

> LC3B-II, is one of the most specific biomarkers of autophagy.... a growing number of studies suggest a link between autophagy and BCSC s [Breast cancer stem cells].... Guan et al. has reported that BCSCs have a higher autophagic flux than non-CSC cells... and Cufí et al. has demonstrated that autophagy positively regulates the CD44+CD24– breast cancer stem-like phenotype... and Maycotte et al. reported that autophagy supports BCSC (stem cell) maintenance by modulating IL6 secretion, and that inhibition of autophagy decreases cell survival, as well as mammosphere forming efficiency.... Here, we report that doxycycline downregulates the autophagy-related protein levels of LC-3BI and LC-3BII, suggesting a role for autophagy in the doxycycline-induced suppression of proliferation, invasion, and self-renewal of breast cancer cells ... Moreover, doxycycline could down regulate the expression of the autophagy marker LC-3BI and LC-3BII, suggesting that inhibiting autophagy may be responsible in part for the observed effects on proliferation, EMT and stem cell markers ... The potent inhibition of EMT and cancer stem-like characteristics in breast cancer cells by doxycycline treatment suggests that this drug can be repurposed as an anti-cancer drug in the treatment of breast cancer patients in the clinic. (45)

Note: LC3 is a light-chain 3 protein associated with microtubules involved with autophagy and a marker to monitor autophagy. (46)

Doxycycline Inhibits NF-kB and IL-6

In 2017, Dr. Xiaoyun Tang et al. studied doxycycline in a mouse model of breast cancer, showing potent anti-inflammatory effects, with a 50% reduction in NF-kB transcriptional activity:

Under basal condition without stimulation, doxycycline was able to decrease the transcriptional activity of nuclear NF-κB by ~50%, which explained the decreased IL-6 mRNA and secretion of IL-6, CCL2 and CXCL2 by doxycycline when LPA and TNFα were absent. (47)

Note: LPA (lysophosphatidate) signaling induces chronic inflammation in the tumor microenvironment, promoting tumor growth, metastasis, and immune evasion. (77)

Doxycycline for various cancer cell types:

- Breast Cancer (47–48)(75–76)
- Melanoma (49)(74)
- Oral Squamous Cell (51)
- Glioblastoma (52)(66)
- Leukemia (53)
- T cell lymphoma (54–56)
- Cervical cancer (57)
- MALT lymphoma (58–65)
- Breast cancer stem cells (67–68)
- Prostate cancer stem cells (69–71)
- Small-cell lung cancer (72)
- Adenocarcinoma of duodenum (73)

As you might expect, doxycycline is more effective when used in combination with drugs that block alternate molecular pathways. One of these drugs is the antibiotic clarithromycin (azithromycin), which inhibits the larger mito-chondrial ribosome, is synergistic with doxycycline and vitamin C as discussed above and in chapter on 35 on clarithromycin.

Doxycycline Has Synergy With

- Exemestane for breast cancer.
- Zolendronic acid for bone metastases.
- Celecoxib in colon cancer.
- Clarithromycin
- IV Vitamin C for cancer stem cells.

Doxycycline Inhibits These Cell Pathways.

- MMP (Matrix Metallo-Proteinase) inhibitor.
- NF-kB inhibitor.

Doxycycline for MALT Lymphoma (Mucosa-Associated Lymphoid Tissue)

MALT lymphoma, a common form of extra-nodal lymphoma, is associated with H. Pylori infections of the stomach and chlamydia infections of the eye. MALT lymphoma of the stomach responds well to antibiotics such as doxycycline and clarithromycin, usually given as triple therapy, along with a proton pump inhibitor antacid (omeprazole). Even when the H. pylori test is negative in gastric MALT lymphomas, some patients may be "cured" by triple therapy antibiotics that include doxycycline.

Dr. Markus Raderer et al. (2015) write:

A relevant percentage of patients with HP [H. Pylori] negative gastric MALT lymphoma may benefit from antibiotic therapy and do not require additional oncological therapies. Our data suggest that the remissions seen in these patients might be durable as evidenced by prolonged follow-up in our series. [MALT=Mucosa-Associated Lymphoma] (59–60)

Ocular adnexal MALT lymphoma is thought to be related to infection with chlamydia psittaci, which is sensitive to doxycycline. Remarkably, treatment with doxycycline may cause MALT lymphoma remission or "cure." Dr. Andrés Ferreri et al. (2006) write that doxycycline is effective treatment even in cases of previous treatment failure with radiotherapy:

> Doxycycline is a fast, safe, and active therapy for Cp DNA-positive OAL [DNA-positive for Chlamydia, Ocular Adnexal Lymphoma] that was effective even in patients with multiple failures involving previously irradiated areas or regional lymphadenopathies. (61–64)

Doxycycline Synergy with Hydroxychloroquine

Coxiella burnetii is an intracellular gram-negative bacterial pathogen which causes Q fever, and is associated with B-cell lymphoma. In 2018, Drs. Cléa Melenotte and Didier Raoult reported a patient whose C. burnetti associated B-cell lymphoma responded to the combination of doxycycline and hydroxychloroquine (autophagy inhibitor). (65)

Conclusion

The old antibiotic doxycycline has been repurposed as a very useful anti-cancer and anti-CSC drug. My hat comes off in admiration and thanks to the Michael Lisanti group. This doxycycline/ vitamin C combination is a dramatic breakthrough in finding an effective, targeted CSC eradication strategy. Hopefully, the

technique of combination drugs to overcome the metabolic plasticity of CSCs will soon be incorporated and routinely used on the oncology wards.

References Chapter 9: Doxycycline Vitamin C Anti Cancer Synergy

1) Satheesh, Noothan Jyothi, Samson Mathews Samuel, and Dietrich Büsselberg. "Combination Therapy with Vitamin C Could Eradicate Cancer Stem Cells." Biomolecules 10.1 (2020): 79.

2) Fiorillo, Marco, et al. "Doxycycline, Azithromycin and Vitamin C (DAV): A potent combination therapy for targeting mitochondria and eradicating cancer stem cells (CSCs)." Aging (Albany NY) 11.8 (2019): 2202.

3) De Francesco, Ernestina Marianna, et al. "Targeting hypoxic cancer stem cells (CSCs) with Doxycycline: implications for optimizing anti-angiogenic therapy." Oncotarget 8.34 (2017): 56126.

4) Sotgia, Federica, Marco Fiorillo, and Michael P. Lisanti. "Hallmarks of the cancer cell of origin: Comparisons with "energetic" cancer stem cells (e-CSCs)." Aging (Albany NY) 11.3 (2019): 1065.

5) De Francesco, Ernestina M., Federica Sotgia, and Michael P. Lisanti. "Cancer stem cells (CSCs): metabolic strategies for their identification and eradication." Biochemical Journal 475.9 (2018): 1611-1634.

6) Scatena, Cristian, et al. "Doxycycline, an inhibitor of mitochondrial biogenesis, effectively reduces cancer stem cells (CSCs) in early breast cancer patients: a clinical pilot study." Frontiers in oncology 8 (2018): 452.

7) Lin, Chang-Ching, et al. "Doxycycline targets aldehyde dehydrogenase-positive breast cancer stem cells." Oncology reports 39.6 (2018): 3041-3047.

8) Lamb, Rebecca, et al. "Mitochondrial mass, a new metabolic biomarker for stem-like cancer cells: Understanding WNT/FGF-driven anabolic signaling." Oncotarget 6.31 (2015): 30453.

9) De Francesco, E. M., Michael Lisanti et al. "Vitamin C and Doxycycline: a synthetic lethal combination

therapy targeting metabolic flexibility in cancer stem cells (CSCs)." Oncotarget (2017).

10) Kawada, Hiroshi, et al. "Phase I Clinical Trial of Intravenous L-ascorbic Acid Following Salvage Chemotherapy for Relapsed B-cell non-Hodgkin's Lymphoma." The Tokai journal of experimental and clinical medicine 39.3 (2014): 111-115.

11) Jhas, Bozhena, et al. "Metabolic adaptation to chronic inhibition of mitochondrial protein synthesis in acute myeloid leukemia cells." PLoS One 8.3 (2013).

12) Horton, Luke A., et al. "Characterization of Dormancy in Doxycycline-resistant MCF-7 Human Breast Carcinoma Cells." (2016).

13) US Patent: Methods of treating cancer with atovaquone-related compounds WO 2015050844 A1

14) Fiorillo, Marco, et al. "Repurposing atovaquone: targeting mitochondrial complex III and OXPHOS to eradicate cancer stem cells." Oncotarget 7.23 (2016): 34084.

15) Patricia Sancho, et al. "MYC/PGC-1a Balance Determines the Metabolic Phenotype and Plasticity of Pancreatic Cancer Stem Cells." Cell Metabolism 22 (2015): 1-16.

16) Amaral, Cristina, et al. "Apoptosis and autophagy in breast cancer cells following exemestane treatment." PLoS One 7.8 (2012): e42398.

17) Koutras, Angelos, et al. "Antiproliferative effect of exemestane in lung cancer cells." Molecular cancer 8.1 (2009): 109.

18) Weinberg, Olga K., et al. "Aromatase inhibitors in human lung cancer therapy." Cancer research 65.24 (2005): 11287-11291.

19) Nuvoli, Barbara, et al. "Exemestane blocks mesothelioma growth through downregulation of cAMP, pCREB and CD44 implicating new treatment option in patients affected by this disease." Molecular cancer 13.1 (2014): 69.

20) Rubins, Jeffrey B., et al. "Inhibition of mesothelioma cell growth in vitro by doxycycline." Journal of Laboratory and Clinical Medicine 138.2 (2001): 101-106.

21) Pomari, Elena, et al. "Intracrine sex steroid synthesis and signaling in human epidermal keratinocytes and dermal fibroblasts." The FASEB Journal 29.2 (2014): 508-524.

22) Nikolakis, Georgios, et al. "Skin steroidogenesis in health and disease." Reviews in Endocrine and Metabolic Disorders 17.3 (2016): 247-258.

23) Hoffmann, Thomas K., et al. "Effects of tamoxifen on human squamous cell carcinoma lines of the head and neck." Anti-cancer drugs 13.5 (2002): 521-531.

24) Cheng, Yi-Shing Lisa, et al. "Aromatase expression in normal human oral keratinocytes and oral squamous cell carcinoma." Archives of oral biology 51.7 (2006): 612-620.

25) Sato, Ryuichiro, et al. "Aromatase in colon carcinoma." Anticancer research 32.8 (2012): 3069-3075.

26) Awada, Ahmad, et al. "The oral mTOR inhibitor RAD001 (everolimus) in combination with letrozole in patients with advanced breast cancer: results of a phase I study with pharmacokinetics." European journal of cancer 44.1 (2008): 84-91.

27) Rudloff, Joëlle, et al. "The mTOR pathway in estrogen response: A potential for combining the rapamycin derivative RAD001 with the aromatase inhibitor Letrozole (Femara®) in breast carcinoma." (2004): 1298-1298.

28) Boulay, Anne, et al. "Dual inhibition of mTOR and estrogen receptor signaling in vitro induces cell death in models of breast cancer." Clinical Cancer Research 11.14 (2005): 5319-5328.

29) Lee, Joycelyn JX, Kiley Loh, and Yoon-Sim Yap. "PI3K/Akt/mTOR inhibitors in breast cancer." Cancer biology & medicine 12.4 (2015): 342.

30) Alizadeh, Javad, et al. "Mevalonate cascade inhibition by simvastatin induces the intrinsic apoptosis pathway via depletion of isoprenoids in tumor cells." Scientific reports 7 (2017): 44841.

31) Qi, X. F., et al. "HMG-CoA reductase inhibitors induce apoptosis of lymphoma cells by promoting ROS generation and regulating Akt, Erk and p38 signals via suppression of mevalonate pathway." Cell Death & Disease 4.2 (2013): e518.

32) Shen, Yuanyuan, et al. "Synergistic effects of combined treatment with simvastatin and exemestane on

MCF-7 human breast cancer cells." Molecular medicine reports 12.1 (2015): 456-462.

33) Duivenvoorden, W. C. M., et al. "Effect of zoledronic acid on the doxycycline-induced decrease in tumour burden in a bone metastasis model of human breast cancer." British journal of cancer 96.10 (2007): 1526.

34) Saikali, Zeina, and Gurmit Singh. "Doxycycline and other tetracyclines in the treatment of bone metastasis." Anti-cancer drugs 14.10 (2003): 773-778.

35) Amaral, Cristina, et al. "Exemestane metabolites suppress growth of estrogen receptor-positive breast cancer cells by inducing apoptosis and autophagy: A comparative study with Exemestane." The international journal of biochemistry & cell biology 69 (2015): 183-195.

36) Wakai, Kae, et al. "Mechanism of inhibitory actions of minocycline and doxycycline on ascitic fluid production induced by mouse fibrosarcoma cells." Life sciences 54.11 (1994): 703-709.

37) Chen, Bo, et al. "Studies on antitumor activity spectrum of doxycycline." Journal of Solid Tumors 6.1 (2016).

38) Barbie, David A., and Brian K. Kennedy. "Doxycycline: new tricks for an old drug." Oncotarget 6.23 (2015): 19336.

39) Pulvino, Mary, et al. "Inhibition of COP9-signalosome (CSN) deneddylating activity and tumor growth of diffuse large B-cell lymphomas by doxycycline." Oncotarget 6.17 (2015): 14796.

40) Lokeshwar, Bal L. "Chemically modified non-antimicrobial tetracyclines are multifunctional drugs against advanced cancers." Pharmacological research 63.2 (2011): 146-150.

41) Markowska, Anna, et al. "Doxycycline, salinomycin, monensin, ivermectin repositioned as cancer drugs." Bioorganic & medicinal chemistry letters (2019).

42) Wan, Liyuan, et al. "Aspirin, lysine, mifepristone and doxycycline combined can effectively and safely prevent and treat cancer metastasis: prevent seeds from germinating on soil." Oncotarget 6.34 (2015): 35157.

43) Onoda, Toshinao, et al. "Tetracycline analogues (doxycycline and COL-3) induce caspase-dependent and-independent apoptosis in human colon cancer cells." International Journal of Cancer 118.5 (2006): 1309-1315.

44) Onoda, Toshinao, et al. "Doxycycline inhibits cell proliferation and invasive potential: combination therapy with cyclooxygenase-2 inhibitor in human colorectal cancer cells." Journal of Laboratory and Clinical Medicine 143.4 (2004): 207-216.

45) Zhang, Le, et al. "Doxycycline inhibits the cancer stem cell phenotype and epithelial-to-mesenchymal transition in breast cancer." Cell Cycle 16.8 (2017): 737-745.

46) Tanida, Isei, Takashi Ueno, and Eiki Kominami. "LC3 and Autophagy." Autophagosome and Phagosome. Humana Press, 2008. 77-88.

47) Tang, Xiaoyun, et al. "Doxycycline attenuates breast cancer related inflammation by decreasing plasma lysophosphatidate concentrations and inhibiting NF-κB activation." Molecular cancer 16.1 (2017): 36.

48) Fife, Rose S., and George W. Sledge Jr. "Effects of doxycycline on in vitro growth, migration, and gelatinase activity of breast carcinoma cells." The Journal of laboratory and clinical medicine 125.3 (1995): 407-411.

49) Sun, Tao, et al. "Doxycycline inhibits the adhesion and migration of melanoma cells by inhibiting the expression and phosphorylation of focal adhesion kinase (FAK)." Cancer letters 285.2 (2009): 141-150.

50) deleted

51) Shen, Ling-Chang, et al. "Anti-invasion and anti-tumor growth effect of doxycycline treatment for human oral squamous-cell carcinoma—in vitro and in vivo studies." Oral oncology 46.3 (2010): 178-184.

52) Wang-Gillam, Andrea, et al. "Anti-tumor effect of doxycycline on glioblastoma cells." Journal of Cancer Molecules 3.5 (2007): 147-153.

53) Tolomeo, Manlio, et al. "Effects of chemically modified tetracyclines (CMTs) in sensitive, multidrug resistant and apoptosis resistant leukaemia cell lines." British journal of pharmacology 133.2 (2001): 306-314.

54) Alexander-Savino, Carolina V., et al. "Doxycycline is an NF-κB inhibitor that induces apoptotic cell death in malignant T-cells." Oncotarget 7.46 (2016): 75954.

55) Iwasaki, Hiromichi, et al. "Doxycycline induces apoptosis by way of caspase-3 activation with inhibition of matrix metalloproteinase in human T-lymphoblastic leukemia CCRF-CEM cells." Journal of Laboratory and Clinical Medicine 140.6 (2002): 382-386.

56) Liu, Jian, Charles A. Kuszynski, and B. Timothy Baxter. "Doxycycline induces Fas/Fas ligand-mediated apoptosis in Jurkat T lymphocytes." Biochemical and biophysical research communications 260.2 (1999): 562-567.

57) Zhao, Yan, et al. "Doxycycline inhibits proliferation and induces apoptosis of both human papillomavirus positive and negative cervical cancer cell lines." Canadian journal of physiology and pharmacology 94.5 (2016): 526-533.

58) Kuo, Sung-Hsin, et al. "Novel Insights of Lymphomagenesis of Helicobacter pylori-Dependent Gastric Mucosa-Associated Lymphoid Tissue Lymphoma." Cancers 11.4 (2019): 547.

59) Raderer, Markus, et al. "Antibiotic treatment as sole management of Helicobacter pylori-negative gastric MALT lymphoma: a single center experience with prolonged follow-up." Annals of hematology 94.6 (2015): 969-973.

60) Kiesewetter, Barbara, and Markus Raderer. "Antibiotic therapy in nongastrointestinal MALT lymphoma: a review of the literature" Blood 122.8 (2013): 1350-1357.

61) Ferreri, Andrés JM, et al. "Bacteria-eradicating therapy with doxycycline in ocular adnexal MALT lymphoma: a multicenter prospective trial." Journal of the National Cancer Institute 98.19 (2006):1375-1382.

62) Han, Jae Joon, et al. "Long-term outcomes of first-line treatment with doxycycline in patients with previously untreated ocular adnexal marginal zone B cell lymphoma." Annals of hematology 94.4 (2015): 575-581.

63) Husain, Amina, et al. "Meta–analyses of the association between Chlamydia psittaci and ocular adnexal lymphoma and the response of ocular adnexal lymphoma to antibiotics." Cancer 110.4 (2007): 809-815.

64) Abramson DH, Rollins I, Coleman M. Periocular mucosa-associated lymphoid/low grade lymphomas: treatment with antibiotics. Am J Ophthalmol. 2005;140:729–730.

65) Melenotte, Cléa, and Didier Raoult. "Pro-apoptotic effect of doxycycline and hydroxychloroquine on B-cell lymphoma induced by C. burnetii." Oncotarget 9.2 (2018): 2726.

66) Tan, Qian, et al. "Induction of mitochondrial dysfunction and oxidative damage by antibiotic drug doxycycline enhances the responsiveness of glioblastoma to chemotherapy." Medical science monitor: international medical journal of experimental and clinical research 23 (2017): 4117.

67) Lin, Chang-Ching, et al. "Doxycycline targets aldehyde dehydrogenase-positive breast cancer stem cells." Oncology reports 39.6 (2018): 3041-3047.

68) Scatena, Cristian, et al. "Doxycycline, an inhibitor of mitochondrial biogenesis, effectively reduces cancer stem cells (CSCs) in early breast cancer patients: a clinical pilot study." Frontiers in oncology 8 (2018): 452.

69) Matsumoto, Takashi, et al. "Doxycycline induces apoptosis via ER stress selectively to cells with a cancer stem cell-like properties: importance of stem cell plasticity." Oncogenesis 6.11 (2017): 1-11.

70) Zhu, Chao, et al. "Doxycycline synergizes with doxorubicin to inhibit the proliferation of castration-resistant prostate cancer cells." Acta biochimica et biophysica Sinica 49.11 (2017): 999-1007.

71) Ogut, Deniz, et al. "Doxycycline down-regulates matrix metalloproteinase expression and inhibits NF-κB signaling in LPS-induced PC3 cells." Folia histochemica et cytobiologica 54.4 (2016): 171-180.

72) Wang, Sheng-Qi, et al. "New application of an old drug: Antitumor activity and mechanisms of doxycycline in small cell lung cancer." International journal of oncology 48.4 (2016): 1353-1360.

73) Galván-Salazar, Hector R., et al. "Preclinical trial on the use of doxycycline for the treatment of adenocarcinoma of the duodenum." Molecular and clinical oncology 5.5 (2016): 657-659.

74) Rok, Jakub, et al. "Cytotoxic and proapoptotic effect of doxycycline—An in vitro study on the human

skin melanoma cells." Toxicology in Vitro (2020): 104790.

75) Zhong, Weilong, et al. "Doxycycline inhibits breast cancer EMT and metastasis through PAR-1/NF-κB/ miR-17/E-cadherin pathway." Oncotarget 8.62 (2017): 104855.

76) Jiang, Xianpeng, et al. "Antibiotics suppress growth of breast cancer cells and synergize cytotoxicity of 2-Deoxy-D-glucose: Treating cancer like an infection." (2019): 3600-3600.

77) Xu, Yan. "Targeting lysophosphatidic acid in cancer: The issues in moving from bench to bedside." Cancers 11.10 (2019): 1523.

Chapter 10

Targeting Cancer Stem Cells with Nontoxic Therapies

Curcumin, Berberine, Pterostilbene, Sulforaphane, Parthenolide, Milk Thistle, ECGC, Allicin

WHEN JIM WAS 36 YEARS old, he was diagnosed with acute myeloblastic leukemia with symptoms of fatigue, anemia, and extremely high white count on his blood panel. Jim received seven chemotherapy treatments over three years, each giving him a temporary remission shorter than the last one. Eventually, the cancer cells became resistant to the chemotherapy, and it was no longer effective. After exhausting all the usual treatments, the doctors offered Jim allogeneic hematopoietic stem cell transplantation, a procedure that obliterates the patient's bone marrow with high-dose chemotherapy. The high-dose chemotherapy produces permanent, irreversible infertility. The patient is then "rescued" with donor bone marrow stem cells from a family member or donor bank. Although potentially curative, bone marrow transplant from a donor is associated with considerable morbidity and mortality from infection and graft vs. host disease. Jim had a successful procedure and is alive and doing well three years later. What can we learn from Jim's story?

Lessons Learned

The first lesson is that hematologic malignancies and all other cancers, for that matter, tend to relapse even after a complete remission induced by cytotoxic chemotherapy. Unknown for many years, the reason for this cancer recurrence has been discovered.

Two Distinct Populations of Cancer Cells

There are actually two distinct populations of cancer cells in the cancer victim. The bulky tumor masses are caused by rapidly replicating cancer cells, highly sensitive to the killing effects of chemotherapy. However, a smaller subset of cancer cells lurks within the tumor mass, hiding in a dormant state and not actively replicating. These are the cancer stem cells (CSCs) that are resistant to conventional cytotoxic chemotherapy, biding their time, waiting for a future opportunity to reactivate and seed metastatic cancer throughout the body.

This explains Jim's futile experience with chemotherapy, which kills off the rapidly replicating leukemia cells while leaving the dormant leukemia stem cells unharmed. This is also true for most other solid-organ cancers. The solution, of course, is to address the dormant CSCs at the same time as the rapidly replicating cancer cells. (1–3)

Oblivious to the Cancer Stem Cell

Unfortunately, modern-day oncology/hematology doctors are oblivious to this important lesson and continue to mindlessly treat their patients with the same chemotherapy protocols as before. Even though this information is in their own journals, they cannot bring themselves to acknowledge it. Sadly, since their doctors will not help them, patients are left to fend for themselves. In order to get off the chemotherapy merry-go-round, the patient must learn about widely available, nontoxic, targeted therapies that kill CSCs. As we will see, some of these therapies are available as supplements at the health food store and some are common drugs requiring a doctor's off-label prescription. Hopefully, with knowledge obtained from this chapter, durable remissions with "curative efficacy" can be achieved.

Many Natural Substance Target Cancer Stem Cells

How many plant species have anti-cancer activity? You might be surprised to know that three thousand plant species have anti-cancer activity according to Dr. Gali-Muhtasib, writing in 2015. (4)

In fact, there are hundreds of nontoxic natural substances available at the health food store targeting CSCs. (4–8)

In 2019, Dr. Liskova reviewed dietary substances targeting CSCs including:

- Diallyl trisulfide (found in garlic)
- Pterostilbene (methylated version of resveratrol)
- Sulforaphane (found in broccoli)
- Resveratrol (from grape skins)
- Curcumin (from turmeric)
- Genistein (phyto-estrogen from soy)
- Epigallocatechin-3-gallate (EGCG) (from green tea)

- Phenethyl isothiocyanate (PEITC) (from cruciferous vegetables)

These compounds demonstrated anti-cancer properties by targeting CSCs-mediated pathways and thus modulating CSCs proliferation, invasiveness, migration, self-renewal, epithelial to mesenchymal transition [EMT], and sensitivity to therapeutic approaches in preclinical research. (8)

In 2015, Dr. Moselhy gave us this list of natural products that target CSCs (6):

- Epigallocatechin-3-gallate [EGCG] – from green tea
- Baicalein – Chinese skullcap
- Curcumin – turmeric
- Cyclopamine – corn lilly
- Flavonoids [genistein] – soy, red clover, coffee
- Isothiocyanates – cruciferous vegetables
- Parthenolide – feverfew
- Quercetin – grapes, plums, berries
- Salinomycin – streptomyces albus
- Silibinin – milk thistle

Too Many Choices

These lists are not complete, as I have left out many substances, concentrating instead on the few discussed in this book. However, now you understand that the problem is not about finding the one elusive anti-cancer drug or botanical substance.

The problem is that we have too many anti-cancer substances to choose from. How do we narrow down the list and use them in an effective combination? Hopefully, this book will give you the information needed to select a few key repurposed drugs and supplements to target CSCs and the important metabolic pathways in a synergistic manner, resulting in the desired curative efficacy.

Curcumin from Turmeric

Isolated from turmeric, curcumin has a two-thousand year history of medicinal use as an anti-oxidant, anti-inflammatory, antimicrobial, anticarcinogenic, thrombus-suppressive, hepatoprotective, cardiovascular-protective, neuroprotective, and anti-arthritic. (9–11)

Curcumin as Anti-Cancer Stem Cell Agent

A massive body of scientific evidence on curcumin shows this natural plant substance kills CSCs while sparing normal cells. The food spice, curcumin (turmeric) is widely available as a nutritional supplement and targets CSCs.

Curcumin Blocks Glutamine Uptake

For example, in 2016, Dr. Y. T. Huang et al. wrote, "Curcumin Induces Apoptosis of Colorectal Cancer Stem Cells by Coupling with CD44 Marker." Dr. Huang and colleagues studied colorectal CSCs and found curcumin couples with the CD44 CSC membrane marker and blocks cell uptake of glutamine, inducing apoptosis in the CSC:

> [Curcumin] might have some blocking effect on the transport of glutamine into the cells, thus decreasing the glutamine content in the CD44+ cells and inducing apoptosis. (12)

Curcumin and EGCG for Breast Cancer Stem Cells

In 2015, Drs. Seyung S. Chung and Jaydutt Vadgama studied breast CSCs and reported synergy with curcumin and EGCG. The combination of curcumin and epigallocatechin gallate from green tea (EGCG) inhibit CSCs via downregulation of STAT3-NF-kB signaling. The CSC marker CD44+ protein, decreased following treatment of the cancer cells with curcumin and EGCG. Drs. Chung and Vadgama write that "the final destination of STAT3 and NF-κB signaling may be the CD44 expression and accompanied cancer stem cell phenotype." (13)

Note: Cancer stem cell "phenotype" accompanies the expression of the CD44 surface marker.

Curcumin Suppresses Cyclin D1 in Mantle Cell Lymphoma

In 2012, Dr. Zainul Hasanali et al. studied curcumin in a B-cell lymphoma (mantle cell) model, finding that curcumin inhibits nuclear factor kappa B (NF-κB) activation and downregulates cyclin D1, thereby inducing apoptosis. There was synergy with bortezomib, a new protease inhibitor drug used for hematologic malignancies. (14)

In 2015, Dr. Shishir Shishodia reported that curcumin inhibits NF-κB activation, induces cell cycle arrest at the G1/S-phase, and induces apoptosis in mantle cell lymphoma. Dr. Shishodia reports as follows:

> The expression of all NF-kappa-B-regulated gene products were downregulated by curcumin leading to the suppression of proliferation, cell cycle arrest at the G1/S-phase

of the cell cycle and induction of apoptosis as indicated by caspase activation. (15)

Making Curcumin More Bio-Available

Although there have been more than 120 clinical trials of curcumin, none have been successful because of poor bio-availability. Only one per cent of oral curcumin is bioavailable due to poor aqueous solubility (in water) and rapid metabolism. Drug inventors have been busy with new ideas to make curcumin more bioavailable and more effective, such as curcumin nanodiscs, and curcumin analogs with structural alterations, such as dimethylcurcumin. (16–21)

Combining curcumin with other synergistic natural substances such as sulforaphane, quercetin, and EGCG (from green tea) has also been suggested to augment activity. (18–21)

Summary of Curcumin's Effects on Cancer Stem Cells

In 2015, Dr. Peter Sordillo wrote an excellent summary of curcumin's ability to kill CSCs in "Curcumin and Cancer Stem Cells" in *Anti-Cancer Research*. Dr. Sordillo reported that curcumin inhibits NF-kB and inhibits the release of cancer-associated cytokines IL-6 and IL-8, resulting in inhibition and suppression of CSCs. (23)

Curcumin Inhibits Wnt and Notch Pathways

Both the Wnt and Notch pathways are important for CSC survival. Curcumin acts to inhibit and block multiple points along the Wnt pathway and Notch pathways, downregulating β-catenin and the genes for vascular endothelial growth factor (VEGF), cyclin D1, and c-Myc. Amazingly, curcumin has no deleterious effects on normal stem cells and targets only the CSCs. (23)

The reason offered for this selectivity is:

1) Curcumin has much greater uptake by cancer cells compared to normal cells.

2) Curcumin affects the micro-environment around the cancer stem cells by suppressing release of pro-inflammatory cytokines IL-6 and IL-8.

3) Curcumin induces cancer stem cells to undergo cell differentiation into a mature cell which then undergoes spontaneous or drug induced apoptosis.

4) Curcumin suppresses the Wnt pathway in cancer stem cells with inhibition of β-catenin, yet has the opposite effect on neural stem cells as it stimulates neurogenesis. (23)

Curcumin is highly lipophilic (oil soluble), crosses the blood-brain barrier easily, and as suggested by Dr. Sordillo, may serve as a "sensitizer" to conventional chemotherapy for treatment of glioblastoma. (24)

Curcumin and Wnt /TCF Beta-Catenin Pathway Inhibition

The key pathway for the CSC is the Wnt pathway, frequently upregulated in cancer cells.

In 2005, Dr. Park studied curcumin's effect on lung cancer stem cells, elucidating curcumin's mechanism of inhibition of Wnt/Beta Catenin pathway. The key signal protein for the Wnt pathway is β-catenin, which enters the nucleus, binds to TCF/LEF which activates expression of Cyclin D1 and c-Myc oncogenes. Dr. Park found no change in cytosolic or membranous B-catenin in curcumin-treated cancer cells. Rather, Dr. Park found decreased B-catenin and TCF-4 in the nucleus of the cancer cells resulting in reduced Wnt transcriptional activity in all cell lines. (25)

Others have confirmed the anti-CSC activity of curcumin via inhibition of the Hedgehog (HH) and Wnt pathways in multiple cancer cell lines. (26–28)

Curcumin Reduces BCL2 in Chemo-Resistant AML Stem Cells

In 2011, Dr. Jia Rao studied the anti-cancer effects of curcumin in nine separate acute myelogenous leukemia (AML) cell lines. Dr. Rao reports that chemotherapy resistance in acute myelogenous leukemia may be due to upregulation of the anti-apoptotic protein Bcl-2 in CD34+ CSCs. Dr. Rao found that treatment of the CSCs with curcumin reduces the Bcl-2 protein levels, leading to apoptosis, while showing no ill effects on normal cells. Dr. Rao writes:

> Curcumin downregulates Bcl-2 and induces apoptosis in DNR-insensitive [chemo-resistant leukemia stem cells], CD34+ AML cell lines and primary CD34+ AML cells. (29–30)

Note: DNR= daunorubicin chemotherapy. AML=acute myelogenous leukemia. Curcumin reduction of the anti-apoptotic protein BCL-2 has been found in other cancer cell types as well.

Curcumin: No Major Toxicities When Using up to 8 Grams per Day

Regarding does escalation studies, Dr. Rao writes: "Curcumin demonstrated **no major toxicities** in phase I and II clinical studies at doses of up to 8 g/day."(29)

Curcumin as Radio-Sensitizer and Radio-Protector

As an adjunct to radiotherapy, curcumin has been suggested as a radio-sensitizer for tumor cells, while it serves as radio-protector for normal cells. (30–33)

Curcumin HK2 and Voltage Dependant Anion Channel (VDAC) on Mitochondrial Membrane

In 2015, Dr. Tewri studied the molecular docking and mutational analysis of curcumin's interaction with human VDAC-1, finding conformational changes restricting movement, an indication that curcumin modulates the VDAC. These are pores on the outer mitochondrial membrane. (34)

Colorectal Cancer

In 2015, Dr. Wang studied the effect of curcumin on colorectal cancer cells, finding curcumin downregulated the expression and activity of Hexokinase 2 (HK2) and induced dissociation of HK2 from the mitochondria resulting in apoptosis. Dr. Wang writes:

> Curcumin downregulated the expression and activity of Hexokinase 2 [HK2] in HCT116 and HT29 [colorectal cancer] cells in a concentration-dependent manner, but

had little effect on the other key glycolytic enzymes…. On the other, **curcumin-induced dissociation of HK2 from the mitochondria, resulting in mitochondrial-mediated apoptosis.** (35)

In 2016, Dr. Bhoi studied a library of phytochemicals and their derivatives for optimal binding to HK2. Dr. Bhoi found a curcumin derivative, 1,2-dihydrobis(de-O-methyl)-curcumin to have "optimal binding affinity" for both HK1 and HK2. (36)

Berberine, "An Epiphany Against Cancer"—A Natural Wnt Pathway Inhibitor

Also called the Oregon grape, berberine is a traditional oriental medicine used for centuries to treat diarrhea and gastroenteritis. Berberine is also a natural Wnt pathway inhibitor, the major pathway for CSC maintenance, and is patented as a CSC agent. (37–52)

In 2019, Dr. Liu summarized the anti-tumor activities of Berberine, writing:

> Berberine affects the development of tumor cells through the inhibition of tumor cell growth…the induction of apoptosis and cell cycle arrest…. berberine can inhibit the migration and invasion of tumor cells… berberine treatment of tumor cells significantly inhibited NF-κB and ultimately decreased the expression of VEGF and IL-8 in tumor cells…ultimately, the antitumor effect of berberine may be related to epigenetic effects… berberine has been found to inhibit the expression of human DNA methyltransferases DNMT1 and DNMT3B in multiple myeloma U266 cells. (53)

An Epiphany Against Cancer

In 2014, Dr. Luis Miguel Guamán Ortiz reviewed the anti-cancer effects of berberine in his article entitled, *Berberine, an Epiphany Against Cancer*. Dr. Ortiz writes:

> Berberine (BBR) treatment promotes cell cycle arrest and death in human cancer cell lines, coupled to an increased expression of apoptotic factors … BBR has the potential to modulate and regulate **Wnt/β-catenin pathway** … regulate the expression of **Bcl-2** ..Berberine alters mitochondrial membrane potential, promotes release of cytochrome C, and triggers apoptosis in the cancer cell. (54)

In 2014, Dr. Park showed that berberine downregulates CSC-associated genes in pancreatic cancer cell lines. (52)

As noted in a previous chapter, berberine and metformin are both OXPHOS inhibitors via inhibition of mitochondrial complex 1 of the electron transport chain (ETC).

Berberine Synergy with Curcumin

In 2015, Dr. Balakrishna found Berberine synergistic when combined with curcumin in various cancer cell lines. (55) Others have found synergy of berberine, curcumin, and resveratrol in combination with chemotherapy drugs. (56–60)

Sulforaphane Anti-Cancer Stem Cell Agent

Sulforaphane and its precursor glucoraphanin, found in broccoli sprouts, is highly bioavailable and has low toxicity. Since the 1990s, there have been over 3000 medical publications on sulforaphane mostly in vitro and in vivo animal models, and over 50 human clinical trials. (61–62)

Mechanism of Action of Sulforaphane

In 2018, Dr. Mokhtari reviewed Sulforaphane in cancer chemoprevention, remarking on three major activities—anti-angiogenesis, anti-metastasis, and activation of protective autophagy—with inhibition of the following metabolic pathways:

> Sulforaphane [SFN] inhibits transcription factors hypoxia-inducible factor [HIF]-1alpha, nuclear factor-kappa-B [NF-kB], and proto-oncogene myc [c-Myc], resulting in the downregulation of key angiogenic and metastatic regulators, vascular endothelial growth factor [VEGF] and matrix metallopeptidase 9 [MMP-9], and thus, the reduction of angiogenic and metastatic potential..... sulforaphane [SFN] induces the recruitment and increases the expression of LC3 to autophagosomes, thus, increasing the activation of the autophagy pathway. (62)

In summary, sulforaphane inhibits the following pathways:

- HIF-1 (Hypoxia-inducible factor).
- NF-kb (Nuclear factor Kappa B—master controller of inflammation).
- C-Myc.
- VEGF (vascular endothelial growth factor).
- MMP (matrix metallo proteinase enzyme degrades extracellular matrix to allow invasion).
- Activates "Protective Autophagy" (survival mechanism).

Eliminates Breast Cancer Stem Cells in Vivo

In 2010, and 2013, Drs. Y. Li and T. Zhang studied sulforaphane in a breast cancer mouse xenograft model in vivo, finding that sulforaphane is "highly potent" for elimination of breast CSCs. Sulforaphane inhibited CSCs at a low concentration of (0.5 to 5 MicroMolar) without affecting the bulk (non-stem cell) cancer cells. Elimination of CSCs in primary xenografts was confirmed by failure of implanted tumors to grow in secondary mice. Beta-Catenin and Cyclin D1 levels were decreased by 80–85%. **Note:** Cyclin D1 is a target gene for Wnt/beta-catenin pathway. (63–64)

Sulforaphane Reaches Therapeutic Levels

In 2007, Dr. Cornblatt did a pilot study of eight healthy women undergoing reduction mammoplasty who were given a single dose of a broccoli sprout preparation containing 200 μmol (MicroMol) of sulforaphane one hour before surgery. When the breast tissue in the removed surgical specimen was examined, sulforaphane metabolites were readily measurable at concentrations effective against breast CSCs, based on the concentrations used in Dr. Li's study above. (65)

Pancreatic Cancer Stem Cells— Sonic Hedgehog Pathway

In 2009, Dr. Kallifatidis studied sulforaphane in a pancreatic cancer cell line, finding efficacy against CSCs:

> Sulforaphane targets pancreatic tumor-initiating cells by NF-kappa-B-induced anti-apoptotic signaling ..." (66)

In 2012, Dr. Rodova studied inhibition of pancreatic CSCs by sulforaphane (SFN), finding inhibition of the sonic hedgehog pathway as the **main mechanism**, writing:

Thus Sulforaphane potentially represents an inexpensive, safe and effective alternative for the management of pancreatic cancer. (67)

Sulforaphane for CSCs: Cancer Cell Types

Sulforaphane has been studied and found effective in preclinical in vitro and in vivo studies in various CSC types, and synergizes with chemotherapy and other natural substances:

- Pancreatic cancer stem cells (67)
- Triple-negative breast cancer stem cells (68–69)
- Lung cancer stem cells (70–71)
- Gastric cancer stem cells (72)
- Oral squamous cancer stem cells (73)
- Chronic leukemia stem cells (74)
- Sulforaphane synergy with Quercetin and EGCG (75–77)

Sulforaphane Depletes Glutathione (GSH) by 90 Per Cent!!

In 2008, Dr. Clarke found that sulforaphane inhibited prostate cancer cells by downregulating intracellular glutathione (GSH) and increasing reactive oxygen species (ROS), causing mitochondrial apoptosis. (78)

In 2005, Dr. Singh reported that sulforaphane caused rapid and marked depletion of intracellular glutathione levels in prostate cancer cells. He writes:

Sulforaphane [SFN] treatment caused a rapid decline in the level of GSH

[Glutathione]. For instance, the GSH levels in PC-3 [Prostate Cancer] cells treated for 3 and 6 h with 40 µm SFN were **reduced by about 90 and 94%,** respectively, compared with controls. (79)

Randomized Trial in Prostate Cancer

In 2015, Dr. Cipolla did a double-blinded, randomized, placebo-controlled trial of sulforaphane in 78 males with rising PSA levels after radical prostatectomy for prostate cancer. Treatment consisted of 60 mg of sulforaphane for 6 months over which time the sulforaphane group had a mean increase in PSA of 0.01 ng/ml compared to a 0.62 ng/ml increase for placebo. PSA doubling time in the sulforaphane group was 28.9 months compared to 15.5 months for the placebo group. Sulforaphane prolonged PSA doubling time, thus delaying "biochemical recurrence." (80)

Pro-Oxidant Sulforaphane Depletes Intracellular Glutathione

In 2017, Dr. DaCosta studied sulforaphane chemoprevention, finding an acute pro-oxidant effect resulting from depletion of intracellular glutathione. He writes:

Sulforaphane [SFN] actually has an acute pro-oxidant effect in cells, largely by depleting intracellular glutathione due to the formation and export of SFN-glutathione complexes [28]. SFN can also increase mitochondrial ROS generation by inhibiting complex III of the mitochondrial respiratory chain, which causes the accumulation of Ubisemiquinone, from which molecular oxygen receives electrons, resulting in the formation of superoxide and hydrogen peroxide. (81)

Others have found similar depletion of intracellular glutathione by sulforaphane, a feature that may be used to overcome resistance to platinum-based chemotherapy, and yet this may impair T cell function, an important part of the immune system. (82–84)

Sulforaphane Inhibits Mitochondrial OXPHOS

Prostate Cancer Studied In Vivo

In 2009, Dr. Xiao studied a sulforaphane in vitro prostate cancer model, finding:

> Sulforaphane statistically significant [sic] inhibited activities of mitochondrial respiratory chain enzymes in LNCaP and PC-3 cells [prostate cancer cell lines]. (85)

Sulforaphane Induces Protective Autophagy—Prostate CA

In 2006, Dr. Herman-Antosiewicz studied sulforaphane in a prostate cancer cell line, finding induction of "protective autophagy," and suggested that the addition of autophagy inhibitor would be synergistic, writing:

> Induction of autophagy represents a defense mechanism against sulforaphane-induced apoptosis in human prostate cancer cells..... It is reasonable to speculate that the cancer chemopreventive activity of sulforaphane may be enhanced by the simultaneous treatment with an inhibitor of autophagy. (86)

Sulforaphane Synergy with Autophagy Inhibitor Chloroquine

In 2013, Dr. Vyas studied sulforaphane in prostate cancer in mouse xenograft model. Previous in vitro studies showed sulforaphane causes induction of "protective autophagy" in prostate cancer cells, which "inhibits apoptotic cell death by delaying release of cytochrome c due to sequestration of mitochondria in autophagosomes."

In other words, the mitochondria cannot release apoptotic proteins freely into the cytoplasm because the mitochondria are sequestered in little bags called autophagosomes. Addition of autophagy inhibitor, chloroquine, significantly augmented the anti-cancer effects of sulforaphane in this animal model. (87) One might speculate about the synergy of sulforaphane with other autophagy inhibitors such as propranolol, thymoquinone, doxycycline etc.

In 2010, Dr. Kanematsu showed that autophagy inhibition **"significantly enhanced"** apoptosis (programmed cell death) when combined with sulforaphane in a breast cancer model, writing:

> These results indicate a cytoprotective role of autophagy against [sulforaphane] SFN-induced apoptosis and that the combination of SFN treatment with autophagy inhibition may be a promising strategy for breast cancer control. (88)

Similarly, in 2010, Dr. Nishikawa found that the addition of autophagy inhibitor "potentiated sulforaphane-induced apoptosis" in a colon cancer model. (89)

In 2010, Dr. Nishiwaka found that the addition of an autophagy inhibitor augmented the anti-angiogenic and apoptotic effects of sulforaphane in vitro in human umbilical vein endothelial cells (HUVECs). (90)

In 2018, Dr. Wilcox Studied the effect of sulforaphane on lung adeno carcinoma (A549) cells in vitro, finding the usually acidic contents of the lysosomes were made more alkaline by the sulforaphane treatment. Lung cancer cell variants with more acidic lysosomes were relatively resistant to the sulforaphane. (91)

Sulforaphane Synergy with Chemotherapy Agents

In 2017 and 2018, studies by Drs. Milczarek and Lee showed sulforaphane synergizes with chemotherapy agents 5-FU in triple-negative breast cancer and cisplatin in mesothelioma. (92–93)

Sulforaphane Neuro Protection, Antidepressant

In 2019, Dr. Klomparens reported on the neuroprotective effects of sulforaphane.

> Animal studies suggest that SFN [sulforaphane] supplementation could be disease-modifying for many common, debilitating central nervous system [CNS] diseases including Alzheimer's disease, Parkinson's disease, epilepsy, stroke, and others. (94)

Sulforaphane also has antidepressant, anxiolytic activities and protects against neurodegenerative disease and chemical induced neurotoxicity, etc. (95–102)

In 2015, Dr. Egea found the combination of melatonin with sulforaphane was synergistic with augmented neuroprotection. (103)

Next, we will discuss another botanical agent, pterostilbene.

Pterostilbene Cancer Stem Cell Agent

Pterostilbene, a methylated version of resveratrol found in blueberries, has greater bio-availability and potency than resveratrol as an anti-CSC agent.

In 2015, Dr. Chi-Hao Wu studied the effect of pterostilbene targeted against breast CSCs (MCF-7 cells) in vitro. His study showed that pterostilbene selectively killed breast CSCs which express the CD44 surface antigen. In addition, pterostilbene increased the sensitivity of breast CSCs to the killing effects of chemotherapy. The underlying mechanism of pterostilbene is degradation of Beta-Catenin via inhibition of Hedgehog/Akt/GSK3β signaling, thus inhibiting downstream expression of cancer growth factors C-Myc and Cyclin D1. (104)

Note: Beta Catenin is the main effector of the Wnt pathway (CSC pathway).

Lung Cancer

In 2013, Dr. Yang studied pterostilbene in adenocarcinoma of the lung, both in vitro and in vivo with mouse tumor xenografts. Dr. Yang showed pterostilbene significantly decreased the mitochondrial membrane potential and increased ROS with depletion of intracellular glutathione in the cancer cells. Expression of apoptosis pathway proteins BAX and Cytochrome C were upregulated. (105)

High Thru-Put Screening

Dr. Papandreou reported in 2015 on their study in which 1,726 small molecules were screened for activation of the Endoplasmic Reticulum (ER) stress response gene. Dr. Papandreou writes:

> Plant stilbenes pterostilbene and piceatannol were the most potent inducers of ER stress from this group. (106)

Pterostilbene Synergy with Autophagy Inhibitor chloroquine

Dr. Papandreou then determined by molecular analysis that pterostilbene blocks the Wnt/B-Catenin pathway and also induces autophagy in acute lymphoblastic leukemia cells. The authors found that

> combining pterostilbene [to induce ER stress] with chloroquine [to inhibit autophagy] leads to significant cellular toxicity in cells from aggressive acute lymphoblastic leukemia [ALL].... toxicity is more pronounced in cancer cells expressing **Wnt growth factors**. The toxicity of stilbenes in these ALL cells can be potentiated by the addition of autophagy inhibitors, suggesting a possible therapeutic application. (106)

For more on this topic, see chapter 16 on pterostilbene.

Parthenolide—Feverfew—Blocks NF-kB, Depletes Glutathione

Parthenolide (PTL) is the major active component in the feverfew plant (Tanacetum parthenium), used for centuries for migraine headache, and more recently for rheumatoid arthritis, due to its anti-inflammatory effects, blocking activation of nuclear factor kappa B (NF-kB). PTL is a member of the sesquiterpene lactone family of over 5,000 natural plant compounds (reported so far), many of which have anti-cancer activity. Many studies show robust anti-cancer activity of PTL, with inhibition of NF-kB, and depletion of intracellular glutathione. Additional studies show PTL to be an excellent agent for eradication of CSCs. (107–128)

In 2005, Dr. Monica Guzmán found that parthenolide, a potent inhibitor of nuclear factor kappa B (NF-kB), induces robust apoptosis in leukemia cells and preferentially targets the CSC population, inhibits NK-kB, activates P53, and increases ROS:

> [Parthenolide PTL] induces robust apoptosis in primary human acute myelogenous leukemia [AML] cells while sparing normal hematopoietic cells. Furthermore, parthenolide **also preferentially targets AML progenitor and stem cell populations.** Notably, in comparison to the standard chemotherapy drug cytosine arabinoside [Ara-C], PTL is much more specific to leukemia cells. The molecular mechanism of PTL-mediated apoptosis is strongly associated **with inhibition of nuclear factor κ B (NF-κB), pro-apoptotic activation of p53, and increased reactive oxygen species (ROS).** (109)

Glutathione Depletion

In 2013, Dr. Shanshan Pei reported that PTL targets the aberrant, upregulated glutathione metabolism in leukemia CSCs by inducing **almost complete glutathione depletion** and severe cell death. At the same time, there was only limited and transient perturbation in normal hematopoietic cells. In addition, the authors tested the combined effects of PTL with commonly used chemotherapy drugs Ara-C and Idarubicin, finding augmented synergistic effects. (110)

In 2017, Dr. Liu studied the anti-cancer effects of PTL in a colorectal cancer cell line, (SW620 in vitro), finding that

> multiple pathways are involved in PTL-induced apoptotic cell death in human cancer cells, including oxidative stress, intracellular thiol [glutathione] depletion, endoplasmic reticulum stress, caspase activation, and mitochondrial dysfunction…. PT exerts antiproliferative effect and induces apoptotic cell death of SW620 cells. In addition, PT prevents cell migration and invasion in a dose-dependent manner. Moreover, PT markedly suppressed migration/invasion-related protein expression, including E-cadherin, β-catenin, vimentin, Snail, cyclo-oxygenase-2 [COX-2], matrix metallo-proteinase-2 [MMP-2], and MMP-9 in SW620 cells. PT also inhibited the expression of anti-apoptotic proteins [Bcl-2 and Bcl-xL] and activated apoptosis terminal factor [caspase-3] in a dose-dependent manner….. The biological activity of PT is related to its ability to **inhibit nuclear factor-κB signaling**… These results suggest that PT treatment inhibits cell migration/invasion via the regulation of EMT markers, MMPs, and COX-2 expressions. (111)

In 1997, Dr. Bork showed that parthenolide completely inhibits activation of nuclear factor kappa B (NF-kB) at low concentrations of 5 micromolar, preventing transcription of the inflammatory cytokine IL-6. Thus, indicating a potent anti-inflammatory mechanism. (108)

Feverfew is active against the following cancer cell types:

- Colorectal Cancer (114–116)
- Melanoma (117)
- Breast cancer stem cells (118–119)
- Multiple myeloma stem cells (120–121)
- Nasopharyngeal cancer (122)
- Prostate cancer stem cells (123)
- Leukemia stem cells (124–129)

As you can see from this list, feverfew is a CSC agent.

Feverfew Therapeutic Blood Levels

In a 1988 *Lancet* article, Dr. Murphy reviewed successful randomized trials of feverfew for prevention of migraine headache, suggesting some level of therapeutic efficacy is obtained from oral ingestion of feverfew. (112)

However, difficulties in demonstrating therapeutic blood levels of feverfew after oral ingestion and concerns of poor bio-availability have spurred interest in derivatives or analogs with greater bio-availability. In 2004, Dr. Curry wrote:

> Feverfew, with up to 4 mg of parthenolide, given daily as an oral tablet is well tolerated without dose-limiting toxicity, but does not provide detectable plasma concentrations. Purification of parthenolide for administration of higher doses will be needed. (113)

The fact that studies like Dr. Murphy's above show feverfew efficacy for migraine headache suggests that Dr. Curry is wrong, and therapeutic blood levels are probably achieved with oral dosing. In the meantime, we await the availability of more bioavailable analogs of PTL. Hopefully these will become commercially available soon. (130–132)

Others - Milk Thistle (Silymarin), ECGC, Allicin (Garlic)

Milk thistle (silybin-phytosome-siliphos), a widely used herbal extract used for liver detoxification, inhibits the Wnt /B-catenin pathway. A number of preclinical studies have shown benefits and promising effects against CSCs. (133–135)

Epigallocatechin-3-gallate (EGCG) from green tea is an anti-CSC agent that works by downregulating NF-kB, showing synergy with quercetin, curcumin, and melatonin. (136–147)

Allicin (garlic) and diallyl disulfide target the Wnt pathway and are CSC agents. (148–157)

Conclusion

Many of the above natural Wnt inhibitors are also OXPHOS inhibitors that target CSCs. Since most of these agents induce protective autophagy, they may synergize with autophagy inhibitors such as propranolol, chloroquine, and thymoquinone. Targeting CSCs with nontoxic therapies is available and hopefully will be incorporated into routine oncology protocols soon, with expected improvement in outcomes. However, it is unlikely your oncologist will recommend or even have knowledge of these nontoxic cancer stem agents.

References Chapter 10: Targeting Cancer Stem Cells with NonToxic Therapies

1) Turdo, Alice, et al. "Meeting the challenge of targeting cancer stem cells." Frontiers in cell and developmental biology 7 (2019): 16.

2) Yan, Yongmin, Xiangsheng Zuo, and Daoyan Wei. "Concise review: emerging role of CD44 in cancer stem cells: a promising biomarker and therapeutic target." Stem cells translational medicine 4.9 (2015): 1033-1043.

3) Yu, Zuoren, et al. "Cancer stem cells." The international journal of biochemistry & cell biology 44.12 (2012): 2144-2151.

4) Gali-Muhtasib, H., et al. "Cell death mechanisms of plant-derived anticancer drugs: beyond apoptosis." Apoptosis: an international journal on programmed cell death 20.12 (2015): 1531-1562

5) Scarpa, E. S., and P. Ninfali. "Phytochemicals as Innovative Therapeutic Tools against Cancer Stem Cells." International journal of molecular sciences 16.7 (2014): 15727-15742.

6) Moselhy, J., et al. "Natural Products That Target Cancer Stem Cells." Anticancer research 35.11 (2015): 5773.

7) Gu, Hao-Feng, Xue-Ying Mao, and Min Du. "Prevention of breast cancer by dietary polyphenols—role of cancer stem cells." Critical Reviews in Food Science and Nutrition (2019): 1-16.

8) Liskova, Alena, et al. "Dietary Phytochemicals Targeting Cancer Stem Cells." Molecules 24.5 (2019): 899.

9) Mbese, Zintle, Vuyolwethu Khwaza, and Blessing Atim Aderibigbe. "Curcumin and Its Derivatives as Potential Therapeutic Agents in Prostate, Colon and Breast Cancers." Molecules 24.23 (2019): 4386.

10) Xiang, De-Biao, et al. "Curcumin: From a controversial "panacea" to effective antineoplastic products." Medicine 99.2 (2020): e18467.

11) Das, Undurti N. "Molecular Mechanisms of Action of Curcumin and Its Relevance to Some Clinical Conditions." Curcumin for Neurological and Psychiatric Disorders. Academic Press, 2019. 325-332.

12) Huang, Yu-Ting, et al. "Curcumin Induces Apoptosis of Colorectal Cancer Stem Cells by Coupling with CD44 Marker." Journal of agricultural and food chemistry (2016).

13) Chung, Seyung S., and Jaydutt V. Vadgama. "Curcumin and Epigallocatechin Gallate Inhibit the Cancer Stem Cell Phenotype via Down-regulation of STAT3–NFκB Signaling." Anticancer research 35.1 (2015): 39-46.

14) Hasanali, Zainul, Kamal Sharma, and Elliot Epner. "Flipping the cyclin D1 switch in mantle cell lymphoma." Best Practice & Research Clinical Haematology 25.2 (2012): 143-152.

15) Shishodia, Shishir, et al. "Curcumin (diferuloylmethane) inhibits constitutive NF-κB activation, induces G1/S arrest, suppresses proliferation, and induces apoptosis in mantle cell lymphoma." Biochemical pharmacology 70.5 (2005): 700-713.

16) Singh, Amareshwar TK, et al. "Curcumin nanodisk-induced apoptosis in mantle cell lymphoma." Leukemia & lymphoma 52.8 (2011): 1537-1543.

17) Tadmor, Tamar, and Aaron Polliack. "Mantle cell lymphoma: curcumin nanodisks and possible new concepts on drug delivery for an incurable lymphoma." Leukemia & lymphoma 52.8 (2011): 1418.

18) Yallapu, Murali M., Meena Jaggi, and Subhash C. Chauhan. "Curcumin nanomedicine: a road to cancer therapeutics." Current pharmaceutical design 19.11 (2013): 1994.

19) Jin, G., et al. "Combination curcumin and (−)-epigallocatechin-3-gallate inhibits colorectal carcinoma microenvironment-induced angiogenesis by JAK/STAT3/IL-8 pathway." Oncogenesis 6.10 (2017): e384-e384.

20) Langner, Ewa, Marta Kinga Lemieszek, and Wojciech Rzeski. "Lycopene, sulforaphane, quercetin, and curcumin applied together show improved antiproliferative potential in colon cancer cells in vitro." Journal of food biochemistry 43.4 (2019): e12802.

21) Negrette-Guzmán, Mario. "Combinations of the antioxidants sulforaphane or curcumin and the conventional antineoplastics cisplatin or doxorubicin as prospects for anticancer chemotherapy." European journal of pharmacology (2019): 172513.

22) Srivastava, Nishtha S., and Rai Ajit K. Srivastava. "Curcumin and quercetin synergistically inhibit cancer cell proliferation in multiple cancer cells and modulate Wnt/β-catenin signaling and apoptotic pathways in A375 cells." Phytomedicine 52 (2019): 117-128.

23) Sordillo, Peter P., and Lawrence Helson. "Curcumin and cancer stem cells: curcumin has asymmetrical effects on cancer and normal stem cells." Anticancer Research 35.2 (2015): 599-614.

24) Sordillo, Laura A., Peter P. Sordillo, and Lawrence Helson. "Curcumin for the treatment of glioblastoma." Anticancer Research 35.12 (2015): 6373-6378.

25) Park, Chi Hoon, et al. "The inhibitory mechanism of curcumin and its derivative against β-catenin/Tcf signaling." FEBS letters 579.13 (2005): 2965-2971.

26) Vallée, Alexandre, Yves Lecarpentier, and Jean-Noël Vallée. "Curcumin: a therapeutic strategy in cancers by inhibiting the canonical WNT/β-catenin pathway." Journal of Experimental & Clinical Cancer Research 38.1 (2019): 323.

27) Zhu, Jian-Yun, et al. "Curcumin suppresses lung cancer stem cells via inhibiting Wnt/β-catenin and sonic hedgehog pathways." Phytotherapy Research 31.4 (2017): 680-688.

28) Li, Xiaoting, et al. "Sonic hedgehog and Wnt/β-catenin pathways mediate curcumin inhibition of breast cancer stem cells." Anti-cancer drugs 29.3 (2018): 208-215.

29) Rao, Jia, et al. "Curcumin reduces expression of Bcl-2, leading to apoptosis in daunorubicin-insensitive CD34+ acute myeloid leukemia cell lines and primary sorted CD34+ acute myeloid leukemia cells." J Transl Med 9.1 (2011): 71.

30) Giordano, Antonio, and Giuseppina Tommonaro. "Curcumin and cancer." Nutrients 11.10 (2019): 2376.

31) Khafif, A. V. I., et al. "Curcumin: a new radio-sensitizer of squamous cell carcinoma cells." Otolaryngology—Head and Neck Surgery 132.2 (2005): 317-321.

32) Khafif, Avi, et al. "Curcumin: A potential radio-enhancer in head and neck cancer." The Laryngoscope 119.10 (2009): 2019-2026.

33) Jagetia GC1. Radioprotection and radiosensitization by curcumin. Adv Exp Med Biol. 2007; 595:301-20.

34) Tewari, Debanjan, et al. "Modulation of the mitochondrial voltage dependent anion channel (VDAC) by curcumin." Biochimica et Biophysica Acta (BBA)-Biomembranes 1848.1 (2015): 151-158.

35) Wang, Ke, et al. "Curcumin inhibits aerobic glycolysis and induces mitochondrial-mediated apoptosis through hexokinase II in human colorectal cancer cells in vitro." Anti-Cancer Drugs 26.1 (2015): 15-24.

36) Bhoi, Sudhir Ranjan, et al. "In silico analysis of hexokinase-I and II as potential drug targets in cancer." Pharm. Biol. Eval 3 (2016): 351-359.

37) Ashrafizadeh, Milad, et al. "Therapeutic and biological activities of berberine: The involvement of Nrf2 signaling pathway." Journal of Cellular Biochemistry 121.2 (2020): 1575-1585.

38) Liu, Jian, et al. "MDM2 inhibition-mediated autophagy contributes to the pro-apoptotic effect of berberine in p53-null leukemic cells." Life Sciences 242 (2020): 117228.

39) Kumar, Ravi, et al. "Berberine induces dose-dependent quiescence and apoptosis in A549 cancer cells by modulating cell cyclins and inflammation independent of mTOR pathway." Life Sciences (2020): 117346.

40) Shinji, Sayaka, et al. "Berberine and palmatine inhibit the growth of human rhabdomyosarcoma cells." Bioscience, Biotechnology, and Biochemistry 84.1 (2020): 63-75.

41) Gong, Chenxue, et al. "Berberine inhibits proliferation and migration of colorectal cancer cells by downregulation of GRP78." Anti-Cancer Drugs 31.2 (2020): 141-149.

42) Kwon, Sohee, and Andrew T. Chan. "Extracting the benefits of berberine for colorectal cancer." The Lancet. Gastroenterology & hepatology (2020).

43) Lin, Yen-Shu, et al. "Different mechanisms involved in the berberine-induced antiproliferation effects in triple-negative breast cancer cell lines." Journal of Cellular Biochemistry 120.8 (2019): 13531-13544.

44) Kaboli, Parham Jabbarzadeh, et al. "Antitumor effects of berberine against EGFR, ERK1/2, P38 and AKT in MDA-MB231 and MCF-7 breast cancer cells using molecular modelling and in vitro study." Pharmacological Reports 71.1 (2019): 13-23.

45) El Khalki, Lamyae, et al. "Berberine Impairs the Survival of Triple Negative Breast Cancer Cells: Cellular and Molecular Analyses." Molecules 25.3 (2020): 506.

46) Zhang, Chaohe, et al. "Effects of Berberine and Its Derivatives on Cancer: A Systems Pharmacology Review." Frontiers in Pharmacology 10 (2019): 1461.

47) Albring, Kai Frederik, et al. "Berberine acts as a natural inhibitor of Wnt/β-catenin signaling—Identification of more active 13-arylalkyl derivatives." Biofactors 39.6 (2013): 652-662.

48) Xie, Dajiang, et al. "Berberine inhibits cell growth via Wnt/beta-catenin signaling in glioma." Int J Clin Exp Med 12.1 (2019): 652-657.

49) Ruan, H., et al. "Berberine binds RXRα to suppress β-catenin signaling in colon cancer cells." Oncogene 36.50 (2017): 6906-6918.

50) Kaboli, Parham Jabbarzadeh, et al. "Targets and mechanisms of berberine, a natural drug with potential to treat cancer with special focus on breast cancer." European Journal of Pharmacology 740 (2014): 584-595.

51) Hsieh, Hsiu-Mei, et al. "Berberine-containing pharmaceutical composition for inhibiting cancer stem cell growth or carcinoma metastasis and application thereof." U.S. Patent Application No. 14/790,154.

52) Park, S. H., J. H. Sung, and Namhyun Chung. "Berberine diminishes side population and down-regulates stem cell-associated genes in the pancreatic cancer cell lines PANC-1 and MIA PaCa-2." Molecular and Cellular Biochemistry 394.1-2 (2014): 209-215.

53) Liu, Da, et al. "A natural isoquinoline alkaloid with antitumor activity: studies of the biological activities of berberine." Frontiers in Pharmacology 10 (2019): 9.

54) Ortiz, Luis Miguel Guamán, et al. "Berberine, an epiphany against cancer." Molecules 19.8 (2014): 12349-12367. Epiphany Against Cancer

55) Balakrishna, Acharya, and M. Hemanth Kumar. "Evaluation of synergetic anticancer activity of berberine and curcumin on different models of A549, Hep-G2, MCF-7, Jurkat, and K562 cell lines." BioMed Research International 2015 (2015).

56) Wang, Kai, et al. "Synergistic chemopreventive effects of curcumin and berberine on human breast

cancer cells through induction of apoptosis and autophagic cell death." Scientific Reports 6 (2016): 26064.

57) Pandey, Arvind, et al. "Berberine and curcumin target survivin and STAT3 in gastric cancer cells and synergize actions of standard chemotherapeutic 5-fluorouracil." Nutrition and Cancer 67.8 (2015): 1295-1306.

58) McCubrey, James A., et al. "Effects of berberine, curcumin, resveratrol alone and in combination with chemotherapeutic drugs and signal transduction inhibitors on cancer cells—Power of nutraceuticals." Advances in Biological Regulation 67 (2018): 190-211.

59) McCubrey, James A., et al. "Effects of resveratrol, curcumin, berberine and other nutraceuticals on aging, cancer development, cancer stem cells and microRNAs." Aging (Albany NY) 9.6 (2017): 1477.

60) Maiti, Panchanan, Alexandra Plemmons, and Gary L. Dunbar. "Combination treatment of berberine and solid lipid curcumin particles increased cell death and inhibited PI3K/Akt/mTOR pathway of human cultured glioblastoma cells more effectively than did individual treatments." PloS One 14.12 (2019).

61) Yagishita, Yoko, et al. "Broccoli or Sulforaphane: Is It the Source or Dose That Matters?" Molecules 24.19 (2019): 3593.

62) Mokhtari, Reza Bayat, et al. "The role of Sulforaphane in cancer chemoprevention and health benefits: a mini-review." Journal of Cell Communication and Signaling 12.1 (2018): 91-101.

63) Li, Yanyan, et al. "Sulforaphane, a dietary component of broccoli/broccoli sprouts, inhibits breast cancer stem cells." Clinical Cancer Research 16.9 (2010): 2580-2590.

64) Li, Y., and T. Zhang. "Targeting cancer stem cells with sulforaphane, a dietary component from broccoli and broccoli sprouts." Future Oncology (London, England) 9.8 (2013): 1097-1103.

65) Cornblatt, Brian S., et al. "Preclinical and clinical evaluation of sulforaphane for chemoprevention in the breast." Carcinogenesis 28.7 (2007): 1485-1490.

66) Kallifatidis G, Rausch V, Baumann B, et al. Sulforaphane targets pancreatic tumour-initiating cells by NF-kappaB-induced antiapoptotic signalling. Gut. 2009; 58:949–63.

67) Rodova, Mariana, et al. "Sonic hedgehog signaling inhibition provides opportunities for targeted therapy by sulforaphane in regulating pancreatic cancer stem cell self-renewal." PloS one 7.9 (2012): e46083.

68) Castro, Nadia P., et al. "Sulforaphane suppresses the growth of triple-negative breast cancer stem-like cells in vitro and in vivo." Cancer Prevention Research 12.3 (2019): 147-158.

69) Burnett, Joseph P., et al. "Sulforaphane enhances the anticancer activity of taxanes against triple negative breast cancer by killing cancer stem cells." Cancer Letters 394 (2017): 52-64.

70) Zhu, Jianyun, et al. "miR-19 targeting of GSK3β mediates sulforaphane suppression of lung cancer stem cells." The Journal of Nutritional Biochemistry 44 (2017): 80-91.

71) Zheng, Zhongnan, et al. "Sulforaphane metabolites inhibit migration and invasion via microtubule-mediated Claudins dysfunction or inhibition of autolysosome formation in human non-small cell lung cancer cells." Cell Death & Disease 10.4 (2019): 1-16.

72) Ge, Miaomiao, et al. "Sulforaphane inhibits gastric cancer stem cells via suppressing sonic hedgehog pathway." International Journal of Food Sciences and Nutrition 70.5 (2019): 570-578.

73) Liu, Chia-Ming, et al. "Sulforaphane targets cancer stemness and tumor initiating properties in oral squamous cell carcinomas via miR-200c induction." Journal of the Formosan Medical Association 116.1 (2017): 41-48.

74) Lin, Li-Ching, et al. "Sulforaphane potentiates the efficacy of imatinib against chronic leukemia cancer stem cells through enhanced abrogation of Wnt/β-catenin function." Journal of Agricultural and Food Chemistry 60.28 (2012): 7031-7039.

75) Srivastava, Rakesh K., et al. "Sulforaphane synergizes with quercetin to inhibit self-renewal capacity of pancreatic cancer stem cells." Frontiers in Bioscience (Elite edition) 3 (2011): 515.

76) Chen, Huaping, et al. "Epigallocatechin gallate and sulforaphane combination treatment induce apoptosis in paclitaxel-resistant ovarian cancer cells through hTERT and Bcl-2 down-regulation." Experimental Cell Research 319.5 (2013): 697-706.

77) Mokhtari, Reza Bayat, et al. "Combination therapy in combating cancer." Oncotarget 8.23 (2017): 38022.

78) Clarke, John D., Roderick H. Dashwood, and Emily Ho. "Multi-targeted prevention of cancer by sulforaphane." Cancer Letters 269.2 (2008): 291-304.

79) Singh, Shivendra V., et al. "Sulforaphane-induced cell death in human prostate cancer cells is initiated by reactive oxygen species." Journal of Biological Chemistry 280.20 (2005): 19911-19924.

80) Cipolla, Bernard G., et al. "Effect of sulforaphane in men with biochemical recurrence after radical prostatectomy." Cancer prevention research 8.8 (2015): 712-719.

81) Dacosta, Christopher, and Yongping Bao. "The role of MicroRNAs in the chemopreventive activity of sulforaphane from cruciferous vegetables." Nutrients 9.8 (2017): 902.

82) Xu, Ying, et al. "Sulforaphane Mediates Glutathione Depletion via Polymeric Nanoparticles to Restore Cisplatin Chemosensitivity." ACS Nano 13.11 (2019): 13445-13455.

83) Liang, Jie, et al. "Sulforaphane inhibits inflammatory responses of primary human T-cells by increasing ROS and depleting glutathione." Frontiers in Immunology 9 (2018): 2584.

84) Kim, Bok-Ryang, et al. "Effects of glutathione on antioxidant response element-mediated gene expression and apoptosis elicited by sulforaphane." Cancer Research 63.21 (2003): 7520-7525.

85) Xiao, Dong, et al. "Cellular responses to cancer chemopreventive agent D, L-sulforaphane in human prostate cancer cells are initiated by mitochondrial reactive oxygen species." Pharmaceutical Research 26.7 (2009): 1729-1738.

86) Herman-Antosiewicz, Anna, Daniel E. Johnson, and Shivendra V. Singh. "Sulforaphane causes autophagy to inhibit release of cytochrome C and apoptosis in human prostate cancer cells." Cancer Research 66.11 (2006): 5828-5835.

87) Vyas, Avani R., et al. "Augmentation of D, L-sulforaphane-mediated prostate cancer chemoprevention by pharmacologic inhibition of autophagy using chloroquine in a transgenic mouse model." Prevention Research (2013): 3695-3695

88) Kanematsu, Sayaka, et al. "Autophagy inhibition enhances sulforaphane-induced apoptosis in human breast cancer cells." Anticancer Research 30.9 (2010): 3381-3390.

89) Nishikawa, Takeshi, et al. "Inhibition of autophagy potentiates sulforaphane-induced apoptosis in human colon cancer cells." Annals of Surgical Oncology 17.2 (2010): 592-602.

90) Nishikawa, Takeshi, et al. "The inhibition of autophagy potentiates anti-angiogenic effects of sulforaphane by inducing apoptosis." Angiogenesis 13.3 (2010): 227-238

91) Wilcox, Alexander, et al. "Sulforaphane Alters the Acidification of the Vacuole to Trigger Cell Death." bioRxiv (2018): 371534.

92) Milczarek, Małgorzata, et al. "Autophagic cell death and premature senescence: New mechanism of 5-fluorouracil and sulforaphane synergistic anticancer effect in MDA-MB-231 triple negative breast cancer cell line." Food and Chemical Toxicology 111 (2018): 1-8.

93) Lee, Yoon-Jin, and Sang-Han Lee. "Pro-oxidant activity of sulforaphane and cisplatin potentiates apoptosis and simultaneously promotes autophagy in malignant mesothelioma cells." Molecular Medicine Reports 16.2 (2017): 2133-2141

94) Klomparens, Eric A., and Yuchuan Ding. "The neuroprotective mechanisms and effects of sulforaphane." Brain Circulation 5.2 (2019): 74-83.

95) Wu, S., et al. "Sulforaphane produces antidepressant-and anxiolytic-like effects in adult mice." Behavioural Brain Research 301 (2015): 55.

96) Sun, Y., et al. "Sulforaphane protects against brain diseases: roles of cytoprotective enzymes." Austin Journal of Cerebrovascular Disease & Stroke 4.1 (2017).

97) Mao, Leilei, et al. "Abstract TP559: Sulforaphane Confers Neuroprotection Against Neuronal Loss, White Matter Injury and BBB Damage Following Experimental Vascular Cognitive Impairment." Stroke 50.Suppl_1 (2019): ATP559-ATP559.

98) Yu, Chang, et al. "Sulforaphane improves outcomes and slows cerebral ischemic/reperfusion injury via inhibition of NLRP3 inflammasome activation in rats." International Immunopharmacology 45 (2017): 74-78.

99) Tarozzi, Andrea, et al. "Sulforaphane as a potential protective phytochemical against neurodegenerative diseases." Oxidative Medicine and Cellular Longevity 2013 (2013).

100) Kim, Hyunjin Vincent, et al. "Amelioration of Alzheimer's disease by neuroprotective effect of sulforaphane in animal model." Amyloid 20.1 (2013): 7-12.

101) Morroni, Fabiana, et al. "Neuroprotective effect of sulforaphane in 6-hydroxydopamine-lesioned mouse model of Parkinson's disease." Neurotoxicology 36 (2013): 63-71.

102) Zhou, Qian, et al. "Sulforaphane protects against rotenone-induced neurotoxicity in vivo: Involvement of the mTOR, Nrf2 and autophagy pathways." Scientific Reports 6.1 (2016): 1-12.

103) Egea, Javier, et al. "Melatonin–sulforaphane hybrid ITH 12674 induces neuroprotection in oxidative stress conditions by a 'drug–prodrug' mechanism of action." British Journal of Pharmacology 172.7 (2015): 1807-1821.

104) Wu, Chi-Hao, et al. "Targeting cancer stem cells in breast cancer: potential anticancer properties of 6-shogaol and pterostilbene." Journal of Agricultural and Food Chemistry 63.9 (2015): 2432-2441.

105) Yang, Yang, et al. "Pterostilbene exerts antitumor activity via the Notch1 signaling pathway in human lung adenocarcinoma cells." PloS one 8.5 (2013): e62652.

106) Papandreou, Ioanna, et al. "Plant stilbenes induce endoplasmic reticulum stress and their anti-cancer activity can be enhanced by inhibitors of autophagy." Experimental Cell Research 339.1 (2015): 147-153.

107) Freund, R. R. A., et al. "Advances in chemistry and bioactivity of parthenolide." Natural Product Reports (2019).

108) Bork, Peter M., et al. "Sesquiterpene lactone containing Mexican Indian medicinal plants and pure sesquiterpene lactones as potent inhibitors of transcription factor NF-κB." FEBS Letters 402.1 (1997): 85-90.

109) Guzman, Monica L., et al. "The sesquiterpene lactone parthenolide induces apoptosis of human acute myelogenous leukemia stem and progenitor cells." Blood 105.11 (2005):

110) Pei, Shanshan, et al. "Targeting aberrant glutathione metabolism to eradicate human acute myelogenous leukemia cells." Journal of Biological Chemistry 288.47 (2013): 33542-33558.

111) Liu, Yu Chuan, et al. "Parthenolide promotes apoptotic cell death and inhibits the migration and invasion of SW620 (colorectal cancer) cells." Intestinal Research 15.2 (2017): 174.

112) Murphy, J. J., S. Heptinstall, and J. R. A. Mitchell. "Randomised double-blind placebo-controlled trial of feverfew in migraine prevention." The Lancet 332.8604 (1988): 189-192.

113) Curry, Eardie A., et al. "Phase I dose escalation trial of feverfew with standardized doses of parthenolide in patients with cancer." Investigational New Drugs 22.3 (2004): 299-305.

114) Zhu, Shi Mao, et al. "Parthenolide inhibits transforming growth factor β1-induced epithelial-mesenchymal transition in colorectal cancer cells." Intestinal Research 17.4 (2019): 527.

115) Kim, Se-Lim, et al. "Parthenolide suppresses tumor growth in a xenograft model of colorectal cancer cells by inducing mitochondrial dysfunction and apoptosis." International Journal of Oncology 41.4 (2012): 1547-1553.

116) Kim, Se-Lim, et al. "Parthenolide exerts inhibitory effects on angiogenesis through the downregulation of VEGF/VEGFRs in colorectal cancer." International Journal of Molecular Medicine 33.5 (2014): 1261-1267.

117) Lesiak, Karolina, et al. "Parthenolide, a sesquiterpene lactone from the medical herb feverfew, shows anticancer activity against human melanoma cells in vitro." Melanoma Research 20.1 (2010): 21-34.

118) Carlisi, D., et al. "Parthenolide and DMAPT exert cytotoxic effects on breast cancer stem-like cells by inducing oxidative stress, mitochondrial dysfunction and necrosis." Cell Death & Disease 7.4 (2016): e2194-e2194.

119) Araújo, Thaise Gonçalves, et al. "Parthenolide and Its Analogues: A New Potential Strategy for the Treatment of Triple-Negative Breast Tumors." Current Medicinal Chemistry (2019).

120) Gunn, Ellen J., et al. "The natural products parthenolide and andrographolide exhibit anti-cancer stem cell activity in multiple myeloma." Leukemia & Lymphoma 52.6 (2011): 1085-1097.

121) Huynh, Daniel T., et al. "Parthenolide and structurally related natural products as anti-cancer stem cell agents: a new era in treatment of multiple myeloma." Tumor Biology (2010): 4292-4292.

122) Liao, Kun, et al. "Parthenolide inhibits cancer stem-like side population of nasopharyngeal carcinoma cells via suppression of the NF-κB/COX-2 pathway." Theranostics 5.3 (2015): 302.

123) Kawasaki, Brian T., et al. "Effects of the sesquiterpene lactone parthenolide on prostate tumor-initiating cells: An integrated molecular profiling approach." The Prostate 69.8 (2009): 827-837.

124) Steele, A. J., et al. "The sesquiterpene lactone parthenolide induces selective apoptosis of B-chronic lymphocytic leukemia cells in vitro." Leukemia 20.6 (2006): 1073-1079.

125) Guzman, Monica L., et al. "An orally bioavailable parthenolide analog selectively eradicates acute myelogenous leukemia stem and progenitor cells." Blood, 110.13 (2007): 4427-4435.

126) Guzman, Monica L., et al. "The sesquiterpene lactone parthenolide induces apoptosis of human acute myelogenous leukemia stem and progenitor cells." Blood 105.11 (2005): 4163-4169.

127) Zong, Hongliang, et al. "In vivo targeting of leukemia stem cells by directing parthenolide-loaded nanoparticles to the bone marrow niche." Leukemia 30.7 (2016): 1582-1586.

128) Diamanti, Paraskevi, et al. "Parthenolide eliminates leukemia-initiating cell populations and improves survival in xenografts of childhood acute lymphoblastic leukemia." Blood, 121.8 (2013): 1384-1393.

129) Pei, Shanshan, et al. "Rational design of a parthenolide-based drug regimen that selectively eradicates acute myelogenous leukemia stem cells." Journal of Biological Chemistry 291.42 (2016): 21984-22000.

130) Wu, C., et al. "Antiproliferative activities of parthenolide and golden feverfew extract against three human cancer cell lines." Journal of Medicinal Food 9.1 (2006): 55-61.

131) Parada-Turska, Jolanta, et al. "Antiproliferative activity of parthenolide against three human cancer cell lines and human umbilical vein endothelial cells." Pharmacological reports 59.2 (2007): 233.

132) Mathema, Vivek Bhakta, et al. "Parthenolide, a sesquiterpene lactone, expresses multiple anti-cancer and anti-inflammatory activities." Inflammation 35.2 (2012): 560-565.

133) Eo, Hyun Ji, Gwang Hun Park, and Jin Boo Jeong. "Inhibition of Wnt signaling by silymarin in human colorectal cancer cells." Biomolecules & Therapeutics 24.4 (2016): 380.

134) Sharifpanah, Fatemeh, et al. "The milk thistle (Silybum marianum) compound Silibinin stimulates leukopoiesis from mouse embryonic stem cells." Phytotherapy Research 33.2 (2019): 452-460.

135) Mao, Jie, et al. "Combined treatment with sorafenib and silibinin synergistically targets both HCC cells and cancer stem cells by enhanced inhibition of the phosphorylation of STAT3/ERK/AKT." European Journal of Pharmacology 832 (2018): 39-49.

136) Das, Plabon K., et al. "Natural Compounds Targeting Cancer Stem Cells: A Promising Resource for Chemotherapy." Anti-Cancer Agents in Medicinal Chemistry (2019).

137) Wei, Ran, et al. "Epigallocatechin-3-Gallate (EGCG) Suppresses Pancreatic Cancer Cell Growth, Invasion, and Migration partly through the Inhibition of Akt Pathway and Epithelial–Mesenchymal Transition: Enhanced Efficacy When Combined with Gemcitabine." Nutrients 11.8 (2019): 1856.

138) Sun, Xianchao, et al. "Epigallocatechin-3-gallate inhibits bladder cancer stem cells via suppression of sonic hedgehog pathway." Oncology Reports 42.1 (2019): 425-435.

139) Chen, Yue, et al. "Epigallocatechin-3-gallate inhibits colorectal cancer stem cells by suppressing Wnt/β-catenin pathway." Nutrients 9.6 (2017): 572.

140) Zhu, Jianyun, et al. "Wnt/β-catenin pathway mediates Epigallocatechin-3-gallate (EGCG) inhibition of lung cancer stem cells." Biochemical and biophysical research communications 482.1 (2017): 15-21.

141) Toden, Shusuke, et al. "Epigallocatechin-3-gallate targets cancer stem-like cells and enhances

5-fluorouracil chemosensitivity in colorectal cancer." Oncotarget 7.13 (2016): 16158.

142) Li, Ya-Jun, et al. "Epigallocatechin-3-gallate inhibits nasopharyngeal cancer stem cell self-renewal and migration and reverses the epithelial–mesenchymal transition via NF-κB p65 inactivation." Tumor Biology 36.4 (2015): 2747-2761.

143) Tang, Su-Ni, et al. "The dietary bioflavonoid quercetin synergizes with epigallocatechin gallate (EGCG) to inhibit prostate cancer stem cell characteristics, invasion, migration and epithelial-mesenchymal transition." Journal of Molecular Signaling 5.1 (2010): 14.

144) Chung, Seyung S., and Jaydutt V. Vadgama. "Curcumin and epigallocatechin gallate inhibit the cancer stem cell phenotype via down-regulation of STAT3–NFκB signaling." Anticancer Research 35.1 (2015): 39-46.

145) Zhang, Lingyun, et al. "Melatonin and (−)-Epigallocatechin-3-Gallate: Partners in Fighting Cancer." Cells 8.7 (2019): 745.

146) Fujiki, Hirota, et al. "Human cancer stem cells are a target for cancer prevention using epigallocatechin gallate." Journal of Cancer Research and Clinical Oncology 143.12 (2017): 2401-2412.

147) Fujiki, Hirota, et al. "Cancer prevention with green tea and its principal constituent, EGCG: From early investigations to current focus on human cancer stem cells." Molecules and Cells 41.2 (2018): 73.

148) Haghi, Atousa, Haniye Azimi, and Roja Rahimi. "A comprehensive review on pharmacotherapeutics of three phytochemicals, curcumin, quercetin, and allicin, in the treatment of gastric cancer." Journal of Gastrointestinal Cancer 48.4 (2017): 314-320.

149) Bhaumik, Ishani, et al. "Natural product inspired allicin analogs as novel anti-cancer agents." Bioorganic Chemistry 86 (2019): 259-272.

150) Li, Chenlong, et al. "Allicin induces apoptosis through activation of both intrinsic and extrinsic pathways in glioma cells." Molecular Medicine Reports 17.4 (2018): 5976-5981.

151) Zhang, Yan, et al. "Phytochemicals of garlic: Promising candidates for cancer therapy." Biomedicine & Pharmacotherapy 123 (2020): 109730.

152) Chan, Marion M., Rensa Chen, and Dunne Fong. "Targeting cancer stem cells with dietary phytochemical-Repositioned drug combinations." Cancer Letters 433 (2018): 53-64.

153) Li, Xiaoting, et al. "Diallyl Trisulfide inhibits breast cancer stem cells via suppression of Wnt/β-catenin pathway." Journal of Cellular Biochemistry 119.5 (2018): 4134-4141

154) Xie, Xinhua, et al. "Diallyl disulfide inhibits breast cancer stem cell progression and glucose metabolism by targeting CD44/PKM2/AMPK signaling." Current Cancer Drug Targets 18.6 (2018): 592-599.

155) Zhang, Qi, et al. "Wnt/β-catenin signaling mediates the suppressive effects of diallyl trisulfide on colorectal cancer stem cells." Cancer Chemotherapy and Pharmacology 81.6 (2018): 969-977.

156) Tao, Qingxia, et al. "Diallyl trisulfide inhibits proliferation, invasion and angiogenesis of glioma cells by inactivating Wnt/β-catenin signaling." Cell and Tissue Research 370.3 (2017): 379-390.

157) Almatroodi, Saleh A., et al. "Garlic and its Active Compounds: A Potential Candidate in The Prevention of Cancer by Modulating Various Cell Signalling Pathways." Anti-Cancer Agents in Medicinal Chemistry 19.11 (2019): 1314-1324.

Chapter 11

Repurposed Drugs Targeting Stem Cells I

THIS CHAPTER LOOKS AT A number of drugs that have been repurposed as CSC agents.

Sulfasalazine

Sulfasalazine (Azulfidine®) is an old drug used for inflammatory bowel disease (Crohn's and ulcerative colitis) and rheumatoid arthritis, psoriasis, and ankylosing spondylitis at a dosage of 2–6 grams per day. The drug is surprisingly well tolerated in many patients suffering from chronic inflammatory conditions requiring long-term use.

Sulfasalazine for Refractory Chronic Urticaria

Urticaria is an unpleasant skin condition characterized by raised itchy welts that is frequently associated with allergic response. Urticaria usually responds promptly to anti-histamines. Sulfasalazine is useful for patients suffering from antihistamine unresponsive (recalcitrant) chronic idiopathic urticaria at a dosage of 2 grams per day. The mechanism is thought to be inhibition of histamine release from mast cells. (1)

Cancer Cell Glutathione— Targeting the xCT Pathway

Sulfasalazine is a cystine/glutamate antiporter inhibitor. Let's translate this into English. The cystine/glutamate antiporter system (also called system Xc- or xCT) is an amino acid transport system involved in transport of cystine into the cell for production of glutathione, the major intracellular anti-oxidant. Glutamate, an excitatory neurotransmitter, is exchanged for the cystine and sent out to the extracellular space. The protein involved in this antiporter transport system is a heterodimer (two subunits), one of which is the light chain, also called xCT. (2)

Note: Cystine is an amino acid.

Depleting Intracellular Glutathione

Sulfasalazine targets CSCs by inhibiting this antiporter system, the xCT pathway for cystine uptake. By starving the CSC of cystine, intracellular glutathione is depleted, rendering the cancer cell defenseless to oxidative stress, ultimately resulting in cell death from oxidative damage. Cancer stem cells can be identified by specific protein surface markers such as CD44 and CD133. The surface marker CD44 is closely associated with the xCT protein, involved in active transport of cystine, and ultimately intracellular glutathione levels.

Gastric Cancer CD44+ Stem Cells

In 2014, Dr. Kohei Shitara's group reported at the ASCO Annual Meeting on the "effect of sulfasalazine (SSZ) on cancer stem-like cells (CSCs) via inhibiting the xCT signal pathway."

Dr. Kohei Shitara et al. reported that the CD44 surface adhesion molecule is expressed in stem-like cancer cells. They found gastric CSCs have a variant marker called CD44v that interacts with xCT, the glutamate-cystine transporter and maintains high levels of the intracellular reduced glutathione (GSH), which is the major intracellular anti-oxidant, rendering the cancer cells resistant to cytotoxic oxidative therapies. In this study, tumor tissues obtained by endoscopic biopsy were studied for CD44v and GSH level before and 2 weeks after escalating doses of oral sulfasalazine. Eleven patients were dosed with from 8–12 grams a day for two weeks. The optimal dose was considered to be 8 grams per day. Dr. Shitara et al. found that

> Sulfasalazine acts as an xCT inhibitor which suppressed CD44v-dependent tumor growth and increased sensitivity to cytotoxic drugs in vivo study. (3)

In 2011, Dr. Takatsugu Ishimoto et al. found sulfasalazine inhibited the xCT membrane transporter of cystine uptake, thereby suppressing CD44-dependent tumor growth in CSCs (in vivo) by depleting glutathione levels and rendering the cancer cell defenseless to ROS (reactive oxygen species). They stated:

> The activity of xCT-mediated cystine uptake in cancer cells is highly associated with cell proliferation, chemoresistance, and tumor growth. Sulfasalazine significantly enhanced the effect of cis-platinum chemotherapy, making the drug effective at low doses. (4)

The cancer cell has upregulated uptake of cystine to maintain anti-oxidant defenses. Blocking the xCT uptake of cystine causes depletion of glutathione which reduces the "ROS defense," leading to a form of "ferropto-

sis" described in chapter 21, on artemisinin. In short, cancer cells contain large amounts of iron, needed for their enhanced metabolic activities. This iron is highly reactive with oxygen molecules in the cell leading to production of massive amounts of ROS, which if unchecked by anti-oxidant defenses will lead to cancer cell damage and death, a process called "ferroptosis". (5–8) (24)

Ferroptosis Synergy with Artemisinin

In 2019, Dr. Xiaojun Xia et al. discussed how xc- inhibitors such as erastin, SAS (sulfasalazine), artesunate and sorafenib bring about ferroptosis by:

> Caus[ing] a significant decrease in the intracellular GSH [glutathione] levels and promotes lethal accumulation of ROS [reactive oxygen species] and iron-dependent cell death due to disruption of cellular redox balance. (9)

In view of the above, one might speculate on a synergistic effect using the combination of both artemisinin (artesunate) and sulfasalazine, which produce ferroptosis by different mechanisms. The peroxide bridge in artemisinin/artesunate reacts with iron in lysosomes to produce ROS. The inhibition of cystine uptake and downregulation of intracellular glutathione strips the cancer cell of anti-oxidant defense, rendering it more vulnerable to ROS. One might then raise a concern about toxicity to normal cells with this combination, a topic for future study with NIH funding. We await these further studies.

Sulfasalazine has been studied in other cancer cell types, including:

- Head and neck cancer (10)
- B-cell lymphoma (11–12)
- Small-cell lung cancer (13)
- Pancreatic cancer (14)
- Breast cancer (15)
- Prostate cancer (16)

Cystine Supplied by Fibroblasts in the Micro-Environment

In 2003, Dr. Peter Gout et al. studied the effect of sulfasalazine on xc– deficient mouse model of T cell lymphoma. These lymphoma cells were genetically modified to knock out the active transport of cystine, and should have been non-viable. However, they grew quite well because of fibroblasts in the micro-environment were "**hijacked**" to feed cystine to the lymphoma cells. The supportive role of the hijacked fibroblasts was inhibited by impairing their cystine uptake by sulfasalazine. Dr. Gout's group found that implanted mouse lymphoma growth was markedly suppressed by low doses of sulfasalazine (0.15 and 0.2 micromolar). They write:

> We found that replication of x(c)- -deficient Nb2–11 lymphoma cells can be sustained in vitro, in the absence of cystine uptake enhancers, by co-culturing with IMR-90 fibroblasts known to secrete cysteine. SASP (sulfasalazine), at 0.15 and 0.2 mM, arrested replication of fibroblast-driven Nb2–11(lymphoma) cells by 93 and 100%, respectively, without impeding fibroblast proliferation. (12)

Inhibition of Nuclear Factor Kappa B

Sulfasalazine is a potent inhibitor of nuclear factor kappa B (NF-kB) accounting for its use as an anti-inflammatory drug. (17–19)

Question of Impairment of T Cell Immunity

The in vitro activation and expansion of T lymphocytes is dependent on xCT, cystine uptake, and glutathione levels. In vitro studies show that sulfasalazine induces apoptosis in T lymphocytes, raising questions about negative effects on the host immune system. (20–23)

In 2019, Dr. Michael Arensman et al. studied this question using an in vitro and in vivo mouse model in which the xCT protein in pancreatic cancer tumor cells was genetically deleted. In addition, xCT knockout mice were also studied. They were quite surprised to find that "knocking out" the xCT cystine importer in genetically modified mice did not impair T cell anti-tumor immunity, writing:

> Surprisingly, T cell proliferation and anti-tumor immunity were not impaired in xCT knockout mice, leading us to evaluate the possibility of combining systemic xCT loss with the immunotherapeutic agent anti–CTLA-4... Surprisingly, although deletion of the xCT led to impaired tumor growth, **T cell proliferation was unaffected**.... The combination of xCT deletion with anti–CTLA-4 resulted in a remarkable increase in durable responses, **suggesting that systemic inhibition of xCT is a viable strategy to expand the efficacy of anti-cancer immunotherapies.** (23)

Thus, in vivo T cell expansion does not require a functioning xCT. This is comforting. However, it would be nice to see additional studies confirming that host anti-cancer immune T cell function is unimpaired by sulfasalazine treatment. Studies showing synergy of sulfasalazine with CAR T cell therapy and checkpoint inhibitor therapy would be a good topic for future study with NIH funding.

Adverse Effects—CNS Toxicity

Although considered safe as a long-term drug treatment in rheumatology patients, sulfasalazine crosses the blood-brain barrier and can result in CNS toxicity, so caution is advised. (25–27) Sulfasalazine is poorly absorbed (3–12%), and has a 5–10 hour half-life.

Conclusion for Sulfasalazine

The elegant 2014 study by Dr. Shitara's group on gastric tumor CD44 markers pre- and post-op shows that sulfasalazine has substantial clinical activity in vivo (in humans). This study suggested therapeutic blood levels are indeed attained at the optimal dosage of 8 grams per day. However, this is a rather large dosage for any drug, which may cause hesitation, especially when there are other more attractive repurposed drug alternatives. Although preclinical studies look promising, I would like to see more data in human clinical trials showing efficacy and low toxicity before becoming more enthusiastic about sulfasalazine. One wonders about combining sulfasalazine with other ferroptosis-inducing agents, such as artesunate, to enhance efficacy. We await these studies as well. (28–36) Next, we discuss Mefloquine as cancer stem cell agent.

Mefloquine as Anti Stem Cell Agent

Chloroquine and mefloquine (Lariam) are old antimalarial drugs, autophagy inhibitors that disrupt lysosomes. In 2013, Dr. Mahadeo Sukhai et al. screened a library of drugs for greatest activity against acute myelogenous leukemia (AML) stem cells. Dr. Sukhai and colleagues found mefloquine was second most active after ivermectin with a half maximal effective concentration (EC50) of less than 8 microMolar.

Mefloquine specifically targets lysosomal function and accumulates in the lysosomes of the malarial parasite. Dr. Sukhai's group found that mefloquine directly disrupted lysosomes of AML cells (and progenitor stem cells) in a dose-dependent manner as measured by release of cathepsins into the cytosol, leaving normal hematopoietic cells unharmed. Serum concentrations of mefloquine up to 5 µM (micromolar) have been reported in individuals receiving 250 mg weekly for malaria prophylaxis. Thus, antileukemia concentrations of mefloquine may be pharmacologically achievable with weekly doses of one 250 mg. tablet, commonly used for malaria prevention. (39)

Synergy of Mefloquine and Artemisinin

The drug displaying the most synergistic activity in combination with mefloquine is artemisinin, identified by Dr. Sukhai and colleagues' drug-screening project. Both are antimalaria drugs. These two drugs are commonly given together in treatment for prevention of malaria. The two in combination synergistically increased ROS production. The anti-cancer effect was reversed by the anti-oxidant vitamin E (tocopherol). (39)

Dr. Sukhai et al. write:

Mefloquine, a quinoline approved for the treatment and prevention of malaria, has toxicity for human AML [acute myelogenous leukemia] cells including AML progenitors [stem cells], while sparing normal human hematopoietic cells treated with the same doses.....antileukemic effects of mefloquine are mediated through disruption of lysosomes, a previously unappreciated mechanism of action of this drug. (39)

Mefloquine in Gastric Cancer

In 2016, Dr. Yanwei Liu et al. studied anti-cancer effect of mefloquine on a gastric cancer cell line in vitro and in vivo mouse xenograft models, finding inhibition at low concentration of 0.5 to 0.7 micromolar. There was enhanced activity in combination with chemotherapy drug, paclitaxel (Taxol).

> Mefloquine potently inhibits proliferation and induces apoptosis of a panel of human gastric cancer cell lines, with EC50 [in the range of] 0.5–0.7 μM. In two independent gastric cancer xenograft mouse models, mefloquine significantly inhibits growth of both tumors. (40)

In 2013, Dr. Kun-Huang Yan et al. studied mefloquine in a prostate cancer cell line in vitro and in vivo finding high cytotoxicity causing cancer cell death, and improved survival of the treated mice. (41)

In 1992, Dr. Hans Glaumann et al. reported on the anti-cancer mechanism of mefloquine in an animal model. Mefloquine caused an expansion of the lysosomal apparatus, earliest seen within 24 hours and lasting for some 7 days. (42)

1) Mefloquine is a lysosomotropic drug that accumulates in lysosomes;

2) Mefloquine impairs lipid degradation with ensuing accumulation of lipids in lysosomes; and

3) Lysosomal trapping explains the high-volume distribution of mefloquine. (42)

Mefloquine has been studied and shows anti-cancer activity in these cancer cell lines:

- Colorectal cancer (43)
- Cervical cancer (44)
- Liver cancer (45)
- Chronic lymphocytic leukemia (CLL) (46)

Mefloquine Neuro-Toxicity

Caution is advised before using mefloquine as well as other quinolones. Although originally marketed as safe for malaria prophylaxis, recent studies show an alarming incidence of neurologic toxicity, which may be "clinically occult," and in some cases, irreversible. (47–48)

A possible mechanism of mefloquine toxicity was elucidated by Dr. Anthony Mawson in his 2013 article, "Mefloquine use, psychosis, and violence: a retinoid toxicity hypothesis." Dr. Mawson wrote:

> The use of mefloquine in the prevention and treatment of malaria has been increasingly linked to a broad range of neuropsychiatric effects, including depression, psychosis, and violence. The symptoms of mefloquine toxicity may result from the spillage of stored retinoids from the damaged liver into the circulation and their transport to the gut and brain, causing the adverse neuropsychiatric and gastrointestinal symptoms as a function of an endogenous form of hypervitaminosis A. (49–50)

Chloroquine Eliminates Cancer Stem Cells

Chloroquine is an antimalaria drug that has been used for over 80 years and was recently repurposed for treatment of auto-immune disease. Chloroquine changes the normally acidic lysosome to a more alkaline pH, thereby inhibiting autophagy in cancer cells. In addition, chloroquine prevents fusion of the lysosome with the autophagosome in the late stage of autophagy.

In 2014, Dr. Dong Soon Choi et al. studied the effects of chloroquine in triple-negative breast cancer cells, finding inhibition of breast CSCs. (51)

Dr. Steve Pascolo et al. (2016) write that chloroquine may be used as an adjuvant to chemotherapy:

> Daily uptake of clinically acceptable doses (less than 10mg/kg) of Chloroquine in addition to chemo-radio-therapy increases the survival of glioblastoma patients. (52)

Chloroquine doubled the median survival time in glioblastoma patients. In a 2006 clinical trial by Dr. Julio Sotelo et al., 30 post-op glioblastoma patients were treated with oral chloroquine, 150 mg per day for 12 months. Median survival after surgery was 24 months for chloroquine-treated patients and 11 months for controls. (53)

Chloroquine is Cancer Stem Cell Agent

Dr. Dong Soon Choi et al. report (2014) that Chloroquine is an effective CSC agent. (51) Chloroquine as an anti-CSC agent has been studied in the following CSCs via inhibition of autophagy:

- Triple-negative breast cancer (51)(54)
- Pancreatic cancer stem cells (55–57)
- Combined with metformin for premalignant lesions (59)
- Leukemia stem cells (60–61)
- Melanoma (62)

Monitor for Retinal Toxicity

Hydroxychloroquine HCQ, a less toxic version of chloroquine, is in common use by rheumatologists (HCQ is Plaquenil) and is considered equally effective. In 2017, Dr. Ciska Verbaanderd et al. reviewed chloroquine (CQ) and HCQ as anti-cancer agents, writing:

> The usual dose for long-term use [rheumatoid arthritis and lupus] is 250 mg of CQ-phosphate per day. For HCQ, doses for long-term use range between 200 and 400 mg per day.

> It is advised that patients receiving chronic CQ or HCQ therapy be monitored through regular ophthalmic examinations [3–6 month intervals], full blood counts and blood glucose level checks.

> Interestingly, CQ and HCQ have already been tested in combination with over 40 other drugs in preclinical cancer research. Both CQ and HCQ can effectively increase the efficacy of various anti-cancer drugs…. in combination with CQ or HCQ include[ing] chemotherapeutic drugs, tyrosine kinase inhibitors, various monoclonal antibodies, hormone therapies and radiotherapy.

> More than 30 clinical studies are currently evaluating HCQ and CQ in different cancers, most of them with the rationale to increase the efficacy of other anti-cancer therapies through inhibition of treatment-induced autophagy. (63)

Long-term use of HC or CQ may cause retinal toxicity, therefore routine patient monitoring for retinal toxicity by an ophthalmologist is recommended. (64)

Ivermectin (Stromectol)

Ivermectin (Stromectol) is a potent blocker of the Wnt pathway at low doses. Ivermectin is an "astonishingly safe" anti-helminthic drug that the FDA-approved in the U.S. for treatment of pediatric scabies. More than 200 million people take the drug globally for prevention or treatment of parasitic disease. There has been extensive use of ivermectin as a veterinary drug for pets and farm animals. (66–77)

Ivermectin Anti-Leukemic Activity

In 2010, Drs. Sumaiya Sharmeen et al. at the University of Toronto screened a library of 100 drugs for activity against a leukemic cell line. They reported ivermectin as the top candidate for inducing leukemic cell death at low micromolar concentrations. Ivermectin also delayed leukemia tumor growth in mouse xenograft models. (78)

Tracking Wnt -TCF Perfectly

In 2014, Dr. Alice Melotti et al. published a study on "Ivermectin inhibition of Wnt - TCF pathway in cancer" in *EMBO Molecular Medicine*. Dr. Melotti and colleagues used a transcriptional reporter assay for TCF activity driven by ß-catenin to test a collection of 1,040 drugs and small molecules (Microsource 1040 library).

Only one agent perfectly tracked the gene expression profile induced by blocking the TCF gene, and therefore blocks the Wnt pathway.

That was ivermectin, the anti-helminthic drug derived from the bacteria strain Streptomyces avermitilis. This has profound significance for anti-CSC therapy, because blocking the Wnt pathway is the key to killing CSCs. (65)

The Wnt PATHWAY—Key to Cancer Stem Cell Destruction

Cancer Cells upregulate the Wnt Pathway— Wnt **ON**: This is BAD.

The Wnt pathway controls embryonic development and cell proliferation and is massively upregulated in CSCs. In 2015, Dr. Mathur reports that inhibiting the Wnt pathway is the key to killing CSCs in a B-cell lymphoma model. (79)

Important!!! Inhibiting the Wnt pathway kills CSCs.

If the Wnt pathway is **ON**, this is BAD. If the Wnt Pathway is **OFF**, this is GOOD, because beta-catenin is degraded.

- Wnt OFF: In the absence of Wnt signals, a cellular complex degrades β-catenin, so there is no entry of the β-catenin protein into the nucleus, the gene TCF/LEF is suppressed, and no nuclear transcription of Cyclin D1 or other growth signals takes place.
- Wnt ON: βeta-catenin is NOT degraded, and instead the accumulated β-catenin enters the nucleus and activates the target genes such as LEF-1, c-Myc and Cyclin D1. (80)

100-Fold Elevated Expression of Wnt Target Genes in Stem Cells

In 2015, Dr. Rohit Mathur et al. from MD Anderson studied B-cell lymphoma, finding that the mantle cell lymphoma (MCL) CSCs have an elevated expression of Wnt target genes **greater than 100-fold** compared with non-stem cells. The authors also reported that blocking the Wnt pathway kills CSCs in MCL. Dr. Mathur et al write:

> The high rate of MCL relapse after initial apparent clinical remissions achieved with conventional chemotherapy… implicates a role for chemo-resistant Mantle Cell Lymphoma – Initiating Cells [stem cells called MCL-ICs] in relapse. Here we showed that MCL-ICs [stem cells] have functional properties of cancer stem cells: high expression of ALDH, anti-oxidant enzymes, chemoresistance-associated genes, and stem cell associated transcription factors, while still retaining [the gene mutation] t(11;14) (q13; q32) and overexpression of cyclin D1 [a proliferation signal]. Our analysis showed that MCL-ICs **overexpress a subset of Wnt ligands** and **FZD receptors** and that **Wnt signaling is activated in MCL-ICs.**… Treatment of primary [mantle cell lymphoma] MCL cells with **Wnt inhibitors preferentially eliminated MCL-ICs [initiating cells, stem cells], which was not achieved with the current chemotherapy** agents vincristine, doxorubicin, or even with the recently FDA-approved agent ibrutinib.

> Burton tyrosine kinase [BTK] has been shown to be a negative regulator of Wnt signaling. Therefore, it is not surprising that ibrutinib [a BTK inhibitor] probably resulted in inducing Wnt signaling rather than inhibiting it and thereby could not eliminate MCL-ICs. **Our results suggest that the inability of conventional chemotherapy to kill MCL-ICs can be overcome by adding inhibitors of Wnt signaling.** (79)

Note: Dr. Mathur's group are reporting that Wnt pathway inhibitors are effective for CSCs while conventional chemotherapy (including the new drug Ibrutinib) are all ineffective for CSCs.

Salinomycin: A Potent Wnt Inhibitor

Salinomycin, a potent Wnt pathway inhibitor that is FDA-approved for veterinary use in animals, has striking activity against CSCs. The chemical structure of salinomycin bears a resemblance to ivermectin. Toxicity is a potential drawback for human use. (81–82) The mechanism is accumulation and sequestration of iron in lysosomes, inducing CSCs death in a process known as ferroptosis, which works by accumulating and sequestering iron in lysosomes. In 2017, Dr. Trang Mai writes:

> In response to the ensuing cytoplasmic depletion of iron, cells triggered the degradation of ferritin in lysosomes, leading to further iron loading in this organelle. Iron-mediated production of reactive oxygen species promoted lysosomal membrane permeabilization, activating a cell death pathway consistent with ferroptosis.(82)

Salinomycin is also a CSC agent. Toxicity limits its use to animals, as salinomycin is not approved for human use. (82–90)

Vitamin A Derivatives—Retinoids ATRA

I was interested in vitamin A derivatives as anti-cancer agents when I learned that Ben Williams survived glioblastoma with a cocktail of repurposed drugs that included 13-cis retinoic acid (Accutane), 160 mg/day on a two week-on one-week-off schedule, over 6 months in 1995. He is still alive and well today.

His inspiring story can be found in his book, *"Surviving Terminal Cancer."* Accutane is a synthetic vitamin A derivative and a well-known acne drug. Since his doctor would not prescribe Accutane, Mr. Williams drove across the border from San Diego to purchase it at a Mexican pharmacy over the counter, no prescription required.

Curative for Pro-Myelocytic Leukemia— Targets Cancer Stem Cells

The vitamin A derivative, all-trans retinoic acid (ATRA), also known as tretinoin (Vesinoid®) is curative for pro-myelocytic leukemia, and has been found to target CSCs in glioblastoma, breast cancer, and head and neck cancer cell lines in vitro. (91–99)

Retinoids, vitamin A and its analogs, are involved in stem cell differentiation, and reduced retinoid signaling is required for cancer development and proliferation. Retinoids may be useful in cancer treatment as they induce differentiation and arrest proliferation. (99–101)

Here is the ATRA dosage according to the FDA package insert:

Vesinoid® [ATRA All-Trans Retinoic Acid] is available by prescription from US Pharmacies as 10 mg gel caps. Dosage for pro-myelocytic leukemia is 45 mg per square meter per day [80–90 mg per day for adult male 160 lbs.] administered as two evenly divided doses until complete remission is documented. [Reference: FDA insert for Vesinoid – ATRA]

Safety of High-Dose Vitamin A

Alternatively, vitamin A can be used instead of a synthetic vitamin A derivative. For example, Dr. Paul Anderson's protocol includes 25,000 IU vitamin A daily. In 2004, Dr. Alberts studied vitamin A dosages up to 75,000 IU per day for a year in subjects with sun-damaged skin and found this dosage efficacious and safe. Doses of vitamin A up to 300,000 IU per day were well tolerated for up to a year. Dr. Alberts writes:

Having previously shown that vitamin A doses as high as 300,000 IU/day were well tolerated for up to 1 year in patients with advanced cancers, we were interested in evaluating the safety and efficacy of retinyl palmitate doses in the intermediate range of 25,000–75,000 IU/day in the treatment of patients with sun-damaged skin. (101)

Vitamin A Derivatives for Nephroblastoma (Wilm's Tumor)

In 2018, Dr. Friesenbichler treated two pediatric patients with Wilm's tumor with 13-cis retinoic acid (isotretinoin, also called Accutane) added on to a chemotherapy protocol with good results and no recurrence.(102)

ATRA Modulates Gene Expression in Cancer Cells

In 2019, Dr. Lara Lima et al. reviewed 31 preclinical "Vesinoid® (ATRA) studies involving nine different human cancer types (neuroblastoma, acute myeloid leukemia, breast cancer, lung cancer, pancreatic cancer, glioma, glioblastoma, embryonal carcinoma, and colorectal cancer) treated with ATRA at concentrations ranging from 10–100 µmol/L for times ranging from 1–21 days. They state:

miRNAs are endogenous, small, noncoding RNAs that **regulate gene expression** by binding to their target mRNAs [messenger RNA], leading to degradation and/or translational repression. (103)

Dr. Lima and colleagues studied the ATRA-induced miRNA expression in cancer cells, finding:

ATRA... was able to modulate the expression of more than 300 miRNAs, and inhibit invasive behavior and deregulated growth of cancer cells, resulting in total tumor remission in some cases. ATRA may thus be broadly effective for neoplasm treatment and prevention.... ATRA has also been shown to function as an anti-cancer agent in several neoplasms, such as gastric cancer, breast cancer, leukemia, nephroblastoma, melanoma, lung cancer, and neuroblastoma (103)

ATRA Markedly Augments Anti-Tumor Immunity

In 2019, Dr. Lu Huang et al. studied ATRA in lung cancer and colon cancer mouse xenografts, finding ATRA markedly upregulated anti-tumor immunity. Dr. Huang's group write:

Flow cytometry assays conducted on intratumoral immune cells revealed that ATRA-treatment decreased the CD8+ T to T-reg cellular ratios while increasing the ratios of CD8+ T to T-reg cells... Taken together, this study uncovered a previously unrecognized role for ATRA in augmenting immunotherapy. These preclinical immunotherapy findings can be translated into the cancer clinic. (104)

It seems that new research on vitamin A derivatives as anti-cancer agents for hepatoma and glioma reveals that Ben Williams was ahead of his time and quite correct to add Accutane to his anti-cancer cocktail. (105–106)

Common Antibiotics—Doxycycline

Doxycycline and other commonly used antibiotics inhibit mitochondrial biogenesis in CSCs and may ultimately find their place in routine use as anti-CSC agents. The common antibiotic doxycycline works by blocking bacterial ribosomal protein production. Mammalian mitochondria are remarkably similar to bacteria. Lynn Margulis theorized (the endo-symbiotic theory) that, in fact, mitochondria evolved from bacteria.

Doxycycline and High-Dose IV Vitamin C - A Lethal Combination for Cancer Stem Cells

Dr. Michael Lisanti's group published a study in *Oncotarget* (June 2017) using an in vitro breast cancer cell model showing that doxycycline and high-dose IV vitamin C are a lethal combination for eradication of CSCs. Indeed, this is a major advance in our understanding of CSC eradication. (107–109)

Additional repurposed drugs will be discussed in the following chapter.

References for Chapter 11: Repurposed Drugs Targeting Cancer Stem Cells

1) McGirt, Laura Y., et al. "Successful treatment of recalcitrant chronic idiopathic urticaria with sulfasalazine." Archives of dermatology 142.10 (2006): 1337-1342.

2) Lewerenz, Jan, et al. "The cystine/glutamate antiporter system xc– in health and disease: from molecular mechanisms to novel therapeutic opportunities." Antioxidants & redox signaling 18.5 (2013): 522-555.

3) Shitara, Kohei, et al. "Effect of sulfasalazine (SSZ) on cancer stem-like cells (CSCs) via inhibiting xCT signal pathway: Phase 1 study in patients with gastric cancer

(EPOC 1205)." ASCO Annual Meeting Proceedings. Vol. 32. No. 15_suppl. 2014.

4) Ishimoto, Takatsugu, et al. "CD44 variant regulates redox status in cancer cells by stabilizing the xCT subunit of system xc– and thereby promotes tumor growth." Cancer cell 19.3 (2011): 387-400.

5) Sehm, Tina, et al. "Sulfasalazine impacts on ferroptotic cell death and alleviates the tumor microenvironment and glioma-induced brain edema." Oncotarget 7.24 (2016): 36021.

6) Kim, Eun Hye, et al. "CISD2 inhibition overcomes resistance to sulfasalazine-induced ferroptotic cell death in head and neck cancer." Cancer letters 432 (2018): 180-190.

7) Abdullah, Md, Do Hyung Kim, and Seung Jin Lee. "System xc-inhibition shares features of necroptosis and ferroptosis in hepatocellular carcinoma cells." (2019): 278-278.

8) Yu, Haochen, et al. "Sulfasalazine-induced ferroptosis in breast cancer cells is reduced by the inhibitory effect of estrogen receptor on the transferrin receptor." Oncology reports 42.2 (2019): 826-838.

9) Xia, Xiaojun, et al. "The Relationship between Ferroptosis and Tumors: A Novel Landscape for Therapeutic Approach." Current gene therapy 19.2 (2019): 117-124.

10) Yoshikawa, M., et al. "xCT inhibition depletes CD44v-expressing tumor cells that are resistant to EGFR-targeted therapy in head and neck squamous cell carcinoma." Cancer research 73.6 (2013): 1855.

11) Bebb, G., et al. "Sulfasalazine, inhibits growth of mantle cell lymphoma (MCL) cell cultures via cyst (e) ine starvation and delays tumour growth in a newly developed murine MCL model." Blood. Vol. 102. No. 11. 2003.

12) Gout, Peter W., Chris R. Simms, and May C. Robertson. "In vitro studies on the lymphoma growth-inhibitory activity of sulfasalazine." Anticancer drugs 14.1 (2003): 21-29.

13) Guan, Jun, et al. "The x c- cystine/glutamate antiporter as a potential therapeutic target for small-cell lung cancer: use of sulfasalazine." Cancer chemotherapy and pharmacology 64.3 (2009): 463-472.

14) Lo, M., et al. "Potential use of the anti-inflammatory drug, sulfasalazine, for targeted therapy of pancreatic cancer." Current Oncology 17.3 (2010): 9-16.

15) Narang, Vishal S., et al. "Suppression of cystine uptake by sulfasalazine inhibits proliferation of human mammary carcinoma cells." Anticancer research 23.6C (2002): 4571-4579.

16) Doxsee, Daniel W., et al. "Sulfasalazine-induced cystine starvation: Potential use for prostate cancer therapy." The Prostate 67.2 (2007): 162-171

17) Wahl, Christian, et al. "Sulfasalazine: a potent and specific inhibitor of nuclear factor kappa B." The Journal of clinical investigation 101.5 (1998): 1163-1174.

18) Gan, Hua-Tian, You-Qin Chen, and Qin Ouyang. "Sulfasalazine inhibits activation of nuclear factor-κB in patients with ulcerative colitis." Journal of gastroenterology and hepatology 20.7 (2005): 1016-1024.

19) Weber, Christoph K., et al. "Suppression of NF-κB activity by sulfasalazine is mediated by direct inhibition of IκB kinases α and β." Gastroenterology 119.5 (2000): 1209-1218.

20) Liptay, Susanne, et al. "Inhibition of nuclear factor kappa B and induction of apoptosis in T-lymphocytes by sulfasalazine." British journal of pharmacology 128.7 (1999): 1361-1369.

21) Liptay, Susanne, et al. "Molecular mechanisms of sulfasalazine-induced T-cell apoptosis." British journal of pharmacology 137.5 (2002): 608-620.

22) Doering, J., et al. "Induction of T lymphocyte apoptosis by sulphasalazine in patients with Crohn's disease." Gut 53.11 (2004): 1632-1638.

23) Arensman, Michael D., et al. "Cystine–glutamate antiporter xCT deficiency suppresses tumor growth while preserving antitumor immunity." Proceedings of the National Academy of Sciences 116.19 (2019): 9533-9542.

24) Bebber, Christina M., et al. "Ferroptosis in Cancer Cell Biology." Cancers 12.1 (2020): 164.

25) Liedorp, M., A. E. Voskuyl, and BW Van Oosten. "Axonal neuropathy with prolonged sulphasalazine use." Clinical & Experimental Rheumatology 26.4 (2008): 671.

26) Chadenat, M. L., Morelon, S., Dupont, C., Dechy, H., Raffin-Sanson, M. L., Dorra, M., & Rouveix, E. (2001, June). Sulfasalazine neurotoxicity. In Annales de medecine interne (Vol. 152, No. 4, pp. 283-284).

27) Mundo, A., et al. "Sulfasalazine: side effects and duration of therapy in patients with rheumatoid arthritis." La Clinica Terapeutica 148.1-2 (1997): 7-13.

28) Lewerenz, Jan, et al. "The cystine/glutamate antiporter system xc− in health and disease: from molecular mechanisms to novel therapeutic opportunities." Antioxidants & redox signaling 18.5 (2013): 522-555.

29) Narang, Vishal S., et al. "Sulfasalazine-induced reduction of glutathione levels in breast cancer cells: enhancement of growth-inhibitory activity of doxorubicin." Chemotherapy 53.3 (2007): 210-217.

30) Wei, Chyou-Wei, et al. "Anti-Cancer Effects of Sulfasalazine and Vitamin E Succinate in MDA-MB 231 Triple-Negative Breast Cancer Cells." International journal of medical sciences 16.4 (2019): 494.

31) Garcia, Carlos Gustavo, et al. "Combination therapy with sulfasalazine and valproic acid promotes human glioblastoma cell death through imbalance of the intracellular oxidative response." Molecular neurobiology 55.8 (2018): 6816-6833.

32) Song, Yeonhwa, et al. "Sulfasalazine attenuates evading anticancer response of CD133-positive hepatocellular carcinoma cells." Journal of Experimental & Clinical Cancer Research 36.1 (2017): 38.

33) Wada, Fumitaka, et al. "High expression of CD 44v9 and xCT in chemoresistant hepatocellular carcinoma: Potential targets by sulfasalazine." Cancer science 109.9 (2018): 2801-2810.

34) Ogihara, Koichiro, et al. "Sulfasalazine could modulate the CD44v9-xCT system and enhance cisplatin-induced cytotoxic effects in metastatic bladder cancer." Cancer science 110.4 (2019): 1431.

35) Mooney, Marie R., et al. "Anti-tumor effect of sulfasalazine in neuroblastoma." Biochemical pharmacology 162 (2019): 237-249.

36) Yoshida, Go J., and Hideyuki Saya. "Therapeutic strategies targeting cancer stem cells." Cancer science 107.1 (2016): 5-11.

37-38) deleted

39) Sukhai, Mahadeo A., et al. "Lysosomal disruption preferentially targets acute myeloid leukemia cells and progenitors." Journal of Clinical Investigation 123.1 (2013): 315.

40) Liu, Yanwei, et al. "Mefloquine effectively targets gastric cancer cells through phosphatase-dependent inhibition of PI3K/Akt/mTOR signaling pathway." Biochemical and biophysical research communications (2016).

41) Yan, Kun-Huang, et al. "Mefloquine induces cell death in prostate cancer cells and provides a potential novel treatment strategy in vivo." Oncology letters 5.5 (2013): 1567-1571.

42) Glaumann, Hans, Anne-Marie Motakefi, and Helena Jansson. "Intracellular distribution and effect of the antimalarial drug mefloquine on lysosomes of rat liver." Liver 12.4 (1992): 183-190.

43) Xu, Xin, et al. "Antimalarial drug mefloquine inhibits nuclear factor kappa B signaling and induces apoptosis in colorectal cancer cells." Cancer science 109.4 (2018): 1220-1229.

44) Li, Hui, et al. "Therapeutic effects of antibiotic drug mefloquine against cervical cancer through impairing mitochondrial function and inhibiting mTOR pathway." Canadian journal of physiology and pharmacology 95.1 (2017): 43-50.

45) Li, Yu-Hui, et al. "Mefloquine targets β-catenin pathway and thus can play a role in the treatment of liver cancer." Microbial pathogenesis 118 (2018): 357-360.

46) Das, Subhadip, et al. "Antimalarial drugs trigger lysosome-mediated cell death in chronic lymphocytic leukemia (CLL) cells." Leukemia research 70 (2018): 79-86.

47) Nevin, Remington L. "A serious nightmare: psychiatric and neurologic adverse reactions to mefloquine are serious adverse reactions." Pharmacology research & perspectives 5.4 (2017): e00328.

48) Nevin, Remington L. "Idiosyncratic quinoline central nervous system toxicity: Historical insights into the chronic neurological sequelae of mefloquine." International Journal for Parasitology: Drugs and Drug Resistance 4.2 (2014): 118-125.

49) Mawson, Anthony. "Mefloquine use, psychosis, and violence: a retinoid toxicity hypothesis." Medical Science Monitor Basic Research 19 (2013): 579-583.

50) Alisky, Joseph M., Elena L. Chertkova, and Kenneth A. Iczkowski. "Drug interactions and pharmacogenetic reactions are the basis for chloroquine and mefloquine-induced psychosis." Medical hypotheses 67.5 (2006): 1090-1094.

51) Choi, Dong Soon, et al. "Chloroquine eliminates cancer stem cells through deregulation of Jak2 and DNMT1." Stem cells 32.9 (2014): 2309-2323.

52) Pascolo, Steve. "Time to use a dose of chloroquine as an adjuvant to anti-cancer chemotherapies." European journal of pharmacology 771 (2016): 139-144.

53) Sotelo, Julio, Eduardo Briceno, and Miguel Angel López-González. "Adding chloroquine to conventional treatment for glioblastoma multiforme: a randomized, double-blind, placebo-controlled trial." Annals of internal medicine 144.5 (2006): 337-343.

54) Liang, Diana H., et al. "The autophagy inhibitor chloroquine targets cancer stem cells in triple negative breast cancer by inducing mitochondrial damage and impairing DNA break repair." Cancer letters 376.2 (2016): 249-258.

55) Balic, Anamaria, et al. "Chloroquine targets pancreatic cancer stem cells via inhibition of CXCR4 and hedgehog signaling." Molecular cancer therapeutics 13.7 (2014): 1758-1771.

56) Frieboes, Hermann B., et al. "Chloroquine-Mediated Cell Death in Metastatic Pancreatic Adenocarcinoma through Inhibition of Autophagy." JOP. Journal of the Pancreas 15.2 (2014): 189-197.

57) Balic, Anamaria, Morten Dræby Sørensen, and Christopher Heeschen. "Old drugs for new purposes-chloroquine targets metastatic pancreatic cancer stem cells & their microenvironment." Cancer Cell Microenviron. 1 (2014): e227.

58) deleted

59) Vazquez-Martin, Alejandro, et al. "Repositioning chloroquine and metformin to eliminate cancer stem cell traits in pre-malignant lesions." Drug Resistance Updates 14.4-5 (2011): 212-223.

60) Calabretta, Bruno, and Paolo Salomoni. "Inhibition of autophagy: a new strategy to enhance sensitivity of chronic myeloid leukemia stem cells to tyrosine kinase inhibitors." Leukemia & lymphoma 52.sup1 (2011): 54-59.

61) Mukhopadhyay, Arunima, et al. "Hydroxychloroquine for chronic myeloid leukemia: complete cure on the horizon?" Expert review of hematology 4.4 (2011): 369-371.

62) Egger, Michael E., et al. "Inhibition of autophagy with chloroquine is effective in melanoma." journal of surgical research 184.1 (2013): 274-281.

63) Verbaanderd, Ciska, et al. "Repurposing Drugs in Oncology (ReDO)—chloroquine and hydroxychloroquine as anti-cancer agents." ecancermedicalscience 11 (2017).

64) Michaelides, Michel, et al. "Retinal toxicity associated with hydroxychloroquine and chloroquine: risk factors, screening, and progression despite cessation of therapy." Archives of ophthalmology 129.1 (2011): 30-39.

65) Melotti, Alice, et al. "The river blindness drug Ivermectin and related macrocyclic lactones inhibit WNT-TCF pathway responses in human cancer." EMBO molecular medicine (2014): e201404084.

66) Chhaiya, Sunita B., Dimple S. Mehta, and Bhaven C. Kataria. "Ivermectin: pharmacology and therapeutic applications." Int J Basic Clin Pharmacol 1.3 (2012): 132.

67) Canga, Aránzazu González, et al. "The pharmacokinetics and interactions of ivermectin in humans—a mini-review." The AAPS journal 10.1 (2008): 42-46.

68) Guzzo, Cynthia A., et al. "Safety, tolerability, and pharmacokinetics of escalating high doses of ivermectin in healthy adult subjects." The Journal of Clinical Pharmacology 42.10 (2002): 1122-1133.

69) Chaccour, Carlos J., et al. "Ivermectin to reduce malaria transmission: a research agenda for a promising new tool for elimination." Malar J 12.153 (2013): 10-1186.

70) Fawcett, Robert S. "Ivermectin use in scabies." American family physician 68.6 (2003): 1089-1092.

71) Draganov, Dobrin, et al. "Modulation of P2X4/P2X7/pannexin-1 sensitivity to extracellular ATP via ivermectin induces a non-apoptotic and inflammatory form of cancer cell death." Scientific reports 5 (2015).

72) Drinyaev, Victor A., et al. "Antitumor effect of avermectins." European journal of pharmacology 501.1 (2004): 19-23.

72A) Navarro, Miriam, et al. "Safety of high-dose ivermectin: a systematic review and meta-analysis." Journal of Antimicrobial Chemotherapy (2020).

73) Markowska, Anna, et al. "Doxycycline, salinomycin, monensin, ivermectin repositioned as cancer drugs." Bioorganic & medicinal chemistry letters (2019).

74) Zhang, Ping, et al. "Ivermectin induces cell cycle arrest and apoptosis of HeLa cells via mitochondrial pathway." Cell proliferation 52.2 (2019): e12543.

75) Diao, Hongxiu, et al. "Ivermectin inhibits canine mammary tumor growth by regulating cell cycle progression and WNT signaling." BMC veterinary research 15.1 (2019): 1-10.

76) Liu, Jingjing, et al. "Ivermectin induces autophagy-mediated cell death through the AKT/mTOR signaling pathway in glioma cells." Bioscience reports 39.12 (2019).

77) Song, Dandan, et al. "Ivermectin inhibits the growth of glioma cells by inducing cell cycle arrest and apoptosis in vitro and in vivo." Journal of cellular biochemistry 120.1 (2019): 622-633.

78) Sharmeen, Sumaiya, et al. "The antiparasitic agent ivermectin induces chloride-dependent membrane hyperpolarization and cell death in leukemia cells." Blood 116.18 (2010): 3593-3603.

79) Mathur, Rohit, et al. "Targeting Wnt pathway in mantle cell lymphoma-initiating cells." Journal of hematology & oncology 8.1 (2015): 63.

80) Han, Jae-Ik, and Ki-Jeong Na. "Wnt/β-Catenin Signaling Pathway in Canine Skin Melanoma and a Possibility as a Cancer Model for Human Skin Melanoma." Melanoma in the Clinic-Diagnosis, Management and Complications of Malignancy. IntechOpen, 2011.

81) Mehrpour, and Raphaël Rodriguez. "Salinomycin kills cancer stem cells by sequestering iron in lysosomes." Ratio 5 (2017): 10.

82) Mai, Trang Thi, et al. "Salinomycin kills cancer stem cells by sequestering iron in lysosomes." Nature chemistry 9.10 (2017): 1025.

83) Chung, Hyewon, et al. "The effect of salinomycin on ovarian cancer stem-like cells." Obstetrics & gynecology science 59.4 (2016): 261-268.

84) Resham, Kahkashan, et al. "Preclinical drug metabolism and pharmacokinetics of salinomycin, a potential candidate for targeting human cancer stem cells." Chemico-biological interactions 240 (2015): 146-152.

85) Boehmerle, Wolfgang, et al. "Specific targeting of neurotoxic side effects and pharmacological profile of the novel cancer stem cell drug salinomycin in mice." Journal of molecular medicine 92.8 (2014): 889-900.

86) Jangamreddy, Jaganmohan R., et al. "Glucose starvation-mediated inhibition of salinomycin induced autophagy amplifies cancer cell specific cell death." Oncotarget 6.12 (2015): 10134.

87) Dewangan, Jayant, Sonal Srivastava, and Srikanta Kumar Rath. "Salinomycin: A new paradigm in cancer therapy." Tumor Biology 39.3 (2017): 1010428317695035.

88) Lu D, Choi MY, Yu J, Castro JE, Kipps TJ, Carson DA. Salinomycin inhibits Wnt signaling and selectively induces apoptosis in chronic lymphocytic leukemia cells. Proc Natl Acad Sci USA. 2011;108:13253–13257.

89) Gupta, Piyush B., et al. "Identification of selective inhibitors of cancer stem cells by high-throughput screening." cell 138.4 (2009): 645-659.

90) Joo, Won Duk, Irene Visintin, and Gil Mor. "Targeted cancer therapy–Are the days of systemic chemotherapy numbered?." Maturitas 76.4 (2013): 308-314.

91) Karsy, Michael, et al. "All-trans retinoic acid modulates cancer stem cells of glioblastoma multiforme in an MAPK-dependent manner." Anticancer research 30.12 (2010): 4915-4920.

92) Zeng, W. G., et al. "All-trans retinoic acid effectively inhibits breast cancer stem cells growth in vitro." Zhonghua zhong liu za zhi [Chinese journal of oncology] 35.2 (2013): 89-93.

93) Herreros-Villanueva, Marta, Tze-Kiong Er, and Luis Bujanda. "Retinoic acid reduces stem cell–like features in pancreatic cancer cells." Pancreas 44.6 (2015): 918-924.

94) Lim, Young Chang, et al. "All-trans-retinoic acid inhibits growth of head and neck cancer stem cells by suppression of Wnt/β-catenin pathway." European Journal of Cancer 48.17 (2012): 3310-3318.

95) Cao, Xin. "Retinoids Induced Cancer Stem Cell Differentiation and Apoptosis for Cancer Therapies." Molecular and Cellular Therapies (2019): 1-8.

96) Cao, Xin, et al. "Retinoids offer new and promising cancer therapeutic avenues." Journal of Molecular and Clinical Medicine 2.2 (2019): 23-27.

97) Li, Dongbei, et al. "All-Trans Retinoic Acid Enhances the Anti-Leukemia Effect of Venetoclax on Acute Myeloid Leukemia Cells." (2019): 5055-5055.

98) Huang, Lu, et al. "All-trans-retinoic acid (ATRA) markedly augments anti-tumor immunity." (2019): 3279-3279.

99) Moreb, Jan S., Deniz A. Ucar-Bilyeu, and Abdullah Khan. "Use of retinoic acid/aldehyde dehydrogenase pathway as potential targeted therapy against cancer stem cells." Cancer chemotherapy and pharmacology 79.2 (2017): 295-301.

100) Tang, Xiao-Han, and Lorraine J. Gudas. "Retinoids, retinoic acid receptors, and cancer." Annual Review of Pathology: Mechanisms of Disease 6 (2011): 345-364.

101) Alberts, David, et al. "Safety and efficacy of dose-intensive oral vitamin A in subjects with sun-damaged skin." Clinical cancer research 10.6 (2004): 1875-1880.

102) Friesenbichler, Waltraud, et al. "Outcome of two patients with bilateral nephroblastomatosis/Wilms tumour treated with an add-on 13-cis retinoic acid therapy–case report." Pediatric hematology and oncology 35.3 (2018): 218-224.

103) Lima, Lara, et al. "Modulation of all-trans retinoic acid-induced MiRNA expression in neoplastic cell lines: a systematic review." BMC cancer 19.1 (2019): 866.

104) Huang, Lu, et al. "All-trans-retinoic acid (ATRA) markedly augments anti-tumor immunity." (2019): 3279-3279.

105) Cui, Jiejie, et al. "All-trans retinoic acid reverses malignant biological behavior of hepatocarcinoma cells by regulating miR-200 family members." Genes & Diseases (2020).

106) Friedman, Marissa D., et al. "Targeting cancer stem cells in glioblastoma multiforme using mTOR inhibitors and the differentiating agent all-trans retinoic acid." Oncology reports 30.4 (2013): 1645-1650.

107) Lamb, Rebecca, et al. "Antibiotics that target mitochondria effectively eradicate cancer stem cells, across multiple tumor types: treating cancer like an infectious disease." Oncotarget 6.7 (2015): 4569.

108) Bonuccelli, Gloria, et al. "NADH autofluorescence, a new metabolic biomarker for cancer stem cells: Identification of Vitamin C and CAPE as natural products targeting "stemness"." Oncotarget 8.13 (2017): 20667.

109) De Francesco, Ernestina Marianna, et al. "Vitamin C and Doxycycline: A synthetic lethal combination therapy targeting metabolic flexibility in cancer stem cells (CSCs)." Oncotarget 8.40 (2017): 67269.

Chapter 12

Repurposed Drugs Targeting Cancer Stem Cells II

The Mitochondrial-Wnt Signaling Axis

In 2019, Drs. Jerry Harb et al. reviewed Wnt pathway drugs as anti-CSC agents, highlighting pyrvinium pamoate, niclosamide, celecoxib, and ethacrynic acid. (1) With the exception of ethacrynic acid, the others are discussed in this book. Not mentioned in Dr. Harb's list are a few other anti-stem cell drugs discussed here, such as ivermectin, salinomycin, mefloquine, hydroxychloroquine, and metformin. (See the chapters on metformin, niclosamide, mefloquine and celecoxib for more on these specific drugs.) In general, all OXPHOS inhibitors are also Wnt pathway inhibitors and therefore may serve as valid anti-CSC agents. This is due to the "mitochondrial-Wnt signaling axis" described in 2019 by Dr. Roberta Costa. (24)

Cancer Stem Cells—Pathways

Blocking the three major CSC pathways serves to eradicate CSCs. Those pathways are:

1) Wnt/Beta-Catenin
2) Sonic hedgehog (Hh)
3) Notch
4) Perhaps NF-kB can be added as a fourth pathway.

Pyrvinium (an OXPHOS Inhibitor) as Anti-Cancer Stem Cell Agent

Pyrvinium (Povan®, Vanquin®, Molevac®) is an FDA-approved antiparasitic drug used since the 1950s to treat pinworm, malaria, and cryptosporidium. Although no longer available in the United States, pyrvinium is available under the trade name Vanquin in Sweden, Denmark, Norway, and Iceland. Pyrvinium is available in other European countries as well (for example, as Molevac in Germany). (2)

Wnt and Hedgehog Pathway Inhibition by Pyrvinium

Pyrvinium pamoate is a potent anti-CSC drug that works by inhibiting the Wnt and Hedgehog pathways. (3–5)

Pyrvinium exhibits potent anti-cancer activity as a Wnt pathway inhibitor against the following CSC lines:

- Breast cancer stem cells (6–7)
- Glioblastoma stem cells (8)
- Lung cancer stem cells (9)
- Ovarian cancer (enhances sensitivity to paclitaxel chemotherapy) (10)
- Blast-phase chronic myeloid leukemia stem cells (11–12)
- Lymphoma (13)
- Multiple myeloma—(inhibits ETC complex I) (14–16)
- Mesothelioma (17)

- B-cell lymphoblastic leukemia (18)
- Wilms tumor (19)
- Intestinal polyposis (20)
- Colon cancer (21)
- Endometriosis (22)

Pyrvinium Inhibits Wnt Pathway and Cancer Stem Cells

In 2016, Drs. Liang and W. Xu et al. studied pyrvinium in a breast cancer cell model, finding pyrvinium inhibited proliferation of breast CSCs in vitro and in vivo related to Wnt pathway inhibition, with measurable reduction of CSC markers. (6–7)

In 2017, Dr. Chongyuan Zhang et al. studied pyrvinium in a chemotherapy resistant ovarian cancer cell model, finding pyrvinium to be a potent Wnt inhibitor, enhancing the efficacy of chemotherapy.

Dr. Zhang and colleagues write:

> Mechanistically, pyrvinium increased the Wnt-negative regulator axin and decreased the Beta-catenin levels in ovarian cancer cells. In addition, pyrvinium suppressed Wnt/β-catenin-mediated transcription, as shown by the decreased mRNA levels of MYC, cyclin D, and BCL-9... pyrvinium acted on ovarian cancer cells via targeting the Wnt/ Beta-catenin signaling pathway. (10)

Note: Wnt pathway inhibition by pyrvinium is related to activation of CK1α which then causes degradation of cytosolic Beta-Catenin, resulting in profound Wnt pathway inhibition.

Dr. Curtis Thorne (2010) studied inhibition of Wnt signaling by pyrvnum in a Xenopus laevis egg extract. Dr. Thorne performed a high throughput screen on a large number of compounds which inhibit the Wnt pathway, finding pyrvinium the best candidate. Pyrvinium binds to and activates casein kinase 1 (CK-1), thus degrading cytosolic Beta-Catenin, resulting in potent inhibition of Wnt signaling at low concentrations (10 nanoMolar). Dr Thorne et al. write:

> We show pyrvinium binds all casein kinase 1 (CK1) family members in vitro at low nanomolar concentrations and pyrvinium selectively potentiates casein kinase 1α (CK1α) kinase activity [which degrades cytosolic Beta-Catenin] ... Our findings reveal allosteric activation of CK1α as an effective mechanism to inhibit Wnt. (34)

In 2018, Dr. Amir Momtazi-Borojeni et al. reviewed the potent anti-CSC activity of pyrvinium, summarizing as follows:

> Pyrvinium acts through the following main mechanisms:
>
> (i) energy and autophagy depletion; and
>
> (ii) inhibition of Akt and Wnt-β-catenin-dependent pathways. Interestingly, pyrvinium has also shown potent anti-cancer stem cell activity. (23)

Wnt Pathway Inhibition- Multiple Myeloma

Multiple myeloma remains incurable in spite of new agents, lenalidamide and bortezomib, which, admittedly, have improved outcomes in the disease.

In 2018, Dr. Fang Xu et al. studied Wnt pathway inhibition by pyrvinium (PP) in a multiple myeloma cell line. They write that pyrvinium inhibits the Wnt/β-catenin pathway, leading to downstream inhibition of axin2, c-Myc and Cyclin D1:

> PP [pyrvinium] potently attenuated growth

and induced apoptosis in MM [Multiple Myeloma] cell lines and primary tumor cells … the induction of apoptosis by PP may be a result of its inhibitory effect on the **Wnt/β-catenin** pathway…. Inhibiting the Wnt/β-catenin pathway will cause a cascade of events; β-catenin levels decrease, as will the expression of downstream target genes, including **axin 2, MYC and cyclin D1.** (14)

Synergy with Dasatinib Targeting Blast-Phase Chronic Leukemia— Inhibiting Mitochondrial Respiration

In 2015, Dr. Wei Xiang et al. studied blast-phase chronic myeloid leukemia, finding pyrvinium synergy with dasatinib, a (TKI) tyrosine kinase inhibitor commonly used in this cell type. Dr. Xiang and colleagues found the CD34+ progenitor cells (cancer stem cells) were selectively targeted while normal hematopoietic stem cells were unaffected. The mechanism was **pyrvinium localization to the mitochondria with inhibition of mitochondrial respiration**, rather than the Wnt pathway inhibition, as usually described for other cancer cell models.

> We show that pyrvinium, a FDA-approved anthelminthic drug, selectively targets BP-CML [Chronic Myelogenous Leukemia] CD34+ progenitor cells. Pyrvinium is effective in inducing apoptosis, inhibiting colony formation and self-renewal capacity of CD34+ cells from [Tyrosine Kinase Inhibitor] TKI-resistant BP-CML patients, while [umbilical] cord blood CD34+ are largely unaffected. The effects of pyrvinium are further enhanced upon combination with dasatinib, a second-generation BCR-ABL1 TKI [B-Cell Receptor Tyrosine Kinase Inhibitor]. In a CML xenograft model pyr-

vinium significantly inhibits tumor growth as a single agent, with complete inhibition in combination with dasatinib … While pyrvinium has been shown to inhibit the Wnt/β-catenin signaling pathway via activation of casein kinase 1α, we find its activity in CML is not dependent on this pathway. Instead, we show that pyrvinium localizes to mitochondria and induces apoptosis by inhibiting mitochondrial respiration. (11)

Pyrvinium: OXPHOS Inhibitor for B-Cell Malignancy

In 2020, Dr. Rajesh Nair et al. studied pyrvinium (PP) in a B-cell lymphoblastic leukemia model, finding impairment of mitochondrial respiration (oxidative phosphorylation—OXPHOS). They write:

> PP's [pyrvinium's] cell death activity was specific for leukemic cells, as primary normal immune cells were resistant to PP-mediated cell death. Metabolic studies indicated that PP, in part, inhibits mitochondrial oxidative phosphorylation. (18)

Similarly, in 2016, Dr. Meifang Xiao et al. studied pyrvinium in T cell lymphoma cell lines, finding impairment of mitochondrial function selectively in malignant T cells, with sparing of normal T cells:

> Pyrvinium impairs mitochondrial functions by inhibiting mitochondrial respiration, suppressing mitochondrial respiratory complex I activity, increasing ROS and decreasing ATP levels. (13)

Mitochondrial OXPHOS Inhibition Causes Wnt Inhibition

In 2019, Dr. Roberto Costa et al. discovered that impaired mitochondrial ATP (energy) production due to **OXPHOS inhibition down-regulates Wnt signaling**. This explains why pyrvinium, as well as other mitochondrial OXPHOS inhibitors, also inhibit the Wnt pathway, serving as an anti-CSC agent.

> The data in the present paper indicate the existence of a mitochondrial-Wnt signaling axis... perturbation of mitochondrial function using a number of inhibitors can cause decreased Wnt activity both in vitro and in vivo. (24)

Important!!! Agents that Inhibit Mitochondrial OXPHOS also inhibit the Wnt Pathway and are potent Anti-Cancer Stem Cell Agents!!!!

This is an important discovery that allows us to label all OXPHOS inhibitors as CSC agents by virtue of Wnt inhibition.

Dr. Xiaonan Zhang et al. (2015) are in agreement with Dr. Costa's group, commenting that OXPHOS Inhibitors are the best candidates discovered on high-throughput drug screens for anti-CSC activity. (33)

Pyrvinium Tumor Microenvironment Agent

In 2012 Drs. Isao Ishii, et al. found that pyrvinium (PP) targets the NADH-fumarate reductase system (complex I and II in the electron transport chain in mitochondrial respiration, writing:

> PP [pyrvinium] suppressed the NADH-fumarate reductase system that mediates a reverse reaction of the mitochondrial electron transport chain complex II in anaerobic organisms such as parasitic helminthes or **mammalian cells under tumor micro-environment-mimicking hypoglycemic/hypoxic conditions, thereby inhibiting efficient ATP production.** (25)

Dr. Chika Sakai et al. note that NADH-fumarate reductase is identical to Complex I and II of the mitochondrial electron transport chain (ETC):

> Mitochondrial NADH-fumarate reductase system (fumarate respiration), which is composed of complex I (NADH–rhodoquinonereductase), rhodoquinone and complex II (rhodoquinol–fumarate reductase. (26)

Disrupts Energy Production from Tumor Micro-Environment

Dr. Eriko Tomitsuka et al. (2012) write:

> PP [pyrvinium] inhibits mitochondrial NADH-fumarate reductase activity and disrupts mitochondrial energy metabolism within the tumor micro-environment.... These results indicate that the NADH-FR [NADH-fumarate reductase] system may be important for maintaining mitochondrial energy production in tumour microenvironments and suggest its potential use as a novel therapeutic target. (27)

Pyrvinium Blocks Glutathione Uptake from Tumor Micro-Environment-Lymphoma

In 2015, Dr. Keiki Sugimoto et al. developed a high through-put drug-screening system using patient-derived xenografts of lymphoma transplanted into immunodeficient mice. Using a library of 2613 off-patent drugs, they found that pyrvinium showed the highest activity with "*strong anti-tumor activity.*" This was confirmed with in vivo studies. The mechanism was related to inhibition of glutathione supply from stromal cells in the micro-environment to the lymphoma cells. Dr. Sugimoto and colleagues write:

We extensively investigated its [pyrvinium's] mechanism of action and found that it inhibited glutathione supply from stromal cells to lymphoma cells. (28)

For more on glutathione depletion, see the discussion in chapter 10 on sulforaphane, pterostilbene and parthenolide, and chapter 11 for sulfasalazine.

Pyrvinium Absorption Zero in 1976 Study

In 1976, Dr. T. C. Smith et al. studied the pharmacokinetics of pyrvinium in healthy volunteers, finding that a single 350 mg/day tablet resulted in no detectable blood level up to four days after ingestion. In other words, oral absorption was virtually zero. (29)

In 2016, Dr. Kamal Ahmed et al. discussed pyrvinium's poor absorption by pointing to the 2009 in vivo anti-cancer study by Dr. Jeremy Jones et al., which required intraperitoneal injection of the pyrvinium into mice to achieve peak levels of 150 nM (nanomolar), well within the effective anti-cancer range of (50–200 nM). However, because this dosage is borderline, with severe toxicity, Dr. Ahmed and colleagues suggested preliminary human studies of toxicity for injected pyrvinium. They write:

> In vitro studies have identified pyrvinium to be effective against the Wnt pathway and cancer cell proliferation within the high-nanomolar range (50–200 nM). When delivered by its standard oral route, pyrvinium's bio-availability is virtually zero, and therefore cannot be employed for in vivo anti-cancer studies. Therefore, it was delivered by daily intraperitoneal injections of 1 mg/kg, which were reported to create acceptable peak plasma levels of 150 nM.

Using this dose, efficient suppression of the Wnt -dependent colon cancer in vivo was achieved. Unfortunately, this dose is borderline with severe toxicity, since any increase resulted in severe toxic effects. Therefore, phase I safety trials should be launched first in order to verify this novel delivery route in patients; no data has been reported so far for any attempts to run such a trial. (4)

In 2017, Dr. Gerhard Hamilton et al. noted that

> The drug [pyrvinium] has no measurable absorption across the gastrointestinal tract and 90% is excreted in feces … At 5 mg/kg/day low amounts appeared in liver and plasma in rats. (3)

However, perhaps Dr. Ahmed and Hamilton are wrong. The finding of zero gastrointestinal absorption of pyrvinium is based on an old study by Dr. T. C. Smith et al. from 1976, and perhaps they are being unduly alarmist about toxicity. More recent in vivo studies in mice with oral gavage of pyrvinium show excellent anti-cancer activity with "minimal or low toxicity."

Pyrvinium Synergy with Chloroquine

For example, in 2013, Dr. Longfei Deng studied pyrvinium (10mg/kg i.g.) by oral gavage once daily in a mouse xenograft 4T1 breast cancer model, with good reduction in tumor volume and enhanced activity (synergy) with the autophagy inhibitor, chloroquine. (30)

Synergy with the autophagy inhibitor chloroquine is not unexpected, since pyrvinium is an OXPHOS inhibitor that stimulates protective autophagy. Other autophagy inhibitors include chloroquine, propranolol, thymoquinone, loratadine (Claritin®), and omeprazole (Prilosec®).

Important!!! OXPHOS inhibitors activate "protective autophagy" and therefore will synergize with autophagy inhibitors.

Effective for Oral Administration

Another example is the 2004 study by Dr. Hiroyasu Esumi et al. in which pyrvinium was found active both by oral gavage and subcutaneous injection in a mouse xenograft model of pancreatic cancer. The in vitro portion of the study showed pyrvinium was extremely toxic to pancreatic cancer cells (in vitro) in a glucose-free medium under conditions of glucose starvation. One might speculate that glucose starvation shifted the cancer cells to OXPHOS metabolism (pyrvinium being effective here), while abundant glucose shifted the cells to GLYCOLYSIS (the Warburg effect), making pyrvinium ineffective.

Regarding the in vivo study, Dr. Esumi et al. write that pyrvinium was effective for both routes of administration in mice:

> Although PP [pyrvinium] has been claimed not to be absorbed by the mammalian intestine, preliminary tests indicated that it is absorbed, because the urine of a human turned red after oral consumption of 100mg of a commercial anthelminthic preparation [our unpublished observation]. We examined the effect of orally administered PP on tumor growth in nude mice bearing PANC-1 tumors. The results clearly demonstrate that PP exerted clear anti-tumor activity on the PANC-1 cells in nude mice…. The dose of PP administered was

100 µg / mouse / day…. PP was also found to exert anti-tumor activity against human pancreatic cancer cell line PANC-1 in nude mice and SCID mice when it was administered subcutaneously or orally. (31)

Dr. Esumi and colleagues were aware of previous claims that pyrvinium is not absorbed and disproved them by showing decreased PBK/AKT phosphorylation (at serine 473) in implanted tumor tissue in their mouse xenograft model after oral drug administration, "indicating that PP had been absorbed and had reached the tumor tissue".

Note: blocking Akt phosphorylation, blocks Akt activation, an anti-cancer effect. Regarding claims of toxicity, Dr. Esumi writes:

> The body weights of animals given vehicle and PP, both 100 and 200 µg /day, did not show any significant differences, indicating low toxicity of PP [data not shown] . (31)

Obviously, Drs. Ahmed and Hamilton are wrong to state in peer reviewed medical literature that pyrvinium has zero absorption and "cannot be employed for in vivo anti-cancer studies." since both Dr. Deng (2013) and Dr. Esumi (2004) and colleagues did exactly that—they used the oral route (oral gavage) in mice with good results. If you have any doubts, just check the urine, which turns red after ingesting pyrvinium, indicating absorption of the drug. They are also wrong about the toxicity issue, as we have shown above.

Pyrvinium for Colonic Polyposis

In 2014, Dr. Bin Li et al. suggested pyrvinium as a Wnt-inhibitor treatment for FAP (familial adenomatous polyposis), which is driven by mutations that upregulate the Wnt pathway and frequently result in colorectal cancer. They write:

> We show that Pyrvinium can function as an **in vivo inhibitor of Wnt-signaling** and polyposis in a mouse model of FAP: APCmin mice [familial polyposis].... Oral administration of Pyrvinium, a CK1α agonist, attenuated the levels of Wnt -driven biomarkers and inhibited adenoma formation in APCmin mice. Considering its well-documented safe use for treating enterobiasis in humans, our findings suggest that Pyrvinium could be repurposed for the clinical treatment of Adenomatous Polyposis Coli APC-associated polyposes. (20)

Pyrvinium is a POTENT Androgen Receptor Blocker

In 2009, Dr. Jeremy Jones et al. found that pyrvinium is a potent androgen receptor blocker, causing prostate atrophy in mice, and suggested pyrvinium would be useful in treatment of androgen receptor mediated disorders such as "female alopecia, female hirsutism, BPH (benign prostatic hyperplasia), and prostate cancer". (32)

Since pyrvinium is a potent androgen receptor blocker, causing prostate atrophy, it may not be suitable in young males who wish to preserve male testosterone function. On the other hand, it may be suitable for females and older males with BPH (benign prostatic hypertrophy). **Note:** BPH responds well to androgen blocker drugs.

Conclusion—Pyrvinium

Pyrvinium satisfies the criteria for a repurposed anti-cancer drug, as both an OXPHOS inhibitor and Wnt pathway inhibitor, and shows potent activity against CSCs. There is evidence that the original 1976 pyrvinium pharmacokinetic study in humans, suggesting zero oral absorption, is inaccurate. There is an urgent unmet need for an updated absorption study using currently available instruments. If this study is ever done, I would expect to find therapeutic blood levels in the 50–150 nanomolar range after pyrvinium oral ingestion.

Other repurposed drugs targeting CSCs—metformin (chapter 14), niclosamide (chapter 23), and celecoxib (chapter 38) —are discussed in their respective chapters. Disulfiram is discussed in the Glossary.

References for Chapter 12: Repurposed Drugs Targeting Cancer Stem Cells Part Two

1) Harb, Jerry, Pen-Jen Lin, and Jijun Hao. "Recent development of Wnt signaling pathway inhibitors for cancer therapeutics." Current oncology reports 21.2 (2019): 12.

2) Beck, J. Walter, et al. "The treatment of pinworm infections in humans (enterobiasis) with pyrvinium chloride and pyrvinium pamoate." The American journal of tropical medicine and hygiene 8.3 (1959): 349-352.

3) Hamilton, Gerhard, and Barbara Rath. "Repurposing of anthelminthics as anticancer drugs." Oncomedicine 2 (2017): 142-149.

4) Ahmed, Kamal, et al. "A second WNT for old drugs: drug repositioning against WNT-dependent cancers." Cancers 8.7 (2016): 66.

5) Li, Bin, et al. "Pyrvinium attenuates Hedgehog signaling downstream of smoothened." Cancer research 74.17 (2014): 4811-4821.

6) Xu, Liang, et al. "WNT pathway inhibitor pyrvinium pamoate inhibits the self-renewal and metastasis of breast cancer stem cells." International journal of oncology 48.3 (2016): 1175-1186.

7) Xu, W., et al. "P1-04-01: The Mechanism of Anti-Breast Cancer TICs Effect of Pyrvinium Pamoate Is through WNT/beta-Catenin Signaling." (2011): P1-04.

8) Venugopal, Chitra, et al. "Pyrvinium targets CD133 in human glioblastoma brain tumor–initiating cells." Clinical Cancer Research 21.23 (2015): 5324-5337.

9) Zhang, Xueyan, et al. "Wnt blockers inhibit the proliferation of lung cancer stem cells." Drug design, development and therapy 9 (2015): 2399.

10) Zhang, Chongyuan, et al. "Targeting of Wnt/β-catenin by anthelmintic drug pyrvinium enhances sensitivity of ovarian cancer cells to chemotherapy." Medical science monitor: international medical journal of experimental and clinical research 23 (2017): 266.

11) Xiang, Wei, et al. "Pyrvinium selectively targets blast phase-chronic myeloid leukemia through inhibition of mitochondrial respiration." Oncotarget 6.32 (2015): 33769.

12) Zhang, Jing, Yanli Jin, and Jingxuan Pan. "Inhibitory effect of the anthelmintic drug pyrvinium pamoate on T315I BCR-ABL-positive CML cells." Molecular medicine reports 16.6 (2017): 9217-9223.

13) Xiao, Meifang, et al. "Pyrvinium selectively induces apoptosis of lymphoma cells through impairing mitochondrial functions and JAK2/STAT5." Biochemical and biophysical research communications 469.3 (2016): 716-722.

14) Xu, Fang, et al. "Anthelmintic pyrvinium pamoate blocks Wnt/β-catenin and induces apoptosis in multiple myeloma cells." Oncology letters 15.4 (2018): 5871-5878.

15) Zeng D, Liu M and Pan J: Blocking EZH2 methylation transferase activity by GSK126 decreases stem cell-like myeloma cells. Oncotarget. 8:3396–3411. 2017.

16) Harada, Yasuo, et al. "Pyrvinium pamoate inhibits proliferation of myeloma/erythroleukemia cells by suppressing mitochondrial respiratory complex I and STAT3." Cancer letters 319.1 (2012): 83-88.

17) Barbarino, Marcella, et al. "Possible repurposing of pyrvinium pamoate for the treatment of mesothelioma: A pre-clinical assessment." Journal of cellular physiology 233.9 (2018): 7391-7401.

18) Nair, Rajesh R., et al. "Pyrvinium Pamoate Use in a B Cell Acute Lymphoblastic Leukemia Model of the Bone Tumor Microenvironment." Pharmaceutical Research 37.3 (2020): 43.

19) Polosukhina, Dina, et al. "Pharmacologic inhibition of β-catenin with Pyrvinium inhibits murine and human models of Wilms tumor." Oncology Research Featuring Preclinical and Clinical Cancer Therapeutics 25.9 (2017): 1653-1664.

20) Li, Bin, et al. "Repurposing the FDA-approved pinworm drug pyrvinium as a novel chemotherapeutic agent for intestinal polyposis." PLoS One 9.7 (2014).

21) Wiegering, Armin, et al. "The impact of pyrvinium pamoate on colon cancer cell viability." International journal of colorectal disease 29.10 (2014): 1189-1198.

22) Karamian, A., et al. "Pyrvinium pamoate inhibits proliferation and invasion of human endometriotic stromal cells." Human & Experimental Toxicology 39.5 (2020): 662-672.

23) Momtazi-Borojeni, Amir A., et al. "The novel role of pyrvinium in cancer therapy." Journal of cellular physiology 233.4 (2018): 2871-2881.

24) Costa, Roberto, et al. "Impaired mitochondrial ATP production downregulates Wnt signaling via ER stress induction." Cell reports 28.8 (2019): 1949-1960.

25) Ishii, Isao, Yasuo Harada, and Tadashi Kasahara. "Reprofiling a classical anthelmintic, pyrvinium pamoate, as an anti-cancer drug targeting mitochondrial respiration." Frontiers in oncology 2 (2012): 137.

26) Sakai, Chika, et al. "Mitochondrial fumarate reductase as a target of chemotherapy: from parasites to cancer cells." Biochimica et Biophysica Acta (BBA)-General Subjects 1820.5 (2012): 643-651.

27) Tomitsuka, Eriko, Kiyoshi Kita, and Hiroyasu Esumi. "An anticancer agent, pyrvinium pamoate inhibits the NADH–fumarate reductase system—a unique mitochondrial energy metabolism in tumour

microenvironments." The Journal of Biochemistry 152.2 (2012): 171-183.

28) Sugimoto, Keiki, et al. "Discovery of a drug targeting microenvironmental support for lymphoma cells by screening using patient-derived xenograft cells." Scientific reports 5 (2015): 13054.

29) Smith, T. C., et al. "Absorption of pyrvinium pamoate." Clinical Pharmacology & Therapeutics 19.6 (1976): 802-806.

30) Deng, Longfei, et al. "Pyrvinium targets autophagy addiction to promote cancer cell death." Cell death & disease 4.5 (2013): e614-e614.

31) Esumi, Hiroyasu, et al. "Antitumor activity of pyrvinium pamoate, 6-(dimethylamino)-2-[2-(2, 5-dimethyl-1-phenyl-1H-pyrrol-3-yl) ethenyl]-1-methyl-quinolinium pamoate salt, showing preferential cytotoxicity during glucose starvation." Cancer science 95.8 (2004): 685-690.

32) Jones, Jeremy O., et al. "Non-competitive androgen receptor inhibition in vitro and in vivo." Proceedings of the National Academy of Sciences 106.17 (2009): 7233-7238.

33) Zhang, Xiaonan, et al. "Targeting mitochondrial function to treat quiescent tumor cells in solid tumors." International journal of molecular sciences 16.11 (2015): 27313-27326.

34) Thorne, Curtis A., et al. "Small-molecule inhibition of Wnt signaling through activation of casein kinase 1α." Nature chemical biology 6.11 (2010): 829.

Chapter 13

Aspirin Targets Cancer Stem Cells

ASA Suppresses GLYCOLYSIS

ASPIRIN (SALICYLIC ACID) IS DERIVED from the bark of the willow tree, and was used medicinally in ancient times by the Sumerians and Egyptians. First synthesized in 1898, aspirin is the most commonly used drug in the world, taken by millions on a regular basis for various ailments, mostly headache and musculoskeletal aches and pains. Both aspirin and the COX-2 inhibitor, celecoxib are nonsteroidal anti-inflammatory drugs (NSAIDs) repurposed as anti-cancer drugs.

You might be surprised to know the bottle of aspirin in your medicine cabinet is actually a stealth anti-cancer stem cell agent. Aspirin inhibits activation of the master inflammatory controller, nuclear factor kappa B (NF-kB) and inhibits its downstream inflammatory effectors, cyclo-oxygenase 1 and 2 (COX-1 and COX-2). (1)

Long-term Aspirin Use Associated with Reduced Cancer Mortality

In 2017, Dr. Yin Cao et al. retrospectively studied a registry of 130,000 people who had been followed for 32 years, writing:

> Long-term aspirin use was associated with reduced risk of total mortality, primarily due to reduced risk of dying from cancers. (2)

In 2013, Dr. Ruth Langley summarized the clinical evidence supporting aspirin both for prevention and treatment of cancer. The mechanism of action seems related to the antiplatelet effect, similar to dipyridamole in which platelet inhibition prevents dissemination of metastatic disease. Like aspirin, Dipyridamole also inhibits the COX enzyme. Dr. Langley writes:

> In summary, data from randomized clinical studies have shown that aspirin prevents the development of malignancy, and it also appears to decrease the development and spread of metastases. (3)

Aspirin as Anti-Cancer Stem Cell Agent in Breast Cancer—Breast Cancer Stem Cells are Glycolytic!!

As discussed in chapter 5 on DCA, in 2014, Dr. Weiguo Feng et al. did transcriptome profiling using RNA sequencing, which revealed that breast cancer stem cells—also called tumor-initiating cells (TICs)—preferentially perform GLYCOLYSIS over mitochondrial OXPHOS compared to non-stem cancer cells. This is due to increased expression and activity of pyruvate dehydrogenase kinase (PDK), which promotes pro-glycolytic phenotype by inhibiting pyruvate dehydrogenase (PDH). They write:

> Glycolysis-associated events/processes, such as glucose uptake, glycolytic enzyme expression, lactate production and ATP

levels, are significantly elevated in CSCs, [cancer stem cells] which is also linked to a decrease in mitochondrial oxidative metabolism. Conversely, inhibition of glycolysis reversely suppresses the CSC maintenance. (4)

The key point here is: Metabolic reprogramming of PDH to force OXPHOS eliminated breast CSCs.

Dr. Feng et al. write: "Metabolic reprogramming via forced activation of PDH preferentially eliminated TICs [tumor initiating cells, also called cancer stem cells] both in vitro and in vivo". (4)

This metabolic programming can be accomplished, for example, with DCA. See the chapter 5 on DCA for more on this topic.

Aspirin is a GLYCOLYSIS Inhibitor

In 2018, Dr. F. Peng et al. studied the effect of aspirin on breast CSCs, finding aspirin restricted tumor GLYCOLYSIS and stemness in vitro and in vivo by significantly decreasing lncRNA H19 and pyruvate dehydrogenase kinase (PDK1). H19 is a long, noncoding RNA oncogene that targets, and increases, PDK1, the master controller for switching between mitochondrial OXPHOS and GLYCOLYSIS. For example, as discussed in chapter 5, DCA (dichloroacetate) inhibits PDK, which then upregulates PDH, which then switches metabolic pathway from GLYCOLYSIS to mitochondrial OXPHOS. Dr. Peng and colleagues summarize their findings:

> Intriguingly, we also uncovered that **aspirin can suppress glycolysis** and BCSC [breast cancer stem cell] maintenance through repressing H19 and PDK1. Taken together,

our studies identify a novel role and regulatory mechanism of PDK1 in BCSC reprogramming, which **provides a promising strategy for breast cancer therapy.** (5)

Aspirin Modulates VDAC

In a previous chapter, we discussed the importance of the attachment of hexokinase 2 (HK-2) to the voltage-dependent anion channel (VDAC), a pore-like structure on the outer mitochondrial membrane. Indeed, this VDAC is the "Achilles Heel" of the cancer cell. In 2017, Dr. Tewari studied aspirin treatment of a HeLa Cell culture (immortalized cervical cancer cell line) in vitro, finding VDAC is a target for aspirin, which closes the VDAC channel and dissociates HK II from the VDAC, promoting cancer cell death. Dr. Debanjan Tewari et al. write:

> In the present study we have identified **VDAC1 as a target for aspirin.** Aspirin induces closing of purified VDAC1… In HeLa cells, aspirin… dissociates HK II from mitochondria and promotes cell death. Possibly, these effects are manifested by the direct aspirin-induced inhibition of VDAC1. (6)

Not only is aspirin a glycolysis inhibitor, it also inhibits the VDAC, a key element of the Warburg Effect in the cancer cell.

Less Cancer in Long-Term Aspirin Users

If aspirin is an anti-cancer agent, then one might expect to find less cancer in registries of patients on long-term aspirin. Has this been studied? And do these people have less cancer?

One such study, done in 2019 by Dr. Kelvin Tsoi et al. in Hong Kong over a ten-year period, found that aspirin users had significant reduction of cancers in liver (RR: 0.49), stomach (RR: 0.42), colorectum (RR: 0.71), lung (RR: 0.65), pancreas (RR: 0.54), oesophagus (RR: 0.59) and leukaemia (RR: 0.67). [**Note:** RR of 0.67 = 33% less cancer, etc. Percent cancer is 1-RR.] (7)

However, breast cancer was not reduced by aspirin in this study.

In 2016, Dr. F. Lapi et al. performed a retrospective study of 13,453 patients, finding that low-dose aspirin use of less than 100 mg per day for five years reduced prostate cancer risk by 57 per cent. (8)

Aspirin after Colorectal Surgery Reduces Mortality

In 2019, Dr. Joseph Sung et al. studied aspirin use after colorectal surgery by 13,528 patients followed over 10 years and found a 31% reduction in colon cancer mortality in continuous aspirin users and a 39% reduction in all-cause mortality. (9)

In 2018, Dr. Kelvin Tsoi et al. studied aspirin use in 612,509 patients over 14 years, finding aspirin users had a 2.5% incidence of colorectal cancer with 1.02% cancer mortality, and non-users had higher 3.27% incidence of colorectal cancer and 1.7% mortality. (10)

There are currently more than ten registered clinical trials evaluating the use of aspirin for patients with colorectal cancer. (1)

Aspirin Combined with Chemotherapy Reduces Cancer Stem Cells

In chapter 2, we discussed unfavorable aspects of chemotherapy, namely the activation of NF-kB and resulting massive inflammation, which leads to an aggressive, drug-resistant, pro-metastatic cancer cell type with the following characteristics:

- More rapid cancer growth (proliferation).
- More resistance to apoptosis (programmed cell death).
- More invasive and metastatic behavior of the cancer.
- Stimulation of tumor angiogenesis (new blood vessel formation).
- Induction of chemo-resistant cancer cell type.
- Greater inhibition of host anti-tumor immunity.

Doxorubicin Increases Cancer Stem Cells

Another unfavorable result of chemotherapy is the increased number of CSCs. In 2019, Dr. Bee Luan Khoo et al. used patient-derived breast cancer cells from blood samples of 68 patients, finding that low-dose aspirin enhanced the cancer-cell-killing effects of the chemotherapy agent doxorubicin by inhibiting IL-6 secretion. When doxorubicin alone was used, this treatment increased the number of CSCs over 7 days. However, when the aspirin was added to the doxorubicin, there was a significant decrease in generation of CSCs.

Dr. Khoo et al. write:

Our findings serve as a basis for optimism regarding... low-dose aspirin in combination with anti-cancer drugs as an effective chemopreventive therapy against breast cancer and potentially other cancer types.... our study is the first to connect the anti-cancer effects of aspirin and anti-cancer drugs with the reduction of CSCs [cancer stem cells]. (11)

This study confirms what we already know about chemotherapy drugs: Not only do they fail to eradicate cancer stem cells, they actually increase numbers of cancer stem cells, caused by increased inflammation. This chemotherapy-induced inflammatory response can be suppressed by aspirin, resulting in reduced numbers of cancer stem cells.

A similar previous study was done in 2015 by Dr. Yiyao Zhang et al. using pancreatic cancer cells from surgical resections of pancreatic cancer. These studies were done using in vitro and in vivo mouse xenografts and found that aspirin decreased the number of cancer stem cells and overcame (gemcitabine) chemotherapy resistance. This is accomplished by disrupting NF-kB/IL6 signaling. (12)

Aspirin is a cancer stem cell agent in the following cancer cell lines:

- Colorectal cancer stem cells (13–15)
- Breast cancer stem cells (4–5)(16–17)
- Glioblastoma stem cells (18)
- Lung cancer stem cells (19–20)

Overcoming Chemotherapy Resistance by Preventing NF-kB Activation

In 2019, Dr. Jonbo Fu et al. found that aspirin overcomes 5-FU chemotherapy resistance in a colorectal cancer cell model by preventing chemotherapy-induced NF-kB activation. (21)

This finding was confirmed in 2020 by Dr. Wei Jiang et al., also in a colon cancer cell model, finding that aspirin prevented binding of NF-kB to the COX-2 promoter. (22)

Aspirin Normalizes EGFR Expression

Epithelial growth factor receptor (EGFR) is a frequently upregulated membrane-bound receptor on cancer cells that transmits the growth signals (epithelial growth factor) into the cancer cell. The new anti-EGFR drugs are EGFR TKIs (tyrosine kinase inhibitors).

In 2019, Dr. Ling LI et al. studied EGFR in lung and breast cancer cell lines, in vitro and in vivo, using the new EGFR drugs gefitinib and osimertinib. Initially the drugs work effectively. However, over time, the cancer cell lines gradually become resistant to the drugs.

Overcoming TKI Resistance

Dr. Li et al. searched a gene signature database to find a drug to overcome TKI drug resistance. The top-ranked candidate was aspirin, which suppresses activation of NF-kB, and suppresses cancer cell "stemness." The concentration of aspirin in the mice was roughly equivalent to a 500 mg dose in a 60 kg male, a commonly used dose considered safe in humans. (23)

Acquired TKI Drug Resistance

In 2019, Drs. H. Yong and H. Rui reported on two patients on osimertinib for non-small-cell lung cancer who unfortunately developed "acquired resistance" to the drug with progressive disease. Both started aspirin for unrelated venous thrombosis, and a "partial anti-tumor response was unexpectedly observed." (24)

Others have studied the ability of aspirin to normalize EGFR expression and its remarkable synergy with EGFR inhibitor drugs in colorectal cancer, epidermoid carcinoma, gastric cancer, ovarian cancer, and lung cancer. (25–30)

Other cancer cell lines in which aspirin shows benefit are:

- Hepatocellular carcinoma (31–32)
- Ovarian and endometrial cancer (33)
- Neuroblastoma (34)

Aspirin Synergy with Metformin

In 2018, in Egypt, Dr. Doaa Ali Abdelmonsif found synergy in the combined use of aspirin and metformin in an HCC (hepatocellular carcinoma) cell line in vitro, with induction of cell cycle arrest and apoptosis, associated with downregulation of AMPK, and mTOR protein expression. In addition, the Wnt pathway was inhibited, with observation of cell-membrane localization of Beta Catenin. (32)

In 2018, Dr. Maria Amaral et al. also found synergy of aspirin with metformin in various breast cancer cell types in vitro. This combination bound to the estrogen receptor and was most effective in cell lines having upregulated COX-2 (cyclo-oxygenase 2 inflammatory pathway). (35)

In 2014 and 2015, Dr. Wen Yue et al. studied the combination of metformin and aspirin in a pancreatic cancer cell line in vitro and in vivo. This combination downregulated the AMPK-mTOR pathway and suppressed the anti-apoptotic protein BCL-2. (36–38)

They then used RNA transcriptome analysis to evaluate the genetic expression of the cancer cells in response to treatment:

> We conducted a transcriptomic analysis using RNA sequencing to assess the differential gene expression induced by metformin (5 milliMolar) and aspirin (2 milliMolar), alone or in combination, after treatment of PANC-1 cells [pancreatic cancer] for 48 hours. (38)

While singly there was only slight change in the genetic expression of the cancer cells, the combination treatment induced a dramatic change, **with over a thousand genes affected**.

While metformin or aspirin alone only slightly changed the transcriptome profile of PANC-1 cells (**149 and 12 genes,** respectively), the combination of metformin and aspirin dramatically affected the transcription of **1,105 genes.** (38)

Aspirin is an Antiplatelet Agent

Additionally, in 2019, Dr. Kelly Johnson et al. found that aspirin inhibits release of platelet factors that activate the Akt pathway. Activation of Akt stimulates breast cancer cells to secrete IL-8, which promotes an invasive, aggressive phenotype. Dr. Johnson and colleagues write:

> Platelets treated with aspirin did not activate the Akt pathway, resulting in reduced IL-8 secretion and impaired tumor cell invasion. Of note, patients with breast cancer receiving aspirin had lower circulating IL-8, and their platelets did not increase tumor cell invasion compared with patients not receiving aspirin. Our data suggest platelets support breast tumor metastasis by inducing tumor cells to secrete IL-8. Our data further support that **aspirin acts as an anti-cancer agent by disrupting the communication between platelets and breast tumor cells.** (38)

In 2019, Drs. Lenard Lichtenberger and K. Vinod Vijayan studied aspirin in a Lewis lung cancer model, finding that the antiplatelet mechanism of aspirin accounts for its anti-cancer activity. Aspirin inhibits COX-1 in platelets. Drs. Lichtenberger and Vijayan write:

> Aspirin, when administered at low doses, has emerged as a powerful anti-cancer drug due to both chemopreventive activity against many forms of cancer and its ability to block metastases when administered post diagnosis. **Platelets, which are often elevated in circulation** during the latter stages of cancer, are known to promote epithelial mesenchymal transition (EMT), cancer cell growth, survival in circulation, and angiogenesis at sites of metastases. Low-dose aspirin has been demonstrated to block this procarcinogenic action of platelets…. aspirin's unique ability to irreversibly inhibit platelet cyclo-oxygenase-1 is a key mechanism by which aspirin exerts anti-cancer activity. (40)

For more on antiplatelet drugs as anti-cancer agents, see chapter 40 on dipyridamole.

Aspirin and the Tumor Micro-environment

Macrophages are the white cells (monocytes) involved in mounting an inflammatory response to bacterial or viral infection. Macrophages do this by secreting a portfolio of inflammatory cytokines such as tumor necrosis factor (TNF), IL-1, IL-6, IL-8, and IL-12. etc. (IL=Interleukin) (41)

Chemokines Attract Macrophages

The recruitment of macrophages by cancer cells in the microenvironment plays a huge role in upregulation of inflammatory pathways to stimulate growth and proliferation. The macrophages are recruited upon secretion by the cancer cells of chemo-attraction chemicals called chemokines. (42–43)

These chemokines are usually written using as abbreviations such as:

- MCP-1 (macrophage chemoattractant protein-1)
- VEGF (vascular endothelial growth factor)
- MCSF (macrophage colony-stimulating factor)

These chemokines induce monocytes to transform into tumor-associated macrophages (TAMs), which support cancer growth. The TAMs secrete cytokines that maintain and heighten a general inflammatory state in the tumor micro-environment. Inflammatory signaling induces aggressive cancer behavior, proliferation, migration, angiogenesis, metastasis, and suppression of anti-tumor immunity. (41)

In 2018, Dr. Chia-Chien Hsieh studied the effect of aspirin on the tumor micro-environment in a triple-negative breast cancer (4T1) cell model in vitro, using a culture medium simulating the macrophage infiltration of the tumor micro-environment. Dr. Hsieh found that aspirin treatment decreased inflammatory cytokines in the tumor microenvironment, writing:

> [the aspirin] interfered with crosstalk between cancer cells and macrophages… and decreased angiogenic and inflammation-associated cytokine VEGF, PAI-1, MCP-1, IL-6, IL-10, and TGF-β production… suggesting that aspirin is a promising agent to prevent tumor progression. (44)

Aspirin Inhibits mTOR and Induces Protective Autophagy

In 2012, Dr. Farhat Din et al., studying a colorectal cancer cell line, found that aspirin activated AMP-kinase, inhibited mTOR signaling, and induced "protective autophagy." As we have discussed elsewhere, mTOR signaling is the master controller for autophagy, and any drug inhibition of mTOR will always stimulate "protective autophagy" and serve as "caloric-restriction mimetic." (45–49)

In 2015, Dr. Muhammad Usman et al. summarized the COX enzyme independent effects of high-dose aspirin, which is paraphrased here:

Aspirin binds to iKB, which inhibits NF-Kb translocation, gene transcription, and inflammatory signaling.

NF-kB inhibits apoptosis by suppressing PTEN. Aspirin reverses this, restoring apoptosis.

Aspirin activates AMP-kinase which inhibits mTOR, which activates "protective autophagy" and mimics caloric restriction. (50)

Note: PTEN is a tumor suppressor gene. (See glossary)

Gastrointestinal Bleeding from Aspirin

Adverse effects of aspirin include: nausea, vomiting, stomach pain, and heartburn. Similar to other NSAIDs, aspirin's major adverse effect is gastrointestinal bleeding, due to a combination of gastroduodenal mucosal injury, erosion, ulceration, and platelet inhibition. The risk of bleeding is higher in the elderly over age 75. Concurrent use of a proton pump inhibitor (PPI) antacid drug reduces the risk of gastro-intestinal bleeding. (1)

In 2018, Dr. Kelvin Tsoi et al. studied GI bleeding in aspirin users, finding more gastrointestinal bleeding in aspirin users (4.64% vs. 2.74%). However, mortality from bleeding only marginally increased in aspirin users: (0.4% aspirin users, and 0.36% non-users). (10)

Conclusion

Aspirin targets the VDAC and detaches HK2 from the VDAC. Aspirin serves as a glycolysis inhibitor and reduces glycolytic cancer stem cells. The aspirin/metformin combination shows striking synergy. Aspirin combined with EGFR-TKIs shows considerable synergy, and ability to overcome TKI drug resistance. Aspirin is beneficial when used with chemotherapy by reducing the activation of NF-kB, thus reducing numbers of cancer stem cells. Aspirin decreases inflammation, decreases cancer stem cells, inhibit platelets and modifies the genetic expression of the cancer cell. Not currently accepted by mainstream oncology for routine use on the oncology wards, aspirin could be incorporated into protocols with anticipated improvement in treatment outcomes.(51)

References for Chapter 13: Aspirin as Anti-Cancer Stem Cell Agent

1) Hua, Hui, et al. "Complex roles of the old drug aspirin in cancer chemoprevention and therapy." Medicinal research reviews 39.1 (2019): 114-145.

2) Cao, Yin, et al. "Long-term aspirin use and total and cancer-specific mortality." Epidemiology Vol.77 (13 Supplement), (2017): 3012-3012.

3) Langley, Ruth E. "Clinical evidence for the use of aspirin in the treatment of cancer." Ecancer medical science 7 (2013).

4) Feng, Weiguo, et al. "Targeting unique metabolic properties of breast tumor initiating cells." Stem Cells 32.7 (2014): 1734-1745.

5) Peng, F., et al. "Glycolysis gatekeeper PDK1 reprograms breast cancer stem cells under hypoxia." Oncogene 37.8 (2018): 1062.

6) Tewari, Debanjan, et al. "Aspirin induces cell death by directly modulating mitochondrial voltage-dependent anion channel (VDAC)." Scientific reports 7.1 (2017): 1-9.

7) Tsoi, Kelvin KF, et al. "Long-term use of low-dose aspirin for cancer prevention: a 10-year population cohort study in Hong Kong." International journal of cancer 145.1 (2019): 267-273.

8) Lapi, F., et al. "Risk of prostate cancer in low-dose aspirin users: A retrospective cohort study." International journal of cancer 139.1 (2016): 205-211.

9) Sung, Joseph JY, et al. "Low-dose aspirin can reduce colorectal cancer mortality after surgery: A 10-year follow-up of 13 528 colorectal cancer patients." Journal of gastroenterology and hepatology 34.6 (2019): 1027-1034.

10) Tsoi, Kelvin KF, et al. "Risk of gastrointestinal bleeding and benefit from colorectal cancer reduction from long-term use of low-dose aspirin: A retrospective study of 612 509 patients." Journal of gastroenterology and hepatology 33.10 (2018): 1728-1736.

11) Khoo, Bee Luan, et al. "Low-dose anti-inflammatory combinatorial therapy reduced cancer stem cell formation in patient-derived preclinical models for tumour relapse prevention." British journal of cancer 120.4 (2019): 407.

12) Zhang, Yiyao, et al. "Aspirin counteracts cancer stem cell features, desmoplasia and gemcitabine resistance in pancreatic cancer." Oncotarget 6.12 (2015): 9999.

13) Dunbar, Karen Jane. "Investigating the effects of aspirin on cell invasion, epithelial-mesenchymal transition and cancer stem cell population in colorectal cancer." (2017).

14) Chen, Zhigang, et al. "Aspirin cooperates with p300 to activate the acetylation of H3K9 and promote FasL-mediated apoptosis of cancer stem-like cells in colorectal cancer." Theranostics 8.16 (2018): 4447.

15) Wang, Hefei, et al. "Reduction of NANOG mediates the inhibitory effect of aspirin on tumor growth and stemness in colorectal cancer." Cellular Physiology and Biochemistry 44.3 (2017): 1051-1063.

16) Tu, L., et al. "Effect of aspirin on breast cancer stem cells and stemness of breast cancer." Zhonghua yi xue za zhi 98.44 (2018): 3598-3602.

17) Saha, Shilpi, et al. "Aspirin suppresses the acquisition of chemoresistance in breast cancer by disrupting an NFκB–IL6 signaling axis responsible for the generation of cancer stem cells." Cancer Research 76.7 (2016): 2000-2012.

18) Pozzoli, Giacomo, et al. "Aspirin inhibits cancer stem cells properties and growth of glioblastoma multiforme through Rb1 pathway modulation." Journal of cellular physiology 234.9 (2019): 15459-15471.

19) Khan, Poulami, et al. "Aspirin enhances cisplatin sensitivity of resistant non-small cell lung carcinoma stem-like cells by targeting mTOR-Akt axis to repress migration." Scientific reports 9.1 (2019): 1-15.

20) Chen, Jinghua, et al. "Aspirin inhibits hypoxia-mediated lung cancer cell stemness and exosome function." Pathology-Research and Practice 215.6 (2019): 152379.

21) Fu, Jinbo, et al. "Aspirin suppresses chemoresistance and enhances antitumor activity of 5-Fu in 5-Fu-resistant colorectal cancer by abolishing 5-Fu-induced NF-κB activation." Scientific reports 9.1 (2019): 1-11.

22) Jiang, Wei, et al. "Aspirin enhances the sensitivity of colon cancer cells to cisplatin by abrogating the binding of NF-κB to the COX-2 promoter." Aging (Albany NY) 12.1 (2020): 611.

23) Li, Ling, et al. "Repositioning Aspirin to Treat Lung and Breast Cancers and Overcome Acquired Resistance to Targeted Therapy." Frontiers in Oncology 9 (2019).

24) Yong, H., and H. Rui. "P1. 03-27 Aspirin Overcomes Acquired Resistance to Osimertinib in Human Lung Cancer Cells via Bim-Dependent Apoptosis Induction." Journal of Thoracic Oncology 14.10 (2019): S428-S429.

25) Patrignani, Paola, and Melania Dovizio. "COX-2 and EGFR: partners in crime split by aspirin." EBioMedicine 2.5 (2015): 372-373.

26) Li, Haitao, et al. "Aspirin prevents colorectal cancer by normalizing EGFR expression." EBioMedicine 2.5 (2015): 447-455.

27) Chiow, Kher Hsin, et al. "SNX3-dependent regulation of epidermal growth factor receptor (EGFR) trafficking and degradation by aspirin in epidermoid carcinoma (A-431) cells." Cellular and Molecular Life Sciences 69.9 (2012): 1505-1521.

28) Becker, J. C., et al. "Acetylsalicylic acid enhances antiproliferative effects of the EGFR inhibitor gefitinib in the absence of activating mutations in gastric cancer." International journal of oncology 29.3 (2006): 615-623.

29) Cho, May, et al. "Aspirin blocks EGF-stimulated cell viability in a COX-1 dependent manner in ovarian cancer cells." Journal of Cancer 4.8 (2013): 671.

30) Hu, Xiu, et al. "Synergistic antitumor activity of aspirin and erlotinib: Inhibition of p38 enhanced aspirin plus erlotinib-induced suppression of metastasis and promoted cancer cell apoptosis." Oncology letters 16.2 (2018): 2715-2724.

31) Huang, Zhenjun, et al. "Aspirin induces BECLIN-1-dependent autophagy of human hepatocellular carcinoma cell." European journal of pharmacology 823 (2018): 58-64.

32) Abdelmonsif, Doaa Ali, et al. "Targeting AMPK, mTOR and β-catenin by combined metformin and aspirin therapy in HCC: an appraisal in Egyptian HCC patients." Molecular diagnosis & therapy 22.1 (2018): 115-127.

33) Verdoodt, F., S. K. Kjaer, and S. Friis. "Influence of aspirin and non-aspirin NSAID use on ovarian and endometrial cancer: summary of epidemiologic evidence of cancer risk and prognosis." Maturitas 100 (2017): 1-7

34) Pozzoli, Giacomo, et al. "Aspirin inhibits proliferation and promotes differentiation of neuroblastoma cells via p21Waf1 protein up-regulation and Rb1 pathway modulation." Journal of cellular and molecular medicine 23.10 (2019): 7078-7087.

35) Amaral, Maria Eduarda Azambuja, et al. "Pre-clinical effects of metformin and aspirin on the cell lines of different breast cancer subtypes." Investigational new drugs 36.5 (2018): 782-796.

36) Yue, Wen, et al. "Repurposing of metformin and aspirin by targeting AMPK-mTOR and inflammation for pancreatic cancer prevention and treatment." Cancer prevention research 7.4 (2014): 388-397.

37) Yue, Wen, et al. "Metformin combined with aspirin significantly inhibit pancreatic cancer cell growth in vitro and in vivo by suppressing anti-apoptotic proteins Mcl-1 and Bcl-2." Oncotarget 6.25 (2015): 21208.

38) Yue, Wen, et al. "Transcriptomic analysis of pancreatic cancer cells in response to metformin and aspirin: an implication of synergy." Scientific reports 5 (2015): 13390.

39) Johnson, Kelly E., et al. "Aspirin inhibits platelets from reprogramming breast tumor cells and promoting metastasis." Blood advances 3.2 (2019): 198-211.

40) Lichtenberger, Lenard M., and K. Vinod Vijayan. "Are Platelets the Primary Target of Aspirin's Remarkable Anticancer Activity?" Cancer research 79.15 (2019): 3820-3823.

41) Vogel, Daphne YS, et al. "Macrophages migrate in an activation-dependent manner to chemokines involved in neuroinflammation." Journal of neuroinflammation 11.1 (2014): 23.

42) Bonecchi, Raffaella, et al. "Chemokines and chemokine receptors: new targets for cancer immunotherapy." Frontiers in immunology 10 (2019): 379.

43) Nagarsheth, Nisha, Max S. Wicha, and Weiping Zou. "Chemokines in the cancer microenvironment and their relevance in cancer immunotherapy." Nature Reviews Immunology 17.9 (2017): 559.

44) Hsieh, Chia-Chien, and Chih-Hsuan Wang. "Aspirin disrupts the crosstalk of angiogenic and inflammatory cytokines between 4T1 breast cancer cells and macrophages." Mediators of Inflammation 2018 (2018).

45) Din, Farhat VN, et al. "Aspirin inhibits mTOR signaling, activates AMP-activated protein kinase, and induces autophagy in colorectal cancer cells." Gastroenterology 142.7 (2012): 1504-1515.

46) Castoldi, Francesca, et al. "Aspirin induces autophagy via inhibition of the acetyltransferase EP300." Oncotarget 9.37 (2018): 24574.

47) Zhao, Qianqian, et al. "Aspirin may inhibit angiogenesis and induce autophagy by inhibiting mTOR signaling pathway in murine hepatocarcinoma and sarcoma models." Oncology letters 12.4 (2016): 2804-2810.

48) Henry, Whitney S., et al. "Aspirin suppresses growth in PI3K-mutant breast cancer by activating AMPK and inhibiting mTORC1 signaling." Cancer research 77.3 (2017): 790-801.

49) Pietrocola, Federico, et al. "Aspirin—another caloric-restriction mimetic." Autophagy 14.7 (2018): 1162-1163.

50) Usman, Muhammad Waqas, et al. "Chemopreventive effects of aspirin at a glance." Biochimica et Biophysica Acta (BBA)-Reviews on Cancer 1855.2 (2015): 254-263.

51) Ai, Guoqiang, et al. "Aspirin and salicylic acid decrease c-Myc expression in cancer cells: a potential role in chemoprevention." Tumor Biology 37.2 (2016): 1727-1738

Chapter 14

Metformin Anti-Cancer Stem Cell Drug

A DERIVATIVE OF THE FRENCH lilac plant, metformin is known as the "the good anti-diabetic drug," taken by 150 million people worldwide for control of blood sugar in type-two diabetes. Metformin is still the best treatment for type-two diabetes. (1–3)

Remarkably, metformin is also an anti-cancer drug. In 2005, Dr. Josie Evans et al. made the observation that diabetic patients on metformin have a 23 per cent reduction in cancer. (4) Others have found a 30–50 per cent reduction in risk for cancer in metformin users. (5) Since 2005, there has been considerable effort to elucidate the anti-cancer mechanism of metformin in both the laboratory and clinical setting. (6–7)

How Does Metformin Work?

Metformin accumulates inside the cancer cell's mitochondria, the microscopic organelles in our cells involved in energy production. Once inside the mitochondria, metformin inhibits complex I of the mitochondrial electron transport chain. This in turn activates AMP-kinase (AMPK), which then inhibits the mTOR signal pathway, which reduces cancer cell proliferation. AMPK activation decreases glucose blood levels by decreasing hepatic glucose output and increasing glucose uptake by muscle and fat tissue. This results in overall increased insulin sensitivity and reduced insulin levels in the type II diabetic.

The inhibition of complex one of the electron transport chain (ETC) in mitochondria appears specific for cancer cells, resulting in a shift toward a glycolytic phenotype with increased glucose consumption and lactate production. (7–9)

Hexokinase 2—A Major Player in the Cancer Cell

As mentioned in chapter 4, "Cancer as a Metabolic Disease," bulk tumor cells proliferate rapidly in an uncontrolled manner. To support this rapid proliferation, their metabolic pathways are massively upregulated. These metabolic variations can be exploited to selectively kill cancer cells, leaving normal cells unharmed. The cancer cell has a voracious appetite for glucose consumption, and accomplishes this by switching to an embryonic form of the hexokinase enzyme called Hexokinase 2 (HK2), which is not present in normal cells. HK2 is the first step in the conversion of glucose to glucose-6-phosphate. Production of HK2 in the cancer cell is upregulated over 100 times by genetic amplification. Another peculiar feature of the cancer cell is the attachment of this hexokinase 2 enzyme to the voltage-dependent anion channel (VDAC) located on the outer mitochondrial membrane of the cancer cell. This unusual attachment of the HK2 to the VDAC supports GLYCOLYSIS and prevents mitochondrial apoptosis, immortalizing the cancer cell. Detachment of HK2 from the VDAC restores mitochondrial apoptosis pathways, allowing the cancer cell to undergo a form of programmed cell death (suicide). (10)

Metformin Docks in Hexokinase 2 Enzyme—A Monkey Wrench for the Cancer Cell

The metformin molecule serves as a "monkey wrench," sabotaging the metabolic machinery of the cancer cell. Separation of the HK2 from the VDAC, and inhibition of the HK-2 enzyme is synonymous with inhibition of GYCOLYSIS.

In 2013, Barbara Salani's group published their in vitro lung cancer cell study, showing that metformin docks in the hexokinase 2 binding site, effectively blocking its function, resulting in separation of hexokinase 2 from the VDAC on the outer mitochondrial membrane. They write:

> This inhibition [of Hexokinase] virtually abolishes cell glucose uptake and phosphorylation as documented by the reduced entrapment of 18F-fluorodeoxy-glucose. [**Note**: this is glucose tagged with a radioactive tracer used for PET imaging]. In-silico models indicate that this action is due to metformin capability to mimic G6P [glucose-6-phosphate] features by steadily binding its pocket in HK2. The impairment of this energy source results in mitochondrial depolarization and subsequent cell death.... metformin is thus prefigured as an uncompetitive and allosteric inhibitor of HK2 as only the enzyme-substrate complex can be bound.... reduced FDG uptake [Flouro-Deoxy-Glucose, the PET Scan Imaging isotope] reflects a selective

metformin-induced impairment of glucose phosphorylation.... **HK2 inhibition by metformin causes release of this enzyme [HK2] from the outer membrane of mitochondria, thus leading to the activation of apoptotic signals [cell death].** (11)

In 2006, Drs. Saroj Mathupala, Young H. Ko, and P. L. Pedersen write separation of HKII from VDAC allows cancer cell apoptosis to proceed:

> When HK [hexokinase] is released from VDAC... tumor cells rapidly undergo apoptosis under a variety of stimuli which were previously ineffective in inducing apoptosis." (10)

Metformin Inhibits Hexokinase Function

In 2013, Drs. Ceclia Marini and Barbara Salani et al., in a follow-up to a previous study, examined the effect of metformin in a triple-negative breast cancer cell model (in vitro) and in mouse xenografts (in vivo). This elegant study used both PET FDG scan imaging and immunofluorescent imaging. Dr. Marini et al. found reduced glucose consumption, which activated AMP-kinase in the cancer cells, thought to be related to inhibition of HK2 function. (11–12)

> [Metformin] **actually inhibits HK function**, resulting in an immediate cytotoxic effect both in vitro and in vivo as well as in a significant reduction of cancer growth rate under chronic treatment... Metformin strikingly impaired glucose consumption of MDA-MB-231[breast cancer cells] in a dose- and time-dependent manner ... that **progressively reduced FDG [PET Scan tracer] uptake down to its minimum values after 48 hours**.... More importantly, metformin treatment had a relevant influence on cancer growth. In fact, weight

of explanted lesions was almost halved in "prolonged" mice treated with metformin for the whole month of study duration, while it was obviously not affected by pulsed treatment... The present study documents that metformin reduces cancer metabolism and growth at least partially via a direct and selective inhibition of HK I and II enzymatic function ... and its interaction with mitochondria hampering a crucial aspect for tumor immortality. (12)

Immunofluorescence Confirms Displacement of HK2 away from Mitochondrial Membrane to the Cytosol

As mentioned above, apoptosis in cancer cells is inhibited by the peculiar placement of HK2 at the VDAC on the outer mitochondrial membrane. Metformin not only inhibits glucose metabolism, it also restores apoptosis (programmed cell death, or suicide) to the cancer cell by displacing HK2 away from the mitochondrial membrane, back to its normal place in the cytosol. Dr. Cecilia Marini et al. write:

> Metformin displaced this [HK2] isoform away from mitochondrial membrane to the cytosol, limiting its preferential access to ATP for glucose phosphorylation and, thus, hampering a major mechanism of cancer growth and immortality... (12)

Metformin Induces Protective Autophagy by Inhibiting mTOR

In 2020, Dr. David Gewirtz defined autophagy:

> Autophagy, a process of cellular self-degradation and cell survival whereby the cell generates energy and metabolic intermediates under conditions of stress [i.e., nutrient deprivation], is also commonly induced in tumor cells in response to chemotherapy and radiation. (13)

Protective autophagy (also called pro-survival autophagy) is an important cell function carried out in the cell by lysosomes, small acid-containing bags used for degradation and digestion of proteins or old organelles earmarked for destruction or recycling. Old cell proteins targeted for recycling are first sequestered into microscopic "bags" called autophagosomes. These are later fused with the acid-containing lysosome, forming the autolysosome that can digest and degrade the cell contents, which are eventually recycled for nutrition or other needed cell activities.

Inner Railroad Microtubule System

The lysosomes are shuttled around the cell on a microtubule system similar to a railroad track. During periods of plentiful nutrients and growth stimulation, AMP-kinase is inhibited and mTOR is activated, directing the lysosomes to re-arrange near the cell periphery at the plasma membrane, ready to work. This is called "lysosomal trafficking." The mTOR pathway is the main gateway and controller of autophagy in the cell.

Perinuclear Clustering

The opposite can also occur with AMP activation. Instead of migrating to the periphery, the lysosomes migrate centrally and cluster around the cell nucleus. For example, AMPK activation from nutrient starvation or drug treatment with metformin inhibits mTOR, which then induces "protective autophagy," a process in which lysosomes assume a peculiar arrangement called "perinuclear clustering." Microscopic observation reveals the lysosomes cluster around the cell nucleus. (13–16)

In chapter 21, on artemisinin, we discuss how microscopic observation of the breast cancer cells reveals perinuclear clustering of lysosomes after artemisinin treatment, a sign of "protective autophagy" induction.

As mentioned above, metformin activates AMP-kinase (AMPK), which inhibits the mTOR signal pathway, which then induces protective autophagy with perinuclear clustering of lysosomes. Similarly, dichloroacetate (DCA) and many other anti-cancer drugs activate protective autophagy, a survival mechanism for the cancer cell. (17)

In this scenario, combination with an autophagy inhibitor such as chloroquine or hydroxychloroquine may prove synergistic. An example of this is the combined use of quercetin, which induces protective autophagy, and chloroquine, the autophagy inhibitor, providing synergistic anti-cancer effects in a gastric cancer cell model studied by Dr. Kui Wang et al. in 2011. (18)

Metformin Synergy with Autophagy Inhibitor chloroquine

Like many mTOR inhibitors, metformin induces protective autophagy, and one might expect that in combination with an autophagy inhibitor such as chloroquine it would provide synergy, with augmented anti-cancer activity. In 2011, Dr. Alelejandro Vasquez-Martin et al. made this same suggestion, proposing the combination of both drugs to eradicate cancer stem cells (CSC) in premalignant lesions, specifically, ductal carcinoma of the breast in situ (DCIS). (19)

Likewise, in 2020, Dr. Bo Li et al. found this combination synergistic in osteosarcoma in vitro. (20)

In 2017, Dr. Remco Molenaar et al. proposed a clinical trial of the metformin/chloroquine combination for solid tumors. (21) We await the results of that investigation. See chapters 32 and 33 on chloroquine and autophagy inhibitors for more on this topic.

Pancreatic Cancer Stems Cell Use OXPHOS

In 2015, Dr. Patricia Sancho et al. studied metformin's effects on pancreatic CSCs, finding that metformin targets pancreatic cancer stem cells (CSCs) but not their differentiated non-cancer stem cells (non-CSCs). Dr. Sancho and colleagues' study of pancreatic cancer demonstrated that tumor bulk, or non CSCs, are highly glycolytic. On the other hand, CSCs use OXPHOS and are dependent on oxidative metabolism with "very limited metabolic plasticity." Thus, mitochondrial inhibition by metformin creates an energy crisis and induces CSC apoptosis. Dr. Sancho et al. state that cancer stem cells are heterogeneous, and become metformin-resistant over time. These resistant cancer stem cells have an intermediate "glycolytic/respiratory phenotype." In other words, they use both the GLYCOLYSIS and OXPHOS pathways. Dr. Sancho et al. write that "resistant Cancer Stem Cell (CSC) clones eventually emerge with intermediate glycolytic/respiratory phenotype."(22) They have replicated the findings of the Lisanti Group, which found that long-term treatment of cancer stem cells (OXPHOS phenotype) with doxycycline resulted in emergence of a doxycycline- resistant (DOX-R) cancer stem cell type, which acquired a purely glycolytic phenotype, also called the Warburg phenotype. (23)

OXPHOS Required for Cancer Stem Cell Functionality

Similarly, Dr. Sancho's group found that cancer stem cells developed resistance to metformin over time, a problem resolved by combining metformin with c-Myc inhibitor drug, overcoming the resistant phenotype. They write that "high OXPHOS activity is mandatory for full cancer stem cell functionality" and that

combining metformin with c-Myc inhibition, prevented or reversed, respectively, resistance to metformin by enforcing their dependence on OXPHOS, suggesting a new multimodal approach for targeting the distinct metabolic features of pancreatic CSCs [cancer stem cells] ... increased MYC expression is indeed the mechanistic link for the altered/distinct metabolic phenotype of resistant CSC with enhanced glycolysis. Notably, MYC inhibition or knockdown also enhanced stemness of resistant CSCs, as evidenced by increased pluripotency gene expression, self-renewal capacity, and CD133+cell content. **These data confirm that high OXPHOS activity is mandatory for full CSC functionality.** (22)

Note: The c-Myc oncogene orchestrates the Warburg Effect (i.e. GLYCOLYSIS). Inhibiting c-Myc will inhibit GYCOLYSIS. C-Myc is also a downstream target of the Wnt/beta-catenin pathway, so all Wnt inhibitors are also c-Myc inhibitors. (24–25) Other C-Myc inhibitors include artesunate, pterostilbene, sulforaphane, and diclofenac.

Artesunate Degrades c-Myc protein

The antimalaria drug artesunate is now a first-line treatment for severe malaria in Third World countries and is commonly infused intravenously in millions of patients with virtually no adverse effects. For more, see chapter 21, "Artemisinin Antimalarial, A Gift from China." Artesunate is also an effective anti-cancer agent that degrades the c-Myc protein. (26–27)

According to Dr. Jin-Jian Lu et al. (2010):

Dihydroartemisinin accelerates c-Myc oncoprotein degradation and induces apoptosis in c-Myc-overexpressing tumor cells ... ARTs [Artemisinin Derivatives] might be useful in the treatment of c-Myc-overexpressing tumors. We also suggest that c-Myc may potentially be a biomarker candidate for prediction of the anti-tumor efficacies of ARTs. (26)

Dr. Lu et al. found that artesunate and dihydro-artemisinin (DHA) induce significant apoptosis in cancer cell lines overexpressing the c-Myc protein. DHA (and artesunate) irreversibly downregulated the protein level of c-Myc and accelerated degradation of c-Myc protein in the cancer cells. Dr. Lu concluded that artesunate would be useful in the treatment of c-Myc-overexpressing cancer cell types, as c-Myc could serve as biomarker candidate for prediction of the anti-tumor efficacy of artesunate. (26–27)

In 2015, Dr. Huabo Wang et al. further discussed c-Myc inhibitors, frequently observing dysregulation and overexpression of the c-Myc oncoprotein in cancer cells. In these overexpressing c-Myc cancers, inhibition of c-Myc leads to cancer cell death. Interestingly, the effects of c-Myc inhibitor can be mimicked by inhibition of the mitochondrial electron transport chain. This is not surprising, as we have already established that OXPHOS inhibitors are also Wnt pathway inhibitors, and since c-Myc is downstream to Wnt, OXPHOS inhibition will also inhibit c-Myc as well. Dr. Wang et al. write:

> All Myc inhibitors, irrespective of class, lead to eventual cellular demise. **This involves the depletion of ATP stores due to mitochondrial dysfunction and the eventual downregulation of Myc protein.** The accompanying metabolic de-regulation causes neutral lipid accumulation, cell-cycle arrest, and an attempt to rectify the ATP deficit by **upregulating AMP-activated protein kinase (AMPK).** These responses are ultimately futile due to the lack of functional Myc to support the requisite **anabolic response.** Finally, the effects of Myc depletion on ATP levels, cell cycle arrest, differentiation and **AMPK activation** can be **mimicked by pharmacologic inhibition of the mitochondrial electron transport chain without affecting Myc levels.** Thus, all Myc inhibitors promote a global energy collapse that appears to underlie many of their phenotypic consequences. (27)

Important! Inhibition of the oncoprotein c-Myc is mimicked by inhibition of the mitochondrial electron transport chain (metformin, doxycycline, pyrvinium, niclosamide etc.); therefore all OXPHOS inhibitors mimic c-Myc inhibition and can lead to "global energy collapse."

Low c-Myc in Cancer Stem Cells, High c-Myc in Glycolytic Cancer Cells

Activation of the c-Myc protein pathway promotes a glycolytic (Warburg-like) cell phenotype. In 2015, Dr. Sancho et al. studied c-Myc in pancreatic cancer stem cells, finding that LOW Myc expression allowed high peroxisome proliferator-activated receptor (PPAR) activity, resulting in increased mitochondrial biogenesis, enhanced mitochondrial activity (OXPHOS), and low mitochondrial reactive oxygen Species (ROS), all prerequisites for cancer cell "stemness." Suppression (or inhibition) of c-Myc to low levels maintained the cancer stem cells, and rendered them unable to switch over to a glycolytic phenotype (the Warburg Effect), thus making the cancer stem cells susceptible to mitochondrial inhibition with metformin and menadione (vitamin K). (22)

Important: Pancreatic cancer stem cells have low c-Myc activity, preventing a switch to the glycolytic phenotype.

Wnt Inhibitors Are Also c-Myc Inhibitors

Other c-Myc inhibitors include all OXPHOS/Wnt inhibitors drugs, such as niclosamide, ivermectin, pyrvinium, aspirin, celecoxib etc. (28)

The signaling proteins c-myc, cyclin D1, and axin are downstream from Wnt pathway signaling, so all Wnt inhibitors also inhibit c-myc and cyclin D1.

Overexpression of C-Myc Associated with Aggressive Biology and Poor Prognosis

The oncogene c-Myc is a transcription factor regulating proliferation, growth, and apoptosis. Overexpression or amplification of the c-Myc oncogene and protein promotes a Warburg-like glycolytic phenotype, associated with aggressive cancer cell biology with poor prognosis, rendering intensive chemotherapy futile, providing brief remission with no survival benefit. In B-Cell lymphoma, Myc gene amplification or overexpression might be related to a more aggressive, blastoid variant. (29)

Indeed, in 2015, Dr. Shuhua Yi et al. studied a series of mantle B-cell lymphoma patients with c-Myc overexpression, writing:

> Intensive chemotherapy, such as HyperCVAD/MA ± R [standard chemotherapy protocol for lymphoma] did not improve the survival of [lymphoma patients] with a c-Myc abnormality, and a new treatment strategy should be developed. (30)

Note: HyperCVAD is an acronym for a routine chemotherapy protocol. "Hyper'" refers to the hyperfractionated nature of the chemotherapy, which is given in smaller doses, or frequently, to minimize side effects. "CVAD" is the acronym of drugs used: cyclophosphamide, vincristine, doxorubicin (trade name, Adriamycin), and dexamethasone. MA=Methotrexate, R=Rituximab.

In patients with c-Myc abnormalities, the cell type is so aggressive that chemotherapy fails to improve survival, and new approaches to treatment are needed. For example, the combination of an OXPHOS inhibitor, such as **metformin** or **doxycycline** (targeting cancer stem cells), along with a c-Myc inhibitor, such as artesunate, might represent such a new treatment strategy. (29–31)

One might suggest the metformin/ menadione (vitamin k) combination as suggested by Dr. Sancho. Another useful combination is DCA / metformin / Poly-MVA, which is discussed in chapter 5, on dichloroacetate (DCA).

Double-Hit Lymphoma

Chemotherapy is futile in another aggressive cell type called "double-hit" lymphoma, which has both c-Myc and BCL-2 (the anti-apoptosis protein) overexpression on immunohistochemistry. The use of OXPHOS inhibitors and c-Myc inhibitors, with the addition of a BCL-2 inhibitor drug such as venetoclax might prove useful. (32)

We await NIH-funded confirmatory studies.

Metformin Synergizes with GLYCOLYSIS Inhibition

As mentioned above, pancreatic cancer stem cells preferentially use mitochondrial OXPHOS (oxidative phosphorylation) pathways for their energetic, migratory, and metastatic capacity. Indeed, Dr. Diana Whitaker-Menezes et al. in *Cell Cycle* (2011) reported that hyperactive oxidative mitochondrial metabolism in cancer stem cells was blocked by metformin, inducing a purely glycolytic phenotype in surviving cancer stem cells, now rendered sensitive to glucose starvation with a second agent such as 2DG or high-dose intravenous vitamin C, creating synthetic lethality. (33–34). Other glycolysis inhibitors, such as DCA or diclofenac might be considered instead of 2DG. For example, in 2018, Dr. Valeria Gerthofer et al. studied the anti-cancer effects of metformin on a glioblastoma cell line. Considerable synergy was observed with the addition of a glycolysis inhibitor, diclofenac. This is expected, since the OXPHOS inhibitor metformin probably induced a glycolytic cell line, now susceptible to inhibition by the diclofenac. (35)

Metformin as an Anti-Cancer Stem Cell Agent

In 2013, Dr. Heather Hirsch et al. studied a breast cancer mouse xenograft model, finding metformin "selectively kills" cancer stem cells by inhibiting NF-kB activation and STAT3 activation. Metformin is also effective as a stem cell agent in mouse xenograft studies involving inflammatory prostate cancer and melanoma cell lines. (9)

Metformin Epigenetic Effects

In 2012, Dr. Bin Bao et al. studied the anti-cancer stem cell ability of metformin in a pancreatic cancer cell line, finding metformin decreased the cancer stem cell markers CD44, EpCAM, EZH2, Notch-1, Nanogand, and Oct4. Metformin also caused:

> re-expression of [micro- RNA's] miRNAs (let-7a ,let-7b, miR-26a, miR-101, miR-200b, and miR-200c) that are typically lost in pancreatic cancer and especially in pancreatospheres [stem cells]. These results clearly suggest that the biologic effects of metformin are mediated through re-expression

of miRNAs and decreased expression of [Cancer Stem Cell] CSC-specific genes, suggesting that metformin could be useful for overcoming therapeutic resistance of pancreatic cancer cells. (36)

Note: Micro RNA (MiRNA) plays a role in the post-transcriptional regulation of protein expression.

In 2017, Dr. Yong Lei et al. reviewed metformin's ability to target and eradicate cancer stem cells in multiple cancer cell types via activation of AMPK and suppression of mTOR, as well as inhibition of NF-kB. (37)

In 2014, Dr. Marta Gritti et al. reported metformin could be repositioned for treatment of glioblastoma cancer stem cells. (39)

In 2017, Dr. Peiguo Shi et al. found metformin suppresses triple-negative breast cancer stem cells. (38)

In 2016, Dr. Fabrizio Marcucci et al. reviewed the current literature on anti-cancer stem cell agents, writing that metformin acts as an endogenous inhibitor of cancer cells, preferentially inhibiting the cancer stem cells rather than bulk tumor by activating AMPK, which leads to inhibition of PI3K/AKT/mTOR signaling and STAT3 signaling. Metformin is currently under investigation in over 100 clinical trials, many involving activity as anti-cancer stem cell agents. We await these results. (40)

In 2019, Dr. Indranil Banerjee et al. studied the combination of metronomic low-dose doxorubicin with metformin in a mouse xenograft breast cancer model, showing a "strong anti-cancer effect," with inhibition of the Wnt/Beta-Catenin pathway and inhibition of cancer stem cells. (41)

Metformin Clinical Trial in Ovarian Cancer

In 2017, Dr. Ronald Buckanovich et al. did a phase II clinical trial of metformin combined with chemotherapy as a cancer stem cell targeting agent in advanced ovarian cancer in 38 patients over 18 months. They found a 3-fold decrease in cancer stem cell markers in the metformin-treated patients:

> Tumors treated with metformin were noted to have a 3-fold decrease in ALDH+ CSC at baseline, increased sensitivity to Cisplatin [chemotherapy] in vitro, and a reduced ability to amplify ALDH+ CSC with passage in vitro. [ALDH+ is a cancer stem cell marker] ... This is the first prospective study of Metformin in EOC [end-stage ovarian cancer] patients. Translational studies confirm an impact of metformin on CSC [cancer stem cells]. Metformin was well tolerated and outcome results were favorable, supporting the use of Metformin in phase-III studies. (42)

In 2017, Dr. Cuyas Elisabet et al. found that metformin inhibits receptor activator of NF-kB ligand (RANKL) and sensitizes breast cancer stem cells to the cancer drug denosumab, a RANKL inhibitor originally developed for treating osteoporosis. (43)

Synthetic Lethality with Glucose Starvation

Chapter 9, "Doxycycline / Vitamin C Anti-Cancer Synergy" discusses the work of the Michael Lisanti Group in Italy. Dr. Lisanti's group showed that converting cancer stem cells to a purely glycolytic phenotype using repeated passages through higher doses of doxycycline renders the cancer stem cells sensitive to synthetic lethality with a second metabolic inhibitor. One such second metabolic inhibitor is high-dose IV vitamin C (ascorbate), which serves as a potent glycolysis inhibitor, 10 times more potent than 2-deoxy-glucose (2-DG). (23)

Synthetic Lethality Metformin/ GLYCOLYSIS Inhibitor

Similarly, synthetic lethality was found with combined use of metformin and the glycolysis inhibitor 2-deoxyglucose (2-DG) in 2016 by Dr. Jie Zhu et al. studying an ovarian cancer cell model, and in 2010 by Dr. Issam Ben Sahra et al. studying a prostate cancer cell model. (44–45)

One might speculate that other glycolysis inhibitors such as DCA, diclofenac or quercetin might serve in place of 2-DG. Indeed, synergy of glycolysis inhibitor DCA with OXPHOS inhibitor metformin has been found, as discussed in Chapter 5 on DCA Dichloroactetate.

Synthetic Lethality with Metformin and Doxycycline

By blocking mitochondrial oxidative phosphorylation, metformin converts cancer stem cells to a purely glycolytic phenotype. One might expect a more robust conversion to glycolytic phenotype with a combination of two OXPHOS inhibitors, doxycycline and metformin. Doxycycline impairs ribosomal protein production in the mitochondria, while, as mentioned above, metformin impairs complex one in the ETC in the mitochondria and blocks the

HK2 enzyme as well. Indeed, two clinical trials of combination doxycycline and metformin are under way at the Sidney Kimmel Cancer Center at Johns Hopkins University. One involves patients with breast or uterine cancer and the second, a randomized phase II trial, involves patients with head-and-neck squamous cell cancer. (46–47)

COC Clinical Trial with Four Drugs

A third study called METRICS, under way by Care Oncology Clinic, London (Health Clinics Limited), will use the combination of four metabolic inhibitors in 207 cancer patients compared to historic controls. (48) These four drugs are:

- Metformin (OXPHOS inhibitor)
- Doxycycline (OXPHOS and Autophagy Inhibitor)
- Mebendazole (microtubule Inhibitor)
- Atorvastatin (HMG-Co reductase/mevalonate inhibitor)

The missing agent, of course is a glycolysis inhibitor drug. One might predict a more robust anti-cancer effect by adding to this protocol a glycolysis inhibitor such as DCA, Quercetin or Diclofenac.

Progression of Chronic Lymphocytic Leukemia (CLL)

CLL cells are usually resting in a quiescent state. However, they can be activated by the immune system to undergo metamorphosis into highly aggressive proliferative cell types. In 2015, Dr. Silvia Bruno et al. studied the effect of metformin administered to quiescent CLL cells as well as stimulated cells in vitro, writing:

> Metformin was administered in vitro either to quiescent cells or during CLL cell activation stimuli, provided by classical co-culturing with CD40L-expressing fibroblasts ... the fraction of Ki-67 positive cells was significantly lower in metformin-treated CLL (cancer) cells than in untreated controls, in a dose-dependent way ... Metformin inhibits cell cycle progression of B-cell chronic lymphocytic leukemia cells (CLL). (49)

Dr. Bruno et al. report that metformin slowed the proliferation rate of the cancer cells, as measured by the Ki-67 index. In addition, the cancer cells stimulated by co-culture with CD40L expressing fibroblasts had a 10-fold increase in glucose uptake compared to quiescent cancer cells. This stimulated rise in glucose uptake, glycolytic ability, and ATP production was remarkably inhibited by metformin. Dr. Bruno's group also studied the combination of metformin with the chemotherapy drug fludarabine, as well as the combination of metformin with a BCL2 inhibitor (ABT-737, similar to venetoclax), finding excellent synergy with augmented cancer cell death for both stimulated and unstimulated CLL cells. (49)

Metformin Inhibits B-Cell Lymphoma

Dr. W.Y. Shi et al. reported in *Cell Death* (2012) that AMPK activity is completely lost in lymphoma cells and is restored by metformin, which blocks lymphoma cell growth via inhibition of the mTOR pathway. Remarkably, metformin blocked tumor growth in murine lymphoma xenografts at a concentration of 10 mM, while leaving normal hematopoietic progenitor cells unharmed. (50)

Metformin for Prostate Cancer

The combination of metformin with the glycolysis inhibitor 2DG was very effective in a prostate cancer cell model studied by Dr. Issam Ben Sahra et al. in 2010 with 96% inhibition of cell viability in prostate cancer cells. (45)

One might expect similar synergy of metformin with other glycolysis inhibitors such as DCA, quercetin, and diclofenac. (18)(51)

In 2013, Dr. Heather Hirsch et al. found metformin effective for inflammatory prostate cancer cell in vitro and in vivo xenografts. The combination of metformin with doxorubicin chemotherapy prevented relapse in a mouse xenograft model of prostate cancer, and also in a lung cancer model. (9)

Retrospective Metformin Study Shows Significant Clinical Benefit in Prostate Cancer

In 2013, Dr. Daniel Spratt et al. did a retrospective study of 2,901 men followed over 9 years after radiation therapy for prostate cancer showing that those patients taking metformin had "significant clinical benefit."

After 9 years of follow-up, mortality from prostate cancer was only 2.7% for metformin users compared to those not using metformin: 22% mortality for diabetics and 8.2% mortality for non-diabetics not using metformin. I thought this was rather impressive. Dr. Spratt et al. write:

Metformin decreased the risk of PSA recurrence, distant metastasis, and PCSM [prostate cancer specific mortality] compared with diabetic non-metformin patients. To our knowledge, this is **the first clinical evidence** that metformin may improve cancer-specific survival outcomes in prostate cancer. Furthermore, metformin strongly decreased the clinically defined transformation from androgen-sensitive prostate cancer to CRPC [castrate-resistant prostate cancer].

Note: PSA = Prostate Specific Antigen, a common marker for prostate cancer. (52)

Metformin Synergy with Rituximab

In routine use since 1997 for B-Cell lymphoma, rituximab (Rituxan®) is a monoclonal antibody directed at the CD-20 protein marker located on the outer membrane surface of the B cells. Rituximab is considered the most significant advance in treatment of B-cell lymphoma since the original introduction of chemotherapy.

In 2015, Dr. Priyank P. Patel et al. studied the combination of metformin and rituximab in vitro and in vivo mouse models of B-cell lymphoma showing good synergy, with enhancement of the anti-tumor activity of rituximab, writing:

Metformin enhanced the antiproliferative effects of [rituximab] mAbs targeting CD20…. Our data suggests that metformin inhibits the proliferation of B-cell lymphoma cell lines and enhances the anti-tumor activity of rituximab. (53)

Metformin as an Immunotherapy Agent

Metformin downregulates inflammatory cytokines used for cancer growth and signaling. Moreover, metformin has a beneficial effect on the immune system by enhancing killer T Cell anti-cancer activity, Dr. Tae Hun Kim et al. report in 2014:

> Metformin has been shown to decrease the production of inflammatory cytokines, including TNF-a, interleukin-6, and vascular endothelial growth factor [VEGF] through the inactivation of **NF-KB** and **HIF-1a**.... Metformin treatment inhibits neoplastic angiogenesis, resulting in the reduction of tumor growth. (54)

Dr. Hirsch et al. write (2013) that "metformin may block a metabolic stress response that stimulates the inflammatory pathway associated with a wide variety of cancers."(9)

Dr. Sara Verdura et al. (2019) consider "metformin as an archetype immuno-metabolic adjuvant for cancer immunotherapy." They write the following about metformin:

> 1) Enhances the anti-tumor functionality of T cells [immune cells].
>
> 2) Downregulates PD-L1 in cancer cells [programmed death ligand which inhibits apoptosis].
>
> 3) Neutralizes immune-inhibitory cell populations residing in the tumor micro-environment [TME]. (55)

In agreement with the concept of metformin as an immunotherapy agent is Dr. Afzal's study in 2018 of a group of metastatic melanoma patients undergoing treatment with new checkpoint inhibitor drugs (anti-PD-1/ anti–CTLA-4 antibodies). Those concurrently taking metformin fared better with prolonged survival. Median overall survival (OS) was 46.7 months (with metformin) versus 28 months, and median progression-free survival PFS 19.8 months (with metformin) versus 5 months. More clinical trials are underway. (56)

Metformin and the Tumor Microenvironment (TME)

In 2019, Dr. Ivana Kurelac et al. reviewed the effects of metformin on the tumor micro-environment, focusing on inhibition of angiogenesis (new blood vessel formation), cancer-associated fibroblasts (CAFs), tumor-associated macrophages, and cancer immunosuppression. Metformin reduces tumor-induced angiogenic signaling by downregulating hypoxia-inducible factor-1-alpha (HIF-1-alpha) and VEGF, resulting in tumor growth retardation, with smaller and less dense tumor micro-vascularity. This is related to the inhibition of complex I of the mitochondrial ETC, producing increased oxygen within the cells. (57–61)

Cancer-Associated Fibroblasts

One of the mechanisms by which the TME is hijacked to stimulate rapid proliferation of the cancer mass is the reprograming of fibroblasts in surrounding tissues into CAFs, which have activated their nuclear factor kappa B (NF-kB) pathway to secrete pro-inflammatory cytokines into the micro-environment that feeds the tumor cells. Metformin directly blocks both CAF and macrophage pro-inflammatory signaling by down- regulating NF-kB in CAFs as well as tumor cells, with decreased IL-6 secretion. Metformin suppresses cancer cell immune evasion and upregulates host anti-cancer immunity. One mechanism of cancer immune evasion is the upregulation of programmed death ligand 1 (PD-L1), which causes cytotoxic T cell exhaustion.

In 2019, Dr. Ivana Kurelac et al. write:

Lymphocyte [T Cell] anti-tumor cytotoxicity is increased upon metformin treatment, both directly and due to reduced PD-L1 expression on cancer cell membrane, or by unlocking cancer immunosuppression by downregulating myeloid-derived suppressor cell [MDSC] functions. Finally, metformin has been associated with inhibition of pro-tumorigenic T-Reg lymphocytes [T-Regulatory]. (57)

In 2016, Dr. Young Kwang Chae et al. reported in *Oncotarget*:

Metformin activates the T-cell-mediated immune response against cancer cells, reduces KI-67 proliferation rate in endometrial cancer and breast cancer patients. (58)

In a 2015 report, Dr. Shingo Eikawa's group studied the immune-mediated anti-tumor effect of metformin using a mouse xenograft model. If the host immune system is functional, the CD8(+) lymphocytes infiltrate the tumor mass and reject (kill) the cancer cells. Dr. Eikawa's group reports that the effect is enhanced by metformin:

Metformin increased the number of CD8(+) tumor-infiltrating lymphocytes [TILs] and protected them from apoptosis and exhaustion characterized by decreased

production of IL-2 [Interleukin-2], TNFa [tumor necrosis factor-alpha], and IFN [interferon]. CD8(+) TILs capable of producing multiple cytokines were mainly PD-1(-)Tim-3(+), an Effector Memory T Cell subset responsible for tumor rejection.(59)

Metformin Synergy with Chemotherapy

In 2009, in a breast cancer xenograft mouse model, Dr. Hirsch et al. observed that metformin acts synergistically with chemotherapy using doxorubicin to block tumor growth and prolong remission in four genetically different breast cancers, concluding that:

The combination of metformin and chemotherapeutic drugs might improve treatment of patients with breast [and possibly other] cancers. (9)

In 2013, Drs. Sherry Bradford and A. Khan observed that the addition of metformin to a chemotherapy regimen resulted in higher sensitivity with a higher cancer cell-kill rate:

Our findings indicate a potential role for metformin.... as a powerful adjuvant to chemotherapy in a wide range of cancer types. (62)

Dr. Rana Sayed et al. (2015) studied the use of chemotherapy in thirty patients suffering from stage IV lung cancer. Fifteen of the patients were randomized to receive metformin in addition to the chemotherapy. Overall survival for the metformin plus chemo group was roughly doubled, to 12.5 months compared to 6.5 months for the chemo-alone group. The metformin group also had less nausea induced by the chemotherapy. (63)

Metformin as a Radiation Sensitizer

Tumor resistance to radiation therapy is thought to be due to tumor hypoxia, or lack of oxygen, in the center of the tumor mass. Metformin reduces oxygen consumption in the tumor mass by inhibition of complex I of the ETC, thus increasing oxygen in the cancer cells and reducing tumor hypoxia. This increased intracellular oxygen (oxidative therapy) makes the tumor cells more sensitive to the killing effects of radiation therapy and the associated increase in reactive oxygen species (ROS). (64–66)

In 2013, Dr. Vanessa Zannella et al. studied two mouse xenograft models, finding that metformin acted as a radio-sensitizer, enhancing the effect of radiation therapy when the mice were given the metformin prior to the radiation therapy. They concluded:

> Our data demonstrate that metformin can improve tumor oxygenation and response to radiotherapy. Our study suggests that metformin may represent an effective and inexpensive means to improve radiotherapy outcome with an optimal therapeutic ratio. (64)

Metformin Degrades Cyclin D1

Overexpression of the cell cycle regulator cyclin D1, a downstream effector of the Wnt pathway, is a frequent feature in cancer and predicts early metastatic spread with poor prognosis. Dr. HyeRan Gwak reports in 2017 that metformin degrades cyclin D1 in ovarian cancer cell models irrespective of p53 status. This is done via metformin's ability to upregu-

late the AMPK/GSK3ß signaling axis. (67)

Metformin Inhibits the Wnt Pathway

In 2016, Dr. Kamal Ahmed et al. reported that metformin inhibits the Wnt pathway in cancer cells at commonly used dosage for type-2 diabetes (500–1000 mg twice a day). The upregulation of AMPK (which inhibits mTOR signaling) by metformin causes indirect inhibition of the Wnt pathway. Downstream mediators of the Wnt pathway are cyclin D1 and C-Myc. As mentoned previously, the Wnt pathway is a cancer stem cell pathway. (28)

Synergy of Metformin and Propranolol

The beta blocker propranolol, widely used in cardiology, has been re- purposed as an anti-cancer drug. Its mode of action is directly on cancer cell metabolism as well as on the cancer micro-environment, disrupting catecholamine cancer signaling. (68–69)

In 2017, Dr. Maria Rico et al. found the combination of metformin and propranolol synergistic in triple-negative breast cancer cell (TNBC) lines studied in vitro and in vivo mouse xenografts. Combining metformin and propranolol strongly inhibited mitochondrial energy production and:

> achieve[d] a complete suppression of the mitochondrial bioenergetics, and drastically activates glycolysis…. recent studies demonstrate that OXPHOS is indispensable for tumor migration and metastasis … Disseminating breast cancer cells indeed display increased levels of mitochondrial respiration. The ability of Met + Prop combination to inhibit rapidly and efficiently

the mitochondrial bioenergetics thus likely underlies the strong antimetastatic properties of the treatment. (70)

DCA is a potent glycolysis inhibitor that synergizes with both metformin and propranolol. One might therefore expect augmented synergy with the metformin/propranolol/DCA combination. We await further NIH-funded studies of this triple combination.

Metformin Synergy with Simvastatin

Statin drugs were originally developed for lowering cholesterol by blocking the enzyme HMG-CoA as well as the mevalonate pathway. Over many years of clinical use, it was discovered that statin drugs have "pleotropic effects," namely anti-inflammatory and antimicrobial effects. Activation of the cellular NF-kB inflammatory pathway is potently inhibited by statin drugs. Recently, there has been interest in statins as repurposed anti-cancer agents. Statin-drug use in combination with metformin prolonged survival in resectable pancreatic cancer patients. (71–73)

In 2019, Dr. Josephine Kim et al. found the simvastatin and metformin combination synergistic in reducing viability of an endometrial cancer cell line, observing "apoptosis and mTOR pathway inhibition." (74)

Metformin Synergy with Curcumin

Curcumin, used for centuries as a spice and anti-inflammatory botanical, has been found synergistic with metformin. In 2017, Dr. Rabah Rashad Falah et al. studied breast cancer in a mouse xenograft model, observing that the metformin plus curcumin combination inhibited angiogenesis, modulated the immune system, and induced apoptosis independent of p53 status. (75)

Metformin Synergy with Dichloroacetate (DCA)

In 2017, Dr. Ward studied the synergistic effects of metformin with the glycolysis inhibitor, dichloroacetate, using the in vitro glioblastoma model. Dr. Ward found increased superoxide production by combining metformin with glycolysis inhibitor DCA, which shunts electron flow into the mitochondrial ETC. The inhibition of complex I of the ETC in the mitochondria by metformin causes superoxide ROS which overwhelms the anti-oxidant defense of the cancer cell, leading to mitochondrial-induced apoptosis. Dr. Ward writes:

> These data suggest that complex I inhibition cooperates with DCA activation of oxidative glucose metabolism to **promote catastrophic oxidative stress in VM-M3 glioblastoma cells.** (52)

See chapter 5 on DCA for more on this topic.

Synergy with Autophagy Inhibitor Chloroquine

As mentioned above, the combination of metformin and chloroquine has been suggested as synergistic, since metformin induces "protective autophagy" via the mTOR pathway, while chloroquine and hydroxychloroquine are autophagy inhibitors. In 2011, Dr. Alenjandro Vasquez-Martin et al. recommended the metformin/ chloroquine combination for eradication of cancer stem cells in premalignant lesions such as ductal carcinoma in situ (DCIS). (76–78)

Other autophagy inhibitors such as thymoquinone (black seed oil), loratadine or clarithromycin (azithromycin) might prove synergistic with metformin. We await results on these additional studies.

Synergy with GLYCOLYSIS Inhibitors

As mentioned above, metformin inhibits OXPHOS by inhibiting complex one of the ETC in mitochondria, which then activates AMPK, which inhibits mTOR, the activator of "protective autophagy." Metformin is considered a "weak" agent when used as monotherapy. It shines best when used in combination, showing synergy with chemotherapy agents and glycolysis inhibitors such as 2-deoxy-glucose (2DG), dichloroactetate (DCA), diclofenac, and quercetin, etc. Dr. Marie Daugan et al. (2016) share these conclusions:

> Nonetheless, although metformin alone displays chemopreventive properties, it does not seem to be sufficient to treat cancer, raising the need to be combined with other drugs (e.g. **chemotherapy or glycolysis inhibitors**) in order to synergistically reveal its cytotoxic action. (79)

Metformin Enhanced by Hyperthermia

According to Dr. Mario Palazzi et al. (2010), hyperthermia is a useful cancer treatment modality in which the body temperature is raised to 42 degrees C. for one hour in a sauna. They write that hyperthermia "appears to be the fourth pillar [of cancer treatment] beside surgery, radiotherapy, and chemotherapy." (80–82)

In 2014, Dr. Hyemi Lee et al. found that hyperthermia treatment increased metformin cytotoxicity against breast cancer cells as well as the CSCs by activating AMPK and inactivating mTOR. Dr. Lee's group concludes that:

> The effects of metformin against cancer cells including CSCs can be markedly enhanced by hyperthermia. (83)

Metformin Use as Adjuvant for Cancer

A number of authors have suggested metformin as an adjuvant for breast cancer and other cancers as well. In view of the studies outlined above, it seems reasonable to offer metformin to the cancer patient as an adjuvant treatment before, during, and after conventional treatment with chemotherapy, surgery, or radiation. (84–86)

Metformin Blood Levels (2.8– 15 µM Micromolar)

Does metformin achieve therapeutic blood levels at standard oral dosing of 500–1000 mg twice a day? Dr. Tae Hun Kim et al. (2014) asked this question, writing that most in vitro studies use metformin concentrations far higher than those achievable with standard oral human dosing:

> In fact, most in vitro studies used doses of metformin between 1 and 40 mM [millimolar], which is well above the feasible therapeutic plasma levels [2.8–15 µM-micromolar] in humans … [using 500–1000

mg per day metformin orally in human dosing]. (54)

Dr. Hannah Bridges et al. (2014) argue that metformin achieves much higher local concentrations in mitochondria than measured in the blood stream by virtue of metformin's accumulation in mitochondria. Dr. Bridges et al. write that:

> the positive charge on the biguanide moiety [of metformin] results in accumulation of biguanides [metformin] in the mitochondrial matrix…. **to concentrations up to 1000-times greater than in the extracellular environment**.

Note: Metformin is a biguanide. (87)

Metformin's Effects on Routine PET SCANS

In 2013, Dr. Peiman Habibollahi et al. studied metformin's effects on PET scan imaging in an animal model of colon cancer. It is well known that metformin increases cellular glucose uptake and decreases serum glucose, accounting for its benefits in diabetes. Similarly, Dr. Habibollahi and colleagues found metformin increased 18F-FDG (radio-labeled glucose) uptake for implanted tumors, indicating increased glucose uptake. Alternatively, when using a thymidine radio-tracer, there was decreased uptake, indicating metformin reduced the rate of cancer-cell proliferation in the tumor. The implication for human medical imaging is that metformin use may paradoxically increase radiotracer activity in the tumor mass on the routine follow-up PET scan, even while producing a clinical benefit. This is important because increased tumor uptake on a PET scan is normally considered prognostic of worsening tumor activity—but not in this scenario. Dr. Habibollahi et al. write:

> Metformin, through activation of the AMPK pathway, produces a dose-dependent increase in tumor glucose uptake while decreasing cell proliferation in human and murine colon cancer cells. (88)

Adverse Side Effects of Metformin

Metformin is usually well tolerated, with occasional reports of diarrhea, bloating, and nausea thought to be related to excessive starting dosage. This can usually be handled by lowering initial dosages and gradually increasing over time to allow the GI tract to acclimate to the drug. (89)

Conclusion

The evidence for metformin as an anti-cancer stem cell drug is overwhelming. Metformin is an OXPHOS inhibitor and best used in combination with glycolysis inhibitors such as DCA (dichloroacetate), diclofenac and quercetin. Metformin also has synergy with propranolol, curcumin, simvastatin, artesunate, doxycycline, and IV vitamin C, creating "synthetic lethality" and overcoming resistant cell types. Metformin can be used in conjunction with radiation therapy, chemotherapy (and rituximab) as a sensitizing agent to augment their effects. Metformin may be considered an adjuvant drug for breast cancer patients and other cancers as well. There is an urgent need for NIH funding for studies confirming this combination approach to eradicating cancer stem cells. Many clinical trials are now underway.

References for Chapter 14: Metformin

1) Saraei, Pouya, et al. "The beneficial effects of metformin on cancer prevention and therapy: a comprehensive review of recent advances." Cancer management and research 11 (2019): 3295.

2) Pryor, Rosina, and Filipe Cabreiro. "Repurposing metformin: an old drug with new tricks in its binding pockets." Biochemical Journal 471.3 (2015): 307-322.

3) Rojas, Lilian Beatriz Aguayo, and Marilia Brito Gomes. "Metformin: an old but still the best treatment for type 2 diabetes." Diabetology & metabolic syndrome 5.1 (2013): 6.

4) Evans, Josie MM, et al. "Metformin and reduced risk of cancer in diabetic patients." Bmj 330.7503 (2005): 1304-1305.

5) Kasznicki, Jacek, Agnieszka Sliwinska, and Józef Drzewoski. "Metformin in cancer prevention and therapy." Annals of translational medicine 2.6 (2014).

6) Sacco, Francesca, et al. "The cell-autonomous mechanisms underlying the activity of metformin as an anticancer drug." British journal of cancer 115.12 (2016): 1451.

7) Chae, Young Kwang, et al. "Repurposing metformin for cancer treatment: current clinical studies." Oncotarget 7.26 (2016): 40767.

8) Chen, Chuan-Mu, et al. "Repurposing Metformin for Lung Cancer Management." A Global Scientific Vision- Prevention, Diagnosis, and Treatment of Lung Cancer. InTech, 2017.

9) Hirsch, Heather A., Dimitrios Iliopoulos, and Kevin Struhl. "Metformin inhibits the inflammatory response associated with cellular transformation and cancer stem cell growth." Proceedings of the National Academy of Sciences 110.3 (2013): 972-977.

10) Mathupala, S. P., Young H. Ko, and P. L. Pedersen. "Hexokinase II: cancer's double-edged sword acting as both facilitator and gatekeeper of malignancy when bound to mitochondria." Oncogene 25.34 (2006): 4777.

11) Salani, Barbara, et al. "Metformin impairs glucose consumption and survival in Calu-1 cells by direct inhibition of hexokinase-II." Scientific reports 3 (2013).

12) Marini, Cecilia, et al. "Direct inhibition of hexokinase activity by metformin at least partially impairs glucose metabolism and tumor growth in experimental breast cancer." Cell Cycle 12.22 (2013): 3490-3499.

13) Gewirtz, David A. "The Switch between Protective and Nonprotective Autophagy; Implications for Autophagy Inhibition as a Therapeutic Strategy in Cancer." Biology 9.1 (2020): 12.

14) Rabanal-Ruiz, Yoana, Elsje G. Otten, and Viktor I. Korolchuk. "mTORC1 as the main gateway to autophagy." Essays in biochemistry 61.6 (2017): 565-584.

15) Paquette, Mathieu, Leeanna El-Houjeiri, and Arnim Pause. "mTOR pathways in cancer and autophagy." Cancers 10.1 (2018): 18.

16) Carroll, Bernadette, and Elaine A. Dunlop. "The lysosome: a crucial hub for AMPK and mTORC1 signalling." Biochemical Journal 474.9 (2017): 1453-1466.

17) Gong, F., et al. "Dichloroacetate induces protective autophagy in LoVo cells: involvement of cathepsin D/thioredoxin-like protein 1 and Akt-mTOR-mediated signaling." Cell Death & Disease 4.11 (2013): e913-e913.

18) Wang, Kui, et al. "Quercetin induces protective autophagy in gastric cancer cells: involvement of Akt-mTOR-and hypoxia-induced factor 1α-mediated signaling." Autophagy 7.9 (2011): 966-978.

19) Vazquez-Martin, Alejandro, et al. "Repositioning chloroquine and metformin to eliminate cancer stem cell traits in pre-malignant lesions." Drug Resistance Updates 14.4-5 (2011): 212-223.

20) Li, Bo, et al. "Metformin induces cell cycle arrest, apoptosis and autophagy through ROS/JNK signaling pathway in human osteosarcoma." International Journal of Biological Sciences 16.1 (2020): 74.

21) Molenaar, Remco J., et al. "Study protocol of a phase IB/II clinical trial of metformin and chloroquine in patients with IDH1-mutated or IDH2-mutated solid tumours." BMJ open 7.6 (2017): e014961.

22) Sancho, Patricia, et al. "MYC/PGC-1a Balance Determines the Metabolic Phenotype and Plasticity of Pancreatic Cancer Stem Cells." Cell Metabolism 22 (2015): 1-16

23) De Francesco, Ernestina Marianna, et al. "Vitamin C and Doxycycline: A synthetic lethal combination therapy targeting metabolic flexibility in cancer stem cells (CSCs)." Oncotarget 8.40 (2017): 67269.

24) Zhang, Shuai, et al. "Wnt/β-catenin signaling pathway upregulates c-Myc expression to promote cell proliferation of P19 teratocarcinoma cells." The Anatomical Record: Advances in Integrative Anatomy and Evolutionary Biology 295.12 (2012): 2104-2113.

25) Yochum, Gregory S., Ryan Cleland, and Richard H. Goodman. "A genome-wide screen for β-catenin binding sites identifies a downstream enhancer element that controls c-Myc gene expression." Molecular and cellular biology 28.24 (2008): 7368-7379.

26) Lu, Jin-Jian, et al. "Dihydroartemisinin accelerates c-MYC oncoprotein degradation and induces apoptosis in c-MYC-overexpressing tumor cells." Biochemical pharmacology 80.1 (2010): 22-30.

27) Wang, Huabo, et al. "Structurally diverse c-Myc inhibitors share a common mechanism of action involving ATP depletion." Oncotarget 6.18 (2015): 15857.

28) Ahmed, Kamal, et al. "A second WNT for old drugs: Drug repositioning against WNT-dependent cancers." Cancers 8.7 (2016): 66.

29) Choe, Ji-Young, et al. "MYC overexpression correlates with MYC amplification or translocation, and is associated with poor prognosis in mantle cell lymphoma." Histopathology 68.3 (2016): 442-449.

30) Yi, Shuhua, et al. "High incidence of MYC and BCL2 abnormalities in mantle cell lymphoma, although only MYC abnormality predicts poor survival." Oncotarget 6.39 (2015): 42362.

31) Nguyen, Lynh, Peter Papenhausen, and Haipeng Shao. "The Role of c-MYC in B-Cell Lymphomas: Diagnostic and Molecular Aspects." Genes 8.4 (2017): 116.

32) Friedberg, Jonathan W. "How I treat" Double Hit" lymphoma." Blood (2017): blood-2017. How I treat Double Hit Lymphoma c-MYC Friedberg Jonathan W Blood 2017

33) Whitaker-Menezes, Diana, et al. "Hyperactivation of oxidative mitochondrial metabolism in epithelial cancer cells in situ: visualizing the therapeutic effects of metformin in tumor tissue." Cell cycle 10.23 (2011): 4047-4064.

34) Menendez, Javier A., et al. "Metformin is synthetically lethal with glucose withdrawal in cancer cells." Cell cycle 11.15 (2012): 2782-2792.

35) Gerthofer, Valeria, et al. "Combined modulation of tumor metabolism by metformin and diclofenac in glioma." International journal of molecular sciences 19.9 (2018): 2586.

36) Bao, Bin, et al. "Metformin inhibits cell proliferation, migration and invasion by attenuating CSC function mediated by deregulating miRNAs in pancreatic cancer cells." Cancer prevention research 5.3 (2012): 355-364.

37) Lei, Yong, et al. "Metformin targets multiple signaling pathways in cancer." Chinese journal of cancer 36.1 (2017): 17.

38) Shi, Peiguo, et al. "Metformin suppresses triple-negative breast cancer stem cells by targeting KLF5 for degradation." Cell discovery 3.1 (2017): 1-13.

39) Gritti, Marta, et al. "Metformin repositioning as antitumoral agent: selective antiproliferative effects in human glioblastoma stem cells, via inhibition of CLIC1-mediated ion current." Oncotarget 5.22 (2014): 11252.

40) Marcucci, Fabrizio, Cristiano Rumio, and François Lefoulon. "Anti-cancer stem-like cell compounds in clinical development–an overview and critical appraisal." Frontiers in oncology 6 (2016): 115.

41) Banerjee, Indranil, et al. "Combination of metformin and metronomic liposomal doxorubicin exerts a robust anticancer effect in triple negative breast cancer by inhibiting breast cancer stem cells & the Wnt/beta-catenin pathway." (2019): 3638-3638.

42) Buckanovich, Ronald J., et al. "A phase II clinical trial of metformin as a cancer stem cell targeting agent in stage IIc/III/IV ovarian, fallopian tube, and primary peritoneal cancer." (2017): 5556-5556.

43) Cuyas, Elisabet, et al. "Metformin inhibits RANKL and sensitizes cancer stem cells to denosumab." Cell Cycle 16.11 (2017): 1022-1028.

44) Zhu, Jie, et al. "Targeting cancer cell metabolism: The combination of metformin and 2-Deoxyglucose regulates apoptosis in ovarian cancer cells via p38 MAPK/JNK signaling pathway." American journal of translational research 8.11 (2016): 4812.

45) Sahra, Issam Ben, et al. "Targeting cancer cell metabolism: the combination of metformin and 2-deoxyglucose induces p53-dependent apoptosis in prostate cancer cells." Cancer research 70.6 (2010): 2465-2475.

46) Clinical Trial: Metformin Hydrochloride and Doxycycline in Treating Patients With Localized Breast or Uterine Cancer . Verified May 2017 by Sidney Kimmel Cancer Center at Thomas Jefferson University. ClinicalTrials.gov Identifier: NCT02874430

47) Clinical Trial: Metformin Hydrochloride and Doxycycline in Treating Patients with Head and Neck Squamous Cell Carcinoma That Can Be Removed by Surgery. NCT03076281

48) Clinical Trial: Study of the Safety, Tolerability and Efficacy of Metabolic Combination Treatments on Cancer (METRICS). Care Oncology Clinic, London (Health Clinics Limited) NCT02201381

49) Bruno, Silvia, et al. "Metformin inhibits cell cycle progression of B-cell chronic lymphocytic leukemia cells." Oncotarget 6.26 (2015): 22624.

50) Shi, W. Y., et al. "Therapeutic metformin/AMPK activation blocked lymphoma cell growth via inhibition of mTOR pathway and induction of autophagy." Cell death & disease 3.3 (2012): e275-e275.

51) Ward, N. P., et al. "Complex I inhibition augments dichloroacetate cytotoxicity through enhancing oxidative stress in VM-M3 glioblastoma cells." PloS one 12.6 (2017): e0180061.

52) Spratt, Daniel E., et al. "Metformin and prostate cancer: reduced development of castration-resistant disease and prostate cancer mortality." European Urology 63.4 (2013): 709-716.

53) Patel, Priyank P., et al. "Metformin enhances the activity of rituximab in B-cell lymphoma pre-clinical models." (2015): e19513-e19513.

54) Kim, Tae Hun, et al. "Metformin against cancer stem cells through the modulation of energy metabolism: special considerations on ovarian cancer." BioMed research international 2014 (2014).

55) Verdura, Sara, et al. "Metformin as an archetype immuno-metabolic adjuvant for cancer immunotherapy." OncoImmunology (2019): 1-10.

56) Afzal, Muhammad Zubair, Rima R. Mercado, and Keisuke Shirai. "Efficacy of metformin in combination with immune checkpoint inhibitors (anti-PD-1/anti-CTLA-4) in metastatic malignant melanoma." Journal for immunotherapy of cancer 6.1 (2018): 64.

57) Kurelac, Ivana, et al. "The multifaceted effects of metformin on tumor microenvironment." Seminars in Cell & Developmental Biology. Academic Press, 2019.

58) Chae, Young Kwang, et al. "Repurposing metformin for cancer treatment: current clinical studies." Oncotarget 7.26 (2016): 40767.

59) Eikawa, Shingo, et al. "Immune-mediated antitumor effect by type 2 diabetes drug, metformin." Proceedings of the National Academy of Sciences 112.6 (2015): 1809-1814.

60) Wang, Jichang, et al. "Suppression of tumor angiogenesis by metformin treatment via a mechanism linked to targeting of HER2/HIF-1α/VEGF secretion axis." Oncotarget 6.42 (2015): 44579.

61) Orecchioni, Stefania, et al. "The biguanides metformin and phenformin inhibit angiogenesis, local and metastatic growth of breast cancer by targeting both neoplastic and microenvironment cells." International Journal of Cancer 136.6 (2015): E534-E544.

62) Bradford, Sherry A., and A. Khan. "Individualizing chemotherapy using the anti-diabetic drug, metformin, as "adjuvant": an exploratory study." J Cancer Sci Ther 5.6 (2013).

63) Sayed, Rana, et al. "Metformin addition to chemotherapy in stage IV non-small cell lung cancer: an open label randomized controlled study." Asian Pac J Cancer Prev 16.15 (2015): 6621-6.

64) Zannella, Vanessa E., et al. "Reprogramming metabolism with metformin improves tumor oxygenation and radiotherapy response." Clinical cancer research 19.24 (2013): 6741-6750.

65) Song, Chang W., et al. "Metformin kills and radio-sensitizes cancer cells and preferentially kills cancer stem cells." Scientific reports 2 (2012): 362.

66) Brown, Stephen L., et al. "A Novel Mechanism of High Dose Radiation Sensitization by Metformin." Frontiers in oncology 9 (2019): 247.

67) Gwak, HyeRan, et al. " Metformin induces degradation of cyclin D1 via AMPK/GSK3ß axis in ovarian cancer. " Molecular carcinogenesis 56.2 (2017): 349-358.

68) Talarico, Giovanna, et al. "Aspirin and atenolol enhance metformin activity against breast cancer by targeting both neoplastic and microenvironment cells." Scientific reports 6 (2016): 18673.

69) Kang, Fei, et al. "Propranolol inhibits glucose metabolism and 18F-FDG uptake of breast cancer through posttranscriptional downregulation of hexokinase-2." Journal of Nuclear Medicine 55.3 (2014): 439-445.

70) Rico, María, et al. "Metformin and propranolol combination prevents cancer progression and metastasis in different breast cancer models." Oncotarget 8.2 (2017): 2874

71) Babcook, Melissa A., et al. "Synergistic simvastatin and metformin combination chemotherapy for osseous metastatic castration-resistant prostate cancer." Molecular cancer therapeutics 13.10 (2014): 2288-2302.

72) Kozak, Margaret M., et al. "Statin and metformin use prolongs survival in patients with resectable pancreatic cancer." Pancreas 45.1 (2016): 64-70.

73) Jian-Yu, E., et al. "Effect of metformin and statin use on survival in pancreatic cancer patients: a systematic literature review and meta-analysis." Current medicinal chemistry 25.22 (2018): 2595-2607.

74) Kim, Josephine S., et al. "Combination simvastatin and metformin synergistically inhibits endometrial cancer cell growth." Gynecologic oncology (2019).

75) Falah, Rabah Rashad, Wamidh H. Talib, and Seba Jamal Shbailat. "Combination of metformin and curcumin targets breast cancer in mice by angiogenesis inhibition, immune system modulation and induction of p53 independent apoptosis." Therapeutic advances in medical oncology 9.4 (2017): 235-252.

76) Wu, Hongqiang, et al. "Metformin promotes the survival of random-pattern skin flaps by inducing autophagy via the AMPK-mTOR-TFEB signaling pathway." International journal of biological sciences 15.2 (2019): 325.

77) Vazquez-Martin, Alejandro, et al. "Repositioning chloroquine and metformin to eliminate cancer stem cell traits in pre-malignant lesions." Drug Resistance Updates 14.4-5 (2011): 212-223.

78) Schwartz, Laurent, et al. "The addition of chloroquine and metformine to Metabloc induces a rapid drop of tumor markers in advanced carcinoma." Cancer Ther 10 (2014): 20-27.

79) Daugan, Marie, et al. "Metformin: An anti-diabetic drug to fight cancer." Pharmacological research 113 (2016): 675-685.

80) Palazzi, Mario, et al. "The role of hyperthermia in the battle against cancer." Tumori Journal 96.6 (2010): 902-910.

81) Jha, Sheetal, Pramod Kumar Sharma, and Rishabha Malviya. "Hyperthermia: role and risk factor for cancer treatment." Achievements in the Life Sciences 10.2 (2016): 161-167.

82) Wust, Peter, et al. "Hyperthermia in combined treatment of cancer." The lancet oncology 3.8 (2002): 487-497.

83) Lee, Hyemi, et al. "Response of breast cancer cells and cancer stem cells to metformin and hyperthermia alone or combined." PloS one 9.2 (2014): e87979.

84) Roshan, Mohsin HK, et al. "Metformin as an Adjuvant in Breast Cancer Treatment." SAGE Open Medicine, Vol.7 (2019): 1 –16.

85) Coyle, C., et al. "Metformin as an adjuvant treatment for cancer: a systematic review and meta-analysis." Annals of Oncology 27.12 (2016): 2184.

86) Heckman-Stoddard, Brandy M., et al. "Repurposing metformin for the prevention of cancer and cancer recurrence." Diabetologia 60.9 (2017): 1639-1647.

87) Bridges, Hannah R., et al. "Effects of metformin and other biguanides on oxidative phosphorylation in mitochondria." Biochemical Journal 462.3 (2014): 475-487.

88) Habibollahi, Peiman, et al. "Metformin—an adjunct antineoplastic therapy—divergently modulates tumor metabolism and proliferation, interfering with early response prediction by 18F-FDG PET imaging." Journal of Nuclear Medicine 54.2 (2013): 252-258.

89) Bonnet, Fabrice, and André Scheen. "Understanding and overcoming metformin gastrointestinal intolerance." Diabetes, Obesity and Metabolism 19.4 (2017): 473-481.

Chapter 15

Targeting Cancer Stem Cells Case Report

Aggressive Metastatic Squamous Cell Skin Cancer in 92-Year-Old Female, with Metastatic Disease to Right Cervical Lymph Node

A 92-YEAR-OLD FEMALE OTHERWISE IN good health presented with a 3-cm mass involving the scalp at the skull vertex growing rapidly and obviously very aggressive. A skin biopsy showed invasive squamous cell carcinoma. The skin lesion was excised with wide margins by a dermatology surgeon using Moh's surgery technique. However, two months later, a large palpable (2–3 cm.) lymph node appeared in the right supraclavicular area, increasing in size rapidly. The patient was scheduled for surgical removal of the neck node about three weeks later allowing time to start a cocktail of five repurposed drugs (listed below).

Repurposed Drug Cocktail

Three weeks later, the patient was taken to the operating room and the enlarged lymph node was removed under local anesthesia. The surgeon remarked that the lymph node felt necrotic in his hand and fell apart. This suggested necrosis of the tumor tissue, indicating the drug cocktail was effective. The pathology report confirmed metastatic squamous cell cancer in the lymph node, indicating a dismal prognosis with metastatic spread.

The patient remained on the repurposed

anti-cancer drug protocol, and 12 weeks later a PET scan showed no evidence of disease, with no abnormal tracer uptake. Although offered by the oncologist, the patient declined radiation therapy. Three years later, in spite of the dismal prognosis of cancer spreading to local lymph nodes, the patient is doing well, with no cancer recurrence.

Treatment Protocol for Aggressive Squamous Cell Cancer

Itraconazole—Clinical trials by Dr. Daniel Kim et al. in 2014 showed the efficacy of itraconazole in basal cell skin cancer; therefore one might expect efficacy in squamous cell cancer as well. Itraconazole disrupts HK2 (Hexokinase 2) from mitochondria and binds to VDAC pores on the mitochondrial membrane. Itraconazole is a 5-LOX, hedgehog (Hh) and Wnt pathway inhibitor and therefore a cancer stem cell agent. Itraconazole suppresses the Akt/mTOR pathway, which stimulates protective autophagy. Itraconazole inhibits VEGF (vascular endothelial growth factor), and has synergy with exemestane. Itraconazole has mineralocorticoid activity that may cause fluid retention. See chapter 28, "Itraconazole." (1–2)

Doxycycline acts as an OXPHOS inhibitor by inhibiting ribosomal protein production in mitochondria. Doxycycline targets hypoxic cancer stem cells. Doxycycline is also an autophagy inhibitor. Doxycycline inhibits the NF-kB pathway, IL-6 and MMP, and has synergy with exemestane for mesothelioma. See Chapter 9, "Doxycycline/Vitamin C Anti-Cancer Synergy." (3)

Mebendazole (MBZ)—MBZ blocks cancer cell replication by inhibiting microtubule spindle formation. MBZ is a potent inhibitor of the Hedgehog cancer stem cell pathway. MBZ restores host anti-cancer immunity and inhibits MMP and Angiogenesis. See Chapter 24 on Mebendazole for more. (4)

Exemestane—Similar to breast tissue, the skin is a "steroidal organ" and estrogenic tumor stimulation is highly probable for most skin cancers. In this case of aggressive squamous cell skin cancer, the intense growth stimulation could be derived from "paracrine" or "incrine" estrogen stimulation, effectively blocked by exemestane, an irreversible aromatase inhibitor which inhibits biosynthesis of estrogen. In addition, exemestane is an OXPHOS inhibitor, and a stand-alone cancer drug by virtue of its metabolites which induce increased ROS (reactive oxygen species), mitochondrial apoptosis, and activation of "protective autophagy". (5–10)

Fenofibrate is a dual GLYCOLYSIS and OXPHOS inhibitor, potentiated by vitamin A derivatives. Fenofibrate accumulates in mitochondria with inhibition of complex one of the ETC, and interrupts the Warburg Effect by disrupting HK-2 from the VDAC, destroys BCL-2, and restores apoptosis. Fenofibrate blocks the activity of FASN (Fatty Acid Synthetase), which deprives the cancer cell of fatty acids used for fuel, and leads to microtubule disruption. Fenofibrate synergizes nicely with microtubule agents such as mebendazole mentioned above. Fenofibrate has potent anti-inflammatory effects with down regulation of NF-kB.

Long-term Remission with Targeted Drug Cocktail

This case was an example of eradication of cancer stem cells leading to a durable long-term remission, or "cure," using only **five** targeted repurposed drugs. Next, we revisit the cancer stem cell hypothesis, metabolic pathways, and characteristics of cancer stem cells.

The Invention of the Cancer Stem Cell

In 1983, Dr. J. Mackillop et al. discovered cancer stem cells and were the first to propose the idea that eradication of cancer stem cells could "cure" cancer, another way of saying "long-term durable remission." (11)

In 1994, Dr. Tsvee Lapidot et al. were the first to characterize cancer stem cell surface markers in an acute myeloid leukemia cell line. They found that the cancer stem cells (called leukemia-initiating cells) were present in the peripheral blood in the ratio of one stem cell per 250,000 cells. (12)

We Need to Rethink the Way We Diagnose and Treat Tumors

In 2006, Dr. M. F. Carke of the American Association for Cancer Research (AACR) accepted the cancer stem cell hypothesis, writing "we need to rethink the way we diagnose and treat cancer":

If cancer stem cells are relatively refractory to therapies that have been developed to eradicate the rapidly dividing cells within the tumor that constitute the majority of the non-stem-cell component of tumors, then they are unlikely to be curative and relapses would be expected. **If correct, the cancer stem cell hypothesis would require that we rethink the way we diagnose and treat tumors.**(13)

The Three Pillars of Cancer Metabolism

- OXPHOS
- GLYCOLYSIS
- Autophagy

Our goal in *Cracking Cancer Toolkit* is to target all three major metabolic pathways, thereby achieving eradication of the cancer stem cells, as well as the bulk tumor cells.

How to Eradicate Cancer Stem Cells

As we have discussed previously, chemotherapy cannot kill cancer stem cells. Paradoxically, chemotherapy increases the numbers of cancer stem cells via activation of nuclear factor kappa B (NF-kB), the inflammatory master controller. In addition, activation of NF-kB leads to an aggressive cancer behavior with greater tendency to metastasize (spread cancer to other parts of the body).

Clearly, eradication of cancer stem cells is required to achieve a durable long-term remission for the cancer patient. Eradication of cancer stem cells depends on inhibition of cancer stem cell metabolic pathways.

Cancer Stem Cell Pathways

In 2019, Dr. Andrea Li Ann Wong et al. described the cancer stem cell pathways as Wnt, Notch and Hedgehog (Hh):

- Wnt/β-catenin (all OXPHOS inhibitors)
- Notch (curcumin, sulindac)
- Hedgehog: (itraconazole, mebendazole) (14)

In previous chapters, we discussed repurposed drugs and natural botanical agents that target these cancer stem cell pathways, thus achieving eradication of cancer stem cells.

A Summary of Cancer Stem Cell Characteristics

In 2019, Dr. Fang-Yu Du et al. commented that significant

crosstalk occurs among differing signaling pathways in the cancer cells leading to compensatory escape, and that conventional chemotherapy can only inhibit tumor growth and lead to drug resistance, but cannot kill cancer stem cells. (15)

Note: The term "compensatory escape" is identical to "metabolic plasticity" of cancer stem cells.

Dr. Du summarized the characteristics of cancer stem cells as:

1) Self-renewal ability to replicate and make new cancer stem cells.

2) Ability to transform into "bulk tumor" cells which are no longer stem cells, and maintain tumor growth.

3) High tumorigenicity, ability to grow new tumors when injected into mouse xenografts.

4) Drug resistance, ability to survive in spite of chemotherapy treatment.

5) Compensatory escape, ability to compensate by switching metabolic pathways, also called "metabolic plasticity."

6) Complexity of crosstalk between stem cell pathways requires multi-targeted therapy and combinations.

7) Cancer stem cells are the cause of chemotherapy and radiotherapy failure.

8) Cancer stem cells have low ROS (reactive oxygen species). (15–17)

Cancer Stem Cell Metabolism: OXPHOS or Glycolysis?

What is the metabolic phenotype of the cancer stem cells? Is it OXPHOS or GLYCOLYSIS? According to Dr. Patricia Sancho et al. in 2015, the metabolic phenotypes vary according to cancer cell type. In breast cancer, they are predominantly GLYCOLYSIS. In pancreatic cancer, glioblastoma, and leukemia, they rely on mitochondrial OXPHOS. Dr. Sancho's group write:

> The metabolic phenotype of CSCs [cancer stem cells] **appears to vary across tumor types.** While in breast cancer and nasopharyngeal carcinoma CSCs were found to be **predominantly glycolytic [GLYCOLYSIS]**.... CSCs in pancreatic cancer, glioblastoma and leukemia appear to rely **on mitochondrial OXPHOS** (18–20)

Hallmarks of Cancer Stem Cell Metabolism

In 2016, Drs. Sancho et al. reviewed the characteristics of cancer stem cells, writing that cancer cells circulating in the bloodstream, also called circulating tumor cells (CTC), are in fact cancer stem cells. Only cancer stem cells have the ability to initiate metastatic lesions at distant sites:

> To date, only arising metastatic CSCs [cancer stem cells] have been shown to initiate secondary lesions... and are traceable as circulating CSCs in the blood. Importantly, these cells must survive the hostile environment of the blood stream, evade immune surveillance and extravasate at a distant location to form metastatic lesions, rendering the process extremely inefficient....

> As opposed to differentiated bulk tumour cells relying on GLYCOLYSIS, CSCs show a distinct metabolic phenotype that, depending on the cancer type, can be highly Glycolytic or OXPHOS dependent.... (30)

Important Point!! Determine for your cancer-cell type whether the cancer stem cells rely on GLYCOLYSIS, OXPHOS, or both!

Cancer Stem Cells are Chameleons!!

In 2019, Dr. Nicole Bezuidenhout and Maria Shoshan studied cancer stem cells (called TICs), writing that the metabolic plasticity they show in switching from OXPHOS to GLYCOLYSIS, and from GLYCOLYSIS to OXPHOS, makes them chameleons!

> TICS [Tumor Initiating Cells, cancer stem cells] are chameleons whose metabolic plasticity appears to support their survival under different conditions of nutrition and other microenvironmental influences ... One might indeed ask whether it is at all possible to ... lasso the elusive unicorn and discern TIC-specific metabolic traits that are not also seen in bulk tumor cells, since the latter can also switch between glycolytic [GLYCOLYSIS] and OXPHOS phe-

notypes as well as show upregulation of FA [fatty acid] and glutamine metabolism.... (21)

DCA Glycolysis Inhibitor

For eradication of the predominantly glycolytic cancer stem cells, the glycolysis inhibitor, dichloroactetate (DCA) is an excellent anti-cancer agent. (22–23)

For the cancer stem cells relying on OXPHOS, the strategy is to first apply an OXPHOS inhibitor (metformin, doxycycline, etc.) which, over time converts the cancer cells from OXPHOS to glycolytic phenotype. Once converted to glycolytic phenotype, the application of a glycolysis inhibitor such as DCA is effective.

The Third Pillar of Metabolism— Autophagy Inhibition

The third pillar of cancer cell metabolism is "protective autophagy." Addition of an autophagy inhibitor (chloroquine, propranolol, thymoquinone, loratadine) augments the anti-cancer program, providing the "final nail in the coffin for the cancer cell." See chapters 31-35 for more on autophagy inhibitors. (24–27)

Targeting Cancer Stem Cells with a Wnt Inhibitor

As mentioned previously, all OXPHOS inhibitors are also Wnt pathway inhibitors that by definition target cancer stem cells. As long as our anti-cancer program contains an OXPHOS inhibitor, we can be assured that cancer stem cells are being targeted. The other cancer stem cell pathway, hedgehog, can be targeted sepa-rately with mebendazole and/or itraconazole. (1–4)

The Notch pathway can be targeted by curcumin and sulindac (an NSAID drug). (28–29)

Conclusion

The above case report is an example demonstrating the principle that targeting cancer stem cell metabolic pathways can result in a durable remission or "cure." A basic idea presented in this book is that we can simplify Weinberg's Ten Hallmarks of Cancer to the *Three Pillars of Cancer Cell Metabolism*:

- OXPHOS
- GLYCOLYSIS
- Autophagy

Blocking all three pathways simultaneously results in "synthetic lethality," eradicates cancer stem cells, and provides a long-term, durable remission for the cancer patient. (31–48)

Important: Always work with a knowledgeable physician who can:

- Monitor the patient for drug toxicities.
- Monitor cancer markers on blood tests.
- Monitor PET-Scan cancer imaging.
- Do appropriate follow-up blood testing to monitor blood counts and liver function.
- Assist with diet and lifestyle modifications.
- Recommend synergistic supplements.
- Coordinate integrative care with conventional care.

References Chapter 15: Targeting Cancer Stem Cells Case Report

1) Kim, Daniel J., et al. "Open-label, exploratory phase II trial of oral itraconazole for the treatment of basal cell carcinoma." J Clin Oncol 32.8 (2014): 745-751.

2) Wei, Xin, et al. ""Hedgehog pathway": a potential target of itraconazole in the treatment of cancer." Journal of Cancer Research and Clinical Oncology 146.2 (2020): 297-304.

3) De Francesco, E. M., Michael Lisanti et al. "Vitamin C and Doxycycline: a synthetic lethal combination therapy targeting metabolic flexibility in cancer stem cells (CSCs)." Oncotarget (2017).

4) Larsen, Andrew R., et al. "Repurposing the anti-helmintic mebendazole as a hedgehog inhibitor." Molecular cancer therapeutics 14.1 (2015): 3-13.

5) Amaral, Cristina, et al. "Exemestane metabolites suppress growth of estrogen receptor-positive breast cancer cells by inducing apoptosis and autophagy: A comparative study with Exemestane." The international journal of biochemistry & cell biology 69 (2015): 183-195.

6) Amaral, Cristina, et al. "Apoptosis and autophagy in breast cancer cells following exemestane treatment." PLoS One 7.8 (2012).

7) Koutras, Angelos, et al. "Antiproliferative effect of exemestane in lung cancer cells." Molecular cancer 8.1 (2009): 109.

8) Sanfilippo, R., et al. "Reversion of resistance to mTOR inhibitors with the addition of exemestane in patients with malignant PEComa." Annals of Oncology 30 (2019): v696-v697.

9) Yang, Juan-Cheng, et al. "Preclinical evaluation of exemestane as a novel chemotherapy for gastric cancer." Journal of cellular and molecular medicine 23.11 (2019): 7417-7426.

10) Liu, Hua, and Paul Talalay. "Relevance of anti-inflammatory and antioxidant activities of exemestane and synergism with sulforaphane for disease prevention." Proceedings of the National Academy of Sciences 110.47 (2013): 19065-19070.

11) Mackillop, W.J., et al. "A stem cell model of human tumor growth: implications for tumor cell clonogenic assays." Journal of the national cancer institute 70.1 (1983): 9-16.

12) Lapidot, Tsvee, et al. "A cell initiating human acute myeloid leukaemia after transplantation into SCID mice." Nature 367.6464 (1994): 645-648.

13) Carke, M. F. "Cancer Stem Cells-Perspectives on current status and future directions." AACR Workshop on Cancer Stem Cells. Cancer Research. Vol. 66. 2006.

14) Wong, Andrea Li Ann, et al. "Understanding the cancer stem cell phenotype: A step forward in the therapeutic management of cancer." Biochemical pharmacology (2019).

15) Du, Fang-Yu, et al. "Targeting cancer stem cells in drug discovery: Current state and future perspectives." World Journal of Stem Cells 11.7 (2019): 398.

16) Diehn, Maximilian, et al. "Association of reactive oxygen species levels and radioresistance in cancer stem cells." Nature 458.7239 (2009): 780-783.

17) Safa, Ahmad R. "Resistance to cell death and its modulation in cancer stem cells." Critical Reviews™ in Oncogenesis 21.3-4 (2016).

18) Sancho, Patricia, et al. "MYC/PGC-1α balance determines the metabolic phenotype and plasticity of pancreatic cancer stem cells." Cell metabolism 22.4 (2015): 590-605.

19) Puigserver, Pere. "PGC1a at the Nexus of Cancer Stem Cell Fates." Free Radical Biology and Medicine 128 (2018): S14.

20) Sun, Haoran, et al. "Therapeutic strategies targeting cancer stem cells and their microenvironment." Frontiers in oncology 9 (2019): 1104.

21) Bezuidenhout, Nicole, and Maria Shoshan. "A Shifty Target: Tumor-Initiating Cells and Their Metabolism." International journal of molecular sciences 20.21 (2019): 5370.

22) Michelakis, E. D., L. Webster, and J. R. Mackey. "Dichloroacetate (DCA) as a potential metabolic-targeting therapy for cancer." British journal of cancer 99.7 (2008): 989-994.

23) Song, Kyoungsub, et al. "Active glycolytic metabolism in CD133 (+) hepatocellular cancer stem cells:

regulation by MIR-122." Oncotarget 6.38 (2015): 40822.

24) Nazio, Francesca, et al. "Autophagy and cancer stem cells: molecular mechanisms and therapeutic applications." Cell Death & Differentiation 26.4 (2019): 690-702.

25) Pagotto, Anna, et al. "Autophagy inhibition reduces chemoresistance and tumorigenic potential of human ovarian cancer stem cells." Cell death & disease 8.7 (2017): e2943-e2943.

26) Yang, Yi, et al. "Autophagy regulates the stemness of cervical cancer stem cells." Biologics: targets & therapy 11 (2017): 71.

27) Bischof, Joachim, et al. "Cancer stem cells: The potential role of autophagy, proteolysis, and cathepsins in glioblastoma stem cells." Tumor Biology 39.3 (2017): 1010428317692227.

28) Sha, Jian, et al. "Curcumin induces G0/G1 arrest and apoptosis in hormone independent prostate cancer DU-145 cells by down regulating Notch signaling." Biomedicine & Pharmacotherapy 84 (2016): 177-184.

29) Hossain, F., et al. "Repurposing sulindac sulfide as a Notch inhibitor to target cancer stem-like cells in triple negative breast cancer." CANCER RESEARCH. Vol. 79. No. 4. AMER ASSOC CANCER RESEARCH, 2019.

30) Sancho, Patricia, David Barneda, and Christopher Heeschen. "Hallmarks of cancer stem cell metabolism." British journal of cancer 114.12 (2016): 1305-1312.

31) Turdo, Alice, et al. "Meeting the challenge of targeting cancer stem cells." Frontiers in cell and developmental biology 7 (2019): 16

32) Zhu, Haitao, et al. "Role of the Hypoxia-inducible factor-1 alpha induced autophagy in the conversion of non-stem pancreatic cancer cells into CD133+ pancreatic cancer stem-like cells." Cancer cell international 13.1 (2013): 119.

33) Feng, Weiguo, et al. "Targeting unique metabolic properties of breast tumor initiating cells." Stem cells 32.7 (2014): 1734-1745.

34) Marcucci, Fabrizio, Cristiano Rumio, and François Lefoulon. "Anti-cancer stem-like cell compounds in clinical development–an overview and critical appraisal." Frontiers in oncology 6 (2016): 115.

35) Renz, Bernhard W., et al. "Repurposing established compounds to target pancreatic cancer stem cells (CSCs)." Medical Sciences 5.2 (2017): 14.

36) Leão, Ricardo, et al. "Cancer stem cells in prostate cancer: Implications for targeted therapy." Urologia internationalis 99.2 (2017): 125-136.

37) Hen, Omri, and Dalit Barkan. "Dormant disseminated tumor cells and cancer stem/progenitor-like cells: similarities and opportunities." Seminars in cancer biology. Academic Press, 2019.

38) Veschi, Veronica, Francesco Verona, and Carol J. Thiele. "Cancer stem cells and neuroblastoma: characteristics and therapeutic targeting options." Frontiers in Endocrinology 10 (2019).

39) Kim, Tae Hun, et al. "Metformin against cancer stem cells through the modulation of energy metabolism: special considerations on ovarian cancer." BioMed research international 2014 (2014).

40) Bost, F., et al. "Energy disruptors: rising stars in anticancer therapy?." Oncogenesis 5.1 (2016): e188. Energy disruptors: rising stars in anticancer therapy?

41) Rodríguez-Lirio, A., et al. "Metformin induces cell cycle arrest and apoptosis in drug-resistant leukemia cells." Leukemia research and treatment 2015 (2015).

42) De Francesco, Ernestina Marianna, et al. "Dodecyl-TPP Targets Mitochondria and Potently Eradicates Cancer Stem Cells (CSCs): Synergy With FDA-Approved Drugs and Natural Compounds (Vitamin C and Berberine)." Frontiers in oncology 9 (2019): 615.

43) Leão, Ricardo, et al. "Cancer Stem Cells in Prostate Cancer: Implications for Targeted Therapy." Urologia Internationalis (2017).

44) Lin, Xiaoping, et al. "Glucose Metabolism on Tumor Plasticity, Diagnosis, and Treatment." Frontiers in Oncology 10 (2020): 317.

45) Lee, Minjong, and Jung-Hwan Yoon. "Metabolic interplay between glycolysis and mitochondrial oxidation: The reverse Warburg effect and its therapeutic implication." World journal of biological chemistry 6.3 (2015): 148.

46) Zhang, Qian, Yunjiang Feng, and Derek Kennedy. "Multidrug-resistant cancer cells and cancer stem cells hijack cellular systems to circumvent systemic

therapies, can natural products reverse this?." Cellular and molecular life sciences 74.5 (2017): 777-801.

47) Moselhy, Jim, et al. "Natural products that target cancer stem cells." Anticancer research 35.11 (2015): 5773-5788.

48) Taylor, Wesley F., and Ehsan Jabbarzadeh. "The use of natural products to target cancer stem cells." American journal of cancer research 7.7 (2017): 1588.

Chapter 16

Pterostilbene

Anti-Cancer Activity from the Natural Plant Pterostilbenes

INTEREST IN THE ANTI-CANCER EFFECTS of everyday foods was stimulated by epidemiology studies showing a reduction in cancer risk with the consumption of fruits and vegetables. (1) In 1997, Dr. Meishiang Jang et al. reported in *Science* that resveratrol from grapes has anti-cancer and anti-inflammatory activity. It may even counteract the effects of aging. (2) Resveratrol is found in the skin of the grape, thought to protect the plant from fungal infection. (3)

Resveratrol Analogs

The methylated analog of resveratrol, called pterostilbene, is more bioavailable and more biologically active. Pterostilbene is a potent anti-fungal, available at the vitamin store as a food supplement, and has considerable anti-cancer activity. (4–7)

USDA Studies of Pterostilbene— Potent and Effective

The USDA and the University of Mississippi have been studying resveratrol analogs for two decades. In 2002, Dr. Agnes M. Rimando et al. reported pterostilbene inhibited breast cancer in a mouse model. (8) In 2013, Drs. Steven Dias and Dr. Kun Li et al. delved into the molecular biology of pterostilbene's anti-cancer activity using prostate cancer in a mouse xeno-graft model and came out with two important papers. The authors showed pterostilbene had higher potency for inhibiting tumor progression than resveratrol. (9–10)

Dr. Diaz concluded:

> 3M-Res [pterostilbene] was the most active in inhibiting [cancer] cell proliferation and suppressing colony formation, and its accumulation in both serum and tumor tissues was the highest … findings offer strong preclinical evidence for the utilization of dietary stilbenes, particularly 3M-Res [pterostilbene], as novel, **potent, effective chemopreventive agents in prostate cancer.** (9)

Pterostilbene, the Most Promising

In 2013, Dr. Kun Li reported that pterostilbene appears to be the most promising of the resveratrol analogs and significantly inhibited tumor growth, progression, local invasion and spontaneous metastasis in a mouse model of prostate cancer by inhibiting MTA1 (metastasis associated protein 1). (10)

Studies have confirmed that pterostilbene exerts antiproliferative and pro-apoptotic effects in various cancer cell types, including lung, gastric, prostate, colon, breast cancers, chronic myelogenous leukemia, and lymphoblastic leukemia and is useful for anti-aging and neuroprotection. (4–7)(11–18)

In 2018, Dr. Rong-Jane Chen et al. reviewed

the anti-cancer effects of pterostilbene, concluding:

> Pterostilbene [PS] has antineoplastic, anti-inflammatory, and anti-oxidant properties and may be useful in prevention of and treatment for cancer, dyslipidemia, diabetes, and cardiovascular and neurological degeneration ... Pterostilbene has inhibitory effects on almost every cellular event that promotes tumor progression toward metastasis ... Most importantly, PS, upon oral administration, is able to simultaneously prevent colonization of CTCs [circulating tumor cells] and diminish the already established secondary tumor masses in distant organs, greatly lowering the risks of patients for metastatic recurrence due to drug resistance ... combining T Cell checkpoint inhibitors might enhance efficacy ... PS inhibits the activation of NF-κB [Nuclear Factor Kappa B] ... PS facilitates both intrinsic and extrinsic apoptotic pathways ... downregulate Bcl-2 [anti-apoptosis protein] ... PS reduces tumor cell adhesion, migration, and intracellular GSG [glutathione] levels while increases the apoptosis index ... PS-**induces protective autophagy** ... Thus, combined **PS with autophagy inhibitor could enhance apoptosis** in bladder cancer cells.... inhibits the human telomerase reverse transcriptase [hTERT] enzyme activity and protein expression, which results in the subsequent induction of DNA damage ... **suppresses Wnt/B-catenin CD133+ stem cells** ... PS has a very safe profile with no toxic effects ... safe for humans at doses up to 250 mg per day. (12)

Other recent revelations about pterostilbene:

1) Synergy in combination with histone deacetylase inhibitor (HDAC) in mouse model of prostate cancer (11)

2) Inhibits MTA-1/HIF-alpha (hypoxia-inducible factor) (11)

3) Inhibition of telomerase activity, induction of cellular senescence (13)

4) Enhances autophagic flux (14)

5) Synergy in combination with astragalus (15)

6) Synergy in combination with quercetin (16)

7) Synergy with glioblastoma drugs, epidermal growth factor receptor (EGFR) inhibitor gefitinib and the antidepressant sertraline (17)

8) Synergy with (EGFR), tyrosine kinase inhibitors (TKIs), and osimertinib for lung cancer (18)

Autophagy Flux Inhibitor— Lysosomal Membrane Disruption

In 2012, Dr. Salvador Mena et al. studied the mechanism of action (MOA) of pterostilbene anti-cancer activity in various cancer cell types with melanoma and lung the most susceptible, and colon and breast most resistant due to the level of heat shock protein. Dr. Mena's group concluded that the main mechanism of cell death is inhibition of autophagy flux and lysosomal membrane rupture with release of contents (enzymes) freely into the cytosol of the cancer cell:

> Results are suggestive of autophagosome accumulation due to inhibited autophagic flux ... lysosomal membrane permeabilization is the main cell death pathway triggered by pterostilbene.... Our results show that Pterostilbene induces destabilization of the lysosomal membranes and release of lysosomal hydrolases into the

cytoplasm, thus leading to the activation of a caspase-independent lysosomal cell death program. (19)

Notice that this mechanism is similar to that of the antimalaria drug mefloquine without its toxicity; mefloquine accumulates in lysosomes and disrupts lysosomal membranes with release of cathepsins (hydrolases) into the cell cytoplasm. While pterostilbene has no adverse effects, mefloquine has the potential for adverse neuropsychiatric events, as well as retinal toxicity. Pterostilbene might serve as an autophagy inhibitor without the adverse effects of mefloquine, chloroquine, and hydroxychloroquine.

Pterostilbene Is NOT an Autophagy Inhibitor

However, as you will read below, later studies show pterostilbene induces "protective autophagy" in many cancer cell lines, and in combination with an autophagy inhibitor such as chloroquine provides synergy. See the discussion below.

Pterostilbene is a PPAR Agonist like Fenofibrate

In 2005, Dr. Agnes Rimando et al. say pterostilbene is a new peroxisome proliferator-activated receptor (PPAR) agonist, similar to fenofibrate. See chapter 37 on Fenofibrate for more on this topic. (20)

Pterostilbene Induces Autophagy— Synergy with Chloroquine

- Induces endoplasmic reticulum (ER) stress

- Blocks Wnt pathway
- Induces protective autophagy

In 2015, Dr. Ioanna Papandreou et al. performed a high-throughput screen of 1,726 small drugs, finding pterostilbene the most potent inducer of ER stress, blocking the Wnt processing pathway, and inducing autophagy in acute leukemia cells. They conclude that combining pterostilbene with chloroquine provides augmented synergy in a lymphoblastic leukemia cell line:

> Combining pterostilbene [to induce ER stress] with chloroquine [to inhibit autophagy] leads to significant cellular toxicity in cells from aggressive acute lymphoblastic leukemia. (21)

Others have observed that pterostilbene induces protective autophagy in cancer cells (22–23)

The addition of an autophagy inhibitor drug (such as chloroquine) promotes the anti-tumor efficacy of pterostilbene. (24–25)

Pterostilbene Anti-Cancer Effects

Numerous studies have been done showing the anti-cancer effects of pterostilbene for:

- Lung cancer (26–29)
- Breast cancer (30–35)
- Skin cancer and cancer protection (36–39)
- Colon cancer (40–44)
- Hepatocellular cancer (45–47)
- Pancreatic cancer (48–49)
- Gastric cancer (50–51)

- Prostate cancer prevention/therapy (52–54)
- Cervical cancer, HPV positive E6 protein (55–58)
- Ovarian cancer (59)
- Leukemia (60–61)
- B-cell (Mantle Cell) and T cell lymphoma (62–66)
- Multiple myeloma (67)
- Glioblastoma (68)

Dr. Shiby Paul et al. (2010) write:

Pterostilbene downregulated the expression of Beta-Catenin and cyclin D1 targets of Wnt pathway.... .pterostilbene reduced the Wnt agonist-induced levels of cyclin D1 and Beta-Catenin in the nucleus ... pterostilbene inhibits colon tumorigenesis by regulating the Wnt/Beta-Catenin-signaling pathway and the inflammatory responses. (44)

Dr. Kamila Siedlecka-Kroplewska et al. (2012) write:

Our results suggest that pterostilbene could serve as a potential additional chemotherapeutic agent for the treatment of leukemia. (60)

Dr. Dandan Yu et al. (2018) write: "Pterostilbene inhibited the PI3K/Akt/mTOR pathway."(62)

Note: Pterostilbene is an OXPHOS inhibitor, and therefore inhibits mTOR as well as the Wnt pathway, and is a cancer stem cell agent.

Mechanism of Action: Acute Myeloid Leukemia Cells

Pterostilbene is an OXPHOS inhibitor that induces Protective Autophagy

Dr. Pei-Ching Hsiao et al. (2014) studied the anti-cancer effects of pterostilbene on various leukemia cell lines. They showed that pterostilbene induced apoptosis in cancer cells via mitochondrial pathways, with activation of the caspase system.

Pterostilbene suppressed cell proliferation in various Leukemia cell lines, and induced G0/G1-phase arrest occurred when expressions of cyclin D3 and cyclin-dependent kinase [CDK] 2/6 were inhibited. Pterostilbene induced cancer cell programmed cell death [apoptosis] through activation of caspases-8–9/-3 [apoptosis cascade], and mitochondrial pathways. (61)

Downregulates the PI3K/Akt/mTOR Pathway

Dr. Dandan Yu (2018) studied the effect of pterostilbene on mantle cell lymphoma cells, finding attenuation of cancer cell progression by downregulation of the PI3K/Akt/mTOR pathway. (62)

Breast Cancer

Dr. Yanshang Wang et al. (2012), showed pterostilbene simultaneously induces apoptosis, cell-cycle arrest and cyto-protective autophagy in breast cancer cells. (32)

Dr. D. Moon et al. (2012), showed that pterostilbene induces apoptosis in breast cancer cell lines via the mitochondrial pathway. (33)

Dr. Julie A. Alosi et al. (2010) studied pterostilbene in breast cancer in vitro showing similar findings with apoptosis induced by mitochondrial pathways. (35)

Wnt/B-catenin-Signaling Pathway—Colon Cancer

Dr. Shiby Paul (2010) et al. reported that pterostilbene inhibits the Wnt/β catenin pathway in colon carcinogenesis in a mouse model. They report that

> pterostilbene reduces the Wnt agonist-induced levels of cyclin D1 and B-catenin in the cancer cell nucleus. Pterostilbene inhibits colon tumorigenesis by regulating the Wnt/b-catenin-signaling pathway and the inflammatory responses. (44)

Pterostilbene for HPV Infection and Cervical Cancer

In 2018–2019, Dr. Kaushiki Chatterjee et al. studied the effect of pterostilbene on HPV- infected cervical cells. They report that pterostilbene is useful in HPV/ cervical cancer chemoprevention by downregulating the E6 oncoprotein:

> E6 is a vital HPV [Human Papilloma Virus] oncoprotein essential for cervical cancer progression. E6 binds to tumor suppressor protein p53 and targets it for degradation by the ubiquitin proteasome pathway, thus causing uncontrolled cell proliferation.... .Resveratrol and to a greater extent pterostilbene downregulates the HPV oncoprotein E6, induces caspase-3 activation, and upregulates p53 protein levels. Results point to a mechanism that may involve the downregulation of the HPV E6 oncoprotein, activation of apoptotic pathways, and

re-establishment of functional p53 protein, with pterostilbene showing greater efficacy than resveratrol.... .This observed suppression of E6 and upregulation of p53 is of paramount importance because HPV infection and cancer progression in cervical cells relies on the expression of the viral E6 oncoprotein which targets p53 for degradation by the ubiquitination. (57–58)

Neuroprotective Effects of Pterostilbene

Dr. Martina La Spina (2019) showed that pterostilbene crosses the blood-brain barrier, attenuates inflammation, and improves cognitive performance in aged rats, suggesting its usefulness in preventing or retarding age-related cognitive loss and dementia in humans. (69–72)

In addition to pterostilbene, Dr. Shibu M. Poulose et al. (2017) listed other nutritional factors inducing adult neurogenesis and improving cognitive function. These agents might be useful in patients after chemotherapy to ameliorate the effects of "chemo brain":

> Curcumin, resveratrol, blueberry polyphenols, sulforaphane, salvionic acid, polyunsaturated fatty acids [PUFAs], and diets enriched with polyphenols and PUFAs, as well as caloric restriction, physical exercise, and learning, have been **shown to induce neurogenesis [regrowth of brain cells] in adult brains**. (73)

Lithium Is Neuroprotective

Lithium is a mineral in the water supply also available as a supplement, (lithium orotate) or a medication (lithium carbonate). Lithium is known to increase hippocampal neurogenesis (regrowth of neurons), and may be useful for neuroprotection and Alzheimer's prevention. (74–75)

Pterostilbene is protective of the following organ systems:

- Liver, from acetaminophen induced toxicity (76)
- Pancreatic beta-cells, from apoptosis in Type I diabetics (77–78)
- Brain from lipo-polysaccharide (LPS) induced brain inflammation and learning/memory impairment. (79)
- Corneal epithelium of the eye from inflammation/oxidation. (80)
- The skin from UV ultraviolet-radiation-induced skin damage and carcinogenesis. (81)(36–37)

Pterostilbene Synergy Combinations:

- HDAC inhibitor (vorinostat) (8)
- Autophagy inhibitor (Chloroquine) (21) (24–25)

Pterostilbene Targets MTA1/HIF-1Alpha

Dr. Nasir Butt et al. (2017) studied a prostate cancer mouse xenograft model, finding synergy of pterostilbene with vorinostat in the inhibition of metastasis-associated protein 1 (MTA1) and hypoxia-inducible factor (HIF-1), decreasing angiogenesis. Dr. Butt's group writes:

> Pterostilbene [Pter] sensitized tumor cells to SAHA [vorinostat HDAC inhibitor] treatment resulting in inhibiting tumor growth and additional decline of tumor progression. These effects were dependent on the reduction of MTA1-associated pro-angiogenic factors HIF-1α, VEGF, and IL-1β leading to decreased angiogenesis. In addition, treatment of PCa [Prostate Cancer] cell lines in vitro with combined Pter and low-dose SAHA resulted in **more potent inhibition** of MTA1/HIF-1α than by high-dose SAHA alone. Our study provides preclinical evidence that Pter/SAHA combination treatment inhibits MTA1/HIF-1α tumor-promoting signaling in PCa [Prostate Cancer]. (11)

Conclusion

Pterostilbene induces ER (endoplasmic reticulum) stress, is an OXPHOS inhibitor that disrupts the mitochondrial membrane leading to mitochondrial apoptosis, inhibits mTOR and induces protective autophagy. There is also inhibition of the Wnt cancer stem cell pathway. Pterostilbene synergizes with the autophagy inhibitor chloroquine and the HDAC inhibitor vorinostat. Pterostilbene inhibits metastasis associated protein (MAP1). Pterostilbene is a compound found in grapes and berries with a wide range of health benefits relating to anti-inflammatory and neuro-protective qualities, with no toxicity. Pterostilbene has striking anti-cancer activity in animal models mediated through well-described molecular pathways. Pterostilbene is not a drug. Rather, it is a safe, nontoxic food supplement available at the vitamin store without a prescription. The lack of toxicity makes pterostilbene a good addition to virtually any anti-cancer program.

References Chapter 16: Pterostilbene

1) Riboli, Elio, and Teresa Norat. "Epidemiologic evidence of the protective effect of fruit and vegetables on cancer risk." The American journal of clinical nutrition 78.3 (2003): 559S-569S.

2) Jang, Meishiang, et al. "Cancer chemopreventive activity of resveratrol, a natural product derived from grapes." Science 275.5297 (1997): 218-220.

3) Roupe, Kathryn A., et al. "Pharmacometrics of stilbenes: seguing towards the clinic." Current clinical pharmacology 1.1 (2006): 81-101.

4) Nutakul, Wasamon, et al. "Inhibitory effects of resveratrol and pterostilbene on human colon cancer cells: a side-by-side comparison." Journal of agricultural and food chemistry 59.20 (2011): 10964-10970.

5) McCormack, Denise, and David McFadden. "Pterostilbene and cancer: current review." Journal of Surgical Research 173.2 (2012): e53-e61.

6) Kapoor, Shailendra. "Pterostilbene and its emerging antineoplastic effects: a prospective treatment option for systemic malignancies." The American Journal of Surgery 205.4 (2013): 483.

7) McCubrey, James A., et al. "Effects of resveratrol, curcumin, berberine and other nutraceuticals on aging, cancer development, cancer stem cells and microRNAs." Aging (Albany NY) 9.6 (2017): 1477.

8) Rimando, Agnes M., et al. "Cancer chemopreventive and antioxidant activities of pterostilbene, a naturally occurring analogue of resveratrol." Journal of agricultural and food chemistry 50.12 (2002): 3453-3457.

9) Dias, Steven J., et al. "Trimethoxy-Resveratrol and Piceatannol Administered Orally Suppress and Inhibit Tumor Formation and Growth in Prostate Cancer Xenografts." The Prostate 73.11 (2013): 1135-1146.

10) Li, Kun, et al. "Pterostilbene acts through metastasis-associated protein 1 to inhibit tumor growth, progression and metastasis in prostate cancer." PloS one 8.3 (2013): e57542.

11) Butt, Nasir A., et al. "Targeting MTA 1/HIF-1α signaling by pterostilbene in combination with histone deacetylase inhibitor attenuates prostate cancer progression." Cancer medicine 6.11 (2017): 2673-2685.

12) Chen, Rong-Jane, et al. "Apoptotic and nonapoptotic activities of pterostilbene against cancer." International journal of molecular sciences 19.1 (2018): 287.

13) Lee, Yu-Hsuan, et al. "Stilbene Compounds Inhibit Tumor Growth by the Induction of Cellular Senescence and the Inhibition of Telomerase Activity." International journal of molecular sciences 20.11 (2019): 2716.

14) Wang, Dong, et al. "Pterostilbene, An Active Constituent of Blueberries, Suppresses Proliferation Potential of Human Cholangiocarcinoma via Enhancing the Autophagic Flux." Frontiers in pharmacology 10 (2019).

15) Huang, Xin-Yan, Song-Zhao Zhang, and Wen-Xi Wang. "Enhanced antitumor efficacy with combined administration of astragalus and pterostilbene for melanoma." Asian Pacific Journal of Cancer Prevention 15.3 (2014): 1163-1169.

16) Ferrer, Paula, et al. "Association between pterostilbene and quercetin inhibits metastatic activity of B16 melanoma." Neoplasia 7.1 (2005): 37-47.

17) Schmidt, Linnéa, et al. "Case-specific potentiation of glioblastoma drugs by pterostilbene." Oncotarget 7.45 (2016): 73200.

18) Bracht, Jillian Wilhelmina Paulina, et al. "Osimertinib and pterostilbene in EGFR-mutation-positive non-small cell lung cancer (NSCLC)." International journal of biological sciences 15.12 (2019): 2607.

19) Mena, Salvador, et al. "Pterostilbene-induced tumor cytotoxicity: a lysosomal membrane permeabilization-dependent mechanism." PLoS One 7.9 (2012): e44524.

20) Rimando, Agnes M., et al. "Pterostilbene, a new agonist for the peroxisome proliferator-activated receptor α-isoform, lowers plasma lipoproteins and cholesterol in hypercholesterolemic hamsters." Journal of agricultural and food chemistry 53.9 (2005): 3403-3407.

21) Papandreou, Ioanna, et al. "Plant stilbenes induce endoplasmic reticulum stress and their anti-cancer activity can be enhanced by inhibitors of autophagy." Experimental cell research 339.1 (2015): 147-153.

22) Wang, Yanshang, et al. "Pterostilbene simultaneously induces apoptosis, cell cycle arrest and cyto-protective autophagy in breast cancer cells." American journal of translational research 4.1 (2012): 44.

23) Ko, Chung-Po, et al. "Pterostilbene induce autophagy on human oral cancer cells through modulation of Akt and mitogen-activated protein kinase pathway." Oral oncology 51.6 (2015): 593-601.

24) Hsieh, Ming-Ju, et al. "A combination of pterostilbene with autophagy inhibitors exerts efficient apoptotic characteristics in both chemosensitive and chemoresistant lung cancer cells." toxicological sciences 137.1 (2014): 65-75.

25) Chen, Wei-Chih, et al. "The anti-tumor efficiency of pterostilbene is promoted with a combined treatment of Fas signaling or autophagy inhibitors in triple negative breast cancer cells." Food & function 5.8 (2014): 1856-1865.

26) Tan, Kok-Tong, et al. "Pterostilbene inhibits lung squamous cell carcinoma growth in vitro and in vivo by inducing S phase arrest and apoptosis." Oncology letters 18.2 (2019): 1631-1640.

27) Schneider, John G., et al. "Pterostilbene inhibits lung cancer through induction of apoptosis." Journal of Surgical Research 161.1 (2010): 18-22.

28) Chen, Rong-Jane, et al. "Chemopreventive effects of pterostilbene on urethane-induced lung carcinogenesis in mice via the inhibition of EGFR-mediated pathways and the induction of apoptosis and autophagy." Journal of agricultural and food chemistry 60.46 (2012): 11533-11541.

29) Yang, Yang, et al. "Pterostilbene exerts antitumor activity via the Notch1 signaling pathway in human lung adenocarcinoma cells." PLoS One 8.5 (2013): e62652.

30) Wakimoto, Rei, et al. "Differential anticancer activity of pterostilbene against three subtypes of human breast cancer cells." Anticancer research 37.11 (2017): 6153-6159.

31) Mak, Ka-Kit, et al. "Pterostilbene, a bioactive component of blueberries, suppresses the generation of breast cancer stem cells within tumor microenvironment and metastasis via modulating NF-κ B/microRNA 448 circuit." Molecular nutrition & food research 57.7 (2013): 1123-1134.

32) Wang, Yanshang, et al. "Pterostilbene simultaneously induces apoptosis, cell cycle arrest and cyto-protective autophagy in breast cancer cells." American journal of translational research 4.1 (2012): 44.

33) Moon, D., et al. "Pterostilbene Induces Mitochondrially-Derived Apoptosis in Breast Cancer in Vitro Via Bax Activation and Cytosolic Calcium Overload." Journal of Surgical Research 172.2 (2012): 342.

34) Pan, Min-Hsiung, et al. "Suppression of heregulin-β1/HER2-modulated invasive and aggressive phenotype of breast carcinoma by pterostilbene via inhibition of matrix metalloproteinase-9, p38 kinase cascade and Akt activation." Evidence-Based Complementary and Alternative Medicine, vol. 2011, Article ID 562187.

35) Alosi, Julie A., et al. "Pterostilbene inhibits breast cancer in vitro through mitochondrial depolarization and induction of caspase-dependent apoptosis." Journal of Surgical Research 161.2 (2010): 195-201.

36) Nagapan, Tava Shelan, et al. "Photoprotective Effect of Stilbenes and its Derivatives Against Ultraviolet Radiation-Induced Skin Disorders." Biomedical and Pharmacology Journal 11.3 (2018): 1199-1208.

37) Li, Huaping, et al. "Pterostilbene protects against UVB-induced photo-damage through a phosphatidylinositol-3-kinase-dependent Nrf2/ARE pathway in human keratinocytes." Redox Report 22.6 (2017): 501-507.

38) Chen, Rong-Jane, et al. "Autophagy-inducing effect of pterostilbene: A prospective therapeutic/preventive option for skin diseases." journal of food and drug analysis 25.1 (2017): 125-133.

39) Tsai, Mei-Ling, et al. "Pterostilbene, a natural analogue of resveratrol, potently inhibits 7, 12-dimethylbenz [a] anthracene (DMBA)/12-O-tetradecanoylphorbol-13-acetate (TPA)-induced mouse skin carcinogenesis." Food & function 3.11 (2012): 1185-1194.

40) Lai, Ching-Shu, et al. "3'-Hydroxypterostilbene Suppresses Colitis-Associated Tumorigenesis by Inhibition of IL-6/STAT3 Signaling in Mice." Journal of agricultural and food chemistry 65.44 (2017): 9655-9664.

41) Tolba, Mai F., and Sherif Z. Abdel-Rahman. "Pterostilbine, an active component of blueberries, sensitizes colon cancer cells to 5-fluorouracil cytotoxicity." Scientific reports 5 (2015): 15239.

42) Cheng, Tzu-Chun, et al. "Potent anti-cancer effect of 3'-hydroxypterostilbene in human colon xenograft tumors." PLoS One 9.11 (2014): e111814.

43) Chiou, Yi-Siou, et al. "Pterostilbene inhibits colorectal aberrant crypt foci (ACF) and colon carcinogenesis via suppression of multiple signal transduction pathways in azoxymethane-treated mice." Journal of agricultural and food chemistry 58.15 (2010): 8833-8841.

44) Paul, Shiby, et al. "Dietary intake of pterostilbene, a constituent of blueberries, inhibits the β-catenin/p65 downstream signaling pathway and colon carcinogenesis in rats." Carcinogenesis 31.7 (2010): 1272-1278.

45) Guo, Liying, et al. "Pterostilbene inhibits hepatocellular carcinoma through p53/SOD2/ROS-mediated mitochondrial apoptosis." Oncology reports 36.6 (2016): 3233-3240.

46) Lee, Chi-Ming, et al. "BlueBerry isolate, pterostilbene, functions as a potential anticancer stem cell agent in suppressing irradiation-mediated enrichment of hepatoma stem cells." Evidence-Based Complementary and Alternative Medicine (2013) Article ID 258425.

47) Pan, Min-Hsiung, et al. "Pterostilbene inhibited tumor invasion via suppressing multiple signal transduction pathways in human hepatocellular carcinoma cells." Carcinogenesis 30.7 (2009): 1234-1242.

48) McCormack, Denise E., Debbie E. McDonald, and David W. McFadden. "Pterostilbene Induces Mitochondrially-Derived Apoptosis in Pancreatic Cancer Cells by Increasing MnSOD Activity and Release of Cytochrome C and Smac/DIABLO." Gastroenterology 140.5 (2011): S-1026.

49) Mannal, Patrick W., et al. "Pterostilbene inhibits pancreatic cancer in vitro." Journal of Gastrointestinal Surgery 14.5 (2010): 873-879.

50) Yunjianan, Feng, et al. "The Induction of Apoptosis in Human Gastric Cancer SGC-7901 Cells by Pterostilbene." Chinese Journal of Cell Biology 3 (2017): 7.

51) Pan, Min-Hsiung, et al. "Pterostilbene induces apoptosis and cell cycle arrest in human gastric carcinoma cells." J. of Agricultural and Food Chemistry 55.19 (2007): 7777-7785.

52) Tsai, Hui-Yun. Growth inhibitory effects of 3'-hydroxypterostilbene in human prostate cancer cells and xenograft mice. Diss. Rutgers University-Graduate School-New Brunswick, 2016.

53) Dhar, Swati, et al. "Dietary pterostilbene is a novel MTA1-targeted chemopreventive and therapeutic agent in prostate cancer." Oncotarget 7.14 (2016): 18469.

54) Kumar, Avinash, Agnes M. Rimando, and Anait S. Levenson. "Resveratrol and pterostilbene as a microRNA-mediated chemopreventive and therapeutic strategy in prostate cancer." Annals of the New York Academy of Sciences 1403.1 (2017): 15-26.

55) Shin, Hee Jeong, et al. "Pterostilbene Suppresses both Cancer Cells and Cancer Stem-Like Cells in Cervical Cancer with Superior Bioavailability to Resveratrol." Molecules 25.1 (2020): 228.

56) Bin, Wu Hong, et al. "Pterostilbene (3', 5'-dimethoxy-resveratrol) exerts potent antitumor effects in HeLa human cervical cancer cells via disruption of mitochondrial membrane potential, apoptosis induction and targeting m-TOR/PI3K/Akt signalling pathway." Journal of BU ON.: official journal of the Balkan Union of Oncology 23.5 (2018): 1384-1389.

57) Chatterjee, Kaushiki, et al. "Dietary polyphenols, resveratrol and pterostilbene exhibit antitumor activity on an HPV E6-positive cervical cancer model An in vitro and in vivo analysis." Frontiers in Oncology 9 (2019): 352.

58) Chatterjee, Kaushiki, et al. "Resveratrol and Pterostilbene Exhibit Anticancer Properties Involving the `Downregulation of HPV Oncoprotein E6 in Cervical Cancer Cells." Nutrients 10.2 (2018): 243.

59) Dong, J., H. Guo, and Y. Chen. "Pterostilbene induces apoptosis through caspase activation in ovarian cancer cells." Eur J Gynaecol Oncol 37.3 (2016): 342-7.

60) Siedlecka-Kroplewska, Kamila, et al. "Pterostilbene induces cell cycle arrest and apoptosis in MOLT4 human leukemia cells." Folia histochemica et cytobiologica 50.4 (2012): 574-580.

61) Hsiao, Pei-Ching, et al. "Pterostilbene simultaneously induced G0/G1-phase arrest and MAPK-mediated mitochondrial-derived apoptosis in human acute myeloid leukemia cell lines." PloS one 9.8 (2014): e105342.

62) Yu, Dandan, et al. "Targeting the PI3K/Akt/mTOR signaling pathway by pterostilbene attenuates mantle

cell lymphoma progression." Acta biochimica et biophysica Sinica 50.8 (2018): 782-792.

64) Kong, Yuanyuan, et al. "Pterostilbene induces apoptosis and cell cycle arrest in diffuse large B-cell lymphoma cells." Scientific Reports 6 (2016): 37417.

65) Peck, Connor J., Michelle H. Townsend, and Kim L. O'Neill. "Resveratrol and pterostibene selectively chemosensitize Burkitt's lymphoma cells to 5-Fluorouracil." (2017): 252-252.

66) Chang, Gaomei, et al. "Pterostilbene induces cell apoptosis and cell cycle arrest in T-cell leukemia/lymphoma by suppressing the ERK1/2 pathway." BioMed research international 2017 (2017).

67) Chen, Gege, et al. "The blueberry component pterostilbene has potent anti-myeloma activity in bortezomib-resistant cells." Oncology reports 38.1 (2017): 488-496.

68) Huynh, Thanh-Tuan, et al. "Pterostilbene suppressed irradiation-resistant glioma stem cells by modulating GRP78/miR-205 axis." The Journal of nutritional biochemistry 26.5 (2015): 466-475.

69) La Spina, Martina, et al. "Pterostilbene Improves Cognitive Performance in Aged Rats: An in Vivo Study." Cell Physiol Biochem 52 (2019): 232-239.

70) Lange, Klaus W., and Shiming Li. "Resveratrol, pterostilbene, and dementia." BioFactors 44.1 (2018): 83-90.

71) Chang, Jaewon, et al. "Low-dose pterostilbene, but not resveratrol, is a potent neuromodulator in aging and Alzheimer's disease." Neurobiology of aging 33.9 (2012): 2062-2071.

72) Liu, Haixiao, et al. "Pterostilbene attenuates astrocytic inflammation and neuronal oxidative injury after ischemia-reperfusion by inhibiting NF-κB phosphorylation." Frontiers in immunology 10 (2019): 2408.

73) Poulose, Shibu M., et al. "Nutritional factors affecting adult neurogenesis and cognitive function." Advances in Nutrition 8.6 (2017): 804-811.

74) Yucel, Kaan, et al. "Bilateral hippocampal volume increase in patients with bipolar disorder and short-term lithium treatment." Neuropsychopharmacology 33.2 (2008): 361.

75) Yan, Xue-Bo, et al. "Lithium regulates hippocampal neurogenesis by ERK pathway and facilitates recovery of spatial learning and memory in rats after transient global cerebral ischemia." Neuropharmacology 53.4 (2007): 487-495.

76) Kang, Ki-Young, Jun-Kyu Shin, and Sun-Mee Lee. "Pterostilbene protects against acetaminophen-induced liver injury by restoring impaired autophagic flux." Food and chemical toxicology 123 (2019): 536-545.

77) Bhakkiyalakshmi, Elango, et al. "Therapeutic potential of pterostilbene against pancreatic beta-cell apoptosis mediated through N rf2." British journal of pharmacology 171.7 (2014): 1747-1757.

78) Sireesh, Dornadula, et al. "Role of pterostilbene in attenuating immune mediated devastation of pancreatic beta cells via Nrf2 signaling cascade." The Journal of nutritional biochemistry 44 (2017): 11-21.

79) Hou, Yue, et al. "Pterostilbene attenuates lipopolysaccharide-induced learning and memory impairment possibly via inhibiting microglia activation and protecting neuronal injury in mice." Progress in Neuro-Psychopharmacology and Biological Psychiatry 54 (2014): 92-102.

80) Li, Jin, et al. "Blueberry component pterostilbene protects corneal epithelial cells from inflammation via anti-oxidative pathway." Scientific Reports 6 (2016): 19408.

81) Sirerol, J. Antoni, et al. "Topical treatment with pterostilbene, a natural phytoalexin, effectively protects hairless mice against UVB radiation-induced skin damage and carcinogenesis." Free Radical Biology and Medicine 85 (2015): 1-11.

82) Wang, H., H. Feng, and Y. Zhang. "Resveratrol inhibits hypoxia-induced glioma cell migration and invasion by the p-STAT3/miR-34a axis." Neoplasma 63.4 (2016): 532-539.

Chapter 17

Boswellia

THE GUM RESIN OF THE boswellia tree (also known as frankincense) has been used medicinally for roughly 5,000 years for just about any ailment you can think of. The main ingredients are boswellic acid, including acetyl keto boswellic acid (AKBA), and their derivatives. (1–5)

Boswellia Is a Plant Steroid 5-LOX Inhibitor

The chemical structure of boswellia contains a steroidal ring that is strikingly similarity to human steroids such as vitamin D3, cardiac glycosides (digoxin), cortisol, testosterone, and estrogen, thus stimulating interest in AKBA as an extremely potent intracellular messenger with anti-inflammatory properties by virtue of its inhibition of 5-lipoxygenase (5-LOX) and downstream leukotriene biosynthesis, a major inflammatory pathway frequently upregulated in cancer cells. The second major inflammatory pathway is the enzyme cyclo-oxygenase-2 (COX-2), nicely inhibited by the commonly used NSAID drug, celecoxib (Celebrex®). Co-administration of both agents (AKBA and celecoxib) was quite effective in a mouse model of LPS induced cognitive impairment, suggesting both COX-2 and 5-LOX inhibition may synergize for anti-cancer treatment. We await NIH-funded studies of this combination. (4)

High Thru-put Screen for Triple-Negative Breast Cancer

In 2017, Dr. Elizabeth Mazzio et al. performed a high thru-put screen of a library of 1,640 plant-derived chemicals and botanical herbs for their cytotoxicity to triple-negative breast cancer (TNBC) cells, in vitro, at low micromolar concentrations. Frankincense (Boswellia serrata extract, or BSE) and 3-O-acetyl-β-boswellic acid (3-OAβBA) were identified as the leading compounds. Dr. Mazzio then did a "whole transcriptome data analysis of RNA" from the breast cancer cells after boswellia treatment, showing that the primary mode of cell death is

> ER [endoplasmic reticulum] stress leading to a UPR [unfolded protein response] … commonly associated with activated cell death. (6)

In recent years, endoplasmic reticulum stress with unfolded protein response has received attention as an important target for cancer treatment. One of the jobs of the endoplasmic reticulum is to fold proteins, as unfolded proteins may create a cell crisis that triggers cancer cell apoptosis. (7–9)

Silver Nanoparticles

Similarly, in 2016, Drs. Jean-Christophe Simard et al. showed that silver nanoparticles also induce "irremediable endoplasmic stress leading to unfolded protein response in breast cancer cells," thereby conferring anti-cancer activity. (10)

The combination of boswellia with silver particles has already been used for other diverse medical indications. One wonders about possible anti-cancer synergy using the combination of boswellia with silver nanoparticles. We await the results of further studies. (11–17)

Gold Nanoparticles

Gold nanoparticles have been studied and found to inhibit cancer and the tumor micro-environment. In 2016, Dr. Sherita L. Moses studied the combination of gold nanoparticles conjugated with boswellia in a breast cancer cell line in vitro, finding good efficacy with no toxicity. (18–22)

Boswellia Effective for Breast Cancer Using In Vivo Mouse Model

Drs. Hiva Alipanah and Parvin Zareian (2018) studied orally administered boswellia extract in a mouse breast cancer xenograft model showing potent anti-cancer activity. The cancer cells stopped dividing, growth of new blood vessels was halted (angiogenesis), and metastatic spread was blocked. (23)

Dr. Yu Shao et al. (1998) studied boswellia in a human leukemia cell model showing reduction of DNA and RNA protein synthesis at low concentrations: "IC50 values ranging from 0.6 to 7.1μM MicroMolar". (24) **Note:** DNA and RNA protein synthesis is a marker for cell proliferation.

Another study by Dr. Shashi Bhusha et al. (2007) showed boswellia- induced apoptosis in leukemia cells at IC50 of 12 mcg/ml. (25)

Boswellia Anti-cancer Effects Reviewed

Boswellia as anti-cancer therapy was reviewed in 2017 by Dr. Manjeet Kumar et al. and in 2019 by Drs. Luay Rashan and Nand Kihor Roy et al. (26–28) Many others have commented on the anti-cancer effects of boswellia. (29–34)

Dr. Kumar and colleagues write (2017) that Boswellia has diverse pharmacological applications, including:

> anti-inflammatory, anti-arthritic, anti-cancer, anti-oxidant, anti-ulcer, anti-bacterial, anti-asthmatic, anti-atherosclerotic, anti-diarrheal, hepatoprotective, renoprotective, anti-hyperglycemic, wound healing, diuretic, analgesic, nervous disorders, neuroprotective. (26)

Boswellia mechanisms of action (MOA) include:

- Inhibitor of 5-lipoxygenase (5-LOX).
- Binds to and inhibits topo-isomerase I and II at 10 mcg/ml.
- Interferes with IκB kinase, which inhibits nuclear factor kappa B (NF-κB).

5-LOX Inhibition Anti-Inflammatory Effects

Leukotrienes are lipids made from white blood cells biosynthesized by the action of the 5-LOX enzyme on arachidonic acid. Drs. Bipin Kumar Nayak and Arun Kumar write (2017) that leukotrienes are involved in various inflammatory disorders, such as:

bronchial asthma, allergic rhinitis, inflammatory bowel and skin diseases, rheumatoid arthritis, cancer, osteoporosis and cardiovascular diseases. (35)

A novel use of boswellia 5-LOX inhibition is in the treatment of anorexia nervosa eating disorders and neurodegenerative diseases. (37–38)

In addition to boswellia, which is a 5-LOX inhibitor, other natural 5-Lox inhibitors include:

- Allicin from allium species (i.e. onions and garlic) (5)
- Thymoquinone (Black Seed Oil) (36)

Topo-Isomerase Inhibitors

Boswellia inhibits topo-isomerase I and II. Discovered by Dr. James Wang in the 1970s, topo-isomerase enzymes are involved in repairing breaks and fixing tangled DNA related to unwinding and overwinding of the double helix during DNA replication. Inhibition of topo-isomerase leads to permanent breaks and damage in DNA, causing apoptosis and cell death.

A major landmark in the pharmacology of chemotherapy agents was the introduction of two topo-isomerase inhibitors, etoposide and doxorubicin, chemotherapy drugs commonly used on the oncology wards.

Topo-isomerase inhibition is also the mechanism of action (MOA) of a major class of antibiotics, the fluoroquinolones—ciprofloxacin (Cipro), levofloxacin (Levaquin), moxifloxacin (Avelox), and ofloxacin (Floxin), which target the bacterial and mitochondrial topo—isomerase, causing bacterial cell death. (39–41) This class of quinolone antibiotics are all mitochondrial toxins, which carry the adverse side effects of peripheral neuropathy and Achilles-tendon rupture. (60–61)

Boswellia Effective for Various Cancer Cell Types

Boswellia has been studied and found effective against the following cancer cell types:

- Breast cancer (6)(23)
- Acute myeloid leukemia (19)(24–25) (43)
- Invasive urothelial (42)
- Pancreatic cancer (44)
- Ileo-cecal adeno carcinoma (45)
- Prostate cancer (46–50)
- Glioblastoma (51–52)
- Cancer-related fatigue (53)
- Melanoma (54)
- Colon cancer (55)
- Hepatocellular cancer (56)
- Meningioma (57)

Boswellia Pharmacokinetics Studies

In 2004, Dr. S. Sharma et al. did a pharmacokinetic study with 12 healthy volunteers, each given 333 mg of boswellia serrata extract (AKBA), with a peak plasma level of 2.7 micromoles per liter attained at 4.5 hours after ingestion. Dr. Sherma's group found an elimination half-life of six hours and suggested oral dosing every 6 hours to attain a drug steady state after 30 hours. (58)

Similarly, in 2004, Dr. Vanessa Sterk et al.

studied the bio-availability of boswellia in healthy volunteers, finding that taking the drug with a high-fat meal increased drug absorption and increased plasma concentration several-fold compared to a fasting state. (59)

Conclusion

Boswellia (frankincense oil) is indeed a potent addition to our anti-cancer armamentarium with 5-LOX inhibition, topo-isomerase inhibition, and endoplasmic stress with unfolded protein response as its main mechanisms. Increased absorption and better blood levels were reported when taken with a fatty meal every 6 hours. Combination with colloidal silver might prove synergistic.

References for Chapter 17: Boswellia

1) Patel, Snehal S., and Jignasha K. Savjani. "Systematic review of plant steroids as potential antiinflammatory agents: Current status and future perspectives." The Journal of Phytopharmacology 4.2 (2015): 121-125.

2) Bishnoi, M., et al. "Analgesic activity of acetyl-11-keto-beta-boswellic acid, a 5-lipoxygenase-enzyme inhibitor." Indian journal of pharmacology 37.4 (2005): 255.

3) Ding, Xiaoling, et al. "Enhancing antitumor effects in pancreatic cancer cells by combined use of COX-2 and 5-LOX inhibitors." Biomedicine & Pharmacotherapy 65.7 (2011): 486-490.

4) Sayed, Aya Shoukry, and Nesrine Salah El Dine El Sayed. "Co-administration of 3-acetyl-11-keto-beta-boswellic acid potentiates the protective effect of celecoxib in lipopolysaccharide-induced cognitive impairment in mice: possible implication of anti-inflammatory and antiglutamatergic pathways." Journal of Molecular Neuroscience 59.1 (2016): 58-67.

5) Werz, Oliver. "Inhibition of 5-lipoxygenase product synthesis by natural compounds of plant origin." Planta medica 73.13 (2007): 1331-1357.

6) Mazzio, Elizabeth A., Charles A. Lewis, and Karam FA Soliman. "Transcriptomic profiling of MDA-MB-231 cells exposed to Boswellia serrata and 3-O-acetyl-B-Boswellic acid; ER/UPR mediated programmed cell death." Cancer Genomics-Proteomics 14.6 (2017): 409-425.

7) Clarke, Robert, et al. "Endoplasmic reticulum stress, the unfolded protein response, autophagy, and the integrated regulation of breast cancer cell fate." Cancer research 72.6 (2012): 1321-1331.

8) Luo, Biquan, and Amy S. Lee. "The critical roles of endoplasmic reticulum chaperones and unfolded protein response in tumorigenesis and anticancer therapies." Oncogene 32.7 (2013): 805-818.

9) Corazzari, Marco, et al. "Endoplasmic reticulum stress, unfolded protein response, and cancer cell fate." Frontiers in Oncology 7 (2017): 78.

10) Simard, Jean-Christophe, Isabelle Durocher, and Denis Girard. "Silver nanoparticles induce irremediable endoplasmic reticulum stress leading to unfolded protein response dependent apoptosis in breast cancer cells." Apoptosis 21.11 (2016): 1279-1290.

11) Khan, Ajmal, et al. "Loading AKBA on surface of silver nanoparticles to improve their sedative-hypnotic and anti-inflammatory efficacies." Nanomedicine 14.21 (2019): 2783-2798.

12) Muralidhar, Yegireddy, et al. "Antibacterial, anti-inflammatory and antioxidant effects of acetyl-11-α-keto-β-boswellic acid mediated silver nanoparticles in experimental murine mastitis." IET Nanobiotechnology 11.6 (2017): 682-689

13) Wang, Ji, et al. "Silica nanoparticles induce autophagosome accumulation via activation of the EIF2AK3 and ATF6 UPR pathways in hepatocytes." Autophagy 14.7 (2018): 1185-1200.

14) Zhang, Rui, et al. "Endoplasmic reticulum stress signaling is involved in silver nanoparticles-induced apoptosis." The international journal of biochemistry & cell biology 44.1 (2012): 224-232.

15) Huo, Lingling, et al. "Silver nanoparticles activate endoplasmic reticulum stress signaling pathway in cell

and mouse models: The role in toxicity evaluation." Biomaterials 61 (2015): 307-315.

16) Sriram, Muthu Irulappan, et al. "Antitumor activity of silver nanoparticles in Dalton's lymphoma ascites tumor model." International journal of nanomedicine 5 (2010): 753.

17) Manjunath, B. N., et al. "New water soluble glyco-sides of 11-keto-β-boswellic acid: A paradigm." Natural product research 32.2 (2018): 154-161.

18) Moses, Sherita L. Citrate reduced gold nanoparti-cles conjugated with Boswellia sacra and Commiphora myrrha to cause cytotoxicity in breast cancer cells without harming health cells:" We three things of Orient are". Diss. Alabama Agricultural and Mechanical University, 2016.

19) Ahmeda, Ahmad, and Mohammad Mahdi Zangeneh. "Novel green synthesis of Boswellia serrata leaf aqueous extract conjugated gold nanoparticles with excellent anti-acute myeloid leukemia property in comparison to mitoxantrone in a leukemic mice model: Introducing a new chemotherapeutic drug." Applied Organometallic Chemistry 34.3 (2020): e5344.

20) Saha, Sounik, et al. "Gold nanoparticle reprograms pancreatic tumor microenvironment and inhibits tumor growth." ACS Nano 10.12 (2016): 10636-10651.

21) Sun, Hainan, et al. "Gold nanoparticle-induced cell death and potential applications in nanomedi-cine." International journal of molecular sciences 19.3 (2018): 754.

22) Melamed, Jilian R., et al. "Using gold nanoparticles to disrupt the tumor microenvironment: an emerg-ing therapeutic strategy." Acs Nano 10.12 (2016): 10631-10635.

23) Alipanah, Hiva, and Parvin Zareian. "Anti-cancer properties of the methanol extract of Boswellia ser-rata gum resin: Cell proliferation arrest and inhibition of angiogenesis and metastasis in BALB/c mice breast cancer model." Physiology and Pharmacology 22.3 (2018): 183-194.

24) Shao, Yu, et al. "Inhibitory activity of boswellic acids from Boswellia serrata against human leukemia HL-60 cells in culture." Planta medica 64.04 (1998): 328-331.

25) Bhushan, Shashi, et al. "A triterpenediol from Boswellia serrata induces apoptosis through both the intrinsic and extrinsic apoptotic pathways in human leukemia HL-60 cells." Apoptosis 12.10 (2007): 1911-1926.

26) Kumar, Manjeet, et al. "Boswellic Acids as Potential Cancer Therapeutics." Cancer Preventive and Therapeutic Compounds: Gift From Mother Nature (2017): 32.

27) Rashan, Luay, et al. "Boswellia Gum Resin and Essential Oils: Potential Health Benefits– An Evidence Based Review." International Journal of Nutrition, Pharmacology, Neurological Diseases 9.2 (2019): 53.

28) Roy, Nand Kishor, et al. "An update on pharma-cological potential of boswellic acids against chronic diseases." International journal of molecular sciences 20.17 (2019): 4101.

29) Mahboubi-Rabbani, Mohammad, and Afshin Zarghi. "Lipoxygenase Inhibitors as Cancer Chemopreventives: Discovery, Recent Developments, and Future Perspectives." Current Medicinal Chemistry (2019).

30) Sharma, Tarun, and Snehasis Jana. "Boswellic Acids as Natural Anticancer Medicine: Precious Gift to Humankind." Journal of Herbal Medicine (2019): 100313.

31) Efferth, Thomas, and Franz Oesch. "Anti-inflammatory and anti-cancer activities of frankin-cense: Targets, treatments and toxicities." Seminars in Cancer Biology. Academic Press, 2020.

32) Efferth, Thomas, and Henry Johannes Greten. "Anti-inflammatory and anti-cancer activity of boswellic acids from frankincense (Boswellia ser-rata Roxb. et Colebr, B. carterii Birdw.)." Forum on Immunopathological Diseases and Therapeutics. Vol. 2. No. 4. Begel House Inc., 2011.

33) Hamidpour, R., et al. "Frankincense (Boswellia Species): The Novel Phytotherapy for Drug Targeting in Cancer." Arch Cancer Res 4.1 (2016): 1-5.

34) Bone, Kerry. "Does Boswellia have a role in cancer therapy." Townsend Letter: The Examiner of Alternative Medicine 277-278 (2006): 41-44.

35) Nayak, Bipin Kumar, and Arun Kumar. "Activity of leukotrienes in inflammation." Eur. J. Pharma. Med. Res 4 (2017): 207-215.

36) Mansour M, Tornhamre S. Inhibition of 5-lipoxygenase and leukotriene C4 synthase in human blood cells by thymoquinone. J Enzyme Inhib Med Chem. 2004; 19 431-6.

37) Brooks, S. J. "Targeting cytokines in the 5-Lox pro-inflammatory pathway for treatment-resistant anorexia nervosa." Journal of Molecular and Genetic Medicine: an international journal of biomedical research 12.4 (2018).

38) Das, Sayanna, and Sudip Kumar Mandal. "Current developments on anti-inflammatory natural medicines." neurodegenerative diseases 23 (2018): 24.

39) Chashoo, Gousia, et al. "A propionyloxy derivative of 11-keto-β-boswellic acid induces apoptosis in HL-60 cells mediated through topoisomerase I & II inhibition." Chemico-biological interactions 189.1-2 (2011): 60-71.

40) Hooper, David C., and George A. Jacoby. "Topoisomerase inhibitors: fluoroquinolone mechanisms of action and resistance." Cold Spring Harbor perspectives in medicine 6.9 (2016): a025320.

41) Nitiss, John L. "Targeting DNA topoisomerase II in cancer chemotherapy." Nature Reviews Cancer 9.5 (2009): 338-350.

42) Xia D, Lou W, Fung KM, Wolley CL, Suhail MM, Lin HK. Cancer chemopreventive effects of Boswellia sacra gum resin hydrodistillates on invasive urothelial cell carcinoma: Report of a Case. Integr Cancer Ther 2017; 16(4):605-611.

43) Xia L, Chen D, Han R, Fang Q, Waxman S, Jing Y. Boswellic acid acetate induces apoptosis through caspase-mediated pathways in myeloid leukemia cells. Mol Cancer Ther 2005; 4:381-388

44) Park B, Prasad S, Yadav V, Sung B, Aggarwal BB. Boswellic acid suppresses growth and metastasis of human pancreatic tumors in an orthotopic nude mouse model through modulation of multiple targets. PLoS One. 2011; 6(10):e26943

45) Xue X, Chen F, Liu A, Sun D, Wu J, Kong F, Luan Y, Qu X, Wang R. Reversal of the multidrug resistance of human ileocecal adenocarcinoma cells by acetyl-11-keto-β-boswellic acid via downregulation of P-glycoprotein signals. Biosci Trends 2016; 10(5):392-399.

46) Liu, Yong-qing, et al. "Acetyl-11-keto-β-boswellic acid suppresses docetaxel-resistant prostate cancer cells in vitro and in vivo by blocking Akt and Stat3 signaling, thus suppressing chemoresistant stem cell-like properties." Acta Pharmacologica Sinica 40.5 (2019): 689-698.

47) Syrovets T, Gschwend JE, Buchele B, Laumonnier Y, Zugmaier W, Genze F, Simmet T. Inhibition of IκB Kinase activity by acetyl-boswellic Acids promotes apoptosis in androgen-independent PC-3 prostate cancer cells in vitro and in vivo. J Biol Chem 2005; 280:6170-6180

48) Schmidt C, Cornelia Loos, Lu Jin, Michael Schmiech, Christoph Q. Schmidt, Menna El Gaafary, Tatiana Syrovets, Thomas Simmet. Acetyl-lupeolic acid inhibits Akt signaling and induces apoptosis in chemoresistant prostate cancer cells in vitro and in vivo Oncotarget 2017; 8(33):55147-55161.

49) Pang, Xiufeng, et al. "Acetyl-11-keto-β-boswellic acid inhibits prostate tumor growth by suppressing vascular endothelial growth factor receptor 2–mediated angiogenesis." Cancer research 69.14 (2009): 5893-5900.

50) Lu, Min, et al. "Acetyl-keto-β-Boswellic acid induces apoptosis through a death receptor 5–mediated pathway in prostate cancer cells." Cancer research 68.4 (2008): 1180-1186.

51) Li, Wan, et al. "3-O-Acetyl-11-keto-β-boswellic acid ameliorated aberrant metabolic landscape and inhibited autophagy in glioblastoma." Acta Pharmaceutica Sinica B (2020).

52) Li, Wan, et al. "3-O-acetyl-11-keto-β-boswellic acid exerts anti-tumor effects in glioblastoma by arresting cell cycle at G2/M phase." Journal of Experimental & Clinical Cancer Research 37.1 (2018): 132.

53) Reis, Debra, and Tisha Throne Jones. "Frankincense essential oil as a supportive therapy for cancer-related fatigue: A case study." Holistic nursing practice 32.3 (2018): 140-142.

54) Hakkim, Faruck L., et al. "Frankincense essential oil suppresses melanoma cancer through down regulation of Bcl-2/Bax cascade signaling and ameliorates

heptotoxicity via phase I and II drug metabolizing enzymes." Oncotarget 10.37 (2019): 3472.

55) Wang, Dan, et al. "Boswellic acid exerts potent anticancer effects in HCT-116 human colon cancer cells mediated via induction of apoptosis, cell cycle arrest, cell migration inhibition and inhibition of PI3K/AKT signalling pathway." J. BUON 23.2 (2018): 340-345.

56) Xu, Chun, et al. "CD8+ T cells mediate the anti-tumor activity of frankincense and myrrh in hepatocellular carcinoma." Journal of translational medicine 16.1 (2018): 132.

57) Park, Yong Seok, et al. "Acetyl-11-Keto-ß-Boswellic Acid (Akba) is Cytotoxic for Meningioma Cells and Inhibits Phosphorylation of the Extracellular-Signal Regulated Kinase 1 and 2." Eicosanoids and Other Bioactive Lipids in Cancer, Inflammation, and Radiation Injury, 5. Springer, Boston, MA, 2002. 387-393.

58) Sharma, S., et al. "Pharmacokinetic study of 11-keto β-Boswellic acid." Phytomedicine 11.2-3 (2004): 255-260.

59) Sterk, Vanessa, Berthold Büchele, and Thomas Simmet. "Effect of food intake on the bioavailability of boswellic acids from a herbal preparation in healthy volunteers." Planta medica 70.12 (2004): 1155-1160.

60) Rosa, Bárbara, et al. "Spontaneous bilateral patellar tendon rupture: case report and review of fluoroquinolone-induced tendinopathy." Clinical case reports 4.7 (2016): 678.

61) Cohen, Jay S. "Peripheral neuropathy associated with fluoroquinolones." Annals of Pharmacotherapy 35.12 (2001): 1540-1547.

inhibit anti-death/survival pathways, suggesting sugar-binding specificity might be one of the main reasons motivating the anti-tumor activity . (15)

Solomon's seal (Polygonatum odoratum and Polygonatum cyrtonema) has been studied and is effective in these cell types:

- Prostate cancer (CAFs = Cancer Associated Fibroblasts) (16)
- Breast cancer (17–18)
- Esophageal cancer (NF-kB pathway) (19)
- Melanoma (20–21)
- Lung cancer (22–24)
- Fibrosarcoma (25)

PCL Accumulates in the Mitochondria and Generates ROS—Downregulates Glutathione

In 2009, Dr. Bo Liu et al. studied PCL in a melanoma model, finding that

The treatment with PCL also abrogated the glutathione anti-oxidant system and induced mitochondria to generate massive ROS accumulation, which subsequently resulted in p38 and p53 activation. (21)

In 2016, Dr. Tao Liu et al. studied PCL in a lung cancer cell model finding "remarkable generation of reactive oxygen species (ROS)" as well as induction of apoptosis and autophagy.

Importantly, we found PCL may bind to the cell surface in a mannose-specific manner, and was then internalized and accumulated primarily onto the mitochondria. (22)

Abrogated GSH Anti-Oxidant System

In 2014, Dr. Chunyang Li et al. studied a non-small-cell lung cancer model using Polygonatum odoratum (POL), finding induction of apoptosis via inhibition of the Akt-NF-kB pathway, while triggering autophagy via suppressing Akt-mTOR pathway. In addition, there was massive accumulation of reactive oxygen species (ROS):

Herein, we demonstrated that nonenzymatic antioxidants GSH [Glutathione] and its partner GPX were decreased with culturing time, indicating that POL might abrogate the GSH anti-oxidant system and result in massive ROS accumulation in A549 cells. (24)

Other agents that downregulate the anti-oxidant system, rendering the cancer cells more sensitive to damaging effects of ROS are: auranofin (inhibits thioredoxin reductase system), celecoxib Cox-2 inhibitor, parthenolide (feverfew), PQQ (pyrroloquinoline-quinine), sulfasalazine (blocks Xct system for cysteine uptake), sulforaphane (downglrulates intracellular glutathione).

Conclusion

The plant lectin, Solomon's seal (PCL), has remarkable anti-cancer activities as a potent EGFR inhibitor. In addition, PCL is taken up and accumulates in mitochondria, depletes glutathione, and generates massive reactive oxygen species (ROS), which then induces both protective autophagy and mitochondrial apoptosis. Solomon 's seal is widely available as a plant extract nutritional supplement.

References for Chapter 18: Solomon's Seal

1) Poiroux, Guillaume, et al. "Plant lectins targeting O-glycans at the cell surface as tools for cancer diagnosis, prognosis and therapy." International journal of molecular sciences 18.6 (2017): 1232.

2) Hashim, Onn Haji, Jaime Jacqueline Jayapalan, and Cheng-Siang Lee. "Lectins: an effective tool for screening of potential cancer biomarkers." PeerJ 5 (2017): e3784.

3) Marvibaigi M, Supriyanto E, Amini N, Abdul Majid FA, Jaganathan SK. Preclinical and clinical effects of mistletoe against breast cancer. Biomed Research International, 2014, 785479 (2014).

4) Yau, Tammy, et al. "Lectins with potential for anti-cancer therapy." Molecules 20.3 (2015): 3791-3810.

5) Zhang, Hong, et al. "Lectin PCL inhibits the Warburg effect of PC3 cells by combining with EGFR and inhibiting HK2." Oncology reports 37.3 (2017): 1765-1771.

6) Sankara Narayanan, Nitin. Role of Epidermal Growth Factor Receptor in Tumor Cell Metabolism. Diss. University of Cincinnati, 2014.

7) Freudlsperger, Christian, et al. "EGFR–PI3K–AKT–mTOR signaling in head and neck squamous cell carcinomas: attractive targets for molecular-oriented therapy." Expert opinion on therapeutic targets 15.1 (2011): 63-74.

8) Bhat, Firdous Ahmad, et al. "Quercetin reverses EGF-induced epithelial to mesenchymal transition and invasiveness in prostate cancer (PC-3) cell line via EGFR/PI3K/Akt pathway." The Journal of Nutritional Biochemistry 25.11 (2014): 1132-1139.

9) Karar, Jayashree, and Amit Maity. "PI3K/AKT/mTOR pathway in angiogenesis." Frontiers in molecular neuroscience 4 (2011): 51.

10) Xu, Qilin, et al. "EGF induces epithelial-mesenchymal transition and cancer stem-like cell properties in human oral cancer cells via promoting Warburg effect." Oncotarget 8.6 (2017): 9557.

11) Jung, Kyung-Ho, et al. "EGF receptor stimulation shifts breast cancer cell glucose metabolism toward glycolytic flux through PI3 kinase signaling." PloS one 14.9 (2019).

12) Lim, Seung-Oe, et al. "EGFR signaling enhances aerobic glycolysis in triple-negative breast cancer cells to promote tumor growth and immune escape." Cancer research 76.5 (2016): 1284-1296.

13) Dykes, Samantha S., Joshua J. Steffan, and James A. Cardelli. "Lysosome trafficking is necessary for EGF-driven invasion and is regulated by p38 MAPK and Na+/H+ exchangers." BMC cancer 17.1 (2017): 672.

14) Sigismund, Sara, Daniele Avanzato, and Letizia Lanzetti. "Emerging functions of the EGFR in cancer." Molecular oncology 12.1 (2018): 3-20.

15) Shi, Zheng, et al. "A novel molecular model of plant lectin-induced programmed cell death in cancer." Biological and Pharmaceutical Bulletin (2017): b17-00363.

16) Han, Shu-Yu, et al. "Polysaccharide from Polygonatum Inhibits the Proliferation of Prostate Cancer-Associated Fibroblasts Cells." Asian Pacific Journal of Cancer Prevention 17.8 (2016): 3829-3833.

17) Tai, Yu, et al. "Effect of Polygonatum odoratum extract on human breast cancer MDA-MB-231 cell proliferation and apoptosis." Experimental and therapeutic medicine 12.4 (2016): 2681-2687.

18) Ouyang, Liang, et al. "Polygonatum odoratum lectin induces apoptosis and autophagy via targeting EGFR-mediated Ras-Raf-MEK-ERK pathway in human MCF-7 breast cancer cells." Phytomedicine 21.12 (2014): 1658-1665.

19) Zhou, Weizheng, et al. "Effects of Polygonatum sibiricum Polysaccharides (PSP) on Human Esophageal Squamous Cell Carcinoma (ESCC) via NF-κB Signaling Pathway." International Journal of Polymer Science 2019 (2019).

20) Luan, Wenkang, et al. "Polygonatum odoratum lectin promotes BECN1 expression and induces autophagy in malignant melanoma by regulation of miR1290." OncoTargets and therapy 10 (2017): 4569.

21) Liu, Bo, et al. "Molecular mechanisms of Polygonatum cyrtonema lectin-induced apoptosis and autophagy in cancer cells." Autophagy 5.2 (2009): 253-255.

22) Liu, Tao, et al. "Role of reactive oxygen species-mediated MAPK and NF-κB activation in polygonatum cyrtonema lectin-induced apoptosis and autophagy in

human lung adenocarcinoma A549 cells." The Journal of Biochemistry 160.6 (2016): 315-324.

23) Wu, Lei, et al. "Polygonatum odoratum lectin induces apoptosis and autophagy by regulation of microRNA-1290 and microRNA-15a-3p in human lung adenocarcinoma A549 cells." International journal of biological macromolecules 85 (2016): 217-226.

24) Li, Chunyang, et al. "Molecular switch role of Akt in Polygonatum odoratum lectin-induced apoptosis and autophagy in human non-small cell lung cancer A549 cells." PloS one 9.7 (2014).

25) Liu, Bo, et al. "Induction of apoptosis by Polygonatum odoratum lectin and its molecular mechanisms in murine fibrosarcoma L929 cells." Biochimica et Biophysica Acta (BBA)-General Subjects 1790.8 (2009): 840-844.

Chapter 19

Cannabidiol and Cannabis Oil

THE CANNABIS PLANT HAS BEEN cultivated for over 6,000 years and has a long history of medicinal use going back to ancient times. However, various misguided government initiatives, such as the 1937 Marijuana Tax Act and the 1970 Controlled Substances Act, banned medical cannabis from doctor's offices and pharmacies, declaring the cannabis plant as having no medicinal value and stigmatizing cannabis as a "Schedule I Drug." Thus, the drug industry effectively manipulated the media and Congress to eliminate any financial competition posed by medical cannabis, a widely available natural remedy. (1–3)

In 1964, while cannabis medical research languished in the United States , Rafael Mechoulaham's group in Israel isolated tetra-hydro-cannabinol (THC), the psychoactive component in cannabis and later, in 1992, discovered the endocannabinoid receptor system and its main neurotransmitter, anandamide (*ananda* means "bliss" in Sanskrit). (4–7)

As of this date, thirty-three states have legalized medicinal cannabis, and 11 states have legalized recreational use. However, at the federal level, cannabis remains illegal, effectively banned as a "Schedule I drug."

Home Use of Medical Cannabis

With widespread use of medical cannabis in the 33 states where it is legal, anecdotal stories of success with cancer patients is commonplace. Some of these case reports have made their way into the medical literature

Highly Aggressive Acute Blastic Leukemia in a 14-Year-Old Girl

In March 2006, a 14-year-old girl suffering from weakness and spontaneous bleeding was diagnosed with acute lymphoblastic leukemia (ALL), with more than 300,000 blast cells present on her peripheral blood smear. Her form of leukemia was highly aggressive, with a positive Philadelphia chromosome. The patient was treated at the Hospital for Sick Children in Toronto, Canada, with bone marrow transplant, aggressive chemotherapy, and radiation therapy.

Acute Lymphoblastic Leukemia Remission with Cannabis Oil

After 34 months, blast cells were again found in the blood, and further treatment was deemed futile. The doctors suspended all treatment and essentially gave up. Her doctors noted the following in the chart:

> The patient suffers from terminal malignant disease…. She has been treated to the limits of available therapy … no further active intervention will be undertaken. (8)

The patient was offered palliative treatment and was sent home to die. While at home, the leukemia blast cell counts continued to increase and frequent blood and platelet transfusions were required.

The family conducted their own research and found Dr. Manuel Guzmán's 2003 article on cannabis as an anti-cancer agent. (9) Cannabis preparations are regarded as relatively safe, without any of the toxic effects of chemotherapy. (10–11)

Finding Rick Simpson and Phoenix Tears

The family then found an organization known as Phoenix Tears, and Rick Simpson, from whom they learned how to prepare their own cannabis oil extract given orally to their daughter. With the introduction of this new cannabis oil treatment, the doctors observed a rapid dose-dependent reduction in leukemic blast cell count. This case is important because it shows the potent anti-cancer effect of cannabis oil in acute leukemia. Dr. Yadvinder Singh and Chamandeep Bali write:

> The results shown here cannot be attributed to the phenomenon of 'spontaneous remission' because a dose response curve was achieved. (8)

Although the treatment was deemed a success, the patient ultimately succumbed to the toxic effects of chemotherapy which had suppressed her immune system, leaving her susceptible to infection. Sadly, the patient died of colon perforation and peritonitis on day 76. This case report by Drs. Singh and Bali appeared in the November 2013 *Journal of Case Reports in Oncology*. (8)

Medical Research on Medicinal Cannabis and Leukemia

There has been abundant research on the effects of medicinal cannabis on leukemic cells. In vitro and in vivo animal and human studies show medicinal cannabis is exceptionally efficacious in killing leukemic cells through signaling pathways that induce cell death (apoptosis). (12–14)

Among the 400 or so various chemical compounds in the cannabis plant, 60 of them are "cannabinoids." THC is the psychoactive component. Cannabidiol (CBD) is considered to be the major medicinal non-psychoactive cannabinoid. In other words, CBD has medicinal value without making you "high" (intoxicated). (15)

CBD Directly Targets VDAC -Induces Apoptosis

In 2013, Dr. N. Rimmerman et al. studied the effects of CBD (cannabidiol) on brain cells (BV-2 microglial cells), finding that CBD binds directly to the voltage-dependent anion channel (VDAC) on the outer mitochondrial membrane. Remember, earlier we discussed Drs. Pederson and Ko proposing to target the VDAC-HK2 as the Achilles heel of the cancer cell. In 2013, Dr. Rimmerman's group found a direct interaction between CBD and the VDAC, suggesting this could account for its anti-cancer and immunomodulatory effects:

> Using microscale thermophoresis, we showed a direct interaction between purified fluorescently labeled VDAC1 and CBD. Thus, VDAC1 seems to serve as a novel mitochondrial target for CBD. The inhibi-

tion of VDAC1 by CBD may be responsible for the immunosuppressive and anti-cancer effects of CBD. (16)

Six years later, in 2019, Dr. Miguel Olivas-Aguirre et al. went further in elucidating the molecular mechanism of cancer cell death caused by CBD in a T Cell lymphoblastic leukemia cell line. Dr. Olivas-Aguirre's group found that the cancer-cell-killing effect of CBD is independent of cannabinoid receptors. Instead, CBD binds directly with the VDAC on the outer mitochondrial membrane, causing increased influx of calcium into the mitochondria which induces release of cytochrome C into the cytosol, which then triggers the caspase cascade and mitochondrial-mediated apoptosis.

> Here we have shown that cell lines derived from acute lymphoblastic leukemia of T lineage [T-ALL], **but not resting healthy T cells,** are highly sensitive to CBD treatment. CBD effect does not depend on cannabinoid receptors…. Instead, CBD directly targets mitochondria and alters their capacity to handle Ca2+ [Calcium]. At lethal concentrations, CBD causes mitochondrial Ca2+ overload, stable mitochondrial transition pore formation and cell death. Our results suggest that CBD is an attractive candidate to be included into chemotherapeutic protocols for T-ALL treatment. (17)

Note: Aspirin is another agent that modulates the VDAC to induce apoptosis in the cancer cell. (18) See the Quick Reference Guide for a list of agents mentioned in this book which target the VDAC and detach HK2, resulting in inhibition of GLYCOLYSIS.

Lung Cancer Remission with CBD Oil

Another case report in 2019 by Dr. Josep Sulé-Suso et al. is an 81-year-old ex-smoker who presented in October 2016 with a 2.5 cm mass in the lung's left-lower lobe. A CAT scan showed metastatic disease involving paratracheal nodes. Endobronchial biopsy of the nodes revealed adenocarcinoma of the lung. The patient declined chemotherapy and radiation, citing his age and desire to maintain quality of life. On his own, the patient began taking CBD oil, two drops daily for a week, then increasing to nine drops daily for a month. A repeat CAT scan at the end of the month November 2017 showed almost complete resolution of the lung mass. The mediastinal nodes were also smaller.

> On further questioning, the patient stated that he had started taking CBD ["MyCBD"] oil 2% [200 mg CBD in 10 mL] from the beginning of September 2017. He took two drops [0.06 mL, 1.32 mg CBD] twice daily for a week and then nine drops [0.3 mL, 6 mg CBD] twice daily until the end of September. Following the November 2017 CT scan, the patient started taking nine drops twice daily. There were no other changes in the patient's diet, medication or lifestyle from September 2017. (19)

Cannabinoids have been studied in these cancer cell lines:

- Gastric cancer (20–21)
- Leukemia (22)
- Mantle cell lymphoma (23)
- Prostate cancer (24)
- Breast cancer (25–33)
- Endometrial cancer (34)

- Non-small-cell lung cancer (35)
- Pancreatic cancer (36)
- Colorectal cancer (37–38)
- Melanoma (39)

Cannabis for Relieving Adverse Effects of Chemotherapy

About twenty years ago, a friend confided in me that she had undergone mastectomy for breast cancer a few years back. She went on to relate her story. During chemotherapy treatments, her nurse quietly entered her room and whispered in her ear the suggestion she should take cannabis, i.e., "smoke pot," to relieve the nausea and loss of appetite, both of which are adverse effects of chemotherapy. Since then, conventional oncology has become more receptive to the idea that cannabis is beneficial for the chemotherapy patient and useful for nausea, appetite, and cancer-related cachexia. (40–44)

Cannabis for Cancer: Where Are We Now?

Recent medical literature is sympathetic to the use of CBD (cannabidiol) by the cancer patient on their own, yet CBD, like all other botanical medicines will probably never find a place in the doctor's oncology bag. The promise of CBD and cannabis medicine has not yet been translated from the "bench to the bedside," and in my opinion, probably never will. (45–55)

In *JAMA Oncology* (2020), Dr. Abrams writes that although there is plenty of favorable preclinical data, there is a paucity of clinical data on humans. In the U.S., cannabis research is hampered by the misguided government classification of cannabis as a Schedule I drug:

> Despite compelling preclinical evidence, data supporting cannabis-based interventions as effective human anti-cancer therapies have yet to accumulate with more investigation certainly warranted, although the schedule I designation of cannabis essentially thwarts therapeutic research worldwide. (56)

Cannabis (CBD/THC) Adverse Effects

Inhibition of Cytochrome P450

In 2020, Drs. Donald Abrams and Manuel Guzmán wrote that CBD is a potent inhibitor of the cytochrome P450 enzyme system:

> CBD is a potent inhibitor of particular cytochrome P450 isoforms, so patients using highly concentrated CBD preparations may risk boosting plasma levels of prescribed pharmaceuticals, thus potentially resulting in increased toxicities. (56)

Anti-Inflammatory Effects and Immune Suppression of Cannabidiol

In 2019, Drs. James Nichols and Barbara Kaplan reviewed the anti-inflammatory properties of cannabidiol (CBD Oil), finding suppression of NF-kB and inhibition of circulating IL-6 inflammatory cytokine. Other immune system effects include induction of apoptosis in lymphocytes and induction of functional T-Reg immune cells. (58–60)

Due to its immune suppressive activities, cannabidiol (CBD) has been suggested as treatment for graft vs. host disease in allogeneic hematopoietic stem cell transplant recipients. (61)

There may be adverse effects on the male reproductive system. (62–63)

Medicinal Cannabis May be Illegal in Your State

As of this writing, 33 states have approved medicinal cannabis, and 11 states have approved recreational use. However, some states still have laws on the books making possession of cannabis a criminal act. At the federal level, the DEA continues to classify cannabis as a Schedule I drug of no medicinal value, and possession and use of cannabis remains a federal crime. *The Boston Globe* reports the DEA has been harassing doctors involved with medical marijuana dispensaries by threatening revocation of their Controlled Substance Prescribing DEA license.

For more on this topic see my 2015 book, with co-authors Elaine A. Moore, and Justin Kander, *Cannabis Extracts in Medicine. The Promise of Benefits in Seizure Disorders, Cancer and Other Conditions* (McFarland, 2015). (64)

Conclusion

Medical cannabis oils and extracts are now widely available, and personal stories of dramatic cancer remissions are circulating on message groups. A few of these, as noted above, are published in the medical literature. In my opinion, a good quality non-psychoactive CBD oil is a good addition to most anti-cancer integrative oncology programs.

References Chapter 19: Cannabidiol and Cannabis Oil

1) Hodroff, Matthew B. "The Controlled Substances Act: Time to Reevaluate Marijuana." Whittier L. Rev. 36 (2014): 117.

2) Ransom, Jesse. """ Anslingerian" Politics: The History of Anti-Marijuana Sentiment in Federal law and How Harry Anslinger's Anti-Marijuana Politics Continue to Prevent the FDA and other Medical Experts from Studying Marijuana's Medical Utility." (1999).

3) McGettigan, Timothy. "The Politics of Marijuana: Truth Regimes and Institutional Ignorance." Available at SSRN 3527126 (2020).

4) Devane, William A., et al. "Isolation and structure of a brain constituent that binds to the cannabinoid receptor." Science 258.5090 (1992): 1946-1949.

5) Mechoulam, Raphael. "Look Back in Ananda—40 Years of Research on Cannabinoids." Endocannabinoids (2005): Chapter 1. in: Onaivi, Emmanuel S., Takayuki Sugiura, and Vincenzo Di Marzo, eds. Endocannabinoids: the brain and body's marijuana and beyond. CRC Press, 2005.

6) Mechoulam, Raphael. Cannabinoids as therapeutic agents. Chapman and Hall/CRC, 2019.

7) Russo, Ethan B. "History of cannabis and its preparations in saga, science, and sobriquet." Chemistry & biodiversity 4.8 (2007): 1614-1648.

8) Singh, Yadvinder, and Chamandeep Bali. "Cannabis extract treatment for terminal acute lymphoblastic leukemia with a Philadelphia chromosome mutation." Case reports in oncology 6.3 (2013): 585-592.

9) Guzmán, Manuel. "Cannabinoids: potential anticancer agents." Nature reviews cancer 3.10 (2003): 745-755.

10) Laezza, Chiara, et al. "The endocannabinoid system: A target for cancer treatment." International Journal of Molecular Sciences 21.3 (2020): 747.

11) Häuser, W., F. Petzke, and M. A. Fitzcharles. "Efficacy, tolerability and safety of cannabis-based medicines for chronic pain management—An overview of systematic reviews." European Journal of Pain 22.3 (2018): 455-470.

12) Wright, Stephen, et al. "Combination of cannabinoids in the treatment of leukaemia." U.S. Patent Application No. 16/488,821.

13) Powles, Thomas, et al. "Cannabis-induced cytotoxicity in leukemic cell lines: the role of the cannabinoid receptors and the MAPK pathway." Blood 105.3 (2005): 1214-1221.

14) Liu, Wai M., et al. "Enhancing the in vitro cytotoxic activity of Δ9-tetrahydrocannabinol in leukemic cells through a combinatorial approach." Leukemia & lymphoma 49.9 (2008): 1800-1809.

15) Atakan, Zerrin. "Cannabis, a complex plant: different compounds and different effects on individuals." Therapeutic advances in psychopharmacology 2.6 (2012): 241-254.

16) Rimmerman, N., et al. "Direct modulation of the outer mitochondrial membrane channel, voltage-dependent anion channel 1 (VDAC1) by cannabidiol: a novel mechanism for cannabinoid-induced cell death." Cell death & disease 4.12 (2013): e949-e949.

17) Olivas-Aguirre, Miguel, et al. "Cannabidiol directly targets mitochondria and disturbs calcium homeostasis in acute lymphoblastic leukemia." Cell death & disease 10.10 (2019): 1-19.

18) Tewari, Debanjan, et al. "Aspirin induces cell death by directly modulating mitochondrial voltage-dependent anion channel (VDAC)." Scientific reports 7.1 (2017): 1-9.

19) Sulé-Suso, Josep, et al. "Striking lung cancer response to self-administration of cannabidiol: A case report and literature review." SAGE open medical case reports 7 (2019): 2050313X19832160.

20) Jeong, Soyeon, et al. "Cannabidiol promotes apoptosis via regulation of XIAP/Smac in gastric cancer." Cell death & disease 10.11 (2019): 1-13.

21) Jeong, Soyeon, et al. "Cannabidiol promotes apoptosis via regulation of XIAP/Smac in gastric cancer." Cell death & disease 10.11 (2019): 1-13.

22) Kampa-Schittenhelm, Kerstin Maria, et al. "Dronabinol has preferential antileukemic activity in acute lymphoblastic and myeloid leukemia with lymphoid differentiation patterns." BMC cancer 16.1 (2016): 25.

23) Flygare, Jenny, et al. "Cannabinoid receptor ligands mediate growth inhibition and cell death in mantle cell lymphoma." FEBS letters 579.30 (2005): 6885-6889.

24) Ruiz, Lidia, Alberto Miguel, and Inés Díaz-Laviada. "Δ9-Tetrahydrocannabinol induces apoptosis in human prostate PC-3 cells via a receptor-independent mechanism." FEBS letters 458.3 (1999): 400-404.

25) Sultan, Ahmed S., Mona A. Marie, and Salah A. Sheweita. "Novel mechanism of cannabidiol-induced apoptosis in breast cancer cell lines." The Breast 41 (2018): 34-41.

26) McAllister, Sean D., et al. "Cannabidiol as a novel inhibitor of Id-1 gene expression in aggressive breast cancer cells." Molecular cancer therapeutics 6.11 (2007): 2921-2927.

27) McAllister, Sean D., et al. "Pathways mediating the effects of cannabidiol on the reduction of breast cancer cell proliferation, invasion, and metastasis." Breast cancer research and treatment 129.1 (2011): 37-47.

28) Shrivastava, Ashutosh, et al. "Cannabidiol induces programmed cell death in breast cancer cells by coordinating the cross-talk between apoptosis and autophagy." Molecular cancer therapeutics 10.7 (2011): 1161-1172.

29) Elbaz, Mohamad, et al. "Modulation of the tumor microenvironment and inhibition of EGF/EGFR pathway: Novel anti-tumor mechanisms of Cannabidiol in breast cancer." Molecular oncology 9.4 (2015): 906-919.

30) Sultan, Ahmed S., Mona A. Marie, and Salah A. Sheweita. "Novel mechanism of cannabidiol-induced apoptosis in breast cancer cell lines." The Breast 41 (2018): 34-41.

31) Caffarel, María M., et al. "Δ9-tetrahydrocannabinol inhibits cell cycle progression in human breast cancer cells through Cdc2 regulation." Cancer research 66.13 (2006): 6615-6621.

32) McKallip, Robert J., Mitzi Nagarkatti, and Prakash S. Nagarkatti. "Δ-9-tetrahydrocannabinol enhances breast cancer growth and metastasis by suppression of the antitumor immune response." The Journal of Immunology 174.6 (2005): 3281-3289.

33) Kisková, Terézia, et al. "Future Aspects for cannabinoids in breast cancer therapy." International journal of molecular sciences 20.7 (2019): 1673.

34) Zhang, Yingzhi, et al. "Δ9-tetrahydrocannabinol inhibits epithelial-mesenchymal transition and metastasis by targeting matrix metalloproteinase-9 in endometrial cancer." Oncology letters 15.6 (2018): 8527-8535.

35) Milian, Lara, et al. "Cannabinoid receptor expression in non-small cell lung cancer. Effectiveness of tetrahydrocannabinol and cannabidiol inhibiting cell proliferation and epithelial-mesenchymal transition in vitro." PloS one 15.2 (2020): e0228909.

36) Sharafi, Golnaz, Hong He, and Mehrdad Nikfarjam. "Potential use of cannabinoids for the treatment of pancreatic cancer." Journal of pancreatic cancer 5.1 (2019): 1-7.

37) Jeong, Soyeon, et al. "Cannabidiol-induced apoptosis is mediated by activation of Noxa in human colorectal cancer cells." Cancer letters 447 (2019): 12-23.

38) Yun, Hye Kyeong, et al. "Cannabidiol-induced apoptosis is mediated by activation of Noxa in human colorectal cancer cells." (2019): 714-714.

39) Simmerman, Erika, et al. "Cannabinoids as a potential new and novel treatment for melanoma: a pilot study in a murine model." Journal of Surgical Research 235 (2019): 210-215.

40) Davis, Mellar P. "Cannabinoids for symptom management and cancer therapy: the evidence." Journal of the National Comprehensive Cancer Network 14.7 (2016): 915-922.

41) Fisher, Emma, et al. "Cannabinoids, cannabis, and cannabis-based medicine for pain management: a protocol for an overview of systematic reviews and a systematic review of randomised controlled trials." Pain reports 4.3 (2019).

42) Blake, Alexia, et al. "A selective review of medical cannabis in cancer pain management." Annals of palliative medicine 6.suppl 2 (2017): s215-s222.

43) Sallan, Stephen E., Norman E. Zinberg, and Emil Frei III. "Antiemetic effect of delta-9-tetrahydrocannabinol in patients receiving cancer chemotherapy." New England Journal of Medicine 293.16 (1975): 795-797.

44) Strasser, Florian, et al. "Comparison of orally administered cannabis extract and delta-9-tetrahydrocannabinol in treating patients with cancer-related anorexia-cachexia syndrome: a multicenter, phase III, randomized, double-blind, placebo-controlled clinical trial from the Cannabis-In-Cachexia-Study-Group." Journal of Clinical Oncology 24.21 (2006): 3394-3400.

45) McAllister, Sean D., Liliana Soroceanu, and Pierre-Yves Desprez. "The antitumor activity of plant-derived non-psychoactive cannabinoids." Journal of neuroimmune pharmacology 10.2 (2015): 255-267.

46) Fowler, Christopher J. "Delta9-tetrahydrocannabinol and cannabidiol as potential curative agents for cancer: A critical examination of the preclinical literature." Clinical Pharmacology & Therapeutics 97.6 (2015): 587-596.

47) Vale, José Sousa. "Cannabis Use in Medical Oncology: A Brief Review." Revista Portuguesa de Farmacoterapia 11.2-3 (2019): 31-38.

48) Kalenderoglou, Nikoletta, Tara Macpherson, and Karen L. Wright. "Cannabidiol Reduces Leukemic Cell Size—But Is It Important?" Frontiers in pharmacology 8 (2017): 144.

49) Moreno, Estefanía, et al. "The endocannabinoid system as a target in cancer diseases: are we there yet?." Frontiers in Pharmacology 10 (2019): 339.

50) Laezza, Chiara, et al. "The Endocannabinoid System: A Target for Cancer Treatment." International Journal of Molecular Sciences 21.3 (2020): 747.

51) Ladin, Daniel A., et al. "Preclinical and clinical assessment of cannabinoids as anti-cancer agents." Frontiers in pharmacology 7 (2016): 361.

52) Almogi-Hazan, Osnat, et al. "The Highs and Lows of Cannabis in Cancer Treatment and Bone Marrow Transplantation." Rambam Maimonides Medical Journal 11.1 (2020).

53) Schwarz, Rico, Robert Ramer, and Burkhard Hinz. "Targeting the endocannabinoid system as a potential anticancer approach." Drug metabolism reviews 50.1 (2018): 26-53.

54) Pellati, Federica, et al. "Cannabis sativa L. and non-psychoactive cannabinoids: their chemistry and role against oxidative stress, inflammation, and cancer." BioMed research international 2018 (2018).

55) Ramer, Robert, and Burkhard Hinz. "Cannabinoids as anticancer drugs." Advances in Pharmacology. Vol. 80. Academic Press, 2017. 397-436.

56) Abrams, Donald I., and Manuel Guzmán. "Can Cannabis Cure Cancer?." JAMA oncology (2020).

57) Nichols, James M., and Barbara LF Kaplan. "Immune Responses Regulated by Cannabidiol." Cannabis and Cannabinoid Research (2019).

58) Rieder, Sadiye Amcaoglu, et al. "Cannabinoid-induced apoptosis in immune cells as a pathway to immunosuppression." Immunobiology 215.8 (2010): 598-605.

59) Wu, Hsin-Ying, et al. "Cannabidiol-induced apoptosis in primary lymphocytes is associated with oxidative stress-dependent activation of caspase-8." Toxicology and applied pharmacology 226.3 (2008): 260-270.

60) Dhital, Saphala, et al. "Cannabidiol (CBD) induces functional Tregs in response to low-level T cell activation." Cellular immunology 312 (2017): 25-34.

61) Yeshurun, Moshe, et al. "Cannabidiol for the prevention of graft-versus-host-disease after allogeneic hematopoietic cell transplantation: results of a phase II study." Biology of Blood and Marrow Transplantation 21.10 (2015): 1770-1775.

62) Machado Bergamaschi, Mateus, et al. "Safety and side effects of cannabidiol, a Cannabis sativa constituent." Current drug safety 6.4 (2011): 237-249.

63) Carvalho, R. K., M. L. Andersen, and R. Mazaro-Costa. "The effects of cannabidiol on male reproductive system: A literature review." Journal of applied toxicology: JAT (2019).

64) Dach, Jeffrey, Elaine A. Moore, and Justin Kander. Cannabis Extracts in Medicine: The Promise of Benefits in Seizure Disorders, Cancer and Other Conditions. McFarland, 2015.

65) Barrie, Allison M., Ariane C. Gushue, and Ramez N. Eskander. "Dramatic response to Laetrile and cannabidiol (CBD) oil in a patient with metastatic low grade serous ovarian carcinoma." Gynecologic oncology reports 29 (2019): 10.

66) Dall'Stella, Paula B., et al. "Case report: Clinical outcome and image response of two patients with secondary high-grade glioma treated with chemoradiation, PCV, and cannabidiol." Frontiers in oncology 8 (2019): 643.

67) Likar, Rudolf, et al. "Concomitant Treatment of Malignant Brain Tumours With CBD–A Case Series and Review of the Literature." Anticancer Research 39.10 (2019): 5797-5801.

68) Kenyon, Julian, W. A. I. Liu, and Angus Dalgleish. "Report of objective clinical responses of cancer patients to pharmaceutical-grade synthetic cannabidiol." Anticancer research 38.10 (2018): 5831-5835.

69) Kis, Brigitta, et al. "Cannabidiol—from Plant to Human Body: A Promising Bioactive Molecule with Multi-Target Effects in Cancer." International journal of molecular sciences 20.23 (2019): 5905.

70) Dall'Stella, Paula B., et al. "Case report: Clinical outcome and image response of two patients with secondary high-grade glioma treated with chemoradiation, PCV, and cannabidiol." Frontiers in oncology 8 (2019): 643.

71) Likar, Rudolf, et al. "Concomitant Treatment of Malignant Brain Tumours With CBD–A Case Series and Review of the Literature." Anticancer Research 39.10 (2019): 5797-5801.

Chapter 20

Cancer as a Parasitic Disease

ON APRIL 16TH, 2016, I attended the 14th Annual International Integrative Oncology Conference in San Diego, California. At the meeting, Dr. Nooshin Darvish presented five case reports of glioblastoma multiforme treated over ten years at her Holistique Clinic in Bellevue, Washington. All five patients underwent surgical biopsy of the tumor mass, and all samples stained positive for the spirochete parasite, Borrelia, the organism found in Lyme disease. (1)

In all cases, the patient's tumor regressed upon treatment for parasitic disease and progressed when treatments were halted. The pathology reports for all cases showed positive for the Borrelia organism (Lyme disease) on FISH (Fluorescent In-Situ Hybridization). This information was new to me, so I wondered if Borrelia had been associated with any other types of cancer. A quick literature search answered the question. In *Blood* (2008), Dr. Claudia Schöllkopf reported that patients who tested positive for Borrelia antibodies had a four times greater risk of mantle cell lymphoma. (2)

Four years previously, in 2004, Borrelia organisms had been identified in two cases of nodal lymphoma. (3)

Cancer as a Parasitic Disease Is an Old Idea

Cancer as a form of parasitic disease is actually an old idea, originally proposed by early microbiologists. They considered the idea self-evident from their microscopic observations of cancer cells.

William Russell Pathologist, 1890

On December 3, 1890, the Scottish pathologist William Russell reported a "cancer microbe" seen under his microscope inside cancer cells. His report in the December 18, 1890, *British Medical Journal* included detailed drawings describing parasitic spores within cancer cells. Since that time, Dr. Russell's hypothesis that cancer is a parasitic disease has been picked up and championed by a long list of impressive scientists. However, all were labeled medical heretics and lived out their careers in obscurity. (4–5)

Cancer as a Placenta—Just Another Parasite?

One hundred years ago, the Scottish biologist John Beard noted that cancer cell behavior was similar to that of the trophoblast cells of the placenta. For more on this topic, see chapter 25, "Cancer as a Trophoblastic Disease."

In 2007, Dr. C. Ferretti et al. reported on the striking similarity of the proliferative, migratory, and invasive features of both cancer and trophoblast cells, which use similar molecular cell pathways with activation of the PI3K/AKT axis to achieve their goals.

Dr. Ferretti et al. write:

An overview of molecular circuitries shared by trophoblast and cancer cells reveals that the activation of the phosphatidylinositol 3'-kinase [PI3K]/AKT axis has recently emerged as a central feature of signaling pathways used by these cells to achieve their proliferative, migratory and invasive processes. (6)

The placenta invades the surrounding uterine tissues and hijacks blood vessels to form its own blood supply. Remember, one of the ten hallmarks of cancer is angiogenesis, the ability to develop new blood vessels. The developing embryo is an implanted organism that, loosely speaking, can be described as "parasite" by virtue of its reliance on the mother's blood supply for nutrition. Is cancer a "placental cell" gone haywire? A few of the speakers at the meeting raised this question. More recently, authors have described cancer as its own parasitic species. Whether cancer is a parasitic disease or something else is yet to be determined. In the meantime, the study of parasitic disease affords us an opportunity to better understand cancer biology. (7–10)

Parasitic Disease in Animals

Parasitic protozoans may invade and hijack cell pathways to enhance survival. In doing so, they may resemble cancer cells. One such example is a tick-borne parasite called

Theileria annulata, affecting South African cattle. Theileria is a protozoan parasite belonging to the Apicomplexa phylum. The invading parasite transforms the animal's lymphocytes into lymphoma cells demonstrating all the usual hallmarks of cancer. Because of the similarity with cancer, this model has been extensively studied, hoping for clues leading to an understanding of cancer biology. (11–17)

Spirochete Parasite Transmitted by Ticks—Resembles Lymphoma

Theileria is an intracellular parasite transmitted by ticks, bearing an uncanny resemblance to the Borrelia Lyme parasite in humans. One species, T. parva, is highly pathogenic for cattle and causes a fatal lymphoproliferative disease known as East Coast fever. Dr. Vishvanath Nene (2016) writes:

Infected cells acquire a metastatic, cancer-like phenotype and are the primary cause of pathology. (18)

Theileria are intracellular protozoan parasites transmitted by ticks. The parasite resides in the cell cytoplasm, where it inhibits host-cell apoptosis pathways to ensure self-survival. The parasites synchronize their replication with that of the host cell, so that daughter cells are also infected. The parasite speeds up cell replication, benefiting its own survival. Cancer cells share many of these same features, such as inhibition of apoptosis (immortalization) and increased speed of replication. The disease is reversible with antiparasitic drug treatment using buparvaquone. (19)

Activation of MAPK and TNF Alpha Pathways

In 2014, Dr. Min Ma and Martin Baumgartner studied Theileria annulata, finding that "host cell motility and invasiveness" was driven by activation of the MAPK pathway by the inflammatory cytokine TNF Alpha, which causes changes in the cytoskeleton of the host cell. This is very similar to many cancers. (20–21) Drs. Ma and Baumgartner write:

> We found that the parasite drives host cell motility and invasiveness through the induction and activation of the host cell protein MAP4K4 [MAPK]. We show that MAP4K4 induction is driven by the inflammatory cytokine TNFα and causes dynamic changes in the cytoskeleton of the host cell that facilitate cell motility. (20)

Cryptosporidium Mouse Model of Colon Cancer

Another animal model of parasitic disease inducing cancer is found in the laboratory of Dr. Sadia Benamrouz et al. (2014) who reported that mice inoculated with the Cryptosporidium parasite quite unexpectedly develop colon cancer. Dr. Benamrouz found histochemical evidence of upregulated Wnt signaling pathways, commonly upregulated in cancer cells. (22)

Since parasitic disease such as cryptosporidium and toxoplasmosis are prevalent in immunosuppressed cancer patients, many are routinely given antiparasitic chemo-prophylaxis by the oncologist. (23–26) In doing so, the oncologist is unwittingly treating the patient with a repurposed anti-cancer drug.

Lymphoma Associated with Coxiella Brunetti, Q Fever

About one fifth of human cancers are linked to infection with a viral or bacterial organism. For example, H. pylori infection is linked to MALT lymphoma. Epstein-Barr virus (EBV) is associated with Burkitt's lymphoma, hepatitis virus with hepatoma, and borrelia and chlamydia with lymphoma. The causative agent for Q fever, Coxiella burnetii, is a gram-negative bacteria which has been associated with Non-Hodgkin's Lymphoma (NHL). Forty cases of NHL associated with Q Fever have been reported in the medical literature. In 2018, Dr. Melenotte reported a patient infected with C. burnetii who shortly thereafter developed B-cell lymphoma. This patient was successfully treated with doxycycline, hydroxychloroquine, and rituximab, with remission of the lymphoma. (27–28)

In 2019, Dr. Cléa Melanotte et al. studied 61 patients with acute Q fever caused by C. burnetii persistent infection, analyzing whole blood samples for changes in gene transcription in peripheral blood monocytes (PBMCs). Dr. Melanotte felt her results indicated that:

> C. burnetii infection triggers the expression of genes implicated in anti apoptotic and proliferative mechanisms.... C. burnetii replicates in a parasitophorous vacuole within human cells and must repress apoptosis of its host to optimally accomplish its life cycle. This is achieved by increasing the expression of the anti-apoptotic BCL2 protein family member Bcl-2-related protein A1 (BCL2A1) and by reducing the expression of the pro-apoptotic BCL2 protein family

members BAX and BAK. Our data strongly suggest that persistent infection with C. burnetii causes alterations in the transcription of genes involved in anti-apoptotic and proliferative process. (27–28)

Antiparasitic Drugs are Anti-Cancer Drugs and Vice Versa

The Nobel Prize in Medicine for 2015 was granted to three doctors for discovery of two antiparasitic drugs, the antimalarial drug artemisinin and the antiparasitic drug ivermectin. (29–33) Although these two drugs were developed and FDA-approved as antiparasitic drugs, both have been extensively studied for their potent anti-cancer effects as outlined in chapters 21 and 22.

Next, let's take a closer look at some of the other antiparasitic drugs repurposed as anti-cancer drugs. (34–36)

Pyrvinium Pamoate

Pyrvinium (Vanquin®) is an old FDA-approved drug for treatment of pinworm in the GI tract, a common parasitic infection in children. The drug is available in Scandinavia and Germany; however Pyrvinium is not available in the U.S. where it has been replaced by mebendazole and pyrantel.

Wnt Pathway Inhibitor--Cancer Stem Cell Agent

By virtue of inhibiting the Wnt pathway, pyrvinium qualifies as a cancer stem cell agent. In 2016, Dr. Thorne did a high-throughput screen for Wnt pathway Inhibition using a Xenopus laevis egg extract, finding pyrvinium a potent Wnt pathway inhibitor at extremely low con-

centrations (EC50 of 10 nanoMolar). Further studies revealed the MOA (mechanism of action) is activation of casein kinase 1-alpha, which degrades cytosolic Beta-Catenin, effectively inhibiting Wnt signaling. (37)

Note: Casein kinase 1 alpha (CK1-alpha) regulates the Wnt/Beta-Catenin and p53 pathways.

Dr. Liang Xu reported in the 2016 *International Journal of Oncology*:

The Wnt pathway inhibitor pyrvinium pamoate inhibits the self-renewal and metastasis of breast cancer stem cells. (38)

Pyrvinium has striking anti-cancer activity, active against blast cell leukemia, lymphoma and breast cancer. (39–42)

Pyrvinium Inhibits NADH-Fumarate Reductase

Not only does pyrvinium inhibit the Wnt pathway via activation of CK1-alpha, it also inhibits mitochondrial respiration in cancer cells. In 2012, Dr. Sakai reported that both parasites and cancer cells share the same energy production pathway, the NADH-fumarate reductase system. Pyrvinium targets this pathway in both parasites and cancer cell mitochondria, explaining the mechanism of pyrvinium anti-cancer activity. (43–44)

For more on this topic, see chapter 12.

Praziquantel

The anti-schistosomal drug, praziquantel (Biltricide) was studied in 2012 by Dr. Zhen Hua Wu et al. Although not effective by itself, praziquantel has synergy with paclitaxel, a commonly used chemotherapy drug. (45)

Niclosamide—Niclocide, Yomesan, Niclosan

Niclosamide (Niclocide) is FDA-approved for the treatment of tapeworm infections (cestodes). Niclosamide targets the Wnt/β-catenin pathway, serving as a potent anti-cancer drug. (46–48)

In 2011, Dr. Takuya Osada et al. reported in *Cancer Research* that orally administered niclosamide is well tolerated, with oral doses achieving therapeutic plasma levels associated with biologic activity, leading to tumor control:

> We found that niclosamide inhibited Wnt/β-catenin pathway activation, downregulated Dvl2, decreased downstream β-catenin signaling, and exerted antiproliferative effects in human colon cancer cell lines and CRC [Colorectal Cancer] cells isolated by surgical resection of metastatic disease, regardless of mutations in APC..... In mice implanted with human CRC xenografts, orally administered niclosamide was well tolerated, achieved plasma and tumor levels associated with biologic activity, and led to tumor control. Our findings support clinical explorations to reposition niclosamide for the treatment of CRC. (46)

In 2014, Dr. Rebecca C. Arend et al. found niclosamide, in combination with cisplatin chemotherapy, effective against ovarian cancer cells isolated from malignant ascites in 34 patients (47).

Niclosamide Wnt Pathway Inhibitor—Cancer Stem Cell Agent

In 2010, Dr. W. Chen et al. did a high-through-put screen of 1,200 drugs from the Prestwick Chemical Library identifying niclosamide as the best drug for Wnt pathway inhibition. (48)

In 2019, Dr. So-Yeon Park et al. found niclosamide effective against colorectal cancer cell lines in vitro and in vivo xenografts, and sensitized colon cancer to chemotherapy and radiotherapy, writing:

> We revealed that niclosamide exerts in vivo effects against both colon carcinogenesis and tumor growth by targeting the Wnt/LEF1/DCLK1-B axis-mediated CSC [Cancer Stem Cell] properties. Niclosamide inhibits certain CSC functions including survival, anti-apoptosis, and self-renewal, resulting in a reduction in CSC populations. Moreover, CSC-targeting niclosamide successfully sensitizes colorectal cancer to chemo-radiation. (49)

In 2015, Dr. Zhan Liao et al. found niclosamide effective against osteosarcoma cells, a form of bone cancer. (50)

In 2013, Dr. Anja Wieland et al. found niclosamide effective against glioblastoma cell lines, a deadly form of brain cancer. This explains the dramatic improvements in five patients with glioblastoma multiforme presented by Dr. Nooshin Darvish et al. when treated with antiparasitic drugs, as described above. (51) Niclosamide was patented in 2012 for treatment of metastatic cancer.

Niclosamide Targets Mitochondria

In a 2014 report in *Cancer Letters*, Dr. Yonghe Li wrote:

> Niclosamide not only inhibits the Wnt/β-catenin, mTORC1, STAT3, NF-κB and Notch signaling pathways, but **also targets mitochondria** in cancer cells to induce cell cycle arrest, growth inhibition and apoptosis. (52)

As we mention elsewhere in this book, in 2019, Dr. Roberto Costa described the mitochondrial/Wnt axis. This implies that all OXPHOS inhibiting agents such as niclosamide and pyrvinium are also Wnt pathway inhibitors and anti-cancer stem cell agents. (53)

Niclosamide Targets NF-κB, Wnt/β-catenin, and Notch Pathways

In a 2012 report, Dr. Jing-Xuan Pan et al. say that niclosamide is a potential anti-cancer stem cell agent by virtue of targeting a number of stem cell pathways, making this drug very promising for eradication of cancer stem cells:

> Because niclosamide targets multiple signaling pathways (e.g., NF-κB, Wnt/β-catenin, and Notch), most of which are closely involved with cancer stem cells, **it holds promise in eradicating cancer stem cells.** (54)

Pork Tapeworm Cysticercosis

Pork Tapeworm, also called cysticercosis, is endemic in developing countries, with over 15% of household workers testing positive for antibodies to the parasite. Seizure disorder and characteristic cerebral calcifications on Brain CAT Scans are typical findings in neurocysticercosis.

Tapeworm in Household Workers

Of 26 housemaids in Lima, Peru, who tested positive for cysticercosis antibodies, half (50 per cent) had characteristic brain calcifications compatible with cysticercosis. (55)

Orthodox Jews living in the United States avoid eating pork for religious reasons; nonetheless tapeworm (cysticercosis) seropositivity was found in 1.3%, indicating cysticercosis has been transmitted to them from their household workers. (56)

Niclosamide Treats Tapeworm

Niclosamide for treatment of tapeworm is listed as an essential medicine by the World Health Organization (WHO). Recommended adult dosage is 2 grams of the drug.

The tablets should be chewed thoroughly before swallowing and washed down with a little water. Adults: 2 g as a single dose. (World Health Organization)

For dwarf tapeworm, dosage is 2 grams daily for seven days and may be repeated a week later. (57)

Nitazoxanide (NTZ)—Alinia—c-Myc Inhibitor

C-Myc Oncogene activation is a "hallmark of cancer initiation and maintenance," a master regulator controlling cell growth, proliferation, and cancer cell metabolism. Although c-Myc is considered "*undruggable*," there is considerable interest in developing a c-Myc inhibitor as a valid anti-cancer strategy. (58–61)

Dr. Lavinia Carabet et al. (2019) write that 40 years of research searching for such a Myc inhibitor has been unsuccessful because of unwanted side effects:

> Myc [avian myelocytomatosis viral oncogene homolog] represents one of the most sought after drug targets in cancer. Myc transcription factor is an essential regulator of cell growth, but in most cancers it is overexpressed and associated with treatment-resistance and lethal outcomes. Over 40 years of research and drug development efforts did not yield a clinically useful Myc inhibitor … A major concern is that Myc

inactivation by any drug may have undesirable side effects on normal cells. (59)

Finding a c-Myc Inhibitor

In 2013, Dr. Fan-Minogue utilized the oncogene c-Myc sensor to establish a cell assay and optimized it to a high-throughput-screening (HTS) format. The authors screened about 5,000 existing bioactive compounds for potential activity as c-Myc inhibitors. Anti-cancer effects of NTZ was validated in various cancer cell lines in vitro and in vivo mouse xenograft models as well. Dr. Hua Fan-Minogue et al. says:

> Among the most potent hits was nitazoxanide (NTZ), a human anti-protozoal drug. (62)

Nitazoxanide is available as Alinia tablets, which have favorable pharmacokinetics with therapeutic serum levels and are considered safe.

Nitazoxanide Inhibits Wnt Pathway and PDI—Protein Folding

Nitazoxanide is an excellent Wnt pathway and IL-6 cytokine inhibitor. (63–64) Wnt inhibition denotes that the drug targets cancer stem cells.

Nitazoxanide also suppresses protein disulfide isomerase (PDI), which is overexpressed in ovarian tumors and other cancers. PDI is a cellular enzyme in the endoplasmic reticulum (ER) involved in protein folding, and a promising target for cancer therapy. (65–70)

Nitazoxanide is OXPHOS Inhibitor— Highest Drug Repositioning Potential

In his PhD dissertation (2017), Dr. Wojciech Senkowski writes that nitazoxanide has the highest drug repositioning potential because of high plasma concentrations and excellent efficacy as an OXPHOS inhibitor. High thru-put screening using tumor spheroids identified nitazoxanide as the best candidate to suppress tumor formation. Dr. Senkowski writes:

> Nitazoxanide reaches high plasma concentrations, persisting for up to a few hours after a single oral dose. Thus, we have chosen nitazoxanide as a molecule with the highest drug repositioning potential. We also identified nitazoxanide, an FDA-approved anthelmintic agent, to act as an OXPHOS inhibitor and to potentiate the effects of standard chemotherapy in vivo. (71)

In 2018, Dr. Anshul Shakya et al. provided an update on nitazoxanide as a multifunctional chemotherapeutic agent:

> NTZ [Nitazoxanide] expresses inhibitory effect on the tumour cell progression by modulating drug detoxification ...unfolded protein response, autophagy, anti-cytokines activities [inhibits IL-6] and c-Myc inhibition. (72)

Broad Spectrum Antiviral Drug

Nitazoxanide is also under study as broad spectrum antiviral agent effective against coronavirus and influenza virus. (73–76)

In 2014, a phase 3 human clinical study by Dr. Jason Haffizulla et al. found that the drug reduces duration of symptoms in patients with influenza, writing:

> Treatment with nitazoxanide 600 mg twice daily for 5 days was associated with a reduction of the duration of symptoms in participants with acute uncomplicated influenza. (76)

Mebendazole—The Antiparasitic Drug Vermox

Of the antiparasitic drugs repurposed for anti-cancer treatment, one of the most promising is mebendazole (Vermox). (77–86)

Although poorly absorbed from the GI tract, therapeutic serum levels are reached with routine antiparasitic dosage of 100 mg twice a day.

In a 2019 review of mebendazole, Dr. Andrea Guerini et al. state:

> Mebendazole meets many of the characteristics desirable for a repurposed drug: good and proven toxicity profile, **pharmacokinetics allowing to reach therapeutic concentrations at disease site**, ease of administration and low price. (87)

Mebendazole is a Microtubule Disruptor and Downregulates B CL-2

Mebendazole is a microtubule-disrupting agent that impairs mitotic spindle formation, preventing cell division and replication. This tubulin disruption also causes downregulation of BCL-2. In 2008, Dr. Nicole Doudican et al. screened 2,000 common drugs for anti-cancer activity against chemo-resistant malignant melanoma. The antiparasitic drug, mebendazole (Vermox), was deemed the most promising agent, finding mebendazole induces apoptosis via BCL-2 inactivation. The BCL-2 is an anti-apoptosis protein frequently upregulated in cancer, preventing apoptosis (programmed cell death) which "immortalizes" the cancer cell. By inactivating BCL-2, mebendazole restores the ability of the cancer cell to commit suicide. For example, a new FDA-approved drug, venetoclax, is a BCL-2 inhibitor used for leukemia and lymphoma. Dr. Doudican's group write:

> Mebendazole treatment induces apoptosis through the intrinsic and extrinsic pathways in melanoma cells but not in melanocytes ... After treatment with 0.5 μmol/L mebendazole for 14 h, we observed overall microtubular network disarray.... mebendazole selectively inhibits growth and induces apoptosis in melanoma cells at clinically achievable doses that are largely nontoxic to melanocytes... **the antineoplastic effects of mebendazole in human melanoma cells result from differential Bcl-2 – mediated cellular responses to mebendazole-induced tubulin disruption**. (88)

Replacement for Vincristine

Recent studies show that mebendazole is a promising agent for a number of cancers including medulloblastoma, a malignant brain tumor in children. Animal xenograft studies show improved survival in mebendazole-treated animals. Indeed, the authors suggested that vincristine, the currently used chemotherapy drug, should be replaced by mebendazole which has better penetration across the blood-brain barrier. (89–90)

Mebendazole More Potent than Chemotherapy

In 2017, Dr. Fugui Zhang et al. studied mebendazole's anti-cancer activity against head-and-neck squamous cell carcinoma cell lines (HNSCC). They found that mebendazole was more potent than the standard chemotherapy drug cisplatin:

> MBZ [Mebendazole] exerts more potent anti-proliferation activity than CIS [cis-

platin] in HNSCC [human head-and-neck squamous cell carcinoma cells].... MBZ effectively inhibits cell proliferation, cell cycle progression and cell migration, and induces apoptosis of HNSCC cells. (91)

Immune System Benefits of Mebendazole

In addition, mebendazole may have a beneficial effect on the immune system with enhanced activation of Killer T Cells responsible for killing tumor cells, as reported by Dr. Jenny Rubin et al. in 2018. (92)

Synergy of Chloroquine with Mebendazole

In 2019, Dr. So Jung Sung et al. reported that the autophagy inhibitor chloroquine synergizes with mebendazole, dramatically augmenting anti-cancer efficacy. (93)

One might expect similar synergy with fenbendazole, another microtubule inhibitor structurally similar to mebendazole in the "azole" drug family. Fenbendazole is a veterinary antiparasitic drug that has been repurposed as an anti-cancer drug. (94)

The Joe Tippens Story

The Joe Tippens story has created considerable interest in fenbendazole as an anti-cancer agent. I had the pleasure of meeting Joe Tippens at the 2020 Annie Appleseed meeting in West Palm Beach, Florida. Joe Tippens grew up on a ranch in western Oklahoma, and was a healthy, successful venture capitalist until 2016, when he was diagnosed with a left-lower lobe asymptomatic lung mass that proved to be small-cell lung cancer with spread to mediastinal nodes. In September 2016, Joe underwent chemotherapy and left lung radio-

therapy at MD Anderson Cancer Center. By December 2016, the left lung mass was gone, yet the cancer was now disseminated widely with metastatic disease. His doctors offered him a clinical trial of Keytruda® (an immune checkpoint inhibitor) and sent him home, with the understanding of a poor prognosis and a three-month life expectancy. Upon returning home, Joe received a telephone call from an old friend, a large-animal veterinarian in western Oklahoma, who told Joe about fenbendazole, a canine dewormer, and suggested he had nothing to lose and should try it. In January of 2017, Joe started the fenbendazole (222 grams per day 3 days a week), which was available online without a prescription at a number of pet medicine online shops. Joe added curcumin (600 mg/day), tocotrienol and tocopheral vitamin E (800mg/day) and "broad spectrum" CBD oil (1–2 droppers/day). In May of 2017, a repeat PET scan was completely clean, showing "no evidence of disease."

Joe writes that when his MD Anderson doctor saw the PET scan, the doctor scratched his head and replied:

> We don't quite know what to make of this as you are the only patient in the clinical trial with this kind of response. [Read the Joe Tippens story at www.mycancerstory-rocks.com.]

Another similar "azole" family drug, flubendazole, has anti-cancer activity, inducing mitotic catastrophe in colon cancer and melanoma cells. (95–96)

Conventional Chemotherapy Drugs As Antiparasitic Drugs

As we have seen above, many antiparasitic drugs have surprising efficacy as anti-cancer drugs. (97) The reverse is also true. Conventional chemotherapy drugs can be repurposed as antiparasitic drugs. (98)

Cancer as a Transmissible Parasite

Pathogenic viruses, bacteria, and fungi may cause infectious disease and are transmissible from one human to another, usually by respiratory droplet, sneezing, coughing, eating contaminated food, etc. The conventional thinking dogmatically states cancer is not a transmissible disease and it is safe to visit a cancer patient without the concern of contracting cancer during the visit.

However, this paradigm was broken in 2004, when Dr. Claudio Murgia et al. reported a type of transmissible cancer in dogs. Dr. Murgia studied genetic markers in the host dog and in the invading cancer cells, showing the cancer "has evolved into a transmissible parasite," representing the oldest known somatic mammalian cell in continuous propagation. Indeed, we now have four examples of transmissible cancer, three in mammals and one in clams. (99–100)

1) Soft shell clam leukemia. (101)
2) Canine transmissible venereal tumor (102–103)
3) Tasmanian devil facial tumor disease. (104)
4) Hamster-induced transmissible sarcoma (105)

Cancer Arising from Tapeworm Infection—Case Report

In 2015, Dr. Atis Muehlenbachs et al. reported a case of cancer in an unfortunate immunosuppressed patient with enlarged lymph nodes that had been invaded by cancer cells. Genomic analysis of lymph node biopsy material revealed tapeworm DNA (Hymenolepis nana) in the cancer cells, indicating "malignant transformation of a tapeworm parasite," apparently indicating the parasitic origin of this patient's cancer. Perhaps the early 1890 microbiologist, William Russell, was right all along, and his hypothesis that cancer is a parasitic disease has a ring of truth to it. (106)

Conclusion

The link between cancer and parasitic disease is intriguing. Animal models in which invading parasites transform normal cells into cancer cells has shed light on this connection. The sheer fact that a wide array of antiparasitic drugs serve as potent anti-cancer agents tends to support the hypothesis that cancer is a form of parasitic disease.

References for Chapter 20: Cancer as a Parasitic Disease

1) Darvish, Nooshin K. ND, "Glioblastoma Linked to Lyme Disease" April 16th, 2016, 14th Annual International Integrative Oncology Conference in San Diego.

2) Schöllkopf, Claudia, et al. "Borrelia infection and risk of non-Hodgkin lymphoma." Blood 111.12 (2008): 5524-5529.

3) Munksgaard, Lars, et al. "Demonstration of B. burgdorferi-DNA in two cases of nodal lymphoma." Leukemia & lymphoma 45.8 (2004): 1721-1723.

4) Cantwell, Alan. The cancer microbe. Aries Rising Press, 1990.

5) Russell, William. "An address on a characteristic organism of cancer." British medical journal 2.1563 (1890): 1356.

6) Ferretti, C., et al. "Molecular circuits shared by placental and cancer cells, and their implications in the proliferative, invasive and migratory capacities of trophoblasts." Human reproduction update 13.2 (2007): 121-141.

7) Parris, George E. "Clinically significant cancer evolves from transient mutated and/or aneuploid neoplasia by cell fusion to form unstable syncytia that give rise to ecologically viable parasite species." Medical hypotheses 65.5 (2005): 846-850.

8) Ujvari, Beata, et al. "Cancer and life-history traits: lessons from host–parasite interactions." Parasitology 143.05 (2016): 533-541.

9) Icard, Philippe, and Hubert Lincet. "The cancer tumor: a metabolic parasite?" Bulletin du Cancer 100.5 (2013): 427-433

10) Oliveira, Guilherme. "Cancer and parasitic infections: similarities and opportunities for the development of new control tools." Revista da Sociedade Brasileira de Medicina Tropical 47.1 (2014): 1-2.

11) Tretina, Kyle, et al. "Theileria-transformed bovine leukocytes have cancer hallmarks." Trends in parasitology 31.7 (2015): 306-314.

12) Wiens, Olga, et al. "Cell cycle-dependent phosphorylation of Theileria annulata schizont surface proteins." PloS one 9.7 (2014): e103821.

13) Kinnaird, Jane H., et al. "A bovine lymphosarcoma cell line infected with Theileria annulata exhibits an irreversible reconfiguration of host cell gene expression." PloS one 8.6 (2013): e66833.

14) Hayashida, K., et al. "Comparative genome analysis of three eukaryotic parasites with differing abilities to transform leukocytes reveals key mediators of Theileria-induced leukocyte transformation." mBio 3.5 (2011): e00204-12.

15) Hayashida, Kyoko, et al. "MDM2 regulates a novel form of incomplete neoplastic transformation of Theileria parva infected lymphocytes." Experimental and molecular pathology 94.1 (2013): 228-238.

16) Nene, Vishvanath, et al. "The biology of Theileria parva and control of East Coast fever—Current status and future trends." Ticks and tick-borne diseases (2016).

17) Dobbelaere, Dirk, and Volker Heussler. "Transformation of leukocytes by Theileria parva and T. annulata." Annual Reviews in Microbiology 53.1 (1999): 1-42.

18) Nene, Vishvanath, et al. "The biology of Theileria parva and control of East Coast fever—Current status and future trends." Ticks and tick-borne diseases (2016).

19) Hayashida, Kyoko, et al. "MDM2 regulates a novel form of incomplete neoplastic transformation of Theileria parva infected lymphocytes." Experimental and molecular pathology 94.1 (2013): 228-238.

20) Ma, Min, and Martin Baumgartner. "Intracellular Theileria annulata promote invasive cell motility through kinase regulation of the host actin cytoskeleton." PLoS Pathog 10.3 (2014): e1004003.

21) D.A. Dobbelaere, V. Heussler. Transformation of leukocytes by Theileria parva and T. annulata. Annu. Rev. Microbiol., 53 (1999), pp. 1–42

22) Benamrouz, Sadia, et al. "Cryptosporidium parvum-induced ileo-caecal adenocarcinoma and Wnt signaling in a mouse model." Disease Models and Mechanisms 7.6 (2014): 693-700.

23) Tamer, Gülden SÖNMEZ, Erdener Balikçi, and Ayşe Erbay. "The prevalence of cryptosporidiosis in children who were diagnosed with leukemia and lymphoma." Turkiye parazitolojii dergisi 32.3 (2008): 192-197.

24) Jiang, CaiXiao, et al. "The seroprevalence of Toxoplasma gondii in Chinese population with cancer: a systematic review and meta-analysis." Medicine 94.50 (2015).

25) Cong, Wei, et al. "Toxoplasma gondii infection in cancer patients: prevalence, risk factors, genotypes and association with clinical diagnosis." Cancer letters 359.2 (2015): 307-313.

26) Tin, Sim Sai, and Viroj Wiwanitkit. "Cryptosporidiosis and Colorectal Cancer." Annals of Colorectal Research 3.3 (2015).

27) Melenotte, Clea, et al. "A transcriptional signature associated with non-Hodgkin lymphoma in the blood of patients with Q fever." PloS one 14.6 (2019): e0217542.

28) Melenotte, Cléa, and Didier Raoult. "Pro-apoptotic effect of doxycycline and hydroxychloroquine on B-cell lymphoma induced by C. burnetii." Oncotarget 9.2 (2018): 2726.

29) Das, A. K. "Anticancer effect of antimalarial artemisinin compounds." Annals of medical and health sciences research 5.2 (2015): 93-102.

30) Melotti, Alice, et al. "The river blindness drug Ivermectin and related macrocyclic lactones inhibit WNT-TCF pathway responses in human cancer." EMBO molecular medicine (2014): e201404084.

31) Draganov, Dobrin, et al. "Modulation of P2X4/P2X7/pannexin-1 sensitivity to extracellular ATP via ivermectin induces a non-apoptotic and inflammatory form of cancer cell death." Scientific reports 5 (2015).

32) Drinyaev, Victor A., et al. "Antitumor effect of avermectins." European journal of pharmacology 501.1 (2004): 19-23.

33) Sharmeen, Sumaiya, et al. "The antiparasitic agent ivermectin induces chloride-dependent membrane hyperpolarization and cell death in leukemia cells." Blood 116.18 (2010): 3593-3603.

34) Albrich, Jennifer. "Helminths and anthelmintics." Professional Nursing Today 13.5 (2009): 8-10.

35) Kucik, Corry Jeb, Gary L. Martin, and Brett V. Sortor. "Common intestinal parasites." American family physician 69.5 (2004).

36) Woodhall, Dana, et al. "Neglected parasitic infections: what every family physician needs to know." Am Fam Physician 89.10 (2014): 803-11.

37) Thorne, Curtis A et al. "Small-Molecule Inhibition of Wnt Signaling through Activation of Casein Kinase 1α." Nature chemical biology 6.11 (2010): 829–836. PMC. Web. 21 Aug. 2016.

38) Xu, Liang, et al. "WNT pathway inhibitor pyrvinium pamoate inhibits the self-renewal and metastasis of breast cancer stem cells." International journal of oncology 48.3 (2016): 1175-1186.

39) Xiao, Meifang, et al. "Pyrvinium selectively induces apoptosis of lymphoma cells through impairing mitochondrial functions and JAK2/STAT5." Biochemical and biophysical research communications 469.3 (2016): 716-722.

40) Xu, Wei, et al. "The antihelmintic drug pyrvinium pamoate targets aggressive breast cancer." PloS one 8.8 (2013): e71508.

41) Ishii, Isao, Yasuo Harada, and Tadashi Kasahara. "Reprofiling a classical anthelmintic, pyrvinium pamoate, as an anti-cancer drug targeting mitochondrial respiration." Frontiers in oncology 2 (2012): 137.

42) Xiang, Wei, et al. "Pyrvinium selectively targets blast phase-chronic myeloid leukemia through inhibition of mitochondrial respiration." Oncotarget 6.32 (2015): 33769-33780.

43) Sakai, Chika, et al. "Mitochondrial fumarate reductase as a target of chemotherapy: from parasites to cancer cells." Biochimica et Biophysica Acta (BBA)-General Subjects 1820.5 (2012): 643-651.

44) Tomitsuka, Eriko, Kiyoshi Kita, and Hiroyasu Esumi. "An anticancer agent, pyrvinium pamoate inhibits the NADH–fumarate reductase system—a unique mitochondrial energy metabolism in tumour microenvironments." Journal of biochemistry 152.2 (2012): 171-183.

45) Wu, Zhen Hua, et al. "Praziquantel Synergistically Enhances Paclitaxel Efficacy to Inhibit Cancer Cell Growth." PLoS ONE 7.12 (2012).

46) Osada, Takuya, et al. "Antihelminth compound niclosamide downregulates Wnt signaling and elicits antitumor responses in tumors with activating APC mutations." Cancer research 71.12 (2011): 4172-4182.

47) Arend, Rebecca C., et al. "Inhibition of Wnt/β-catenin pathway by niclosamide: A therapeutic target for ovarian cancer." Gynecologic oncology 134.1 (2014): 112-120.

48) Chen, W., M. Chen, and L. S. Barak. "Development of small molecules targeting the Wnt pathway for the treatment of colon cancer: a high-throughput screening approach." American journal of physiology.

Gastrointestinal and liver physiology 299.2 (2010): G293.

49) Park, So-Yeon, et al. "Inhibition of LEF1-mediated DCLK1 by niclosamide attenuates colorectal cancer stemness." Clinical Cancer Research 25.4 (2019): 1415-1429.

50) Liao, Zhan, et al. "The anthelmintic drug niclosamide inhibits the proliferative activity of human osteosarcoma cells by targeting multiple signal pathways." Current cancer drug targets 15.8 (2015): 726-738.

51) Wieland, Anja, et al. "Anticancer effects of niclosamide in human glioblastoma." Clinical Cancer Research 19.15 (2013): 4124-4136.

52) Li, Yonghe, et al. "Multi-targeted therapy of cancer by niclosamide: A new application for an old drug." Cancer letters 349.1 (2014): 8-14.

53) Costa, Roberto, et al. "Impaired mitochondrial ATP production downregulates Wnt signaling via ER stress induction." Cell reports 28.8 (2019): 1949-1960.

54) Pan, Jing-Xuan, Ke Ding, and Cheng-Yan Wang. "Niclosamide, an old antihelminthic agent, demonstrates antitumor activity by blocking multiple signaling pathways of cancer stem cells." Chinese journal of cancer 31.4 (2012): 178.

55) Huisa, Branko N., et al. "Taeniasis and cysticercosis in housemaids working in affluent neighborhoods in Lima, Peru." The American journal of tropical medicine and hygiene 73.3 (2005): 496-500.

56) Schantz, Peter M., et al. "Neurocysticercosis in an orthodox Jewish community in New York City." New England Journal of Medicine 327.10 (1992): 692-695.

57) World Health Organization. "WHO model prescribing information: drugs used in parasitic diseases." (1995).

58) Chen, Hui, Hudan Liu, and Guoliang Qing. "Targeting oncogenic Myc as a strategy for cancer treatment." Signal transduction and targeted therapy 3.1 (2018): 1-7.

59) Carabet, Lavinia A., Paul S. Rennie, and Artem Cherkasov. "Therapeutic inhibition of Myc in cancer. Structural bases and computer-aided drug discovery approaches." International journal of molecular sciences 20.1 (2019): 120.

60) Gabay, Meital, Yulin Li, and Dean W. Felsher. "MYC activation is a hallmark of cancer initiation and maintenance." Cold Spring Harbor perspectives in medicine 4.6 (2014): a014241.

61) Miller, Donald M., et al. "c-Myc and cancer metabolism." (2012): 5546-5553.

62) Fan-Minogue, Hua, et al. "A c-Myc activation sensor-based high throughput drug screening identifies an anti-neoplastic effect of Nitazoxanide." Molecular cancer therapeutics 12.9 (2013): 1896.

63) Qu, Yi, et al. "Small molecule nitazoxanide (NTZ), promotes [beta]-catenin citrullination and inhibits Wnt signaling in cancer." Nature Chemical Biology (2017).

64) Hong, Seong Keun, et al. "Nitazoxanide suppresses IL-6 production in LPS-stimulated mouse macrophages and TG-injected mice." International immunopharmacology 13.1 (2012): 23-27.

65) Di Santo, Nicola, and Jessie Ehrisman. "Research perspective: potential role of nitazoxanide in ovarian cancer treatment. Old drug, new purpose?" Cancers 5.3 (2013): 1163-1176.

66) Lee, Eunyoug, and Do Hee Lee. "Emerging roles of protein disulfide isomerase in cancer." BMB reports 50.8 (2017): 401.

67) Xu, Shili, Saranya Sankar, and Nouri Neamati. "Protein disulfide isomerase: a promising target for cancer therapy." Drug discovery today 19.3 (2014): 222-240.

68) Kuo, T. F., et al. "Protein disulfide isomerase a4 acts as a novel regulator of cancer growth through the procaspase pathway." Oncogene (2017). Oncogene. 2017 Sep 28; 36(39):5484-5496.

69) Badolato, Mariateresa, et al. "Synthesis and Experimental Validation of New PDI Inhibitors with Antiproliferative Activity." Journal of Chemistry 2017 (2017).

70) Di Santo, Nicola, and Jessie Ehrisman. "A functional perspective of nitazoxanide as a potential anticancer drug." Mutation Research/Fundamental and Molecular Mechanisms of Mutagenesis 768 (2014): 16-21.

71) Senkowski, Wojciech. High-throughput screening using multicellular tumor spheroids to reveal

and exploit tumor-specific vulnerabilities. Diss. Acta Universitatis Upsaliensis, 2017.

72) Shakya, Anshul, Hans R. Bhat, and Surajit Kumar Ghosh. "Update on nitazoxanide: a multifunctional chemotherapeutic agent." Current drug discovery technologies 15.3 (2018): 201-213.

73) Rossignol, Jean-François. "Nitazoxanide: a first-in-class broad-spectrum antiviral agent." Antiviral research 110 (2014): 94-103.

74) Rossignol, Jean-François. "Nitazoxanide, a new drug candidate for the treatment of Middle East respiratory syndrome coronavirus." Journal of infection and public health 9.3 (2016): 227-230.

75) Koszalka, Paulina, Danielle Tilmanis, and Aeron C. Hurt. "Influenza antivirals currently in late-phase clinical trial." Influenza and Other Respiratory Viruses 11.3 (2017): 240.

76) Haffizulla, Jason, et al. "Effect of nitazoxanide in adults and adolescents with acute uncomplicated influenza: a double-blind, randomised, placebo-controlled, phase 2b/3 trial." The Lancet Infectious Diseases 14.7 (2014): 609-618.

77) Dobrosotskaya, I. Y., et al. "Mebendazole monotherapy and long-term disease control in metastatic adrenocortical carcinoma." Endocrine practice: 17.3 (2011): e59.

78) Bai, Ren-Yuan, et al. "Antiparasitic mebendazole shows survival benefit in 2 preclinical models of glioblastoma multiforme." Neuro-oncology (2011): nor077.

79) Nygren, Peter, and Rolf Larsson. "Drug repositioning from bench to bedside: Tumour remission by the antihelmintic drug mebendazole in refractory metastatic colon cancer." Acta Oncologica 53.3 (2014): 427-428.

80) Larsen, Andrew R., et al. "Repurposing the antihelmintic mebendazole as a hedgehog inhibitor." Molecular cancer therapeutics 14.1 (2015): 3-13.

81) Pinto, Laine Celestino, et al. "The anthelmintic drug mebendazole inhibits growth, migration and invasion in gastric cancer cell model." Toxicology in vitro 29.8 (2015): 2038-2044.

82) Pantziarka, Pan et al. "Repurposing Drugs in Oncology (ReDO)—mebendazole as an Anti-Cancer Agent." ecancermedicalscience 8 (2014): 443. PMC. Web. 13 Jan. 2015.

83) Popović, Dušica J., et al. "Application of a widely-used tropical anti-worm agent, mebendazole, in modern oncology." Tropical Journal of Pharmaceutical Research 16.10 (2017): 2555-2562.

84) Popović, Dušica J., et al. "Effect of mebendazole on fibrosarcoma in hamsters." Tropical Journal of Pharmaceutical Research 16.10 (2017): 2445-2451

85) He, Licai, et al. "Mebendazole exhibits potent anti-leukemia activity on acute myeloid leukemia." Experimental cell research 369.1 (2018): 61-68.

86) Zhang, Le, et al. "Mebendazole Potentiates Radiation Therapy in Triple-Negative Breast Cancer." International Journal of Radiation Oncology, Biology, Physics. 103.1 (2019): 195-207.

87) Guerini, Andrea Emanuele, et al. "Mebendazole as a Candidate for Drug Repurposing in Oncology: An Extensive Review of Current Literature." Cancers 11.9 (2019): 1284.

88) Doudican, Nicole, et al. "Mebendazole induces apoptosis via Bcl-2 inactivation in chemoresistant melanoma cells." Molecular Cancer Research 6.8 (2008): 1308-1315.

89) Gamble, Alex, et al. "ATPS-83 Repurposing Mebendazole as a Replacement for Vincristine for the Treatment of Brain Tumors." Neuro-Oncology 17.suppl 5 (2015): v36-v36.

90) Bodhinayake, Imithri, Marc Symons, and John A. Boockvar. "Repurposing Mebendazole for the Treatment of Medulloblastoma." Neurosurgery 76.2 (2015): N15-N16.

91) Zhang, Fugui, et al. "Anthelmintic mebendazole enhances cisplatin's effect on suppressing cell proliferation and promotes differentiation of head and neck squamous cell carcinoma (HNSCC)." Oncotarget 8.8 (2017): 12968.

92) Rubin, Jenny, et al. "Mebendazole stimulates CD14+ myeloid cells to enhance T-cell activation and tumour cell killing." Oncotarget 9.56 (2018): 30805.

93) Sung, So Jung, et al. "Autophagy Is a Potential Target for Enhancing the Anti-Angiogenic Effect of Mebendazole in Endothelial Cells." Biomolecules & therapeutics 27.1 (2019): 117.

94) Dogra, Nilambra, Ashok Kumar, and Tapas Mukhopadhyay. "Fenbendazole acts as a moderate microtubule destabilizing agent and causes cancer cell death by modulating multiple cellular pathways." Scientific reports 8.1 (2018): 11926.

95) Králová, Věra, et al. "Flubendazole induces mitotic catastrophe and senescence in colon cancer cells in vitro." Journal of Pharmacy and Pharmacology 68.2 (2016): 208-218.

96) Čáňová, K., et al. "Flubendazole induces mitotic catastrophe and apoptosis in melanoma cells." Toxicology in Vitro 46 (2018): 313-322.

97) Hamilton, Gerhard, and Barbara Rath. "Repurposing of Anthelminthics as Anticancer Drugs."Mutat Res. 2014 Oct; 768:16-21.

98) Klinkert, M-Q., and V. Heussler. "The use of anti-cancer drugs in antiparasitic chemotherapy." Mini reviews in medicinal chemistry 6.2 (2006): 131-143.

99) Murgia, Claudio, et al. "Clonal Origin and Evolution of a Transmissible Cancer." Cell 126.3 (2006): 477.

100) Trends Genet. 2016 Jan; 32(1):1-15. Transmissible Tumors: Breaking the Cancer Paradigm. Ostrander EA1, Davis BW2, Ostrander GK3.

101) Metzger, Michael J., et al. "Horizontal transmission of clonal cancer cells causes leukemia in soft-shell clams." Cell 161.2 (2015): 255-263.

102) Murchison, Elizabeth P., et al. "Transmissible dog cancer genome reveals the origin and history of an ancient cell lineage." Science 343.6169 (2014): 437-440.

103) Decker, Brennan, et al. "Comparison against 186 canid whole-genome sequences reveals survival strategies of an ancient clonally transmissible canine tumor." Genome research 25.11 (2015): 1646-1655.

104) Murchison, Elizabeth P., et al. "The Tasmanian devil transcriptome reveals Schwann cell origins of a clonally transmissible cancer." Science 327.5961 (2010): 84-87.

105) Tissot, Tazzio, et al. "Host manipulation by cancer cells: Expectations, facts, and therapeutic implications." BioEssays (2016).

106) Muehlenbachs, Atis, et al. "Malignant Transformation of Hymenolepis nana in a Human Host." New England Journal of Medicine 373.19 (2015): 1845-1852.

Chapter 21

Artemisinin, Our Gift from China

SUSAN WAS A 56-YEAR-OLD HOMEMAKER in good health, until one day she noticed pain in her left abdomen and a change in bowel habits. Her doctored ordered an X-ray test of her colon called a barium enema, which revealed that she had colon cancer, with a typical apple core appearance on the barium X-ray of the colon. Colonoscopy and biopsy confirmed the diagnosis. Susan was sent to a colon cancer surgeon who performed a "curative resection."

Artemisinin Prospective Randomized Trial in Colon Cancer

After the operation, it seemed the cancer was gone. However, Susan was worried about recurrence, which can happen because microscopic cancer cells may have already spread outside the colon. While reading the newspaper, Susan saw a news story about Dorothy B., a colon cancer patient who participated in a clinical study with Dr. Sanjeev Krishna at St George University London in 2010. (1–2)

In the study, Dorothy B. took a new anti-cancer tablet, called artesunate (an artemisinin derivative), for two weeks before her colon resection. Five years later, she is alive and well. Susan called me to ask if artemisinin could improve her chances of beating cancer recurrence after surgery. I said to Susan, "Artemisinin is our ultimate weapon against cancer, a gift from China."

This 2015 randomized study by Dr. Sanjeev Krishna et al. included 20 colon cancer patients awaiting "curative resection" for colon cancer. (1–2) Half received the artesunate pill for two weeks prior to surgery, and the other half a placebo. Five years later, there were 6 cancer recurrences in the placebo group, but only one in the artesunate (artemisinin) group. There were no deaths in the artesunate group, compared to three deaths in the placebo group. I was very impressed by this.

Ridiculing Chinese Herbs

In the old days, when I worked as a hospital-based physician, we took lunch in the doctor's dining room where conversation included amazement and ridicule at the stories of patients who took Chinese herbs for their medical condition. The surgeons had a good laugh, expressing amazement that any intelligent American would choose to take a Chinese herb for a medical condition.

Artemisinin—A Gift from the Chinese Government

During the Vietnam War, in the 1960s, the North Vietnamese soldiers succumbed to malaria in great numbers. This loss of military readiness prompted the Chinese government to develop better and more effective antimalarial drugs. China enlisted the help of a young medical student named Tu YouYou. She uncovered an ancient Chinese medical text in an archaeological excavation written by Ge Hong (281–340 AD), which describes an herbal tea, sweet wormwood, to treat fevers and chills. This tea was later mentioned in the 1596 *Compendium of Materia Medica* by Li Shizen. Dr. Youyou ultimately isolated the active molecule in the tea, called artemisinin, an effective antimalaria drug, for which she received the 2015 Nobel Prize in Medicine. Artemisinin, and derivatives like artesunate, are now lifesaving drugs used by millions to treat malaria. Who's laughing at Chinese herbs now?

Antimalarial Drugs Are Also Anti-Cancer Drugs

Over the years, it was discovered that artemisinin is also a very effective anti-cancer drug. In 2015, Dr. A. K. Das reported that artemisinin (and its derivatives) are effective against 55 cancer cell lines with inhibitory effects against pancreatic cancer, osteosarcoma, lung cancer, colon, melanoma, breast, ovarian, prostate, central nervous system, lymphoma, leukemia and renal cancer cells. In addition, artesunate potentiated the effect of the common chemotherapy drug doxorubin in a drug-resistant leukemia line. (3)

Cancer Cells Contain Massive Amounts of Iron (Fe)

The molecular mechanism by which artemisinin compounds serve as effective anti-cancer agents can be found in a feature of its molecular structure, the endoperoxide bridge, which reacts with the iron molecule producing a Fenton reaction, in which reactive oxygen species (ROS) are generated.

What is the targeted nontoxic approach to cancer treatment? As discussed in chapter 4, "Cancer as a Metabolic Disease." The nontoxic approach to treating cancer is to exploit key metabolic differences between cancer cells and normal cells, to devise ways to kill cancer cells while leaving normal cells unharmed. One key metabolic difference is the higher Fe content of cancer cells. The Endoperoxide Bridge (oxygen) in artemisinin attaches to the Fe in the cancer cell, setting off a chemical reaction that ultimately kills the cancer cell. (3–5)

Cancer Cells Contain Massive Amounts of Iron in Lysosomes

The rapid metabolic rate and rapid proliferation of cancer cells requires a large amount of iron. For this purpose, cancer cells express high levels of the transferrin receptors needed for internalizing iron (Fe) at a tremendous rate. (6) This is a useful difference when compared to normal cells. (7)

In fact, a correlation between expression of transferrin membrane receptor and Ki-67 (a marker of tumor proliferation) has also been reported. The more aggressive the tumor, the greater the number of transferrin receptors. (8)

This difference in iron content and iron transport is one of the reasons why artemisinin compounds kill cancer cells selectively while sparing normal cells.

Addition of Iron Enhances the Killing Effect of Artemisinin

Since the anti-cancer effects of artemisinin rely on the presence of iron in the cancer cell, its effects are upregulated 1.5–10 fold by ingestion of iron supplements, as you might expect. (9)

Dr. Jigang Wang (2017) found enhancement of anticancer activity and synergy of artemisinin with the porphyrin precursor amino levulinic acid (ALA), used by the cell to make the porphyrin ring in hemoglobin, the scaffolding that surrounds the iron molecule. (10)

ALA is available as GleoLan®, an optical imaging agent used by the neurosurgeon in the operating room to visualize brain tumors, making resection more accurate, thus sparing normal tissue. (11)

However, considering the high cost of GleoLan, $4,000 per vial, perhaps the ingestion of liquid chlorophyll would provide similar synergy. Available at the health food store for a few dollars, Chlorophyll is effective for increasing heme production in anemic dialysis patients and contains a porphyrin ring, providing similar ALA precursors for increasing heme synthesis at lower cost. (12)

Artemisinin Mechanism of Action

Artemisinin enters the cancer cell lysosomes, which already contain iron as a degradation product from ferritin (an iron-storage product). The endoperoxide oxygen bridge in artemisinin reacts with the iron causing a "Fenton Reaction" producing hydroxyl radicals. (13–14)

Fenton Reaction in Lysosomes—Ferroptosis

Lysosomes are the cell organelles, "microscopic bags" that contain acid used for digestion and degradation of unwanted intracellular debris and endocytosed bacteria and protein in a process called autophagy. For example, our white cells, called neutrophils, kill bacteria in our bloodstream by eating them, engulfing them in a process called macropinocytosis. Once eaten by the white cell, these unwanted proteins are digested in lysosomes. The acid in the lysosome is produced by a molecular machine called the V-ATPase, a molecular pump for acid production. Lysosomes often accumulate large amounts of iron, especially in cancer cells, which may then react with oxygen in the Fenton reaction, causing release of hydroxyl radicals. This compromises the lysosomal membrane, disrupts membrane integrity, and causes the membrane to release its acid contents freely into the cell cytosol, initiating a form of cell death called "ferroptosis" (as opposed to apoptosis), as we will detail below. (15–16)

Mode of Action of Artemisinin Cancer Cell Death

Perhaps the best understanding of the mechanism action of artemisinin comes from Dr. Nai-Di Yang in 2014, who used a blue fluorescent tag on the artemisinin molecule to follow its location in the cancer cell. (13)

In this scenario, artesunate induces cell death in human cancer cells via enhancing lysosomal function and lysosomal degradation of ferritin. Artemisinin enters cancer cells along with iron-loaded ferritin. Both enter the lysosome, which then triggers ROS in mitochondria and caspase-3 programmed cell death. This is further explained below.

Cancer-Cell-Killing Mechanism

Firstly, Artemisinin (ART) accumulates in the lysosomes. Secondly, ART increases lysosomal acidification, cathepsin enzyme activity, and protein degradation via promoting lysosomal V-ATPase assembly. ART induces autophagy, based on the observations that ART increases autophagosome formation and enhances autophagic flux. (13) Stimulation of autophagy is related to suppression of nuclear factor kappa B (NF-kB), the master inflammatory controller. (14–16)

Perinuclear Clustering of Lysosomes—Autophagy

In 2014, Dr. Nai-Di Yang et al. observed a peculiar perinuclear clustering of lysosomes in the artemisinin-treated cancer cells, writing this is an indication of autophagy induction (protective autophagy):

> We believe that this perinuclear clustering of lysosomes is, in fact, an indication of autophagy induction. We observed increase of mitochondrial ROS implicating lysosomal iron as a critical mediator in ART-induced mitochondrial ROS production and cell death. It is possible that enhanced lysosomal degradation of ferritin induced by ART leads to the transient increase of cytosolic ferrous iron, which then affects the mitochondria, leading to enhanced mitochondrial ROS production. (13)

Note: another possible mechanism of action of artesunate is direct involvement with iron molecules within components of the mitochondrial ETC (electron transport chain), such as cytochrome C, which contains a central iron molecule within a porphyrin ring, similar to hemoglobin. Obviously, this will acting as OXPHOS inhibitor causing mitochondrial dysfunction.

V-ATPase Inhibitors Interfere with Artesunate

V-ATPase is the acid pumping protein assembly that pumps acid into the lysosomes. Inhibiting lysosomal acid production with bafilomycin, a lysosomal V-ATPase inhibitor drug, effectively blocked cancer cell death induced by artemisinin. Dr. Yang writes:

> Ferritin delivery and degradation in lysosomes is required for the toxicity of ART. Therefore, lysosomal inhibitors significantly protect the cells from ART-induced cell death via blockage of ferritin degradation. (13)

Another class of drugs that inhibits V-ATPase are the proton pump inhibitors (PPI) such as omeprazole. Like bafilomycin, these PPI drugs would be expected to interfere with the anti-cancer activity of artesunate, and it is advisable to avoid PPI drugs while using ART.

Chloroquine Inhibits Ferritin Degradation and Cell Death Induced by ART

Dr. Yang et al. found the autophagy inhibitor chloroquine, like bafilomycin, blocked the anti-cancer effects of artemisinin. They wrote:

> In fact, we also found that chloroquine inhibited the ferritin degradation and cell death induced by ART as efficiently as BAF. (13)

The iron chelator, deferoxamine (DFO),

binds iron, making it unavailable. Since iron is needed for artemisinin to kill cancer cells, as one might expect, DFO inhibited cell death by artemisinin. The anti-oxidant n-acetyl cysteine which inhibits ROS, also inhibits cell death from artemisinin. (17–19)

Perinuclear Clustering of Lysosomes

In 2010, studying MCF-7 breast cancer cells in vitro, Dr. Anne Hamacher-Brady et al. observed that artemisinin causes a peculiar re-arrangement of the lysosomes and mito-chondria in a pattern typical for autophagy. (20)

Perinuclear clustering of lysosomes is an indication of autophagy induction and may be caused by cell starvation or anti-cancer drug treatment, which activates the mTOR pathway, inducing "protective autophagy," a survival mechanism. Quite the opposite is "lysosomal trafficking," in which lysosomes migrate to the cell surface near the cell membrane. Lysosomal trafficking is associated with plentiful nutrients in the micro-environment and a more aggressive, invasive, and metastatic behavior of the cancer cell. In lysosomal trafficking, lysosomes are positioned near the cell membrane for bi-directional activity. The lysosomes can deliver acidic contents to the micro-environment or receive exogenous nutrients, which are delivered to the interior of the cancer cell, via macropinocytosis (21–23)

Artemisinin Derivatives

The efficacy of artemisinin may be impaired by poor drug absorption, resulting in low blood levels. How can the potency and efficacy of artemisinin be increased? This can be done by making a derivative such as artemether, or artesunate, which are modified artemisinin compounds possessing greater bio-availability and potency. Care needs to be taken here, however, because greater bio-availability and potency may be associated with increased toxicity, which we will discuss below.

Transferrin-Tagged Artemisinin

Another technique to improve efficacy is to tag the artemisinin molecule with transferrin, the iron carrier protein. In 2008, Dr. Ikuhiko Nakase et al. found that this transferrin conjugate had greater anti-cancer potency. Perhaps in the future, such a molecule could be commercially developed. (24)

Many Antimalaria Drugs Serve as Anti-Cancer Drugs

In 2015, Dr. Chanakya Nath Kundu et al. reported that many antimalarial drugs serve as effective anti-cancer drugs and vice versa. Artemisinin and its derivatives act as radiosensitizers, making cancer cells more sensitive to radiotherapy and work in synergy with many natural anti-cancer substances. (25)

Other Anti-Cancer Treatments Work in Synergy

Intracellular iron is required for artemisinin to kill the cancer cell. Ingesting an Iron supplement increases the effect of the artemisinin. However, one should be careful to take the iron supplement at a different time from the arte-

avoid reacting directly with the iron GI tract. Most artemisinin practitioners will use a schedule to allow "rest days." The artemisinin is taken 14 days on, then 4 days off. This is thought to improve GI absorption.

Anti-Cancer Supplements Synergistic With Artemisinin

Many natural substances work together in synergy with Artemisinin. These include:

- Curcumin (26–30)
- Berberine (31)
- Resveratrol (32)
- Pterostilbene (33–35)
- Allicin (36–37)
- Melatonin (38–41)
- Vitamin C (42)
- Sulforaphane (43)
- Butyrate (44–47)
- HDAC Inhibitor (48)

Synergy of High-Dose IV Vitamin C with Artemisinin

The suppressed knowledge of IV vitamin C as an effective anti-cancer treatment is finally coming to light with new research over the last decade. High-dose IV vitamin C (ascorbate) 50–75 grams produces blood levels producing pro-oxidant effects acting in synergy with the oxidizing effects of artemisinin, making both treatments more effective in killing cancer cells selectively without harming normal cells, according to Dr. Thomas Gerhardt (2015). (42)

Since both high-dose IV vitamin C and artemisinin are extremely safe, this highly effective treatment may be useful as an anti-cancer pro-tocol. This IV vitamin C bag may be followed by IV alpha lipoic acid (300 mg IV), which shunts cancer cell metabolism toward utilizing oxygen (OXPHOS metabolism) in the mitochondria. The alpha lipoic acid heightens the vitamin C effect as explained in chapter 7, on alpha lipoic acid. IV artesunate (available as first-line therapy for severe malaria) is commonly given just before the IV vitamin C, augmenting the pro-oxidative effect.

Artemisinin-Curcumin Synergy

In a 2006 study by Dr. Nandakumar using malaria-infected cultured RBCs, the combination of artemisinin with curcumin was found to synergize. (26)

This combination showed greater malaria-killing activity than the individual compounds. The molecular pathways were not elucidated. However, since the mechanism for artemisinin action in both malaria parasites and cancer cells is similar, one might anticipate a synergistic effect for this combination. However, to my knowledge, this has not yet been studied and would be a good topic for NIH funding for future research.

Artemisinin-Allicin (Garlic) Synergy

Allicin (diallyl thiosulfinate) the active ingredient in garlic, has known anti-cancer effects. Allicin induces caspase-mediated apoptosis in lymphoma and other cancers. Dr. Wei Jiang et al. reported in 2013 on the synergistic combination of artesunate (artemisinin derivative) with allicin, which increased the anti-cancer effect on osteosarcoma cell lines in vitro and in vivo. Dr. Jiang's group also reported on mouse tumor xenograft studies; these in vivo studies showed enhanced synergy for the combination of Allicin and Artesunate. (36)

Platelet Inhibition

Allicin and thiosulfinates are potent platelet-aggregation inhibitors that can aggravate bleeding, so caution is advised when used with other platelet inhibitors, such as feverfew, aspirin, vitamin E, fish Oil, gingko, and ibrutinib (Imbruvica, Bruton's kinase inhibitor).

Synergy of Artemisinin with Resveratrol

The synergic effect of artemisinin and resveratrol in cancer cells was reported in 2014 by Dr. Peichun Li with the combination of artemisinin and resveratrol in hepatoma (HepG2) and cervical cancer (HeLa) cell lines. The combination significantly reduced cell migration, increased ROS, and increased apoptosis and necrosis of the two cancer cell lines. (32)

Pterostilbene is a methylated derivative of resveratrol, chemically similar but with better bio-availability. A 2005 study by Dr. Tolomeo showed the 3-hydroxy-pterostilbene to be 50–100 times stronger than resveratrol in killing multidrug-resistant leukemia cells. One might expect pterostilbene to demonstrate even greater synergy with artemisinin compared to resveratrol. We await these future studies. (35)

Synergy of Artemisinin with Butyrate

Drs. Narendra Singh and Henry Lai report in 2005 that the cancer-cell-killing effect of artemisinin is enhanced with the addition of butyrate, a short-chain fatty acid. Their study used a lymphoblastic leukemia cell line, treated with a combination of dihydroartemisinin and butyrate. (44)

In a 2007 report, Dr. B. Pajak et al. outlined the molecular basis of the anti-cancer effects of butyrate. A small four-carbon chain fatty acid, butyrate is a normal product of large-bowel microbial fermentation of dietary fiber. Butyrate inhibits (HDAC) histone deacetylase activity, allowing DNA binding of several transcription factors, which increases the expression of pro-apoptotic genes and results in amplification of apoptotic pathways (programmed cell suicide) in the cancer cell, while sparing normal cells. (45)

In a 2013 report, Dr. Jane Fauser studied the anti-cancer effects of butyrate and coconut oil (lauric acid) on a colon cancer cell line. Dr. Fauser reported butyrate induces apoptosis by

inhibiting histone deacetylase activity, inducing cell cycle arrest, promoting differentiation, activating NF-κB, downregulating α 2 β 1, modifying glucose availability, and inducing caspase activation in colon cancer cell. (46)

In 2006, Dr. Choi reported on the anti-cancer effects of butyrate on a leukemia cell line. Dr. Choi found that butyrate induced apoptosis of human leukemic cells by inhibition of telomerase activity. In addition, butyrate served as a histone deacetylase (HDAC) inhibitor, resulting in dose-dependent apoptosis associated with upregulation in pro-apoptotic Bax protein expression and downregulation of the anti-apoptotic proteins, Bcl-2 and Bcl-XL. (47)

In a 2006 report, Dr. Ulrike Heider et al. studied the effect of sodium butyrate on three

...ll Lymphoma types. Dr. Heider's ... reported that butyrate induced potent ...ogrammed cell death (apoptosis) of all three mantle cell lymphoma types in a dose-dependent manner. (48)

Butyrate is available as a supplement, or as a butyrate-producing probiotic, both available at the health food store. A probiotic named clostridium butyricum is known to produce butyrate. This is available from Japan in a product called Miyarisan, available over the counter (OTC). It is also contained in Probiotic 3 from Advanced Orthomolecular Research (AOR).

Targeting (Progenitor) Cancer Stem Cells

Cytotoxic chemotherapy may be quite useful for controlling hematologic cancers such as lymphoma and leukemia. Although highly toxic, and frequently associated with adverse effects, chemotherapy drugs may induce complete remission (CR), with the disappearance of tumor masses and clearing of radionuclide activity on follow-up PET scan. In more aggressive cell types, relapse with metastatic disease is inevitable. Relapse is thought to be caused by cancer stem cells (progenitor cells), which are dormant and not actively replicating. Cancer stem cells are insensitive (resistant) to cytotoxic chemotherapy, which is not effective for dormant, non-replicating cancer stem cells. (49–51)

Since there are no FDA-approved oncology drugs specifically approved to target cancer stem cells, the next logical question is: Are there natural nontoxic targeted therapies that target cancer stem cells? Yes, berberine (51), and sulforaphane (43) are only two of many. For more

on this topic, see chapter 10, Targeting Cancer Stem Cells with Nontoxic Therapies.

FeverFew—Targeting Cancer Stem Cells, Depleting Glutathione

The well-known anti-migraine botanical, feverfew (parthenolide) has been found to target cancer stem cells. In 2005, Dr. Monica Guzmán et al. studied the effect of parthenolide on acute myelogenous leukemia (AML) stem cells. Dr. Monica Guzmán writes:

> Parthenolide preferentially targets AML progenitor and stem cell populations.... The molecular mechanism of Parthenolide mediated apoptosis is strongly associated with inhibition of NF-κB [nuclear factor Kappa B], pro-apoptotic activation of p53, and increased reactive oxygen species [ROS]. On the basis of these findings, we propose that the activity of Parthenolide triggers Cancer Stem Cell-specific apoptosis and as such represents a potentially important new class of drugs for Cancer Stem Cell-targeted therapy. (52)

Feverfew (parthenolide) is a widely used botanical that exerts potent anti-cancer effects by blocking activation of nuclear factor kappa B (NF-kB) and depleting the cancer cell of glutathione, rendering it sensitive to ROS, which triggers apoptotic pathways. Parthenolide shares some chemical structure similarities with artemisinin. Both are "sesquiterpene lactones." One might speculate that the two agents might work synergistically together with enhanced cancer-cell-killing effects and that this would be a good topic for NIH funding and future study. (52–60)

Sulforaphane—Targeting Cancer Stem Cells and Depleting Glutathione

The active ingredient in broccoli is sulforaphane, a widely used nutritional supplement with no adverse effects. Sulforaphane has been widely studied as an effective anti-cancer agent that targets cancer stem cells and depletes glutathione in the cancer cell, thus rendering it more sensitive to oxidative damage. (61–66)

In 2010, Dr. Yanyan Li et al. reported that sulforaphane eliminated breast cancer stem cells in vivo in a mouse xenograft model. Tumor-bearing primary mice were treated with sulforaphane. The tumor cells from the primary mice were then re-implanted into secondary mice, showing no growth of tumor cells, indicating the cancer stem cells had been eradicated. Dr. Li's group writes:

> Sulforaphane decreased the protein level of βeta-catenin by up to 85% in MCF7 and SUM159 [breast cancer] cells; and the expression of cyclin D1, one of the Wnt/β-catenin target genes, declined by up to 77% as well. (64–65)

A 2012 study by Dr. Mariana Rodova et al. showed that sulforaphane is effective as anti-cancer treatment for pancreatic cancer stem cells via the blockade of hedgehog signaling. (66)

Other Repurposed Drugs That May Work with Artemisinin

Sulfasalazine (Azulfadine), an old anti-inflammatory drug widely used in rheumatology, inhibits the active transport of cystine into the cancer cell. Sulfasalazine comes in a 500-mg oral tablet started at a dose of 500 mg per day and increased gradually to 2,000 mg per day while watching for adverse effects. For most adults with rheumatoid arthritis, the maintenance dose is 2 to 3 grams daily.

Sulfasalazine—Glutathione Depletion

When the cancer cell is deficient in cystine, it cannot make glutathione, the intracellular anti-oxidant. Lack of anti-oxidant protection leads directly to "ferroptosis" in cancer cell studies. (67–68)

Sulfasalazine has a long history of use for inflammatory bowel disease and rheumatoid arthritis. Its benefits are thought to arise from its ability to suppress nuclear factor kappa B. Sulfasalazine is also a potent suppressor of lymphoma cells on the basis of suppression of cystine uptake, which impairs anti-oxidant defense.

Sulfasalazine Lymphoma Model in Mice

Dr. Bebb reported in 2003 that sulfasalazine inhibits growth of B-Cell lymphoma in a murine mantle cell lymphoma (MCL) model. (75)

In 2003, Drs. Peter Gout, Chris Simms, and May Robertson found that sulfasalazine suppressed 90% of lymphoma xenografts in mice, a remarkable finding. (76)

Since ferroptosis is also seen when cancer cells are treated with artemisinin, one might logically assume the two drugs artemisinin and sulfasalazine would be synergistic, augmenting cancer cell death. Unfortunately, the appropriate cell culture studies (in vitro or in vivo) have not yet been done. We await future research.

...loroquine Antimalarial
Autophagy Inhibitor

Hydroxychloroquine (Plaquenil®) and chloroquine (Avelan), are old antimalarial drugs. They serve as lysosomal inhibitors and autophagy inhibitors. The chloroquine becomes trapped within the acidic vacuoles of the lysosomes, causing increased pH (loss of acidity), inactivating the lysosomes and inhibiting autophagy.

Concurrent Chloroquine and Artemisinin, Yes or No?

Since artemisinin and derivatives like artesunate activate protective autophagy, one might speculate that addition of an autophagy inhibitor would be synergistic, augmenting the cancer-cell-killing effects.

Quite the contrary. In 2014, Dr. Nai-Di Yang found that chloroquine inhibited the effect of artemisinin in his study, similar to the inhibitory activity of the lysosomal V-ATP-ase inhibitor, baflinomycin. (13)

Similarly, in 2010 Dr. Hamacher-Brady found that chloroquine administered concurrent with the artemisinin impaired cancer-cell-killing activity. (20)

Pretreatment Rather Than Co-Treatment

In 2014, Dr. Arnab Ganguli et al. studied a non-small-cell lung cancer cell model using the combination of artemisinin with the autophagy inhibitor chloroquine. While co-treatment was not helpful, pretreatment with chloroquine was synergistic and augmented the cancer-killing effect of artemisinin. They write:

Pretreatment with chloroquine [CQ] and followed by ART treatment had synergistic combination index [CI] for cell death. Inhibition of autophagy by CQ pretreatment led to accumulation of acidic vacuoles [lysosomes] which acquainted with unprocessed damage mitochondria that subsequently promoted ROS [reactive oxygen species] generation, and resulted releases of Cyt C [cytochrome C] in cytosol that caused caspase-3 dependent apoptosis cell death in ART-treated A549 [lung cancer] cells ... pretreatment of CQ was found to be more effective to increase the potency of artemisinin than co-treatment. (79)

So, it is clear that simultaneous or concurrent use of chloroquine together with artemisinin should be avoided, as this inhibits the cell-killing effects. Rather, as suggested by Dr. Ganguli, it might be appropriate to use the chloroquine drug as a pretreatment. In other words, take the chloroquine during one of the off-days, when the patient is not taking the artemisinin. A typical artemisinin schedule is 14 days on and 4 days off (although this may vary). So, taking the chloroquine during the days off would serve as a pretreatment for the next artemisinin cycle, as suggested by Dr. Ganguli and colleagues. Obviously, this strategy needs more study.

Chloroquine May Augment Standard Chemo-radiation

In 2016, Dr. Steve Pascolo and others suggested that the addition of chloroquine to standard chemo-radiation protocols would potentiate current anti-cancer treatments. (80–83)

Safety and Toxicity of Chloroquine

Used for over 80 years as a treatment for malaria, chloroquine has a long track record of safety in the treatment of rheumatoid arthritis at a dosage of 250 mg daily over a period of years. (84)

The most worrisome toxicity relates to ocular and macular toxicity at high doses over long periods of time. Examination by an eye specialist (ophthalmologist) every 6–12 months is recommended. The eye exam should include testing color vision and visual fields. (85)

The use of a small dose of 250 mg of chloroquine once a week prior to the start of a 5-day course of artemisinin is considerably less than usual chloroquine dosage for rheumatologic disease, and therefore considered safe. Usual chloroquine dosage for traveler's prevention of malaria is one 500 mg tablet once a week starting one week before departure and continuing for 4 weeks after returning. Although higher doses may have retinal toxicity, typical prophylactic doses are considered not harmful to the retina. (86)

Sequential, Not Concurrent

Sequential, and not concurrent, use of chloroquine might ultimately prove to be effective for augmenting the anti-cancer effect of artemisinin. I would like to see mouse xenograft tumor-validation studies of this combination. However, as far as I know, these types of in vivo studies have not been done. This would be a good subject for NIH funding of future research. (79–83)

Mefloquine (Lariam)

In 1992, Drs. Hans Glaumann, Anne-Marie Motakefi, and Helena Jansson studied the intracellular distribution of mefloquine in rat liver. Mefloquine caused expansion of lysosomes in rat livers starting at 24 hours after administration and lasting for 7 days. The lysosomes later harbored multi-lamellar bodies that disappeared after 7–10 days. Dr. Hans Glaumann et al. concluded:

1) mefloquine is a lysosomotropic drug that accumulates in lysosomes;

2) mefloquine impairs lipid degradation with ensuing accumulation of lipids in lysosomes; and

3) lysosomal trapping explains the high-volume distribution of mefloquine. (87)

Mefloquine Superiority to Chloroquine

In a 2012 breast cancer cell study, Dr. Natasha Sharma et al. found mefloquine superior to chloroquine for causing cancer cell death. (88)

In 2013, Dr. Mahdeo Sukhai et al. screened a library of 100 drugs (on- and off-patent) for activity against AML. At the top of the activity list was ivermectin; the second most active was the antimalarial drug mefloquine, which selectively killed a panel of leukemia cells and leukemia stem cells in mice. Dr. Sukhai et al. wrote:

Mefloquine specifically targets lysosomal function. This finding is consistent with mefloquine's known ability to preferentially accumulate in lysosomes of the malarial parasite…. Mefloquine directly disrupted lysosomes isolated from AML [Acute Myelogenous Leukemia] cell lines

...ary AML patients' samples. AML ...ave increased lysosomal mass com-...ared with normal hematopoietic cells.... Serum concentrations of mefloquine up to 5 μM have been reported in individuals receiving 250 mg weekly for malaria prophylaxis. Thus, antileukemia concentrations of mefloquine may be pharmacologically achievable.... as it involves induction of lysosome disruption, the mechanism of action of mefloquine appears distinct from that of chloroquine and other inhibitors of autophagy. (89)

Mefloquin-Malaria Prophylaxis for Travelers

Mefloquin is currently recommended for malaria prophylaxis in travelers. Dosage is usually a 250 mg tablet per week for a few weeks prior to the trip.

Toxicity

Mefloquin may be associated with neuro-psychiatric adverse effects. Artemisinin in combination with mefloquine has been effective antimalaria treatment for decades; however long-term use can result in neurotoxicity, so caution is advised. (90–91)

The antimalaria combination of chloroquine and artesunate (artemisinin derivative), although considered safe, was found to provide no benefit above chloroquine monotherapy and is no longer considered useful in this combination. (92)

Artemisinin Synergy with Rituximab, Lenalidamide

The anti-CD-20 monoclonal antibody, rituximab, has revolutionized the treatment of lymphoma by targeting the CD20 protein on B-cell lymphoma membranes and increasing response and survival rates. Most lymphoma patients receive rituximab, either combined with chemotherapy or as a stand-alone treatment at some point. Artemisinin has good synergism with rituximab, with increased anti-cancer activity. Dr. Sebastian Seiber et al. (2009) write that "both agents act synergistically by activating at least partially converging signaling pathways." (93)

Artemisinin Synergy with Lenalidamide and Venetoclax

In 2011, Drs. W. M. Liu, et al. reported impressive enhancement of anti-cancer activity with the combination of artesunate and the new immunomodulatory drug lenalidamide. (94)

In 2017, working with leukemia in vitro and in vivo, Dr. Bijender Kumar et al. found artemisinin synergy with the BCL-2 inhibitor venetoclax (ABT-199). **Note:** BCL-2 is the anti-apoptotic protein that immortalizes the cancer cell. (95)

Combination of Artesunate and Captopril Synergistic

Captopril is an old, off-patent anti-hypertensive (blood pressure) pill that inhibits the angiotensin I-converting enzyme (ACE), also called an ACE inhibitor. In 2013, Dr. Krusche found synergistic inhibition of angiogenesis by artesunate and captopril, inhibiting growth of new blood vessels in the tumor micro-environment. (96)

Artemisinin Safety and Toxicity

In 2008, Dr. Uma Malhotra et al. reported that a 52-year-old male developed drug induced hepatitis with marked elevation of liver enzymes after taking an herbal capsule of artemisinin 200 mg, three times a day for 10 days. Although this appears to be a rare complication, it would be prudent to monitor liver enzymes in patients on long-term treatment. (97)

Neurotoxicity of the more potent artemisinin derivatives has been reported in studies using animals (dogs and mice). Anecdotal reports of cerebellar toxicity (ataxia and slurred speech) have been reported in humans. (98–99)

In spite of this, the remarkable safety of artemisinin was demonstrated in the year 2000 with a study of 242 Vietnamese human subjects who showed no brain stem adverse effects after multiple courses of artemisinin (or its derivatives) for malaria treatment. (100)

Another study, looking at post mortem neuropathology, also found no evidence of neurotoxic effects. (101)

Toxicity in Combination with DCA Dichloroacetate

In 2016, Dr. Martin Uhl et al. reported a case of a glioblastoma patient with fatal liver failure and bone marrow toxicity after combined use of DCA with artesunate. (102) Since this is only one case report, it is difficult to say if this combination should be avoided altogether or if one should simply use more caution when using this combination. Hopefully, further studies of the DCA / artesunate combination will answer this question. See chapter 5 on Dichloroacetate.

Reproductive Toxicity of Artesunate

In a 2011 study by Dr. Stephen Olumide, long-term administration to mice of the more potent artemisinin derivative, artesunate, induced reversible infertility, with reduced sperm counts. Another study in 2015 by Dr. Supriya Singh showed artesunate caused DNA sperm damage. (103–104)

Cannabinoid Extracts Have Anti-Cancer Activity

Cannabis extracts have a long history of beneficial use in chemotherapy patients for relief of nausea and stimulation of appetite effects. There is also a pain relief effect from cannabis extracts. Is there synergism and augmentation of anti-cancer effects with cannabis extracts and artemisinin compounds? Taken in combination, would cannabis extracts increase the anti-cancer effect of artemisinin? This would be a good topic for NIH funding of future research. For more on Cannabis, see Chapter 19. (105)

Ivermectin (Stromectol for Humans and Ivomec for Dogs)

The 2015 Nobel Prize in Medicine was awarded to William C. Campbell and Satoshi Ōmura for discovery of the "wonder drug from Japan," ivermectin, a well-known antiparasitic agent used to treat billons of pets and livestock around the world. In humans, ivermectin is well known as a treatment for lice (pediculosis) and scabies (mites). Ivermectin also treats

.ch as nematodes, onchocerciasis, ...oidiasis, ascariasis, cutaneous larva ...rans, filariases, gnathostomiasis, and trichuriasis. (106)

In 2010, Dr. Sumaiya Sharmeen et al. screened a library of drugs for cytotoxicity to leukemia cells, finding that ivermectin was a promising anti-leukemic agent producing cell death at low micromolar concentrations. Dr. Sharmeen then studied three mouse models of leukemia showing that tumor growth was delayed "at drug concentrations that appear pharmacologically achievable." Dr. Sharmeen and colleagues reported that ivermectin blocks the glutamate-gated chloride channels, increases intracellular chloride ion concentrations, and increases the size of leukemia cells. This causes plasma membrane hyperpolarization. Ivermectin also increased ROS in cancer cells, which is functionally important for ivermectin-induced cell death. Finally, ivermectin synergized with conventional chemotherapy agents, cytarabine (ara-C) and Adriamycin (the anthracycline drug Daunorubicin) to increase ROS production. (107–108)

Dr. Dobrin Draganov et al. reported in 2015 that ivermectin

> kills mouse and human triple-negative breast cancer [TNBC] cells through augmented P2X7-dependent purinergic signaling associated with caspase-1 and caspase-3 activation.... also involved is the recruitment and activation of T cells, macrophages and dendritic cells, a form of immunomodulation and cancer immunotherapy. (109)

In 2014, Dr. Alice Melotti reported that ivermectin inhibits the Wnt -TCF pathway in cancer cells, further elucidating the molecular mechanism of cancer cell death. Targeting the Wnt pathway successfully eliminated cancer stem cells in a mantle cell lymphoma cell line. (110-111)

In 2014, Dr. Melotti et al. studied ivermectin in a colon cancer cell model, finding it effective at micromolar concentrations against both tumor bulk as well as cancer stem cells. The authors suggested that ivermectin might be useful as a routine prophylactic agent—for instance, against colon cancer in familial polyposis or to prevent nascent cancer in the general aging population. (111)

In 2009, Dr. Hisashi Hashimoto et al. showed ivermectin effective against ovarian cancer cell lines. (112)

Safety and Dosage of Ivermectin

About 200 million people are currently taking ivermectin for the treatment or prevention of a disease called river blindness (onchocerciasis) caused by parasitic worms. In 2011, Drs. Andy Crump and Satoshi Omura wrote that ivermectin is

> astonishingly safe for human use.... Indeed, it is such a safe drug, with minimal side effects, that it can be administered by non-medical staff and even illiterate individuals in remote rural communities. (106)

In 2002, Dr. Cynthia Guzzo studied escalating doses of ivermectin in healthy volunteers, finding no CNS toxicity for Ivermectin doses up to 10 times the highest FDA-approved dose of 200 microg/kg. (120 mg single dose which is

10 times the 12 mg recommended dose). There is better absorption of the drug with higher plasma levels when taken with food. (113)

Ivermectin (Stromectol®) is available in the US in tablet sizes of both 3 mg and 6 mg. Dosage for treatment of head lice (pediculosis) is 200 mcg/kg (12 mgs for a 60kg male).) (114)

Dr. Menno Smit (2016) writes:

Ivermectin has a wide therapeutic index and previous studies have shown doses up to 2000 mcg/kg (ie, 10 times the US Food and Drug Administration approved dose) are well tolerated and safe; the highest dose used for onchocerciasis is a single dose of 800 mcg/kg. (115)

Ivermectin Synergy with Artemisinin?

Ivermectin and artemisinin have been used safely in a treatment for malaria called artemisinin combination therapy (ACT). (116)

Would ivermectin combined with artemisinin provide synergy as anti-cancer treatment? The two agents use differing mechanisms to selectively increase ROS inside the cancer cell. The artemisinin works via the Fenton reaction, the oxidation reaction with iron, while the ivermectin acts on chloride ion channels. Would the two agents enhance each other's cell-killing effects, working in synergy? This would be an excellent topic for future study with NIH funding.

Artemisinin Synergy with Alpha Lipoic Acid?

Alpha lipoic acid (ALA) and artemisinin infusions are commonly given together as part of a comprehensive cancer treatment. Alpha lipoic acid may work in synergy with the artemisinin, causing oxidative damage to mitochondria and inducing mitochondrial apoptosis in the cancer cell.

Artemisinin Wnt Pathway Inhibitor— Targets Cancer Stem Cells

Two studies suggest artemisinin compounds downregulate the Wnt pathway and target cancer stem cells in lung cancer and brain glioma cell models. (117–119)

In a 2007 colorectal cancer cell study by Dr. Lin-Na Li et al., artesunate was found to strongly inhibit the Wnt /Beta-Catenin pathway, suggesting utility as a cancer stem cell agent. (119)

In 2016, Dr. Amit Subedi et al. used high thruput screening to identify artesunate as selective inhibitor of cancer stem cells. Artesunate was found to strongly inhibit the Wnt /Beta-Catenin pathway, suggesting utility as a stem cell agent. Indeed, in 2016, Dr. Subedi and colleagues reported:

High-throughput screening identifies artesunate as selective inhibitor of cancer stemness.... Artesunate induced mitochondrial dysfunction that selectively inhibited cancer stemness of iCSCL [induced cancer stem-like] cells, indicating an essential role of mitochondrial metabolism in cancer stemness. (120)

Again, this suggests a mitochondrial/Wnt pathway/stem cell interaction as described by Dr. Roberto Costa (2019) in *Cell Reports.*

...e (ART) Inhibits Wnt Pathway-...uces SKM Apoptosis ß-catenin

In 2015 Dr. Na Xu et al. studied the effect of artesunate on SKM-1 cells in vitro, a model for myelodysplastic syndrome, and a pre-leukemic condition. Dr. Na Xu's group found that

ART treatment inhibited Wnt/β-catenin downstream expression of targets such as c-myc and cyclinD1. (124)

When SKM-1 cells were treated with artesunate, both β-catenin and E-cadherin translocated from the nucleus to the cell membrane, thereby forming the Beta-Catenin/E-cadherin complex and strengthening cell-cell adhesion. Similar translocation of Beta-Catenin from cell nucleus to outer membrane was seen in a colorectal cancer model after treatment with artesunate as reported by Dr. Lin-Na Li and colleagues in their 2007 study:

Artesunate [ART] attenuates the growth of human colorectal carcinoma and inhibits hyperactive Wnt/Beta-Catenin pathway.... This suggests the anti-cancer activity of Artesunate correlates with inhibition of the hyperactive Wnt /Beta-Catenin pathway.... These results and the known low toxicity are clues that ART might be a promising candidate drug for the treatment of colorectal carcinoma. (125)

Artemisinin—A Potent Anti-Inflammatory Drug

Downregulates Nuclear Factor Kappa B and Inflammatory Cytokines-PI3 kinase/Akt Signal Pathway

Artemisinin is also a potent anti-inflammatory drug with potential use in rheumatoid arthritis and other inflammatory diseases. A number of studies show striking downregulation and inhibition of the major inflammatory transcription factor, NF kappa B (NF-kB) and its downstream signaling proteins, c-Myc and Cyclin D1.

Dr. H. Xu et al. (2007) showed that artesunate

inhibits TNF-α-induced production of pro-inflammatory cytokines IL-1β, IL-6 and IL-8 via inhibition of NF-κB and PI3 kinase/Akt signal pathways in human rheumatoid arthritis fibroblast-like synoviocytes. (121)

A number of new anti-cancer drugs in development, such as buparlisib and Idelalisib target this same PI3 kinase/Akt signal pathway inhibited nicely by artesunate. (122)

Dr. Xu et al. write:

Our results indicate that artesunate **exerts an anti-inflammatory effect** in RA [rheumatoid arthritis] FLS [fibroblast-like synoviocytes] and provide the evidence that artesunate may have therapeutic potential for RA. (121)

Note: FLS = the cells in the lining of the joint which are the target of inflammation in rheumatoid arthritls. (121)

In 2014, Dr. Kalvin Q. Tran et al. studied an endometrial cancer cell model, revealing the exact mechanism of NF-kB inhibition by artemisinin, with prevention of nuclear translocation of NF-kB. The p65 and p50 are subunits of the NF-kB protein residing in the cytosol. Artemisinin prevents p65 and p50 nuclear translocation by interacting with IkB-alpha, the NF-kB inhibitor, leading to a loss of CDK4 gene expression. (123)

Note: CDK4 is Cyclin Dependent Kinase-4, a member of the Cyclin D1 family downstream from Wnt pathway and involved in cell cycle progression. Inhibition of CDK4 blocks rapid cancer cell proliferation and is a valid anticancer strategy.

Artemisinin Anti-Inflammatory Agent

In 2017, Dr. Ka Se Wang et al. also studied the anti-inflammatory effects of artemisinin using a TPA-induced skin inflammation model in mice, showing inhibition of NF-kB. Dr. Wang concluded that "artemisinin may be a potentially useful therapeutic agent for inflammatory-related diseases." (126)

Note: TPA is 12-O-tetradecanoylphorbol-13-acetate, a carcinogenic chemical applied topically to induce skin cancer in mice.

Inflammatory Signals from the Micro-Environment in Mantle Cell Lymphoma

In *Blood* 2012, Dr. Liang Zhang et al. studied the role of the micro-environment in mantle cell lymphoma (MCL). Dr. Zhang's group found that the inflammatory cytokine IL-6 secreted by stromal cells in the micro-environment activated the Jak2/STAT3 and PI3K/Akt pathways in MCL. Downstream from NF-kB, IL-6 is a key cytokine for MCL growth and survival,

and inhibiting NF-kB with ART serves to inhibit IL-6 production by stromal cells in the TME. This provides a beneficial anticancer effect, with inhibition of cancer cell growth, increase in apoptosis, and greater chemo-sensitivity of cancer cells. (127)

Dr. Raymond Lai et al. report in *J Pathology* (2003) that STAT3 (signal transducer and activator of transcription 3) is the signal transducer of IL-10, another cytokine that is upregulated in the tumor micro-environment, and this STAT3/IL-10 increases proliferation in mantle cell lymphoma. Since STAT3 is a downstream effector of IL-6, inhibiting NF-kB/IL-6 (with ART), also inhibits STAT3. (128)

ART enhanced Natural Killer Cell Activity

In 2017, Dr. Youn Kyung Houh found that artemisinin exerts potent anti-cancer effects by upregulating the host immune system by "enhancing human NK (Natural Killer) cell cytotoxicity and degranulation."(129)

Artesunate Best Inhibitor of STAT3

In 2016, Dr. Ilamathi et al. studied the effects of artesunate on a hepatocellular cancer line, finding inhibition of STAT3. (130)

In 2017, Dr. Mei Tan et al. wrote in *Leukemia Research*: "Artesunate induces apoptosis via inhibition of STAT3 in THP-1 (leukemia) cells." (131)

In 2017, Dr. Mei Tan and colleagues found that 30 leukemia patients had significantly increased STAT3 protein levels compared to controls. Artesunate downregulated STAT3, increased apoptosis, and significantly inhibited

...tion of leukemia cells in a mouse ...ic model. (131)

...imilarly, in a hepatocellular cancer mouse model, Artesunate obliterated the cancer by suppressing IL-6-JAK-STAT signaling. (132–133)

FDA Restricting Artesunate in the U.S.

Although IV artesunate 60 mg vials are widely used as first-line malaria treatment in Third World areas, inside the U.S. this drug is neither FDA approved nor commercially available. The drug has been made available, however, through an investigational new drug application (IND). Drs. Phillip Rosenthal and Katherine Tan discuss the distress and confusion encountered by physicians in the U.S. when trying to treat a malaria patient with IV artesunate in a timely fashion: (134)

> Not having artesunate as a readily available first-line treatment for severe malaria caused some distress and confusion among American providers, who questioned why the international standard of care to treat severe malaria was not routinely available in the United States ... The availability of intravenous artesunate for all patients with severe malaria through an IND represents a step in the right direction. It is reassuring that the international standard is now also the clear standard of care in the United States. However, availability through an IND is not a long-term solution. Ideally, commercial availability will allow U.S. hospitals to stock this now first-line treatment. This will require a manufacturer of intravenous artesunate bringing the drug to the FDA for approval. Approval can be anticipated, as the drug has an excellent record

of efficacy and safety around the world. Ultimately, achieving routine availability of intravenous artesunate will improve our ability to treat severe malaria in the United States. (134)

Artesunate for malaria treatment in the U.S. is available by calling the CDC Malaria Hotline (770–488–7788) to request IV artesunate, which will then be sent by overnight air to the patient's hospital. (135) According to the CDC website:

> In the United States, an average of 1,700 cases of malaria are imported each year, of which 300 are severe. As of April 1, 2019, IV artesunate, the WHO-recommended first-line treatment for severe malaria, will become the first-line drug for treatment of severe malaria in the United States. Because IV artesunate is neither FDA-approved nor commercially available in the United States, CDC has made IV artesunate available under an expanded access investigational new drug [IND] protocol. Starting on April 1, 2019, all U.S. clinicians must call CDC [Malaria Hotline] to obtain IV artesunate to treat cases of severe malaria. (136)

Obviously, this "IND protocol" arrangement makes it virtually impossible to treat cancer patients in the U.S. with IV artesunate, a promising nontoxic drug that competes with chemotherapy. A skeptic might suggest this is an intentional effort by the FDA to remove a safe, effective repurposed anti-cancer drug (artesunate) from competing with the chemotherapy paradigm, thus protecting the profits of the pharmaceutical industry. (They would never do that, would they?) Hopefully, in the near future, a public clamor will force the FDA,

CDC, and other government agencies to make artesunate commercially available for acute malaria and allow "off-label use" of artesunate in cancer treatment.

Note: Off-label use is a common prescribing practice by physicians in which FDA approved drugs are prescribed for a medical indication other than originally designated for FDA approval, based on the physician's judgment that the drug is medically appropriate.

Conclusion

In my opinion, with the state of our knowledge of nontoxic targeted agents, malignant cancer is now a curable disease, and suffering or death from cancer should become a thing of the past. We have discussed artemisinin, the Chinese antimalaria drug, which is also a targeted nontoxic anti-cancer agent. The artemisinin Endoperoxide Bridge reacts with iron in the cancer cell to produce oxidative-free radicals, which induce apoptotic pathways. Downregulating the glutathione system with sulfasalazine, allicin (from garlic), feverfew (parthenolide), or sulforaphane (from broccoli) renders the cancer cell more susceptible to oxidative damage from artemisinin and augments the cancer-cell-killing effects. Another useful effect of artesunate is downregulation of NF-kB inflammatory pathways needed for cancer cell proliferation. We have discussed ivermectin, an astonishingly safe drug taken by 200 million people, with potent anti-cancer effects, at micromolar concentrations, for both tumor bulk as well as cancer stem cells. Combinations of these agents may prove useful, and should be funded for future NIH research. The cancer patient of today may not have the luxury of time, and may be inclined to proceed before prospective randomized studies are completed. Indeed, prospective randomized trials may never be forthcoming due to the nature of the drug discovery and approval system in the U.S. (137-160)

Even though artemisinin and co-agents are considered relatively safe, there may be toxicity at higher dosage, and the user must remain vigilant and reduce dosage should toxicity occur. It is recommended that you work closely with a knowledgeable clinician.

Credit and thanks go to Robert Jay Rowen, MD, who brought artemisinin to my attention in a 2002 article in *Townsend Letter*: "Artemisinin: From Malaria to Cancer Treatment."

Thanks also to Stephen Levine, PhD, founder of Allergy Research Group for introducing high-quality artemisinin products for the general public.

References for Chapter 21: Artemisinin

1) Krishna, Sanjeev, et al. "A randomised, double blind, placebo-controlled pilot study of oral artesunate therapy for colorectal cancer." EBioMedicine 2.1 (2015): 82-90.

2) Augustin, Yolanda, et al. "The wisdom of crowds and the repurposing of artesunate as an anticancer drug." ecancermedicalscience 9 (2015).

3) Das, A. K. "Anticancer effect of antimalarial artemisinin compounds." Annals of medical and health sciences research 5.2 (2015): 93-102.

4) Mercer, Amy E., et al. "The role of heme and the mitochondrion in the chemical and molecular mechanisms of mammalian cell death induced by

the artemisinin antimalarials." Journal of Biological Chemistry 286.2 (2011): 987-996.

5) Robert, Anne, Jérôme Cazelles, and Bernard Meunier. "Characterization of the alkylation product of heme by the antimalarial drug artemisinin." Angewandte Chemie International Edition 40.10 (2001): 1954-1957.

6) Kwok, Juliana C., and Des R. Richardson. "The iron metabolism of neoplastic cells: alterations that facilitate proliferation?" Critical Reviews in Oncology/Hematology 42.1 (2002): 65-78.

7) Lepelletier, Yves, et al. "Prevention of mantle lymphoma tumor establishment by routing transferrin receptor toward lysosomal compartments." Cancer research 67.3 (2007): 1145-1154.

8) Obrador-Hevia, Antònia, et al. "Molecular biology of mantle cell lymphoma: from profiling studies to new therapeutic strategies." Blood reviews 23.5 (2009): 205-216.

9) Efferth, Thomas, et al. "Enhancement of cytotoxicity of artemisinins toward cancer cells by ferrous iron." Free Radical Biology and Medicine 37.7 (2004): 998-1009.

10) Wang, Jigang, et al. "Mechanistic investigation of the specific anticancer property of artemisinin and its combination with aminolevulinic acid for enhanced anticolorectal cancer activity." ACS central science 3.7 (2017): 743-750.

11) Haider, Sameah A., et al. "The impact of 5-aminolevulinic acid on extent of resection in newly diagnosed high grade gliomas: a systematic review and single institutional experience." Journal of neuro-oncology 141.3 (2019): 507-515.

12) Xu, X. F., et al. "Effects of sodium ferrous chlorophyll treatment on anemia of hemodialysis patients and relevant biochemical parameters." Journal of biological regulators and homeostatic agents 30.1 (2016): 135-140.

13) Yang, Nai-Di, et al. "Artesunate induces cell death in human cancer cells via enhancing lysosomal function and lysosomal degradation of ferritin." Journal of Biological Chemistry 289.48 (2014): 33425-33441.

14) Hu, Wei, et al. "Dihydroartemisinin induces autophagy by suppressing NF-κB activation." Cancer letters 343.2 (2014): 239-248.

15) Wang, Zeng, et al. "Dihydroartemisinin induces autophagy and inhibits the growth of iron-loaded human myeloid leukemia K562 cells via ROS toxicity." FEBS open bio 2 (2012): 103-112.

16) Chen, Kai, et al. "Artesunate induces G2/M cell cycle arrest through autophagy induction in breast cancer cells." Anti-cancer drugs 25.6 (2014): 652-662.

17) O'Neill, Paul M., Victoria E. Barton, and Stephen A. Ward. "The molecular mechanism of action of artemisinin—the debate continues." Molecules 15.3 (2010): 1705-1721.

18) Xie, Y., et al. "Ferroptosis: process and function." Cell Death & Differentiation (2016).

19) Ooko, E., et al. "Artemisinin derivatives induce iron-dependent cell death (ferroptosis) in tumor cells." Phytomedicine: international journal of phytotherapy and phytopharmacology 22.11 (2015): 1045.

20) Hamacher-Brady, Anne, et al. "Artesunate Activates Mitochondrial Apoptosis in Breast Cancer Cells via Iron-catalyzed Lysosomal Reactive Oxygen Species Production." J. Biol. Chem 2011.286 (2010): 6587-6601.

21) Korolchuk, Viktor I., et al. "Lysosomal positioning coordinates cellular nutrient responses." Nature cell biology 13.4 (2011): 453-460.

22) Piao, Shengfu, and Ravi K. Amaravadi. "Targeting the lysosome in cancer." Annals of the New York Academy of Sciences 1371.1 (2016): 45.

23) Davidson, Shawn M., and Matthew G. Vander Heiden. "Critical functions of the lysosome in cancer biology." Annual review of pharmacology and toxicology 57 (2017): 481-507.

24) Nakase, Ikuhiko, et al. "Anticancer properties of artemisinin derivatives and their targeted delivery by transferrin conjugation." International journal of pharmaceutics 354.1-2 (2008): 28-33.

25) Kundu, Chanakya Nath, et al. "Anti-malarials are anti-cancers and vice versa—One arrow two sparrows." Acta tropica 149 (2015): 113-127.

26) Nandakumar, Dalavaikodihalli Nanjaiah, et al. "Curcumin-artemisinin combination therapy for malaria." Antimicrobial agents and chemotherapy 50.5 (2006): 1859-1860.

27) Hasanali, Zainul, Kamal Sharma, and Elliot Epner. "Flipping the cyclin D1 switch in mantle cell lymphoma." Best Practice & Research Clinical Haematology 25.2 (2012): 143-152.

28) Vallianou, Natalia G., et al. "Potential anticancer properties and mechanisms of action of curcumin." Anticancer research 35.2 (2015): 645-651.

29) Shanmugam, Muthu K., et al. "The multifaceted role of curcumin in cancer prevention and treatment." Molecules 20.2 (2015): 2728-2769.

30) Willenbacher, Ella, et al. "Curcumin: new insights into an ancient ingredient against cancer." International journal of molecular sciences 20.8 (2019): 1808.

31) Guamán Ortiz, Luis Miguel, et al. "Berberine, an epiphany against cancer." Molecules 19.8 (2014): 12349-12367.

32) Li, Peichun, et al. "Synergic effects of artemisinin and resveratrol in cancer cells." Journal of cancer research and clinical oncology 140.12 (2014): 2065-2075.

33) Chen, Rong-Jane, et al. "Apoptotic and nonapoptotic activities of pterostilbene against cancer." International journal of molecular sciences 19.1 (2018): 287.

34) Zhang, Lingling, et al. "Targeting cancer stem cells and signaling pathways by resveratrol and pterostilbene." Biofactors 44.1 (2018): 61-68.

35) Tolomeo, Manlio, et al. "Pterostilbene and 3'-hydroxypterostilbene are effective apoptosis-inducing agents in MDR and BCR-ABL-expressing leukemia cells." The international journal of biochemistry & cell biology 37.8 (2005): 1709-1726.

36) Jiang, Wei, et al. "The synergistic anticancer effect of artesunate combined with allicin in osteosarcoma cell line in vitro and in vivo." Asian Pacific Journal of Cancer Prevention 14.8 (2013): 465-4619.

37) Padilla-Camberos, Eduardo, et al. "Antitumoral activity of allicin in murine lymphoma L5178Y." Asian Pac J Cancer Prev 11.5 (2010): 1241-4.

38) Talib, Wamidh H. "Melatonin and cancer hallmarks." Molecules 23.3 (2018): 518.

39) Di Bella, Giuseppe, et al. "Melatonin anticancer effects." International journal of molecular sciences 14.2 (2013): 2410-2430.

40) Trubiani, Oriana, et al. "Melatonin provokes cell death in human B-lymphoma cells by mitochondrial-dependent apoptotic pathway activation." Journal of pineal research 39.4 (2005): 425-431.

41) Sánchez-Hidalgo, Marina, et al. "Melatonin inhibits cell proliferation and induces caspase activation and apoptosis in human malignant lymphoid cell lines." Journal of pineal research 53.4 (2012): 366-373.

42) Gerhardt, Thomas, et al. "Effects of antioxidants and pro-oxidants on cytotoxicity of dihydroartemisinin to Molt-4 human leukemia cells." Anticancer research 35.4 (2015): 1867-1871.

43) Li, Yanyan, et al. "Sulforaphane, a dietary component of broccoli/broccoli sprouts, inhibits breast cancer stem cells." Clinical Cancer Research 16.9 (2010): 2580-2590.

44) Singh, Narendra, and Lai, Henry. "Synergistic cytotoxicity of artemisinin and sodium butyrate on human cancer cells." Anticancer research 25.6B (2005): 4325-4331.

45) Pajak, B., A. Orzechowski, and B. Gajkowska. "Molecular basis of sodium butyrate-dependent proapoptotic activity in cancer cells." Advances in Medical Sciences (De Gruyter Open) 52 (2007).

46) Fauser, Jane Kathryn. Medium Chain Fatty Acids and Wnt/β-Catenin Inhibitors as Adjunctive Colorectal Cancer Chemotherapeutic Agents. Diss. The University of Adelaide, 2012.

47) Choi, Yung Hyun. "Apoptosis of U937 human leukemic cells by sodium butyrate is associated with inhibition of telomerase activity." International journal of oncology 29.5 (2006): 1207-1213.

48) Heider, Ulrike, et al. "Histone deacetylase inhibitors reduce VEGF production and induce growth suppression and apoptosis in human mantle cell lymphoma." European journal of haematology 76.1 (2006): 42-50.

49) Yu, Zuoren, et al. "Cancer stem cells." The international journal of biochemistry & cell biology 44.12 (2012): 2144-2151.

50) Pardal, Ricardo, Michael F. Clarke, and Sean J. Morrison. "Applying the principles of stem-cell biology to cancer." Nature Reviews Cancer 3.12 (2003): 895.

51) Hsieh, Hsiu-Mei, et al. "Berberine-containing pharmaceutical composition for inhibiting cancer stem cell growth or carcinoma metastasis and application thereof." U.S. Patent Application No. 14/790,154.

52) Guzman, Monica L., et al. "The sesquiterpene lactone parthenolide induces apoptosis of human acute myelogenous leukemia stem and progenitor cells." Blood 105.11 (2005): 4163-4169.

53) Li, Xue, et al. "Parthenolide inhibits ubiquitin-specific peptidase 7 (USP7), Wnt signaling, and colorectal cancer cell growth." Journal of Biological Chemistry 295.11 (2020): 3576-3589.

54) Araújo, Thaise Gonçalves, et al. "Parthenolide and Its Analogues: A New Potential Strategy for the Treatment of Triple-Negative Breast Tumors." Current medicinal chemistry (2020).

55) Dawood, Mona, Edna Ooko, and Thomas Efferth. "Collateral sensitivity of parthenolide via NF-κB and HIF-α inhibition and epigenetic changes in drug-resistant cancer cell lines." Frontiers in pharmacology 10 (2019): 542.

56) Gunn, Ellen J., et al. "The natural products parthenolide and andrographolide exhibit anti-cancer stem cell activity in multiple myeloma." Leukemia & lymphoma 52.6 (2011): 1085-1097.

57) Pajak, Beata, Barbara Gajkowska, and Arkadiusz Orzechowski. "Molecular basis of parthenolide-dependent proapoptotic activity in cancer cells." Folia histochemica et cytobiologica 46.2 (2008): 129-135.

58) Pei, Shanshan, et al. "Targeting aberrant glutathione metabolism to eradicate human acute myelogenous leukemia cells." Journal of Biological Chemistry 288.47 (2013): 33542-33558.

59) Bennaceur-Griscelli, Annelise, et al. "High level of glutathione-S-transferase π expression in mantle cell lymphomas." Clinical cancer research 10.9 (2004): 3029-3034.

60) Zhou, Jianbiao, and Wee-Joo Chng. "Identification and targeting leukemia stem cells: The path to the cure for acute myeloid leukemia." World J Stem Cells 6.4 (2014): 473-484.

61) Sestili, Piero, and Carmela Fimognari. "Cytotoxic and Antitumor Activity of Sulforaphane: The Role of Reactive Oxygen Species." BioMed Research International 2015 (2015).

62) Fimognari C., Turrini E., Sestili P., et al. Antileukemic activity of sulforaphane in primary blasts from patients affected by myelo- and lympho-proliferative disorders and in hypoxic conditions. PLoS ONE. 2014; 9(7)

63) Shang, Hung-Sheng, et al. "Sulforaphane-induced apoptosis in human leukemia HL-60 cells through extrinsic and intrinsic signal pathways and altering associated genes expression assayed by cDNA microarray." Environmental toxicology (2016).

64) Li, Yanyan, et al. "Sulforaphane, a dietary component of broccoli/broccoli sprouts, inhibits breast cancer stem cells." Clinical Cancer Research 16.9 (2010): 2580-2590.

65) Li, Y., and T. Zhang. "Targeting cancer stem cells with sulforaphane, a dietary component from broccoli and broccoli sprouts." Future oncology (London, England) 9.8 (2013): 1097-1103.

66) Rodova, Mariana, et al. "Sonic hedgehog signaling inhibition provides opportunities for targeted therapy by sulforaphane in regulating pancreatic cancer stem cell self-renewal." PloS one 7.9 (2012): e46083.

67) Ishimoto, Takatsugu, et al. "CD44 variant regulates redox status in cancer cells by stabilizing the xCT subunit of system xc– and thereby promotes tumor growth." Cancer cell 19.3 (2011): 387-400.

68) Lewerenz, Jan, et al. "The cystine/glutamate antiporter system xc– in health and disease: from molecular mechanisms to novel therapeutic opportunities." Antioxidants & redox signaling 18.5 (2013): 522-555.

71) Gout, P. W., et al. "Sulfasalazine, a potent suppressor of lymphoma growth by inhibition of the x c-cystine transporter: a new action for an old drug." Leukemia (08876924) 15.10 (2001).

70) Doxsee, Daniel W., et al. "Sulfasalazine-induced cystine starvation: Potential use for prostate cancer therapy." The Prostate 67.2 (2007): 162-171.

71) Chung, W. Joon, and Harald Sontheimer. "Sulfasalazine inhibits the growth of primary brain tumors independent of nuclear factor-κB." Journal of neurochemistry 110.1 (2009): 182-193.

72) Guan, Jun, et al. "The x c– cystine/glutamate antiporter as a potential therapeutic target for small-cell lung cancer: use of sulfasalazine." Cancer chemotherapy and pharmacology 64.3 (2009): 463-472.

73) Dixon, Scott J., et al. "Pharmacological inhibition of cystine–glutamate exchange induces endoplasmic reticulum stress and ferroptosis." Elife 3 (2014): e02523.

74) Narang, Vishal S., et al. "Sulfasalazine-induced reduction of glutathione levels in breast cancer cells: enhancement of growth-inhibitory activity of doxorubicin." Chemotherapy 53.3 (2007): 210-217

75) Bebb, G., et al. "Sulfasalazine, inhibits growth of mantle cell lymphoma (MCL) cell cultures via cyst (e) ine starvation and delays tumour growth in a newly developed murine MCL model." BLOOD. Vol. 102. No. 11. (2003).

76) Gout, Peter W. "In vitro studies on the lymphoma growth-inhibitory activity of sulfasalazine." Anticancer drugs 14.1 (2003): 21-29.

77) Guan, Jun, et al. "The x c– cystine/glutamate antiporter as a potential therapeutic target for small-cell lung cancer: use of sulfasalazine." Cancer chemotherapy and pharmacology 64.3 (2009): 463-472.

78) Lo, M., et al. "Potential use of the anti-inflammatory drug, sulfasalazine, for targeted therapy of pancreatic cancer." Current Oncology 17.3 (2010): 9-16.

79) Ganguli, Arnab, et al. "Inhibition of autophagy by chloroquine potentiates synergistically anti-cancer property of artemisinin by promoting ROS dependent apoptosis." Biochimie 107 (2014): 338-349.

80) Solomon, V. Raja, and Hoyun Lee. "Chloroquine and its analogs: a new promise of an old drug for effective and safe cancer therapies." European journal of pharmacology 625.1 (2009): 220-233.

81) Kimura, Tomonori, et al. Chloroquine in cancer therapy: a double-edged sword of autophagy." Cancer research 73.1 (2013): 3-7.

82) Pascolo, Steve. "Time to use a dose of chloroquine as an adjuvant to anti-cancer chemotherapies." European journal of pharmacology 771 (2016): 139-144.

83) Geng, Ying, et al. "Chloroquine-induced autophagic vacuole accumulation and cell death in glioma cells is p53 independent." Neuro-oncology 12.5 (2010): 473-481.

84) Bagnall, Arthur W. "The value of chloroquine in rheumatoid disease: a four-year study of continuous therapy." Canadian Medical Association Journal 77.3 (1957): 182.

85) Marmor MF, Kellner U, Lai TY, Melles RB, Mieler WF, American Academy of Ophthalmology. Recommendations on Screening for Chloroquine and Hydroxychloroquine Retinopathy (2016 Revision). Ophthalmology. 2016 Jun. 123 (6):1386-94

86) Juckett, Gregory. "Malaria prevention in travelers." American family physician 59.9 (1999): 2523-30.

87) Glaumann, Hans, Anne-Marie Motakefi, and Helena Jansson. "Intracellular distribution and effect of the antimalarial drug mefloquine on lysosomes of rat liver." Liver 12.4 (1992): 183-190.

88) Sharma, Natasha, et al. "Inhibition of autophagy and induction of breast cancer cell death by mefloquine, an antimalarial agent." Cancer letters 326.2 (2012): 143-154.

89) Sukhai, Mahadeo A., et al. "Lysosomal disruption preferentially targets acute myeloid leukemia cells and progenitors." Journal of Clinical Investigation 123.1 (2013): 315.

90) Hoglund, Richard M., Ronnatrai Ruengweerayut, and Kesara Na-Bangchang. "Population pharmacokinetics of mefloquine given as a 3-day artesunate–mefloquine in patients with acute uncomplicated Plasmodium falciparum malaria in a multidrug-resistant area along the Thai–Myanmar border." Malaria journal 17.1 (2018): 322.

91) de Lima, Daniely Alves, et al. "Safety assessment of MEFAS: an innovative hybrid salt of mefloquine and artesunate for malaria treatment." Drug and chemical toxicology (2019): 1-6.

92) Kofoed, Poul-Erik, et al. "No benefits from combining chloroquine with artesunate for three days

for treatment of Plasmodium falciparum in Guinea-Bissau." Transactions of the Royal Society of Tropical Medicine and Hygiene 97.4 (2003): 429-433.

93) Sieber, Sebastian, et al. "Combination treatment of malignant B cells using the anti-CD20 antibody rituximab and the anti-malarial artesunate." International journal of oncology 35.1 (2009): 149-158.

94) Liu, W. M., A. M. Gravett, and A. G. Dalgleish. "The antimalarial agent artesunate possesses anticancer properties that can be enhanced by combination strategies." International journal of cancer 128.6 (2011): 1471-1480.

95) Kumar, Bijender, et al. "Antileukemic activity and cellular effects of the antimalarial agent artesunate in acute myeloid leukemia." Leukemia Research (2017).

96) Krusche, Benjamin, Joachim Arend, and Thomas Efferth. "Synergistic inhibition of angiogenesis by artesunate and captopril in vitro and in vivo." Evidence-Based Complementary and Alternative Medicine. (2013).

97) Malhotra, U., et al. "Hepatitis temporally associated with an herbal supplement containing artemisinin-Washington, 2008." Morbidity and Mortality Weekly Report 58.31 (2009): 854-856.

98) Brewer, Thomas G., et al. "Fatal neurotoxicity of arteether and artemether." The American journal of tropical medicine and hygiene 51.3 (1994): 251-259.

99) Miller, Loren G., and Claire B. Panosian. "Ataxia and slurred speech after artesunate treatment for falciparum malaria." New England Journal of Medicine 336.18 (1997): 1328-1329.

100) Kissinger, E., et al. "Clinical and neurophysiological study of the effects of multiple doses of artemisinin on brain-stem function in Vietnamese patients." The American journal of tropical medicine and hygiene 63.1 (2000): 48-55.

101) Hien, T. T., et al. "Neuropathological assessment of artemether-treated severe malaria." The Lancet 362.9380 (2003): 295-296.

102) Uhl, Martin, Stefan Schwab, and Thomas Efferth. "Fatal liver and bone marrow toxicity by combination treatment of dichloroacetate and artesunate in a glioblastoma multiforme patient: case report and review of the literature." Frontiers in oncology 6 (2016): 204.

103) Olumide, Stephen Akinsomisoye, and Yinusa Raji. "Long-term administration of artesunate induces reproductive toxicity in male rats." Journal of reproduction & infertility 12.4 (2011): 249.

104) Singh, Supriya, Anirudha Giri, and Sarbani Giri. "The antimalarial agent artesunate causes sperm DNA damage and hepatic antioxidant defense in mice." Mutation Research/Genetic Toxicology and Environmental Mutagenesis 777 (2015): 1-6.

105) Chakravarti B, Ravi J, Ganju RK. Cannabinoids as therapeutic agents in cancer: current status and future implications. Oncotarget. 2014; 5(15):5852-5872.

106) Crump, Andy, and Satoshi Omura. "Ivermectin, 'Wonder Drug'from Japan: the human use perspective." Proceedings of the Japan Academy, Series B 87.2 (2011): 13-28.

107) Sharmeen, Sumaiya, et al. "The antiparasitic agent ivermectin induces chloride-dependent membrane hyperpolarization and cell death in leukemia cells." Blood 116.18 (2010): 3593-3603.

108) Furusawa, Shinobu, et al. "Potentiation of Doxorubicin-Induced Apoptosis of Resistant Mouse Leukaemia Cells by Ivermectin." Pharmacy and Pharmacology Communications 6.3 (2000): 129-134.

109) Draganov, Dobrin, et al. "Modulation of P2X4/P2X7/pannexin-1 sensitivity to extracellular ATP via ivermectin induces a non-apoptotic and inflammatory form of cancer cell death." Scientific reports 5 (2015).

110) Mathur, Rohit, et al. "Targeting Wnt pathway in mantle cell lymphoma-initiating cells." Journal of hematology & oncology 8.1 (2015): 63.

111) Melotti, Alice, et al. "The river blindness drug Ivermectin and related macrocyclic lactones inhibit WNT-TCF pathway responses in human cancer." EMBO molecular medicine (2014): e201404084.

112) Hashimoto, Hisashi, et al. "Ivermectin inactivates the kinase PAK1 and blocks the PAK1-dependent growth of human ovarian cancer and NF2 tumor cell lines." Drug discoveries & therapeutics 3.6 (2009). Ivermectin inactivates blocks kinase PAK1 Ovarian Cancer Hashimoto 2009

113) Guzzo, Cynthia A., et al. "Safety, tolerability, and pharmacokinetics of escalating high doses of

ivermectin in healthy adult subjects." The Journal of Clinical Pharmacology 42.10 (2002): 1122-1133.

114) Chhaiya, Sunita B., Dimple S. Mehta, and Bhaven C. Kataria. "Ivermectin: pharmacology and therapeutic applications." Int J Basic Clin Pharmacol 1.3 (2012): 132-139.

115) Smit, Menno R., et al. "Efficacy and safety of high-dose ivermectin for reducing malaria transmission (IVERMAL): protocol for a double-blind, randomized, placebo-controlled, dose-finding trial in Western Kenya." JMIR research protocols 5.4 (2016): e213.

116) Chaccour, Carlos J., et al. "Ivermectin to reduce malaria transmission: a research agenda for a promising new tool for elimination." Malaria journal 12.1 (2013): 153.

117) Tong, Yunli, et al. "Artemisinin and its derivatives can significantly inhibit lung tumorigenesis and tumor metastasis through Wnt/β-catenin signaling." Oncotarget 7.21 (2016): 31413.

118) Cao, Liu, et al. "Dihydroartemisinin exhibits anti-glioma stem cell activity through inhibiting p-AKT and activating caspase-3." Die Pharmazie-An International Journal of Pharmaceutical Sciences 69.10 (2014): 752-758.

119) Li, Lin-Na, et al. "Artesunate attenuates the growth of human colorectal carcinoma and inhibits hyperactive Wnt/β-catenin pathway." International journal of cancer 121.6 (2007): 1360-1365.

120) Subedi, Amit, et al. "High-throughput screening identifies artesunate as selective inhibitor of cancer stemness: Involvement of mitochondrial metabolism." Biochemical and Biophysical Research Communications 4.477 (2016): 737-742.

121) Xu, H., et al. "Anti-malarial agent artesunate inhibits TNF-α-induced production of proinflammatory cytokines via inhibition of NF-κB and PI3 kinase/Akt signal pathway in human rheumatoid arthritis fibroblast-like synoviocytes." (2007): 920-926.

122) Massacesi, Cristian, et al. "PI3K inhibitors as new cancer therapeutics: implications for clinical trial design." OncoTargets and therapy 9 (2016): 203.

123) Tran, Kalvin Q., Antony S. Tin, and Gary L. Firestone. "Artemisinin triggers a G1 cell cycle arrest of human Ishikawa endometrial cancer cells and

inhibits Cyclin Dependent Kinase-4 promoter activity and expression by disrupting NF-kB transcriptional signaling." Anti-cancer drugs 25.3 (2014): 270.

124) Xu, Na, et al. "Artesunate Induces SKM-1 Cells Apoptosis by Inhibiting Hyperactive β-catenin Signaling Pathway." International journal of medical sciences 12.6 (2015): 524.

125) Li, Lin-Na, et al. "Artesunate attenuates the growth of human colorectal carcinoma and inhibits hyperactive Wnt/β-catenin pathway." International journal of cancer 121.6 (2007): 1360-1365.

126) Wang, Ke Si, et al. "Artemisinin inhibits inflammatory response via regulating NF-κB and MAPK signaling pathways." Immunopharmacology and immunotoxicology 39.1 (2017): 28-36.

127) Zhang, Liang, et al. "Role of the microenvironment in mantle cell lymphoma: IL-6 is an important survival factor for the tumor cells." Blood 120.18 (2012): 3783-3792.

128) Lai, Raymond, et al. "Expression of STAT3 and its phosphorylated forms in mantle cell lymphoma cell lines and tumours." The Journal of Pathology: A Journal of the Pathological Society of Great Britain and Ireland 199.1 (2003): 84-89.

129) Houh, Youn Kyung, et al. "The Effects of Artemisinin on the Cytolytic Activity of Natural Killer (NK) Cells." International Journal of Molecular Sciences 18.7 (2017): 1600.

130) Ilamathi, M., S. Santhosh, and V. Sivaramakrishnan. "Artesunate as an Anti-Cancer Agent Targets Stat-3 and Favorably Suppresses Hepatocellular Carcinoma." Current topics in medicinal chemistry 16.22 (2016): 2453-2463.

131) Tan, Mei, et al. "Artesunate induces apoptosis via inhibition of STAT3 in THP-1 cells." Leukemia Research (2017).Leuk Res. 2017 Nov; 62:98-103.

132) Ilamathi, M., et al. "Artesunate obliterates experimental hepatocellular carcinoma in rats through suppression of IL-6-JAK-STAT signalling." Biomedecine & pharmacotherapie 82 (2016): 72.

133) Ilamathi, M., S. Santhosh, and V. Sivaramakrishnan. "Artesunate as an Anti-Cancer Agent Targets Stat-3 and Favorably Suppresses Hepatocellular Carcinoma."

Current topics in medicinal chemistry 16.22 (2016): 2453-2463.

134) Rosenthal, Philip J., and Kathrine R. Tan. "Expanded Availability of Intravenous Artesunate for the Treatment of Severe Malaria in the United States." The American journal of tropical medicine and hygiene 100.6 (2019): 1295.

135) Centers for Disease Control and Prevention. "Notice to readers: new medication for severe malaria available under an investigational new drug protocol." MMWR Morb Mortal Wkly Rep 56.30 (2007): 769-770.

136) Guidance for Using Intravenous Artesunate for Treating Severe Malaria in the United States. The Centers for Disease Control and Prevention. Content source: Center for Preparedness and Response (CPR) Page last reviewed: March 6, 2019

137) Våtsveen, Thea Kristin, et al. "Artesunate shows potent anti-tumor activity in B-cell lymphoma." Journal of hematology & oncology 11.1 (2018): 23.

138) Lam, Nelson Siukei, et al. "Artemisinin and its derivatives: a potential treatment for leukemia." Anti-cancer drugs 30.1 (2019): 1-18.

139) Greenshields, Anna L., Wasundara Fernando, and David W. Hoskin. "The anti-malarial drug artesunate causes cell cycle arrest and apoptosis of triple-negative MDA-MB-468 and HER2-enriched SK-BR-3 breast cancer cells." Experimental and molecular pathology 107 (2019): 10-22.

140) Cheng, Zhiyong, et al. "Artesunate affects proliferation, apoptosis, cell cycle and PTEN/FAK signaling in multiple myeloma RPMI 8226 cells." Int J Clin Exp Med 12.4 (2019): 3641-3649.

141) Ma, Ling, and Honghua Fei. "Antimalarial drug artesunate is effective against chemoresistant anaplastic thyroid carcinoma via targeting mitochondrial metabolism." Journal of Bioenergetics and Biomembranes (2020): 1-8.

142) Jiang, Feng, et al. "Artesunate induces apoptosis and autophagy in HCT116 colon cancer cells, and autophagy inhibition enhances the artesunate-induced apoptosis." International journal of molecular medicine 42.3 (2018): 1295-1304.

143) Dou, Cui-Yun, et al. "Cytotoxic effect of Artesunate on myeloid leukemia cell lines through up-regulating

miR-29c expression." Translational Cancer Research 7.6 (2018): 1748-1750.

144) Greenshields, Anna L., Trevor G. Shepherd, and David W. Hoskin. "Contribution of reactive oxygen species to ovarian cancer cell growth arrest and killing by the anti-malarial drug artesunate." Molecular carcinogenesis 56.1 (2017): 75-93.

145) Zheng, Lei, and Jingxuan Pan. "The anti-malarial drug artesunate blocks Wnt/β-catenin pathway and inhibits growth, migration and invasion of uveal melanoma cells." Current cancer drug targets 18.10 (2018): 988-998.

146) Xiao, Qingfeng, et al. "Artesunate targets oral tongue squamous cell carcinoma via mitochondrial dysfunction-dependent oxidative damage and Akt/AMPK/mTOR inhibition." Journal of Bioenergetics and Biomembranes (2020): 1-9.

147) Cheng, Zhiyong, et al. "Artesunate affects proliferation, apoptosis, cell cycle and PTEN/FAK signaling in multiple myeloma RPMI 8226 cells." Int J Clin Exp Med 12.4 (2019): 3641-3649.

148) Chen, Li, et al. "Artesunate enhances adriamycin cytotoxicity by inhibiting glycolysis in adriamycin-resistant chronic myeloid leukemia K562/ADR cells." RSC advances 9.2 (2019): 1004-1014.

149) Yao, Zhihan, et al. "Dihydroartemisinin potentiates antitumor activity of 5-fluorouracil against a resistant colorectal cancer cell line." Biochemical and biophysical research communications 501.3 (2018): 636-642.

150) Li, Hao, et al. "Artesunate and sorafenib: Combinatorial inhibition of liver cancer cell growth." Oncology letters 18.5 (2019): 4735-4743.

151) Zhao, Xinying, et al. "Artemether suppresses cell proliferation and induces apoptosis in diffuse large B cell lymphoma cells." Experimental and therapeutic medicine 14.5 (2017): 4083-4090.

152) Konstat-Korzenny, Enrique, et al. "Artemisinin and its synthetic derivatives as a possible therapy for cancer." Medical Sciences 6.1 (2018): 19.

153) Da Eun Jeong, Hye Jin Song, et al. Repurposing the anti-malarial drug artesunate as a novel therapeutic agent for metastatic renal cell carcinoma due to its

attenuation of tumor growth, metastasis, and angiogenesis." Oncotarget 6.32 (2015): 33046.

154) Chen, Cai-Ping, et al. "Synergistic antitumor activity of artesunate and HDAC inhibitors through elevating heme synthesis via synergistic upregulation of ALAS1 expression." Acta Pharmaceutica Sinica B 9.5 (2019): 937-951.

155) Aktaş, İ., et al. "Artemisinin attenuates doxorubicin induced cardiotoxicity and hepatotoxicity in rats." Biotechnic & Histochemistry 95.2 (2020): 121-128.

156) Savage, Ruth L., et al. "Suspected Hepatotoxicity With a Supercritical Carbon Dioxide Extract of Artemisia annua in Grapeseed Oil Used in New Zealand." Frontiers in Pharmacology 10 (2019).

157) Kumar, Shiva. "Cholestatic liver injury secondary to artemisinin." Hepatology 62.3 (2015): 973-974.

158) Ruperti-Repilado, Francisco Javier, et al. "Danger of herbal tea: a case of acute cholestatic hepatitis due to Artemisia annua tea." Frontiers in medicine 6 (2019).

159) Zaki, Ahmed, et al. "Protective Effect of Dietary Vitamin E (a Tocopherol) on Artemisinin Induced Oxidative Liver Tissue Damage in Rats." International Journal of Morphology 38.2 (2020).

160) Eid, Refaat A., et al. "Vitamin C Administration Attenuated Artemether-Induced Hepatic Injury in Rats." International Journal of Morphology 38.1 (2020).

Chapter 22

Ivermectin—One of the Greatest Medical Accomplishments of the 20th Century

THE 2015 NOBEL PRIZE IN Medicine was awarded to William C. Campbell and Satoshi Ōmura for the 1981 discovery of Ivermectin. Dr. Andy Crump (2012) describes Ivermectin is an "astonishingly safe ... wonder drug ... one of the greatest medical accomplishments of the 20th century."

Ivermectin is a member of the avermectin family, first isolated in 1967 from the bacteria Streptomyces avermitilis, found in a single Japanese soil sample. Throughout the next decade, two hundred million people globally, many of them poor, will take the drug for prevention or treatment of parasitic disease. Ivermectin is dispensed without payment in a global campaign to eliminate river blindness (onchocerciasis) and lymphatic filariasis (elephantiasis). In addition, the drug treats strongyloidiasis, ascariasis, cutaneous larva migrans, gnathostomiasis and trichuriasis, as well as pediculosis (lice) and scabies (mites) in humans. (1–2)

Ivermectin has extensive global veterinary use as an antiparasitic drug for billions of pets, horses, and farm animals. For dogs, ivermectin prevents heartworm (Dirofilaria immitis). (3)

Ivermectin Antiparasitic Drug Repurposed as Anti-cancer Drug

While originally developed as an antiparasitic drug, FDA-approved for human use in 1987, ivermectin has been repurposed as an effective anti-cancer drug at low micromolar concentrations. (4–5)

In 2018, Dr. Mandy Juarez reviewed the anti-cancer activity of Ivermectin, finding several targets, including:

- Multidrug resistance protein (MDR)
- Akt/mTOR and Wnt -TCF pathways
- Purinergic P2X receptors (ATP sensitive receptors)
- PAK-1 protein (P21-activated kinase)
- Cancer-related epigenetic deregulators such as SIN3A and SIN3B, RNA helicase
- Chloride channel receptors
- Cancer stem cells. (5)

Anti-Cancer Effect Achievable at Antiparasitic Dosage

Dr. Mandy Juarez writes (2018) that the anti-cancer activity of Ivermectin is pharmacologically achievable at the same dosage used for human parasitic disease:

Importantly, the in vitro and in vivo anti-tumor activities of ivermectin are achieved at concentrations that can be clinically reachable based on the human pharmacokinetic studies done in healthy and parasited patients. Thus, existing information on ivermectin could allow its rapid move into clinical trials for cancer patients. (5)

Ivermectin Most Promising

In 2010, Dr. Sumaiya Sharmeen et al. at the University of Toronto screened a library of 100 drugs for activity against a leukemic cell line and reported ivermectin as the most promising, inducing leukemic cell death at low micromolar concentrations, while sparing normal cells. Ivermectin was also effective against leukemia mouse xenografts, synergizing with the chemotherapy drugs cytarabine and daunorubicin. (6)

Dr. Hisashi Hashimoto et al. reported (2009) that Ivermectin is effective against ovarian cancer cell lines by blocking PAK1 kinase. (7)

Ivermectin does not cross the blood-brain barrier, accounting for the absence of adverse neurologic effects.

Ivermectin Wnt Pathway Cancer Stem Cell Agent

In *EMBO Molecular Medicine* (2014), Dr. Alice Melotti et al. reported ivermectin as an inhibitor of the Wnt-TCF (Wnt/T Cell Factor) pathway, a critical pathway in cancer stem cells. Dr. Melotti used a transcriptional reporter assay for TCF activity driven by Beta-Catenin to test a collection of 1,040 drugs and small molecules. Only one agent, ivermectin, perfectly tracked the gene expression profile induced by blocking the TCF gene and therefore inhibited the Wnt pathway. (8)

This has profound significance for anti-cancer stem cell therapy, because blocking the Wnt pathway is the key to eradicating cancer stem cells and solving the problem of cancer recurrence after chemotherapy. For example, blocking the Wnt pathway in mantle cell lymphoma preferentially kills the cancer stem cells. (9–10)

In 2012, Dr. Robin Hallet et al. reported that blocking the Wnt /Beta-Catenin signaling pathway in a breast cancer model eradicated cancer stem cells. (11)

Other useful inhibitors of the Wnt pathway listed by Dr. Pay-Chin Leow (2010) targeting cancer stem cells include curcumin and the small molecule PKF118–310, a fungal product. In addition to curcumin, other natural dietary Wnt inhibitors include sulforaphane, ECGC (green tea), resveratrol (pterostilbene), and retinoids (vitamin A derivatives). See the Quick Reference Guide for a list of Wnt inhibitors discussed in this book. (12–13)

Structurally Similar to Salinomycin

In 2018, Dr. Guadalupe Dominguez-Gomez et al. studied ivermectin as a cancer stem cell agent, finding it structurally similar to salinomycin, another well-known anti-cancer stem cell drug:

Ivermectin exhibits a high degree of [structural] similarity with salinomycin [antiparasitic drug for veterinary use only] and preferentially inhibited the CSC [cancer stem cell] subpopulation in a breast cancer model. (14)

Ivermectin Effective Against Triple-Negative Breast Cancer Cells (TNBC)

In 2015, Dr. Dobrin Dragonov et al. reported in *Scientific Reports* on the mechanism of cancer-cell-killing by ivermectin. Dr. Dragonov's lab was heavily involved in studying P2X receptors, a family of ATP-gated cation channels. These are cell-membrane pores that open in response to ATP in the micro-environment.

Dr. Dragonov's group makes the observation that tumors have upregulated P2X7 receptors, which are involved with regulation of high ATP concentrations in the tumor micro-environment, promoting tumor progression. The application of ivermectin sensitizes the cation channels to ATP, further opening the channel pores, allowing an influx of large cations causing cancer cell death. They write:

> Ivermectin kills mouse and human triple-negative breast cancer [TNBC] cells through augmented P2X7-dependent purinergic signaling associated with caspase-1 and caspase-3 activation. [**Note:** caspase activation means apoptotic programmed cell death controlled by mitochondria]. (15–17)

Dr. Kshitija Dhuna et al. report (2019) that the natural botanical compound gensenoside (ginseng) also modulates P2X receptors in a manner similar to ivermectins inducing of cancer cell death. Therefore, synergy of ginseng with ivermectin might be expected. (18)

Effective at Low Concentration

Dr. Dragonov reports that mouse and human TNBC (triple negative breast cancer) cells are sensitive to ivermectin, with IC50 values as low as 2 µM with 24 hour exposure time. In addition, Dr. Dragonov hypothesized that ivermectin kills cancer cells by enhancing receptor P2X7 sensitivity to extracellular ATP. In doing so, ivermectin induces both an apoptotic and a non-apoptotic, inflammatory type of cell death. The inflammatory cell death stimulates the immune system, an added beneficial effect, so

that the patient's own immune system will kill new cancer cells in the future.

Ivermectin Synergy with Chemotherapy

Dr. Dragonov reports that ivermectin has cancer-cell-killing effects synergistic with chemotherapeutic agents such as doxorubicin (Adriamycin) and paclitaxel (Taxol), which induce reactive oxygen species (ROS).

Ivermectin Induces Immunogenic Cell Death

Dr. Dragonov reports that beneficial long-term clinical response after chemotherapy involves stimulation of a robust anti-cancer immune response, also called induction of "immunogenic cell death (ICD)." Ivermectin is one agent that induces ICD immunogenic cancer cell death, and therefore may induce long-term or permanent remission after treatment. (15)

Ivermectin – Mitochondrial Apoptosis

In 2019, Dr. Ping Zhang studied the effect of Ivermectin (IVM) on cervical cancer cells (HeLa cell line) producing cell-cycle arrest via mitochondrial apoptosis pathways, with inhibition of BCL2 (the anti-apoptosis protein) and upregulation of Bax (the pro-apoptotic protein). Dr. Zhang's group describes the cervical cancer cells after treatment with ivermectin (IVM):

> The content of cytochrome c in cytoplasm increases indicating mitochondrial-mediated apoptosis signal transduction pathway ... IVM inhibited the expression of apoptosis protein Bcl-2, increased the expression of apoptosis protein Bax , and

further activated the downstream apoptosis-inducing caspase-3/-9, and cleaved PARP [poly ADP-ribose polymerase-1] which eventually led to apoptosis.

Note: Detection of cleaved PARP is a used as marker for apoptosis. (19)

Glioma Cells

In 2019, Dr. Dandan Song et al. showed that ivermectin inhibited growth of glioma cells by inducing apoptosis and cell-cycle arrest in vitro and in vivo. However, since ivermectin does not cross the blood-brain barrier, clinical utility for glioblastoma is limited. (20)

Ivermectin Effective for Canine Breast Cancer

In 2019, Dr. Hongxiu Diao et al. studied ivermectin's inhibitory effect on canine breast cancer cells involved in regulating cell-cycle progression, and Wnt signaling. Dr. Diao reported cell-cycle arrest at G1 phase via downregulation of CDK4 and cyclin D1 expression. However, unlike the 2019 study of HeLa cervical cancer cells by Dr. Zhang, there was no significant induction of apoptosis. Dr. Diao et al. observed significantly reduced Beta-Catenin nuclear translocation after treatment with ivermectin, resulting in the inactivation of Wnt signaling. Significant suppression of tumor growth by ivermectin was observed in canine mammary tumor xenografts. (21)

Ivermectin Inhibits Complex I ETC in CML—Synergy with Tyrosine Kinase Inhibitors

In 2018, Dr. Jiaqiao Wang et al. studied the effect of ivermectin on chronic myeloid leukemia (CML). Ivermectin kills CML cells by targeting mitochondrial respiration and inhibiting complex I activity, thereby producing mitochondrial dysfunction and resulting in inhibition of OXPHOS. Ivermectin is therefore an OXPHOS inhibitor. All OXPHOS inhibitors activate autophagy and target the Wnt cancer stem cell pathway. Ivermectin synergizes with standard CML tyrosine kinase inhibitors, augmenting their activity. (22)

Ivermectin Reverses Drug Resistance

In 2019, using breast cancer and colorectal cancer cell lines, Dr. Lu Jiang et al. showed that ivermectin reverses cancer cell drug resistance to chemotherapy by reducing expression of P-glycoprotein (P-gp). This is done by inhibiting the epidermal growth factor receptor (EGFR) and its downstream signaling cascade ERK/Akt/NF-kB, not by directly inhibiting P-gp activity. Dr. Jiang and colleagues write that ivermectin could be useful in drug-resistant cancers:

> Thus, ivermectin, a FDA-approved antiparasitic drug, could potentially be used in combination with chemotherapeutic agents to treat cancers and in particular, the drug-resistant cancers. (23)

Ivermectin mTOR Inhibitor— Induces Autophagy

Ivermectin degrades the PAK protein, which then inhibits mTOR, which activates autophagy. **Note**: PAK1 is P21-activated kinase (see Glossary). In 2016, Dr. Kui Wang et al. studied the effect of ivermectin in a breast cancer cell line in vitro and in vivo, writing:

> Ivermectin markedly inhibits the growth of breast cancer cells by stimulating cytostatic macroautophagy/autophagy in vitro and in vivo. (24)

In 2020, Dr. Jian Liu et al. studied the anti-tumor molecular mechanism of ivermectin, writing:

> Ivermectin causes cell death in cancer cell lines by inducing PAK1-mediated cytostatic autophagy, caspase-dependent apoptosis and immunogenic cell death [ICD] through the modulation of some pathways, including the Wnt -T cell factor [TCF], Hippo and Akt/mTOR pathways. (25)

Ivermectin degrades PAK1 protein, which then inhibits mTOR, which leads to increased autophagic flux. Dr. Qianhui Dou et al. (2016) write:

> Iivermectin-induced autophagy is cytostatic in breast cancer cells, and suppression of autophagy may attenuate the anti-cancer effect of ivermectin (26)

Thus, the addition of autophagy inhibitor chloroquine failed to increase (attenuates) the effectiveness of ivermectin in Dr. Dou's breast cancer model. (24–26)

As mentioned above, ivermectin degrades P21-activated kinase (PAK1), which is upreg-ulated in many cancers. In 2011, Dr. Christy Ong et al. found genomic amplification of the PAK1 protein in breast cancer and squamous cell lung cancer, writing:

> Breast cancer cells with PAK1 genomic amplification rapidly underwent apoptosis after inhibition of this kinase. (27)

PAK1 signaling is overexpressed and highly activated in lymphomas, and its inhibition significantly inhibits cancer cell viability. (27–28)

Ivermectin Activates Protective Autophagy Synergy with Autophagy Inhibitor

In 2019, Dr. Faming Deng et al. studied the anti-cancer effects of ivermectin in a melanoma cell line, finding that ivermectin increases autophagy and that inhibiting autophagy enhances ivermectin-induced apoptosis in human melanoma cells. (29)

Similarly, in 2019, Dr. Lingjing Liu et al. studied ivermectin in a glioblastoma cell line in vitro and in vivo mouse xenografts, finding inhibition of mTOR, which stimulated "protective autophagy." The combination of ivermectin with autophagy inhibitor Chloroquine co-treatment was synergistic both in vitro and in vivo, augmenting the anti-cancer effects. (30)

Ivermectin Antiviral Effects

Ivermectin has antiviral activity against many RNA viruses (adenovirus, coronavirus, yellow fever virus, dengue fever) thought to be related to inhibition of nuclear transport performed by the importin $\alpha/\beta1$ heterodimer. In 2020, Dr. Leon Caly et al. reported that a single treatment with ivermectin reduced viral RNA 5,000 fold after 48 hours in a cell culture infected with SARS-coV-2 virus in vitro. Others have suggested prophylaxis or treatment using the synergistic combination of ivermectin, hydroxychloroquine and azithromycin for RNA viruses such as SARS-coV-2 (COVID-19). (43–48)

In 2020, Dr. Mohammed Tarek Alam et al. from Bangaldesh treated 100 patients with the combination of Ivermectin (0.2mg/kg single dose) and Doxycycline (100 mg daily for 10 days). All patients had mild to moderate severity of disease and inititally tested positive for Covid-19 by RT-PCR test. All patients reported symptom improvement within 72 hours. All patients converted to a negative PCR test within 4-18 days of starting treatment, with no noticeable side effects. Dr. Alam writes:

> Combination of Ivermectin and doxycycline was found to be very effective in viral clearance in mild and moderately sick COVID-19 patients. (49)

Although results above of Dr. Alam's study appeared promising, a follow up study by Dr Podder (2020), this time with a randomized trial (with a control group) showed the similar recovery from the disease in both control and Ivermectin treated group, indicating good recovery without Ivermectin treatment. (50)

Ivermectin for Rosacea of Face

Rosacea is a common dermatologic disorder with characteristic red patches on the face. Ivermectin 1% topical cream has now proven to be the most effective dermatologic treatment available. Whether mode of action (MOA) for rosacea is antiparasitic or anti-inflammatory has yet to be determined. (31–32)

Ivermectin Toxicity Attenuated by Supplements

Although considered remarkably safe, ivermectin at high dosage can cause bone marrow and neurologic toxicity. In 2018, Dr. Ahmad Khalil et al. showed that bone marrow cytotoxicity of ivermectin could be attenuated by aged garlic, vitamins A, C, E and grape seed oil. (33–37)

Summary

The antiparasitic "wonder drug," ivermectin has been repurposed as an anti-cancer drug effective at doses commonly used for parasites. Ivermectin is remarkably safe and works through multiple pathways. Ivermectin induces mitochondrial dysfunction and apoptosis, inhibits mTOR, activates autophagy and targets the Wnt pathway (cancer stem cell agent). Ivermectin augments the effects of chemotherapy. (38)

Dr. Jian Liu concludes by writing in 2020:

> To manage patients with cancer in a more effective way, ivermectin can be adopted together with other medications... currently being used ... For example, when combined with daunorubicin/cytarabine, tamoxifen, paclitaxel.... ivermectin exhibits a more powerful anti-cancer effect against leukaemia, TNBC [breast cancer], EOC [epithelial ovarian cancer] and melanoma ... at clinical doses for the treatment of human parasitic infections. (25)

References for Chapter 22: Ivermectin

1) Crump, Andy, and Satoshi Omura. "Ivermectin, Wonder Drug from Japan: the human use perspective." Proceedings of the Japan Academy, Series B 87.2 (2011): 13-28.

2) Fawcett, Robert S. "Ivermectin use in scabies." American Family Physician 68.6 (2003): 1089-1092.

3) Khan Sharun, T. S., et al. "Current therapeutic applications and pharmacokinetic modulations of ivermectin." Veterinary World 12.8 (2019): 1204.

4) Antoszczak, Michał, et al. "Old wine in new bottles: Drug repurposing in oncology." European journal of pharmacology 866 (2020): 172784.

5) Juarez, Mandy, Alejandro Schcolnik-Cabrera, and Alfonso Dueñas-Gonzalez. "The multitargeted drug ivermectin: from an antiparasitic agent to a repositioned cancer drug." American journal of cancer research 8.2 (2018): 317.

6) Sharmeen, Sumaiya, et al. "The antiparasitic agent ivermectin induces chloride-dependent membrane hyperpolarization and cell death in leukemia cells." Blood 116.18 (2010): 3593-3603.

7) Hashimoto, Hisashi, et al. "Ivermectin inactivates the kinase PAK1 and blocks the PAK1-dependent growth of human ovarian cancer and NF2 tumor cell lines." Drug discoveries & therapeutics 3.6 (2009).

8) Melotti, Alice, et al. "The river blindness drug Ivermectin and related macrocyclic lactones inhibit WNT-TCF pathway responses in human cancer." EMBO molecular medicine 6.10 (2014): 1263-1278.

9) Kimura, Yoshizo, et al. "The Wnt signaling pathway and mitotic regulators in the initiation and evolution of mantle cell lymphoma: Gene expression analysis." International journal of oncology 43.2 (2013): 457-468.

10) Mathur, Rohit, et al. "Targeting Wnt pathway in mantle cell lymphoma-initiating cells." Journal of hematology & oncology 8.1 (2015): 63.

11) Hallett, Robin M., et al. "Small molecule antagonists of the Wnt/beta-catenin signaling pathway target breast tumor-initiating cells in a Her2/Neu mouse model of breast cancer." PloS one 7.3 (2012): e33976.

12) Leow, Pay-Chin, et al. "Antitumor activity of natural compounds, curcumin and PKF118-310, as Wnt/β-catenin antagonists against human osteosarcoma cells." Investigational new drugs 28.6 (2010): 766-782.

13) Tarapore, Rohinton S., Imtiaz A. Siddiqui, and Hasan Mukhtar. "Modulation of Wnt/β-catenin signaling pathway by bioactive food components." Carcinogenesis 33.3 (2012): 483-491.

14) Dominguez-Gomez, Guadalupe, et al. "Ivermectin as an inhibitor of cancer stem-like cells." Molecular medicine reports 17.2 (2018): 3397-3403.

15) Draganov, Dobrin, et al. "Modulation of P2X4/P2X7/pannexin-1 sensitivity to extracellular ATP via ivermectin induces a non-apoptotic and inflammatory form of cancer cell death." Scientific reports 5 (2015).

16) Mackay, Laurent, et al. "Deciphering the regulation of P2X4 receptor channel gating by ivermectin using Markov models." PLoS computational biology 13.7 (2017): e1005643.

17) Latapiat, Verónica, et al. "P2X4 receptor in silico and electrophysiological approaches reveal insights of ivermectin and zinc allosteric modulation." Frontiers in pharmacology 8 (2017): 918.

18) Dhuna, et al. "Ginsenosides act as positive modulators of P2X4 receptors." Molecular pharmacology 95.2 (2019): 210-221.

19) Zhang, Ping, et al. "Ivermectin induces cell cycle arrest and apoptosis of HeLa cells via mitochondrial pathway." Cell proliferation 52.2 (2019): e12543.

20) Song, Dandan, et al. "Ivermectin inhibits the growth of glioma cells by inducing cell cycle arrest and apoptosis in vitro and in vivo." Journal of cellular biochemistry 120.1 (2019): 622-633.

21) Diao, Hongxiu, et al. "Ivermectin inhibits canine mammary tumor growth by regulating cell cycle progression and WNT signaling." BMC Veterinary Research 15.1 (2019).

22) Wang, Jiaqiao, et al. "Antibiotic ivermectin selectively induces apoptosis in chronic myeloid leukemia through inducing mitochondrial dysfunction and oxidative stress." Biochemical and biophysical research communications 497.1 (2018): 241-247.

23) Jiang, Lu, et al. "Ivermectin reverses the drug resistance in cancer cells through EGFR/ERK/Akt/NF-KB pathway." Journal of Experimental & Clinical Cancer Research 38.1 (2019): 265.

24) Wang, Kui, et al. "Ivermectin induces PAK1-mediated cytostatic autophagy in breast cancer." Autophagy 12.12 (2016): 2498-2499.

25) Liu, Jian, et al. "Progress in Understanding the Molecular Mechanisms Underlying the Antitumour Effects of Ivermectin." Drug Design, Development and Therapy 14 (2020): 285.

26) Dou, Qianhui, et al. "Ivermectin induces cytostatic autophagy by blocking the PAK1/Akt axis in breast cancer." Cancer research 76.15 (2016): 4457-4469.

27) Ong, Christy C., et al. "Targeting p21-activated kinase 1 (PAK1) to induce apoptosis of tumor cells." Proceedings of the National Academy of Sciences 108.17 (2011): 7177-7182.

28) Tian, Tian. "Role of Rac1-Pak pathway in aggressive b-cell lymphoma." (2019).

29) Deng, Faming, et al. "Suppressing ROS-TFE3-dependent autophagy enhances ivermectin-induced apoptosis in human melanoma cells." Journal of cellular biochemistry 120.2 (2019): 1702-1715.

30) Liu, Jingjing, et al. "Ivermectin induces autophagy-mediated cell death through the AKT/mTOR signaling pathway in glioma cells." Bioscience reports 39.12 (2019).

31) Mendieta Eckert, Marta, and Nerea Landa Gundin. "Treatment of rosacea with topical ivermectin cream: a series of 34 cases." Dermatology online journal 22.8 (2016).

32) Husein-ElAhmed, Husein, and Martin Steinhoff. "Efficacy of topical ivermectin and impact on quality of life in patients with papulopustular rosacea: A systematic review and meta-analysis." Dermatologic Therapy.

33) Khalil, Ahmad M., and Hadeel M. Abu Samrah. "In vivo combined treatment of rats with ivermectin and aged garlic extract attenuates ivermectin-induced cytogenotoxicity in bone marrow cells." Research in veterinary science 120 (2018): 94-100.

34) Omshi, Fatemeh Sadat Hosseini, et al. "Effect of vitamin A and vitamin C on attenuation of ivermectin-induced toxicity in male Wistar rats." Environmental Science and Pollution Research 25.29 (2018): 29408-29417.

35) Ahmed, Salama Ameera, et al. "Protective effects of vitamin E and grape seed oil against acute hepatorenal ivermectin toxicity in mice: biochemical and histopathological studies." GSC Biological and Pharmaceutical Sciences 7.2 (2019): 087-094.

36) Trailović, Saša M., and Jelena Trailović NEDELJKOVIĆ. "Central and peripheral neurotoxic effects of ivermectin in rats." Journal of Veterinary Medical Science (2010): 1012080409-1012080409.

37) Guzzo, Cynthia A., et al. "Safety, Tolerability, and Pharmacokinetics of Escalating High Doses of Ivermectin in Healthy Adult Subjects." Journal of Clinical Pharmacology 42 (2002): 1122-1133.

38) Zhang, Xiaohong, et al. "Ivermectin Augments the In Vitro and In Vivo Efficacy of Cisplatin in Epithelial Ovarian Cancer by Suppressing Akt/mTOR Signaling." The American Journal of the Medical Sciences 359.2 (2020): 123-129.

39) Guilford, Frederick T., and Simon Yu. "Antiparasitic and Antifungal Medications for Targeting Cancer Cells Literature Review and Case Studies." synthesis 9 (2019):

40) Canga, Aránzazu González, et al. "The pharmacokinetics and interactions of ivermectin in humans—a mini-review." The AAPS journal 10.1 (2008): 42-46.

41) Guzzo, Cynthia A., et al. "Safety, tolerability, and pharmacokinetics of escalating high doses of ivermectin in healthy adult subjects." The Journal of Clinical Pharmacology 42.10 (2002): 1122-1133.

42) Jung, Chang Hwa, et al. "mTOR regulation of autophagy." FEBS letters 584.7 (2010): 1287-1295.

43) Caly, Leon, et al. "The FDA-approved drug ivermectin inhibits the replication of SARS-CoV-2 in vitro." Antiviral research (2020): 104787.

44) Bray, Mike, et al. "Ivermectin and COVID-19: a report in Antiviral Research, widespread interest, an FDA warning, two letters to the editor and the authors' responses." Antiviral Research (2020).

45) Yang, Sundy NY, et al. "The broad spectrum antiviral ivermectin targets the host nuclear transport

importin α/β1 heterodimer." Antiviral research (2020): 104760.

46) Rizzo, Emanuele. "Ivermectin, antiviral properties and COVID-19: a possible new mechanism of action." Naunyn-schmiedeberg's Archives of Pharmacology (2020): 1.

47) Patrì, Angela, and Gabriella Fabbrocini. "Hydroxychloroquine and ivermectin: A synergistic combination for COVID-19 chemoprophylaxis and treatment?" Journal of the American Academy of Dermatology 82.6 (2020): e221.

48) Choudhary, Renuka, and Anil K. Sharma. "Potential use of hydroxychloroquine, ivermectin and azithromycin drugs in fighting COVID-19: trends, scope and relevance." New Microbes and New Infections (2020): 100684.

49) Alam, Mohammed Tarek, et al. "A case series of 100 COVID-19 positive patients treated with combination of Ivermectin and Doxycycline." Journal of Bangladesh College of Physicians and Surgeons (2020): 10-15.

50) Podder, Chinmay Saha, et al. "Outcome of ivermectin treated mild to moderate COVID-19 cases: a single-centre, open-label, randomised controlled study." IMC J Med Sci (2020). 14(2)

Chapter 23

Niclosamide Antiparasitic Drug

Niclosamide (Niclocide) Antiparasitic Blocks Wnt pathway

THE OLD ANTIPARASITIC ORAL DRUG niclosamide (Niclocide, Yomesan) was discovered in 1953 by Bayer. Even though it has been used since 1962 to treat tapeworm, FDA approval for this indication was only granted in 1982. (1) Typical treatment of H. nana (dwarf tapeworm) uses a 2 Gram oral dose for 7 days. (30)

Niclosamide for Other Clinical Applications

Dr. Wei Chen et al. (2019) reviewed the broader clinical applications of niclosamide, other than as an antiparasitic drug, which include a long list of indications:

Cancer, bacterial and viral infection, metabolic diseases such as Type II diabetes, nonalcoholic steatohepatitis [NASH], nonalcoholic Fatty Liver Disease [NAFLD], artery constriction, endometriosis, neuropathic pain, rheumatoid arthritis, sclerodermatous graft-versus-host disease, systemic sclerosis. (1)

Repurposing Niclosamide for Cancer

A large volume of medical research suggests niclosamide can be repurposed as a potent anti-cancer drug targeting the Wnt/β-catenin pathway.

One potential drawback to systemic use is lack of water solubility, with poor gastrointes-

tinal (GI) absorption, as a result of which very low blood concentrations achieved. Although this can be perceived as a benefit in the treatment of intraluminal GI parasites, it represents a problem as a repurposed cancer drug. We will examine the question of obtaining therapeutic blood levels with oral administration. See chapter 20, Cancer as a Parasitic Disease.

Potent Anti-Cancer Stem Cell Agent— Inhibitor of Wnt/β-catenin Pathway

In 2012, Drs. Jing-Xuan Pan et al. reported in *Chinese Journal of Cancer* that Niclosamide serves as an anti-cancer drug targeting multiple pathways. Earlier in 2009, Dr. Chen used a high-throughput screening method to identify niclosamide as a potent inhibitor of the Wnt/Beta-Catenin pathway, downregulating the Nuclear Factor Kappa B (NF-κB) inflammatory pathway, as well as potent anti-cancer stem cell agent. (3–4) Dr. Pan et al. write:

Niclosamide targets multiple signaling pathways [NF-κB, Wnt/β-catenin, Notch, ROS, mTORC1, and Stat3], most of which are closely involved with cancer stem cells....., and holds promise in eradicating cancer stem cells. (3)

Degrades the LRP6 CoReceptor at One Micromolar

In 2011, Dr. Lu found that niclosamide inhibited the Wnt pathway by targeting the LRP6-

Wnt co-receptor on the cancer cell surface, degrading the LRP6 protein. This was found at low concentrations of the drug with IC50 values less than 1 micromolar for prostate and breast cancer cells. (5)

Studying colorectal cancer cells, in 2019, Dr. Jiangbo Wang et al. found that autophagosome formation (autophagy) is required for niclosamide inhibition of Wnt signaling. In other words, niclosamide- resistant cancer cells had deficient autophagy. (6)

Niclosamide Inhibits Antegrade Lysosome Trafficking

In a previous chapter on artemisinin, we discussed the post-treatment observation of the peculiar re-arrangement of lysosomes in breast cancer cells called "perinuclear clustering." The back and forth movement of lysosomes from central to peripheral locations in the cell is mediated by the microtubule system and motor proteins, subject to various stimuli (nutrient starvation) and pro-apoptotic drugs. (7)

In cancer cells, antegrade trafficking, or movement of lysosomes to the cell periphery near the cell membrane, is associated with aggressive behavior, and tumor cell invasion. The opposite, called perinuclear clustering of lysosomes (i.e. inhibition of antegrade trafficking), is associated with a more benign state, with inhibition of tumor invasion.

In 2016, Dr. Magdalena Circu et al., working with a prostate cancer cell line, used a high-content imaging system to screen 2,210 repurposed and natural products for "antegrade lysosome trafficking inhibition" (i.e., perinu-

clear clustering), identifying niclosamide as the best candidate. The mechanism has to do with action on lysosomal pH. Lysosomal acidity is lost, and instead, the acid is released into the cytosol. (8–9)

Dual Targeting Mitochondria and Lysosomes

This was confirmed in 2019 by Drs. Uyen Thi Tran and Toshimori Kitami. In 2019, they used a high-throughput screening technique to identify niclosamide as activator of the NLRP3 inflammasome through two targets. First, the lysosomal acid is transferred out to the cytosol, causing intracellular acidification and inhibition of glycolysis. Second, niclosamide is a mitochondrial uncoupling agent inhibiting mitochondrial production of ATP (OXPHOS inhibitor). This produces dual targeting of lysosomes and mitochondrial OXPHOS inhibition. Furthermore, release of the acidic contents of lysosomes into the cytosol inhibits GLYCOLYSIS. Drs. Tran and Kitami write:

> We find that niclosamide engages two targets, mitochondria and acidic organelles [lysosomes], both of which are necessary to induce NLRP3 inflammasome activation. Niclosamide transfers protons from acidic organelles to cytosol, leading to intracellular acidification and suppression of glycolysis. Glycolytic inhibition, combined with mitochondrial inhibitory action of niclosamide, decreases intracellular ATP level, leading to intracellular potassium loss, a key event to NLRP3 inflammasome activation. (10)

Niclosamide Synergy with Chloroquine

In 2015, Dr. Xiang et al. studied a T cell leukemia model, finding the combination of niclosamide with the autophagy inhibitor chloroquine (which blocks fusion of the autophagosome with the lysosome) was synergistic, with augmented anti-cancer activity. (11)

Niclosamide for Ovarian Cancer

Ovarian cancer (CA) is the deadliest gynecological malignancy, with 14,000 deaths annually in the U.S. Ovarian cancer typically presents late in the disease course, with metastatic spread. There may be malignant ascites (fluid in the abdomen) from peritoneal seeding. Although many cases will achieve remission with platinum-based chemotherapy, ultimately 75% will recur within 5 years, perhaps with a chemo-resistant cell type. Recurrence is thought to be due to ovarian cancer stem cells resistant to chemotherapy.

Niclosamide for Ovarian Cancer

In 2012, searching for a more effective drug to treat ovarian cancer, Dr. Yi-Te Yo et al. used high-throughput screening of more than 1,200 clinically approved drugs. The anthelmintic drug, niclosamide was identified as the most promising candidate, selectively targeting ovarian cancer stem cells in vitro and in vivo. Niclosamide was not only effective as monotherapy against ovarian cancer cell lines, it was also effective in combination with conventional chemotherapy drugs, enhancing the ovarian cancer-cell-killing effect. (12)

Niclosamide Synergy with Chemotherapy

In 2014, Dr. Rebecca Arend et al. isolated ovarian cancer cells from 34 patients' malignant ascites. The cancer cells were treated in vitro with a combination of niclosamide (0.1 to 5 micromolar) and chemotherapy agent carboplatin (5–150 micromolar), showing synergy with the combination in 32/34 patient samples. Additionally, Dr. Arend and colleagues' 2014 study showed that niclosamide is a potent Wnt/Beta-Catenin inhibitor, leading to decreased proliferation and cancer cell death. (13)

In 2016, Dr. Arend et al. again studied ovarian cancer, reporting that upregulated pathways associated with recurrence and chemoresistance are the Wnt, mTOR, and STAT3 (the Wnt/Beta-Catenin signaling pathway, the mammalian target of rapamycin [mTOR] pathway, and the signal transducer and activator of transcription-3 [STAT3 pathway]). In vitro ovarian cancer cell studies show all three pathways are inhibited by niclosamide. In addition, niclosamide effectively targeted CD133+ cancer stem cells as well as chemotherapy resistant ovarian cancer cells. (14)

Water-Soluble Analogs

One problem with niclosamide is its poor water solubility. To address this issue, Dr. Arend's group developed more water-soluble analogs of niclosamide with greater anti-cancer efficacy. (15)

In 2016, Dr. Chi Kang Lin et al. developed a nano-formulated version of niclosamide (nano-NI) with improved absorption and bio-availability. They write:

Nano-NI effectively inhibited the growth of ovarian cancer cells in which it induced a metabolic shift to glycolysis at a concentration of less than 3 µM in vitro and suppressed tumor growth without obvious toxicity at an oral dose of 100 mg/kg in vivo. (16)

Dr. Deng in 2019 showed niclosamide effective for ovarian cancer with augmented efficacy when IGF-R signaling is blocked. (2) **Note:** The metabolic shift to GLYCOLYIS in the above study is due the fact that Niclosamide is an OXPHOS inhibitor. IGF-R is insulin-like growth factor receptor, a marker for growth hormone.

Niclosamide for Ovarian Cancer, Case Report

A 45-year-old yoga teacher on thyroid pills had a pelvic sonogram showing a large ovarian mass, for which a total hysterectomy was performed. The pathology report revealed ovarian cancer with peritoneal spread. After surgery, the patient was scheduled for platinum-based chemotherapy—cisplatin combined with the taxane paclitaxel (Taxol). **Note**: taxanes are microtubule inhibitors that prevent cancer cell replication. Prior to and during chemotherapy, the patient took 2 grams of niclosamide daily every other week for 8 weeks. The patient also took many of the anti-cancer stem cell supplements listed in this book—berberine, curcumin, sulforaphane, etc. Five years later, the patient is cancer free, and remains in remission with no further treatment.

Niclosamide is a Mitochondrial Uncoupler

The "tumor suppressor protein" P-53 has been dubbed the guardian of the genome, because any DNA damage will activate P-53 DNA repair functions. If the DNA cannot be repaired, then P-53 will induce the cell to commit suicide, i.e. undergo apoptosis, thus protecting the host from cancerous tumor formation. Loss of P53 due to mutation is present in about 50% of all cancers, usually predictive of treatment failure and poor prognosis with shortened survival. Immunohistochemically detected p53 and p21 staining on biopsy slides is sufficient to determine mutated P53 status with disrupted function in lymphoma cases. (17–20)

In 2018, Dr. R. Kumar et al. studied P53 deficient ovarian cancer cell lines and xenografts. Dr. Kumar's group performed a high-throughput screen of "1,600 FDA-approved compounds from the PHARMAKON Library," finding niclosamide the most potent drug against P53-deficient cancer cells, effective at the low dose of 2.0 micromolar. Further studies of this model with metabolic profiling (the study of small-molecule metabolites of the cancer cell, providing a functional readout of the cancer cell metabolism) showed uncoupling of mitochondrial OXPHOS, which means no ATP production even though electrons are flowing through the ETC electron transport chain. Some anti-cancer drugs (such as fenbendazole) depend on a functioning P53. In the event of a non-functioning, defective P53, Dr. Kumar et al. write niclosamide is the drug of choice:

Niclosamide induces **mitochondrial uncoupling**, which renders mutant p53 cells susceptible to mitochondrial-dependent apoptosis through preferential accumulation of AA [arachidonic acid], and represents a first-in-class inhibitor of p53 mutant tumors. Wild-type p53 evades the cytotoxicity by promoting the transcriptional induction of two key lipid oxygenation genes, ALOX5 and ALOX12B, which catalyzes the dioxygenation and breakdown of AA. Therefore, we propose a new paradigm for targeting cancers defective in the p53 pathway, by exploiting their vulnerability to mitochondrial uncoupling. (21)

What is a mitochondrial uncoupler? Dr. James Figarola et al. (2018) explain:

Mitochondria uncouplers exert their effects by dissipating the proton gradient formed by the electron transport chain, thus uncoupling ATP production and causing energetic stress…. the antiproliferative and anti-tumor effects of niclosamide in vitro and in mice xenograft studies result from uncoupling of mitochondrial OXPHOS that induces energetic stress on cells, consequently leading to AMPK activation and mTOR inhibition.(22)

Note: AMPK activation/mTOR inhibition is also achieved by metformin and itraconazole, and many other anti-cancer drugs.

Mitochondrial Uncoupling for Colon Cancer

Dr. Amer Alasadi et al. (2018) studied the effect of mitochondrial uncoupler niclosamide on hepatic metastasis in colon cancer. Dr. Alasadi 's group writes:

Mitochondrial uncoupling is a process that facilitates proton influx across the mitochondrial inner membrane without generating ATP, stimulating a futile cycle of acetyl- CoA oxidation.

Dr. Alasadi's study used niclosamide in cultured colon cancer cells, and colon cancer xenografts showed that mitochondrial uncoupling:

promotes pyruvate influx to mitochondria and reduces various anabolic pathway activities, inhibits cell proliferation and reduces clonogenicity of cultured colon cancer cells. Furthermore, oral treatment with mitochondrial uncoupler [niclosamide] reduces intestinal polyp formation in APCmin/+ mice [genetically modified mice having familial polyposis of the colon], and diminishes hepatic metastasis of colon cancer cells transplanted intrasplenically. (23)

The use of niclosamide for colon cancer has been extensively studied. The mechanism of action, as described by Dr. Mohammed Suliman et al. in 2016, is downregulation of Notch pathway and upregulation of tumor suppressor gene miR-200. (24)

Downregulating the Wnt Pathway

Perhaps, the highest level of interest is devoted to niclosamide's ability to downregulate the Wnt/Beta-Catenin signaling pathway, a pathway activated by mutations in colonic polyps in 80% of colon cancer cases. (25)

In 2011, Dr. Takuya Osada et al. found:

In mice implanted with human CRC [ColoRectal Cancer] xenografts, orally administered niclosamide was well tolerated, achieved plasma and tumor levels associated with biologic activity, and led to tumor control. Our findings support clinical explorations to reposition niclosamide for the treatment of CRC. (26)

Potent Wnt Inhibitor

In 2019, Dr. So-Yeon Park et al. investigated the molecular mechanism by which niclosamide is a potent Wnt inhibitor and anti-cancer stem cell agent in colon cancer. Dr. Park's study concluded that niclosamide

> exerts in vivo effects against both colon carcinogenesis and tumor growth by targeting the Wnt/LEF1/DCLK1-B axis-mediated CSC [cancer stem cell] properties. Niclosamide inhibits certain CSC functions including survival, anti-apoptosis, and self-renewal, resulting in a reduction in CSC populations. Moreover, CSC-targeting niclosamide successfully sensitizes colorectal cancer to chemo-radiation. These findings provide a preclinical rationale to broaden the clinical evaluation of niclosamide for colorectal cancer treatment. (27)

Wnt/B-catenin/S100A4 Pathway

The downstream signaling protein induced by Wnt pathway activation at the cell membrane is Beta-Catenin, which then localizes to the nucleus and activates transcription of the S100A4 gene and protein. This is the subject of a 2016 study by Dr. Mathias Dahlman et al., finding that elevated levels of S100A4 protein predicted metastatic behavior with poor prognosis in mouse xenograft studies, as well as in human colon cancer cases. (28)

Dr. Susen Burock's group performed a high-throughput screen identifying niclosamide as an inhibitor of S100A4 gene expression. (29)

Niclosamide Human Clinical Trials

In view of the above excellent results with in vitro and in vivo studies, two human clinical trials of niclosamide in colon cancer are underway. The first is sponsored by Michael A Morse, MD, at Duke University, a phase 1 study of 18 patients given niclosamide for 7 days prior to surgical resection of their colon cancer (clinical trial NCT02687009). The study completion date is July 2022.

The second is a phase 2 trial led by Dr. Burock in Charite University, Berlin, Germany (NCT02519582) in which 37 patients with progressive metastatic colon cancer are treated with oral niclosamide (2 grams daily) until disease progression or unacceptable toxicity. Measurement of S100A4 protein levels will be done (see Dr. Mathias Dahlman et al. above); the estimated study completion date was August 2020. (As of this writing, no results have been posted.) I would assume the 2 gram per day dosage was chosen because it is the same dosage for dwarf hookworm, and provides serum concentrations of 0.25–6.0 micrograms per milliliter, corresponding with effective anti-cancer activity in many of the in vitro and in vivo studies. (29)

Niclosamide Targets Mitochondria, Inhibits Wnt, STAT, NF-kB, and Notch Pathways

Dr. Yonghe Li in et al. (2014) in *Cancer Letters* report that:

Niclosamide not only inhibits the Wnt/β-catenin, mTORC1, STAT3, NF-κB and Notch signaling pathways, but also targets mitochondria in cancer cells to induce cell-cycle arrest, growth inhibition and apoptosis. (30)

Niclosamide Effective for Lymphoma

In 2015, Dr. Junaid Ansari et al. studied the effect of niclosamide on a panel of aggressive B-Cell lymphoma cell lines (in vitro), finding effective inhibition of proliferation and induction of apoptosis at low concentrations of 0.1 microMolar, while sparing normal lymphocytes that are not affected by the drug. Dr. Ansari et al. write:

> Treatment with niclosamide at doses **as low as 0.1 μM** resulted in time- and dose-dependent apoptosis, cytotoxicity and inhibition of proliferation in aggressive lymphoma cell lines. The 50% inhibitory concentration in a proliferation assay [0.5 to 0.7 microMolar].... niclosamide showed significant cytotoxicity in a patient with mantle cell lymphoma [MCL]. (31)

Niclosamide for Multiple Myeloma Better than Chemotherapy

In 2011, Dr. F. L. Khanim et al. screened 100 off-patent oral drugs for anti-myeloma activity, finding that niclosamide:

> at clinically achievable nontoxic concentrations, killed Multiple Myeloma cell lines **as efficiently or better than chemotherapy and anti-myeloma drugs** with little impact on normal cells. More importantly there was rapid reduction in light chain production [the clonal antibodies which cause amyloid deposits and renal impairment]. (32)

Dr. Khanim's group showed the anti-Myeloma activity was due to rapid loss of mitochondrial membrane potential, uncoupling of oxidative phosphorylation (OXPHOS) and production of mitochondrial superoxide (a potent form of ROS). The peak serum concentration (3.2 μM) of niclosamide used in Dr. Khanim's study correlates with clinically achievable levels with standard anthelminthic dosing: **"Micromolar concentrations are achieved in serum after a single oral dose in animals or humans."** Significant antiproliferative activity was seen with niclosamide concentrations as low as 0.5 to 1.0 micromolar. These levels are nontoxic to normal bone marrow. (32)

Niclosamide for Breast Cancer Stem Cells

In 2013, Dr. Yu-Chi Wang et al. screened the LOPAC chemical library of 1,258 compounds, identifying niclosamide as the best inhibitor of breast cancer stem cells. (33) In 2014, Dr. Tinghong Ye et al. studied the effect of niclosamide on breast cancer cells in vitro, and in vivo with a mouse breast cancer model, showing

> dramatic growth inhibition, and apoptosis in a dose-dependent manner.... Apoptosis was associated downregulation of Bcl-2, Mcl-1 and Survivin..... Niclosamide blocked cancer cell migration and invasion [properties of cancer stem cells] ... reduced STAT3 [a cancer stem cell pathway], ... without detectable toxicity.(34)

Dr. Ye et al. report on histological and immunohistochemical analyses in the mouse breast cancer model. After niclosamide treatment, Dr. Ye observed:

decrease in Ki67-positive cells, VEGF-positive cells and microvessel density [MVD] and an increase in cleaved caspase-3-positive cells upon niclosamide.....Notably, niclosamide reduced the number of myeloid-derived suppressor cells [MDSCs] in tumor tissues and blocked formation of pulmonary metastases. (34)

Note: MDSCs suppress anti-tumor immune function, so decreasing MDSCs helps to restore anti-tumor immunity. Dr. Ye's group also state:

> Niclosamide is a potent Stat3 inhibitor, and also targets other multiple signaling pathways [NF-kB, ROS, Notch, Wnt/β-catenin and mTOR]. (34)

In 2011, Dr. Wenyan Lu et al. showed niclosamide inhibited the Wnt/ Beta-Catenin pathway by targeting and degrading the LR6 protein, the key Wnt co-receptor. (35)

Micro-Environment Study of Breast Cancer

The tumor micro-environment (TME) is composed of cells and tissues around the cancer mass, playing a supportive role in feeding the cancer mass with nutrients and growth factors. According to Drs. Freja Venning et al. (2015), the tumor micro-environment includes:

> immune cells, fibroblasts, pericytes, endothelial cells, adipocytes, and mesenchymal stem cells, and also the interstitial fluids and the extracellular matrix [ECM]. (36)

EMT Transition in Breast Cancer

A 2019 study by Dr. Jones Gyamfi et al. examined the micro-environment of breast cancer, composed predominantly of adipocytes, or fat cells. Dr. Gyamfi's group says these adipocytes surrounding the cancer mass induce "epithelial mesenchymal transition (EMT) of breast cancer cells through paracrine IL-6/Stat3 signaling." (37)

What does this mean in English? What is the EMT? This is the process that changes a well-behaved epithelial cell, attached to a fixed place at the basement membrane, into a more aggressive "mesenchymal cell," no longer attached and now able to migrate freely around the body. In other words, this describes the transition from a sedentary cancer cell into a more aggressive cell type capable of metastasizing throughout the body. According to Drs. Kalluri and Weinberg in 2009 JCI:

> EMT is a process that allows an epithelial cell, which normally interacts with basement membrane via its basal surface, to undergo multiple biochemical changes that enable it to assume a mesenchymal cell phenotype, which includes **enhanced migratory capacity, invasiveness, elevated resistance to apoptosis, and greatly increased production of ECM [extracellular matrix] components.** (38)

What is paracrine signaling? Paracrine signaling is cell-to-cell hormone signaling. For example, a cytokine (IL-6), a hormone (estradiol), or a growth factor (EGF, VEGF) is released by cells in the micro-environment, binding to and stimulating nearby cancer cells.

Dr. Gyamfi and colleagues write:

> During tumour progression induction of EMT occurs via paracrine signals from cells in the tumour micro-environment, allowing tumour cells to infiltrate surrounding tissue

and metastasize to distant sites.... Several growth factors, including TGF-β, Wnt and IL-6 have been shown to trigger EMT in transformed cell lines... Thus, the potential of blocking IL-6 and STAT3 activity has emerged as a potential therapeutic strategy. (37)

Previous high-throughput screening using adrenocortical carcinoma and prostate cancer cells identified niclosamide as a potent STAT3 inhibitor. Dr. Gyamfi's breast cancer cell study found that the Niclosamide inhibition of IL-6/STAT3 reversed adipocyte-induced EMT. They state:

> Niclosamide inhibited adipocyte-induced effects and significantly decreased cell motility in a dose-dependent manner.... . niclosamide reversed adipocyte-induced EMT with a correlated inhibition of IL-6/Stat3 activation and downregulation of EMT-TFs TWIST and SNAIL. Moreover, niclosamide markedly impaired MDA-MB-468 and MCF-7 [breast cancer cells] migration and invasion. (37)

Squamous Cell Cancer

Oral squamous cell cancer is especially difficult to treat and carries a poor prognosis with a 50%, 5-year survival. In 2018, Dr. Lin-Hong Wang et al. studied the effect of niclosamide on oral cancer cell lines, showing

> inhibition of the Wnt/β-catenin signaling pathway by targeting multiple components of this pathway, including downregulating the expression of β-catenin, Disheveled 2 [DVL2], phosphorylated glycogen synthase kinase-3β [p-GSK3β] and Cyclin D1.... as well as reduced the formation of primary and secondary tumorspheres. (39)

In 2018, Dr. Zewen Han et al. found a novel mechanism of niclosamide anti-cancer effect on head-and-neck squamous cell cancer. Dr. Han's group studied the micro RNA let-7, which functions as a tumor suppressor. Many cancers downregulate let-7. Dr. Han's group found that niclosamide restores and upregulates let-7, which then "restricted tumor cell proliferation and induced G1 phase cell cycle arrest."(40)

Similarly, using an in vitro model, Dr. Xiaoxu Li et al. (2017) found that niclosamide-induced cell cycle arrest (G1 phase) via the let-7/STAT3 pathway in oral squamous cell cancer, which inhibited proliferative, migratory, and invasive properties. (41) Dr. Li et al. also found that niclosamide inhibited "vasculogenic mimicry" formation of new blood vessels, using oral cancer cell lines in vitro and in vivo. (42) They conclude that niclosamide is preferred therapy for oral squamous cell cancer, yet voice concern over the issue of poor bio-availability that has yet to be addressed:

> Niclosamide exerts its anti-OSCC [oral squamous cell cancer] effects by cell cycle arrest through regulating cell cycle-related proteins, inhibits migration and invasion by upregulation of let-7a and downregulation of STAT3 in two OSCC cell lines. Considering that niclosamide inhibits the growth, migration and invasion of OSCC cells, it perhaps to be a preferred therapeutic candidate for improving treatment of OSCC patients in future. However, the development of poor bio-availability, the safety needs for cancer patients, and the functional mechanisms analysis of niclosamide are required to be elucidated. (41)

Platinum Chemo-Resistant Lung Cancer

Non-small-cell lung cancer (adenocarcinoma) is the most common lung cancer cell type, usually aggressive and with a high mortality rate. Although remissions can be obtained with platinum-based chemotherapy drugs (e.g., cisplatin, also called DDP), the duration of the response is short, and chemo—resistant recurrence is common. In 2018, Dr. Yufang Zuo et al. examined the effect of niclosamide, combined with platinum-based chemotherapy (DDP) on chemo-resistant lung cancer cells, finding that the two agents had a synergistic effect and:

> directly induced apoptosis, which may be associated with caspase-3 activation … niclosamide decreased the expression level of c-myc protein…. and may present as a promising drug candidate in lung cancer therapy. (43)

Immunotherapy with Checkpoint Blockade—One of the Most Important Advances in the History of Cancer Treatment

Cancer cell immune evasion is due in part to inhibition of T cells, the working cells of our immune system that attack and destroy cancer cells. Cytotoxic T lymphocyte-associated protein 4 (CTLA-4) and the programmed cell death 1 (PD-1) receptor are the two proteins targeted by checkpoint inhibitor antibodies. Antibodies directed at these two proteins will unleash the power of our T cells, freeing them to proliferate and attack the invading cancer cells. According to Dr. Antoni Ribas and Jedd D. Wolchok in 2018,

therapeutic blockade of the PD-1 pathway is arguably one of the most important advances in the history of cancer treatment…..Inflammation induced PDL1 expression in the micro-environment results in PD-1 mediated T cell exhaustion, inhibiting the anti-tumor cytotoxic T cell response … blockade [of PD-1] results in preferential stimulation of anti-tumor T cells. (44)

Although there have been durable remissions with checkpoint blockade, (anti-PD1/PD-L1 and anti–CTLA-4), overall results have been disappointing, with either primary failure or recurrence of resistant cell type after initial remission. Dr. Valsamo Anagnostou et al. write in 2019:

> Despite the durable clinical benefit observed with immune checkpoint inhibitors for patients with NSCLC [non–small-cell lung cancer], the majority of patients are either refractory or eventually develop acquired resistance after an initial response. (45)

Niclosamide Synergistic with Checkpoint Inhibitors

In 2019, Dr. Fan Luo et al. studied the use of niclosamide combined with checkpoint blockade drugs in an in vitro and in vivo lung cancer cell model. Dr. Luo et al. reports the two agents are synergistic with augmented anti-cancer activity involving blockage of STAT3 binding to promoter of PD-L1 with downregulation of PD-L1 expression. This resulted in "enhanced cancer cell lysis mediated by T cells in presence of PD-L1 blockade."(46)

In view of the above findings, one wonders

about possible synergism between checkpoint blockade and other repurposed anti-cancer drugs, such as ivermectin, mebendazole, and fenbendazole, etc. as mentioned in other chapters of this book. This would be a good topic for future NIH funding and study.

Combining HDAC Inhibitor with Niclosamide in Lung Cancer

The nuclear DNA is wrapped around a histone protein core, forming a structure called chromatin. When histones are treated with histone de-acetylase (HDACs), this results in more tightly packed chromatin and suppression of gene transcription (gene silencing). In a cancer cell, there is dysregulation of this process, with silencing of genes that restrict growth and proliferation and overexpression of genes involving unrestricted growth, proliferation, and inflammation. HDAC inhibitors have been shown to reverse this process, having anti-cancer activity. (47–53)

Valproic acid is an old anti-seizure drug FDA-approved for epilepsy and repurposed as a histone deacetylase (HDAC) inhibitor.

In a 2019 study by Drs. Oguzhan Akgun et al. the combination of HDAC inhibitor valproic acid with niclosamide was studied in a lung cancer cell line. Dr. Akgun and colleagues:

> observed that combination therapy initiates the activation of tumor necrosis receptors and causes apoptosis by activated caspase.... .the extrinsic apoptotic pathway was activated on the mitochondrial pathway.... ER [endoplamic reticulum] stress and mitochondrial membrane potential loss associated with increased

ROS [reactive oxygen species] levels induce cell death.... combination therapy caused a dramatic decrease in cell viability by inducing the extrinsic apoptotic pathway in lung cancer cell line. (51)

One might wonder about synergy of niclosamide with other natural HDAC inhibitors such as curcumin, sulforaphane, and butyrate. (52–53) We await further studies to confirm this.

Niclosamide for Other Cancers

Niclosamide anti-cancer studies include:

- Lymphoma (17)(31)
- Glioblastoma (54)
- Acute myeloid leukemia (AML) (55–57)
- Renal cell carcinoma (58),
- Hepatocellular carcinoma (59)
- Melanoma (60–61)
- Osteosarcoma (62)
- Adrenocortical carcinoma (63)
- Prostate cancer (8)(64)

Other indications include:

- Inflammatory airway disease (65)
- Endometriosis (66–67)
- Amyotrophic lateral sclerosis (ALS) (68)
- Psoriasis (69)
- Diabetes and diabetic kidney disease(70–71)
- Broad antiviral effects (72–74)
- Clostridia difficile enterocolitis (75–76)
- H. Pylori gastric infection (77)
- Vancomycin resistant enterococci (78)

- MRSA methicillin resistant staph aureus (79)
- Synergy with chloroquine (11)
- Inhibits antegrade lysosome trafficking (8–9)

Niclosamide Autophagy Inhibitor

The mTORC1 pathway plays an important role in the control of autophagy. During nutrient deprivation (starvation), mTOR is suppressed and autophagy is activated (antegrade trafficking). During nutrient excess, mTOR is activated, triggering cell proliferation, and autophagy is inactivated (perinuclear clustering). Cancer cells have upregulated the mTOR pathway, triggering increasing metabolic activity to support rapid proliferation. Many anti-cancer drugs downregulate mTOR, which activates "protective autophagy," explaining the observation of "perinuclear clustering of lysosomes."

In 2009, Dr. Aruna Balgi et al. screened more than 3,500 compounds and:

identified three approved drugs [perhexiline, niclosamide, amiodarone] and one pharmacological reagent [rottlerin] **capable of rapidly increasing autophagosome content.** Biochemical assays showed that **the four compounds stimulate autophagy and inhibit mTORC1** signaling in cells maintained in nutrient-rich conditions. (80)

Niclosamide Blocks Late-Stage Autophagy

In 2014, Dr. Ying Gao et al. studied the effect of Niclosamide on lysosomes, finding niclosamide blocked late-stage autophagy:

After Niclosamide treatments [there was] impaired lysosome function. In addition, both LC-II and P62 proteins accumulated significantly when treated by Niclosamide suggesting the late stage of autophagy was blocked ... increased pH of lysosomes and release of cathepsins from lysosome to cytosol resulted from membrane permeabilization ... Niclosamide not only inhibited mTOR activity, but also strongly blocked autophagy via lysosomal dysfunction. (81)

Note: LC3-II, written above as LC-II, (light chain microtubule-associated protein) and P62 protein are both commonly used to monitor autophagic activity.

Notice that niclosamide inhibits mTOR activity, which normally activates "protective autophagy", yet at the same time niclosamide blocks late-stage autophagy, making this a "double whammy" to kill the cancer cell. We will discuss the importance of this later in the autophagy inhibitors chapters (chapters 31–33).

Palladium Complex in Breast Cancer

In 2015, Dr. Didem Karakas et al. studied palladium complex in a breast cancer stem cell model finding enhanced cytotoxicity with the addition of niclosamide. Dr. Karakas's group report that niclosamide (1.5 micromolar) suppresses autophagy (with decreased ATG5 gene levels) and enhanced cytotoxic activity of the palladium complex:

Importantly, the addition of niclosamide resulted in the **suppression of autophagy** [proved by the decrease in ATG5 gene levels] that might have contributed to the enhanced cytotoxicity. In conclusion, the application of this combination may be regarded as a novel and effective approach for the treatment of breast cancer due to its promising cytotoxic effect on cancer stem cells that cause recurrence of the disease. (82)

Note: The ATG5 gene makes the autophagy-related 5 (ATG5) protein.

Note: Another palladium containing anti-cancer compound is poly-MVA (palladium, thiamine, alpha lipoic acid) in a liquid mineral polymer developed by Merrill Garnett. (83–85)

Synergy of Niclosamide with 2-DG GLYCOLYSIS Inhibitor

In 2019, Dr. Lili Liu et al. studied lung cancer cells in vitro, finding marked synergy with dual inhibition of S100A4 (a downstream Wnt pathway protein) by niclosamide, and inhibition of GLYCOLYSIS with 2 DG (2-deoxy-glucose). One might speculate similar synergy with Niclosamide and other glycolysis inhibitors such as DCA (dichloroacetate), Diclofenac and Quercetin. We await these future studies. (86)

Niclosamide Prevents Conversion of Non-Stem cells to Stem Cells

In 2013, Dr. Seog-Young Kin et al. studied how IL-6/STAT3 signaling transforms breast cancer cells into breast cancer stem cells, finding that niclosamide effectively prevents this conversion by blocking OCT-4 gene expression.

Data from cytokine array assay show that IL-6 was secreted from non-CSCs when cells were cultured in ultra-low attachment plates. IL-6 regulates CSC-associated OCT-4 gene expression through the IL-6-JAK1-STAT3 signal transduction pathway in non-CSCs. Inhibiting this pathway by treatment with anti-IL-6 antibody (1 µg/ml) or **niclosamide (0.5–2 µM)**/LLL12 (5–10 µM) effectively prevented OCT-4 gene expression. (87)

Niclosamide Dosing

In 2018 Dr. Susen Burock et al. studied oral niclosamide in patients with metastatic colorectal cancer, writing:

Niclosamide has only little side effects and seems to be well tolerated even when applied over a long period. The oral dose of niclosamide for adults in anti-helminthic treatments is 2 g on day one followed by 1 g daily for 6 consecutive days. The serum concentration of niclosamide after a single dose of 2 g leads to maximal serum concentrations of 0.25–6.0 µg/ml which corresponds to the concentration used on the above mentioned models. (29)

In Dr. Burdock's group Nicolo Trial, currently underway, patients will be treated with 2 grams niclosamide daily with a meal. (29)

Typical Dosing for Adult Tapeworm Treatment

Typical niclosamide treatment dosage for dwarf tapeworm: Adults—2 grams a day for seven days. Treatment may be repeated in seven to fourteen days if needed. (30)(88) The 2005 WHO safety report on niclosamide found no toxicities, and it was deemed generally safe for use in pregnant women and children. (89)

Niclosamide for Clostridia Difficile Enterocolitis

Clostridia difficile enterocolitis is a growing problem in hospital wards due to the frequent use of high-dose IV antibiotics in the oncology patient for febrile neutropenia after chemotherapy. Relapse of C. Diff after conventional antibiotic treatment with vancomycin and flagyl is quite common, and carries a high mortality rate. Niclosamide could be a good solution, having been repurposed as an effective treatment for C. Diff. enterocolitis. Niclosamide eradicates the spore form of the organism, preventing recurrence. (92–93)

Niclosamide for H. Pylori

Niclosamide is also effective for H. Pylori gastric infection. (94)

Niclosamide as an Antiviral Drug

Niclosamide has broad antiviral activity, including COVID-19 (corona virus) by virtue of its effects on lysosomal function, very similar to other autophagy inhibitors such as hydroxychloroquine and azithromycin, discussed in more detail in the chapters on autophagy inhibitors, chapters 31–34. (95–102) In 2020, Dr. Jimin Xu et al. write:

> Through a series of drug repurposing screening campaigns, niclosamide, an FDA-approved anthelminthic drug, was found to be effective against various viral infections with nanomolar to micromolar potency such as SARS-CoV, MERS-CoV, ZIKV, HCV, and human adenovirus, indicating its potential as an antiviral agent. (96)

Conclusion

Niclosamide is a remarkable repurposed anti-cancer drug, achieving therapeutic levels at doses commonly used for treating parasites, with no toxicity. The major anti-cancer mechanisms are firstly, mitochondrial uncoupling, which serves as an OXPHOS inhibitor, which triggers "protective autophagy," and secondly, inhibition of late-phase autophagy that augments the cancer cell-killing effect.

The effect of niclosamide on cancer cell lysosomes leads to release of acid into the cytosol with acidification of the cancer cell, which actually inhibits GLYCOLYSIS in the cytoplasm. Therefore niclosamide is also a GLYCOLYSIS inhibitor. However, niclosamide is synergistic with other GLYCOLYSIS inhibitors such as 2-DG. Synergy with DCA is expected, yet requires confirmation with further study.

As mentioned above, niclosamide targets all three pillars of cancer-cell metabolism: OXPHOS, GLYCOLYSIS, and autophagy. In addition, niclosamide targets the Wnt and Notch cancer stem cell pathways, serving as cancer stem cell agent. Will niclosamide revolutionize cancer treatment and make conventional chemotherapy a relic for the medical museum? I hope so.

References for Chapter 23: Niclosamide

1) Chen, Wei, et al. "Niclosamide: beyond an antihelminthic drug." Cellular Signaling 41 (2018): 89-96.

2) Deng, Youlin, et al. "A blockade of IGF signaling sensitizes human ovarian cancer cells to the anthelmintic niclosamide-induced anti-proliferative and anticancer

activities." Cellular Physiology and Biochemistry 39.3 (2016): 871-888.

3) Pan, Jing-Xuan, Ke Ding, and Cheng-Yan Wang. "Niclosamide, an old antihelminthic agent, demonstrates antitumor activity by blocking multiple signaling pathways of cancer stem cells." Chinese journal of cancer 31.4 (2012): 178.

4) Chen M, Wang J, Lu J, et al. The anti-helminthic niclosamide inhibits Wnt/Frizzled1 signaling. Biochemistry. 2009;48:10267–10274.

5) Lu, Wenyan, et al. "Niclosamide suppresses cancer cell growth by inducing Wnt co-receptor LRP6 degradation and inhibiting the Wnt/β-catenin pathway." PloS one 6.12 (2011): e29290.

6) Wang, Jiangbo, et al. "Niclosamide-induced Wnt signaling inhibition in colorectal cancer is mediated by autophagy." Biochemical Journal 476.3 (2019): 535-546.

7) Pu, Jing, et al. "Mechanisms and functions of lysosome positioning." Journal of cell science 129.23 (2016): 4329-4339.

8) Circu, Magdalena L., et al. "A Novel High Content Imaging-Based Screen Identifies the Anti-Helminthic Niclosamide as an Inhibitor of Lysosome Anterograde Trafficking and Prostate Cancer Cell Invasion." PLoS ONE 11.1 (2016).

9) Circu, Magdalena L., et al. "Correction: A Novel High Content Imaging-Based Screen Identifies the Anti-Helminthic Niclosamide as an Inhibitor of Lysosome Anterograde Trafficking and Prostate Cancer Cell Invasion." PloS one 11.3 (2016).

10) Tran, Uyen Thi, and Toshimori Kitami. "Niclosamide activates the NLRP3 inflammasome by intracellular acidification and mitochondrial inhibition." Communications biology 2.1 (2019): 1-14.

11) Xiang, Di, et al. "Niclosamide, an anti-helminthic molecule, downregulates the retroviral oncoprotein Tax and pro-survival Bcl-2 proteins in HTLV-1-transformed T lymphocytes." Biochemical and biophysical research communications 464.1 (2015): 221-228.

12) Yo, Yi-Te, et al. "Growth Inhibition of Ovarian Tumor–Initiating Cells by Niclosamide." Molecular Cancer Therapeutics 11.8 (2012): 1703-1712.

13) Arend, R. C., et al. "Inhibition of Wnt/β-catenin pathway by niclosamide: a therapeutic target for ovarian cancer." Gynecologic oncology 134.1 (2014): 112.

14) Arend, Rebecca C., et al. "Niclosamide and its analogs are potent inhibitors of Wnt/β-catenin, mTOR and STAT3 signaling in ovarian cancer." Oncotarget 7.52 (2016): 86803.

15) Haygood, Christen L. Walters, et al. "Niclosamide analogs for treatment of ovarian cancer." International Journal of Gynecologic Cancer 25.8 (2015): 1377-1385.

16) Lin, Chi Kang, et al. "Preclinical evaluation of a nanoformulated antihelminthic, niclosamide, in ovarian cancer." Oncotarget 7.8 (2016): 8993-9006.

17) Møller, Michael B., et al. "Disrupted p53 function as predictor of treatment failure and poor prognosis in B-and T-cell non-Hodgkin's lymphoma." Clinical Cancer Research 5.5 (1999): 1085-1091.

18) Toufektchan, Eléonore, and Franck Toledo. "The guardian of the genome revisited: p53 downregulates genes required for telomere maintenance, DNA repair, and centromere structure." Cancers 10.5 (2018): 135.

19) Patel, K. R., and H. D. Patel. "p53: An Attractive Therapeutic Target for Cancer." Current medicinal chemistry (2019).

20) Mantovani, Fiamma, Licio Collavin, and Giannino Del Sal. "Mutant p53 as a guardian of the cancer cell." Cell Death & Differentiation 26.2 (2019): 199-212.

21) Kumar, R., et al. "Mitochondrial uncoupling reveals a novel therapeutic opportunity for p53-defective cancers." Nature Communications 9 (2018).

22) Figarola, James L., et al. "Bioenergetic modulation with the mitochondria uncouplers SR4 and niclosamide prevents proliferation and growth of treatment-naïve and vemurafenib-resistant melanomas." Oncotarget 9.97 (2018): 36945.

23) Alasadi, Amer, et al. "Effect of mitochondrial uncouplers niclosamide ethanolamine (NEN) and oxyclozanide on hepatic metastasis of colon cancer." Cell death & disease 9.2 (2018): 215.

24) Suliman, Mohammed A., et al. "Niclosamide inhibits colon cancer progression through downregulation of the Notch pathway and upregulation of the tumor

suppressor miR-200 family." International journal of molecular medicine 38.3 (2016): 776-784.

25) Monin, Malte B., et al. "The anthelmintic niclosamide inhibits colorectal cancer cell lines via modulation of the canonical and noncanonical Wnt signaling pathway." Journal of Surgical Research 203.1 (2016): 193-205.

26) Osada, Takuya, et al. "Antihelminth compound niclosamide downregulates Wnt signaling and elicits antitumor responses in tumors with activating APC mutations." Cancer research 71.12 (2011): 4172-4182.

27) Park, So-Yeon, et al. "Inhibition of LEF1-mediated DCLK1 by niclosamide attenuates colorectal cancer stemness." Clinical Cancer Research 25.4 (2019): 1415-1429.

28) Dahlmann, Mathias, et al. "S100A4 in cancer metastasis: Wnt signaling-driven interventions for metastasis restriction." Cancers 8.6 (2016): 59.

29) Burock, Susen, et al. "Phase II trial to investigate the safety and efficacy of orally applied niclosamide in patients with metachronous or sychronous metastases of a colorectal cancer progressing after therapy: the NIKOLO trial." BMC Cancer 18 (2018).

30) Li, Yonghe, et al. "Multi-targeted therapy of cancer by niclosamide: A new application for an old drug." Cancer letters 349.1 (2014): 8-14.

31) Ansari, Junaid, et al. "Potent Inhibition of the Growth and Induction of Apoptosis in Lymphoma by the Anthelminthic Drug Niclosamide: In Vitro Data. Blood (2015) 126 (23): 5131-5131.

32) Khanim, F. L., et al. "Redeployment-based drug screening identifies the anti-helminthic niclosamide as anti-myeloma therapy that also reduces free light chain production." Blood cancer journal 1.10 (2011): e39.

33) Wang, Yu-Chi, et al. "Drug screening identifies niclosamide as an inhibitor of breast cancer stem-like cells." PloS one 8.9 (2013): e74538.

34) Ye, Tinghong, et al. "The anthelmintic drug niclosamide induces apoptosis, impairs metastasis and reduces immunosuppressive cells in breast cancer model." PloS one 9.1 (2014): e85887.

35) Lu, Wenyan, et al. "Niclosamide suppresses cancer cell growth by inducing Wnt co-receptor LRP6 degradation and inhibiting the Wnt/β-catenin pathway." PloS one 6.12 (2011): e29290.

36) Venning, Freja A., Lena Wullkopf, and Janine T. Erler. "Targeting ECM disrupts cancer progression." Frontiers in oncology 5 (2015): 224.

37) Gyamfi, Jones, et al. "Niclosamide reverses adipocyte induced epithelial-mesenchymal transition in breast cancer cells via suppression of the interleukin-6/STAT3 signalling axis." Scientific reports 9.1 (2019): 1-14.

38) Kalluri, Raghu, and Robert A. Weinberg. "The basics of epithelial-mesenchymal transition." The Journal of clinical investigation 119.6 (2009): 1420-1428.

39) Wang, Lin-Hong, et al. "The antihelminthic niclosamide inhibits cancer stemness, extracellular matrix remodeling, and metastasis through dysregulation of the nuclear β-catenin/c-Myc axis in OSCC." Scientific reports 8.1 (2018): 12776.

40) Han, Zewen, et al. "Niclosamide induces cell cycle arrest in G1 phase in head and neck squamous cell carcinoma through let-7d/CDC34 axis." Frontiers in pharmacology 9 (2019): 1544.

41) Li, Xiaoxu, et al. "Targeting of cell cycle and let-7a/STAT3 pathway by niclosamide inhibits proliferation, migration and invasion in oral squamous cell carcinoma cells." Biomedicine & Pharmacotherapy 96 (2017): 434-442.

42) Li, Xiaoxu, et al. "Niclosamide acts as a new inhibitor of vasculogenic mimicry in oral cancer through upregulation of miR-124 and downregulation of STAT3." Oncology reports 39.2 (2018): 827-833.

43) Zuo, Yufang, et al. "Niclosamide enhances the cytotoxic effect of cisplatin in cisplatin-resistant human lung cancer cells via suppression of lung resistance-related protein and c-myc." Molecular medicine reports 17.3 (2018): 3497-3502.

44) Ribas, Antoni, and Jedd D. Wolchok. "Cancer immunotherapy using checkpoint blockade." Science 359.6382 (2018): 1350-1355.

45) Anagnostou, Valsamo, et al. "Dynamics of Tumor and Immune Responses during Immune Checkpoint

Blockade in Non–Small Cell Lung Cancer." *Cancer research* 79.6 (2019): 1214-1225.

46) Luo, Fan, et al. "Niclosamide, an antihelmintic drug, enhances efficacy of PD-1/PD-L1 immune checkpoint blockade in non-small cell lung cancer." Journal for immunotherapy of cancer 7.1 (2019): 1-13.

47) Ropero, Santiago, and Manel Esteller. "The role of histone deacetylases (HDACs) in human cancer." Molecular oncology 1.1 (2007): 19-25.

48) Chen, Hong Ping, Yu Tina Zhao, and Ting C. Zhao. "Histone deacetylases and mechanisms of regulation of gene expression." Critical Reviews™ in Oncogenesis 20.1-2 (2015).

49) Atadja, Peter W. "HDAC inhibitors and cancer therapy." Epigenetics and Disease. Springer, Basel, 2011. 175-195.

50) Li, Yixuan, and Edward Seto. "HDACs and HDAC inhibitors in cancer development and therapy." Cold Spring Harbor perspectives in medicine 6.10 (2016): a026831.

51) Akgun, Oguzhan, Merve Erkisa, and Ferda Ari. "Effective and new potent drug combination: Histone deacetylase and Wnt/β-catenin pathway inhibitors in lung carcinoma cells." Journal of cellular biochemistry (2019).

52) Soflaei, Sara S., et al. "Curcumin: a natural pan-HDAC inhibitor in cancer." Current pharmaceutical design 24.2 (2018): 123-129.

53) Yoon, Somy, and Gwang Hyeon Eom. "HDAC and HDAC inhibitor: from cancer to cardiovascular diseases." Chonnam medical journal 52.1 (2016): 1-11.

54) Wieland, Anja, et al. "Anticancer effects of niclosamide in human glioblastoma." Clinical Cancer

55) Jin, Yanli, et al. Antineoplastic mechanisms of niclosamide in acute myelogenous leukemia stem cells: inactivation of the NF-κB pathway and generation of reactive oxygen species. Cancer research 70.6 (2010): 2516-2527.

56) Jin, Bei, et al. "Anthelmintic niclosamide suppresses transcription of BCR-ABL fusion oncogene via disabling Sp1 and induces apoptosis in imatinib-resistant CML cells harboring T315I mutant." Cell death & disease 9.2 (2018): 68.

57) Chae, Hee-Don, et al. "Niclosamide suppresses acute myeloid leukemia cell proliferation through inhibition of CREB-dependent signaling pathways." Oncotarget 9.4 (2018): 4301.

58) Zhao, Juan, et al. "Niclosamide suppresses renal cell carcinoma by inhibiting Wnt/β-catenin and inducing mitochondrial dysfunctions." SpringerPlus 5.1 (2016): 1436.

59) Chen, Bin, et al. "Computational discovery of niclosamide ethanolamine, a repurposed drug candidate that reduces growth of hepatocellular carcinoma cells in vitro and in mice by inhibiting cell division cycle 37 signaling." Gastroenterology 152.8 (2017): 2022-2036.

60) Zhou, Jingfeng, et al. "The antihelminthic drug niclosamide effectively inhibits the malignant phenotypes of uveal melanoma in vitro and in vivo." Theranostics 7.6 (2017): 1447.

61) Figarola, James L., et al. "Bioenergetic modulation with the mitochondria uncouplers SR4 and niclosamide prevents proliferation and growth of treatment-naïve and vemurafenib-resistant melanomas." Oncotarget 9.97 (2018): 36945.

62) Liao, Zhan, et al. "The anthelmintic drug niclosamide inhibits the proliferative activity of human osteosarcoma cells by targeting multiple signal pathways." Current cancer drug targets 15.8 (2015): 726-738.

63) Satoh, Kei, et al. "Identification of niclosamide as a novel anticancer agent for adrenocortical carcinoma." Clinical Cancer Research 22.14 (2016): 3458-3466.

64) Sobhani, Navid, et al. "Current status of androgen receptor-splice variant 7 inhibitor niclosamide in castrate-resistant prostate-cancer." Investigational new drugs 36.6 (2018): 1133-1137.

65) Cabrita, Inês, et al. "Niclosamide repurposed for the treatment of inflammatory airway disease." JCI insight 4.15 (2019).

66) Prather, Genna R., et al. "Niclosamide as a potential nonsteroidal therapy for endometriosis that preserves reproductive function in an experimental mouse model." Biology of reproduction 95.4 (2016): 74-1.

67) Sekulovski, Nikola, et al. "Endometriotic inflammatory microenvironment induced by macrophages can

be targeted by niclosamide." Biology of reproduction 100.2 (2018): 398-408.

68) Serrano, Alessia, et al. "The S100A4 Transcriptional Inhibitor Niclosamide Reduces Pro-Inflammatory and Migratory Phenotypes of Microglia: Implications for Amyotrophic Lateral Sclerosis." Cells 8.10 (2019): 1261.

69) Thatikonda, Sowjanya, Venkatesh Pooladanda, and Chandraiah Godugu. "Repurposing an old drug for new use: Niclosamide in psoriasis-like skin inflammation." Journal of Cellular Physiology (2019).

70) Tao, Hanlin, et al. "Niclosamide ethanolamine–induced mild mitochondrial uncoupling improves diabetic symptoms in mice." Nature medicine 20.11 (2014): 1263.

71) Han, Pengxun, et al. "Niclosamide ethanolamine improves diabetes and diabetic kidney disease in mice." American journal of translational research 10.4 (2018): 1071.

72) Jurgeit, Andreas, et al. "Niclosamide is a proton carrier and targets acidic endosomes with broad antiviral effects." PLoS pathogens 8.10 (2012): e1002976.

73) Marrugal-Lorenzo, José A., et al. "Repositioning salicylanilide anthelmintic drugs to treat adenovirus infections." Scientific reports 9.1 (2019): 17.

74) Huang, Lu, et al. "Niclosamide inhibits lytic replication of Epstein-Barr virus by disrupting mTOR activation." Antiviral research 138 (2017): 68-78.

75) Misch, Elizabeth Ann, and Nasia Safdar. "Clostridioides difficile Infection in the Stem Cell Transplant and Hematologic Malignancy Population." Infectious Disease Clinics 33.2 (2019): 447-466.

76) Tam, John, et al. "Host-targeted niclosamide inhibits C. difficile virulence and prevents disease in mice without disrupting the gut microbiota." Nature communications 9.1 (2018): 5233.

77) Tharmalingam, Nagendran, et al. "Repurposing the anthelmintic drug niclosamide to combat Helicobacter pylori." Scientific reports 8.1 (2018): 3701.

78) Mohammad, Haroon, et al. "Repurposing niclosamide for intestinal decolonization of vancomycin-resistant enterococci." International journal of antimicrobial agents 51.6 (2018): 897-904.

79) Rajamuthiah, Rajmohan, et al. "Repurposing salicylanilide anthelmintic drugs to combat drug resistant Staphylococcus aureus." PloS one 10.4 (2015): e0124595.

80) Balgi, Aruna D., et al. "Screen for chemical modulators of autophagy reveals novel therapeutic inhibitors of mTORC1 signaling." PloS one 4.9 (2009).

81) Gao, Ying, et al. "Niclosamide blocks autophagy via lysosomal dysfunction (663.18)." The FASEB Journal 28.1_supplement (2014): 663-18.

82) Karakas, Didem, et al. "Addition of niclosamide to palladium (II) saccharinate complex of terpyridine results in enhanced cytotoxic activity inducing apoptosis on cancer stem cells of breast cancer." Bioorganic & medicinal chemistry 23.17 (2015): 5580-5586.

83) Garnett, Merrill, and Joy Garnett. First Pulse. First Pulse Projects, 1998.

84) Corduneanu, Oana, et al. "Lipoic acid–palladium complex interaction with DNA, voltammetric and AFM characterization." Talanta 77.5 (2009): 1843-1853.

85) Sridharan, Vijayalakshmi, et al. "Late administration of a palladium lipoic acid complex (POLY-MVA) modifies cardiac mitochondria but not functional or structural manifestations of radiation-induced heart disease in a rat model." Radiation research 187.3 (2017): 361-366.

86) Liu, Lili, et al. "S100A4 alters metabolism and promotes invasion of lung cancer cells by up-regulating mitochondrial complex I protein NDUFS2." Journal of Biological Chemistry 294.18 (2019): 7516-7527.

87) Kim, Seog-Young, et al. "Role of the IL-6-JAK1-STAT3-Oct-4 pathway in the conversion of non-stem cancer cells into cancer stem-like cells." Cellular signalling 25.4 (2013): 961-969.

88) Li, Min, et al. "Suppression of lysosome function induces autophagy via a feedback down-regulation of MTOR complex 1 (MTORC1) activity." Journal of Biological Chemistry 288.50 (2013): 35769-35780.

89) Gilles, H. M. "Diseases of the alimentary system: Treatment of intestinal worms." British medical journal 2.6047 (1976): 1314.

90) Ofori-Adjei, D., et al. "A review of the safety of niclosamide, pyrantel, triclabendazole and

oxamniquine." International Journal of Risk & Safety in Medicine 20.3 (2008): 113-122.

91) Gohil, Vishal M., et al. "Nutrient-sensitized screening for drugs that shift energy metabolism from mitochondrial respiration to glycolysis." Nature biotechnology 28.3 (2010): 249-255.

92) Tam, John, et al. "Host-targeted niclosamide inhibits C. difficile virulence and prevents disease in mice without disrupting the gut microbiota." Nature communications 9.1 (2018): 1-11.

93) Gooyit, Major, and Kim D. Janda. "Reprofiled anthelmintics abate hypervirulent stationary-phase Clostridium difficile." Scientific reports 6 (2016): 33642.

94) Tharmalingam, Nagendran, et al. "Repurposing the anthelmintic drug niclosamide to combat Helicobacter pylori." Scientific reports 8.1 (2018): 3701.

95) Jurgeit, Andreas, et al. "Niclosamide is a proton carrier and targets acidic endosomes with broad antiviral effects." PLoS pathogens 8.10 (2012).

96) Xu, Jimin, et al. "Broad Spectrum Antiviral Agent Niclosamide and Its Therapeutic Potential." ACS infectious diseases (2020).

97) Marrugal-Lorenzo, José A., et al. "Repositioning salicylanilide anthelmintic drugs to treat adenovirus infections." Scientific reports 9.1 (2019): 1-10.

98) Wu, Chang-Jer, et al. "Inhibition of severe acute respiratory syndrome coronavirus replication by niclosamide." Antimicrobial agents and chemotherapy 48.7 (2004): 2693-2696.

99) Chang, Yi-Wei, et al. "Pharmacokinetics of anti-SARS-CoV agent niclosamide and its analogs in rats." Journal of Food and Drug Analysis 14.4 (2006).

100) Gautret, Philippe, et al. "Hydroxychloroquine and azithromycin as a treatment of COVID-19: results of an open-label non-randomized clinical trial." International Journal of Antimicrobial Agents (2020): 105949.

101) Yang, Naidi, and Han-Ming Shen. "Targeting the Endocytic Pathway and Autophagy Process as a Novel Therapeutic Strategy in COVID-19." Int J Biol Sci 16.10 (2020): 1724-1731.

102) Nujić, Krunoslav, et al. "Impairment of lysosomal functions by azithromycin and chloroquine contributes to anti-inflammatory phenotype." Cellular immunology 279.1 (2012): 78-86.

Chapter 24

Mebendazole and Fenbendazole

MEBENDAZOLE (VERMOX®) IS AN OLD anti-parasitic drug for whipworm, pinworm, roundworm, and hookworm, used for decades with no known clinical toxicity. First synthesized by Janssen Pharmaceutical in 1968 and FDA-approved in 1972, Mebendazole is an inexpensive generic drug available through compounding pharmacies in the U.S.

There is considerable Interest in mebendazole as a repurposed anti-cancer drug serving as a microtubule inhibitor, similar to the taxane class of chemotherapy drugs derived from the Pacific Yew Tree (taxane, paclitaxel, docetaxel, etc.). Mebendazole also shares similarity with other microtubule-destabilizing drugs—vinblastine, vincristine, nocodazole, and colchicine, which interfere with microtubule polymerization.

This feature is useful for cancer treatment because microtubules are components of the "spindle structures" used in cell division, mitosis, and other important cell functions. Inhibiting the spindle formation by the microtubule system prevents the two-cell nuclei from dividing and separating to form two new cells, thus preventing uncontrolled cell division, one of Weinberg's ten hallmarks of cancer.

The usual dosage for mebendazole is 100 mg caps, one cap twice a day. To increase bio-availability, mebendazole should be taken with a fatty meal (whole milk or ice cream). The

Benzimidazole class of drugs includes albendazole, fenbendazole, flubendazole, mebendazole, oxibendazole, and thiabendazole, all used as veterinary anthelminthics (antiparasitic drugs). (1–5)

Abnormal Spindle Formation in Mouse Cancer Model

In 2002, Dr. Ji-ichiro Sasaki et al. studied mebendazole in a lung cancer mouse xenograft model, finding a strong anti-tumor effect with reduction in metastatic lesions, surprisingly, without any toxicity compared to the chemotherapy drug paclitaxel (taxane). Dr. Sasaki and colleagues write:

> We speculate that tumor cells may be defective in mitotic checkpoint function and sensitive to the spindle inhibitor MZ [Mebendazole]. Abnormal spindle formation may be the key factor determining whether a cell undergoes apoptosis, whereas strong microtubule inhibitors [Taxane chemotherapy] elicit toxicity even in normal cells... (6)

Review of the Literature

In 2019, Dr. Andrea Emanuele Guerini et al. reviewed all the available medical literature on mebendazole as a repurposed anti-cancer drug, writing that mebendazole (MBZ) has many desirable characteristics:

> MBZ meets many of the characteristics

desirable for a repurposed drug: good and proven toxicity profile, pharmacokinetics allowing to reach therapeutic concentrations at disease site, ease of administration and low price. (7)

Anti-cancer characteristics of mebendazole (MBZ):

- Inhibits tubulin polymerization
- Inhibits tumor angiogenesis
- Inhibits matrix metalloproteinases (MMP)
- Inhibits multidrug resistance (MDR)
- Synergy with radiation and chemotherapy
- Stimulates host anti-tumor immune response
- May reduce or arrest tumor growth
- Decrease metastatic spread
- Improved survival

Mebendazole Synergy with Autophagy Inhibitors—Pronounced Induction of Protective Autophagy

Like many other anti-cancer drugs, mebendazole causes "pronounced induction of protective autophagy" in cancer cells. In 2019, Dr. So Jung Sung et al. studied the anti-angiogenic effect of mebendazole on endothelial cells (EC), finding synergy with autophagy inhibitors such as the antimalarial, chloroquine:

> Treatment of endothelial cells with mebendazole induced cell shrinkage, cell cycle arrest, apoptosis, nuclear fragmentation, p53 expression, and pronounced induction of **protective autophagy**.... Treatment with **autophagy inhibitors** such as 3-methyladenine and **chloroquine** resulted in

marked enhancement of antiproliferative and pro-apoptotic effects of MBZ [Mebendazole]. (8)

Other autophagy inhibitors mentioned in this book include:

- Mefloquine/chloroquine/hydroxychloroquine
- Thymoquinone (black seed oil)
- Loratadine
- Clarithromycin (Azithromycin)
- Propranolol
- Niclosamide
- Proton Pump Inhibitor Antacids (PPI's)

Metastatic Adrenocortical Cancer

In 2011, Dr. I. A. Dobrosotskaya et al. reported a remarkable case of mebendazole inducing long-term disease control in a 48-year-old male with metastatic adrenocortical carcinoma. After unsuccessful conventional chemo-radiation treatments, the patient was given only a 100 mg capsule of mebendazole twice daily. The metastatic disease initially regressed and then remained stable over 19 months, finally progressing after 24 months of mebendazole as sole treatment. (9)

One might wonder if the addition of one of the autophagy inhibitors, such as hydroxychloroquine (Plaquenil®), or chloroquine in synergy with mebendazole, would have controlled the disease for a longer time, perhaps indefinitely.

In 2008, Dr. Daniele Martiarelli et al. showed inhibition of adrenocortical carcinoma in a mouse xenograft model, in vivo:

Mebendazole significantly inhibited cancer cells growth, both in vitro and in vivo, the effects being due to the induction of apoptosis. Moreover, mebendazole inhibited invasion and migration of cancer cells in vitro, and metastases formation in vivo. (10)

Case Report: Metastatic Colon Cancer Remission

In 2014, Drs. Peter Nygren and Rolf Larsson reported a case of a 74-year-old male with metastatic colon cancer refractory to chemotherapy. The patient was started on mebendazole 100 mg oral capsule twice a day, after which CAT Scans showed near complete remission of metastatic lung lesions, and partial remission of liver lesions and nodes, with no reported adverse effects. However, the drug did cause liver enzyme elevation. (11)

High Through-Put Screen Identifies Mebendazole for Leukemia

In 2018, Dr. Licai He et al. did a high through-put screen of more than 1,000 FDA-approved drugs, finding mebendazole the best candidate to inhibit growth of acute myeloid leukemia (AML) cell lines at pharmacologically achievable concentrations, with no toxicity to normal cells. Dr. He et al. write:

> MBZ [Mebendazole] repressed the progression of leukemic cells in vivo and prolonged survival in AML xenograft mouse model. Taken together, our results suggest that MBZ could be a potential new therapeutic agent for the treatment of AML patients. (12)

Immune Modulation Anti-Tumor Effects of Mebendazole

In 2017, Dr. Kristin Blom et al. found that mebendazole is associated with monocyte/macrophage activation, serving to upregulate host anti-tumor immune function. (13)

A follow-up study in 2017 by Dr. Jenny Rubin et al. showed mebendazole potentiated the anti-cancer effects of the immune cells, activated peripheral blood monocytes (PBMCs), explaining their augmented anti-cancer activity. (14)

Synergy with oncology drugs and radiation:

- Sorafenib for hepatocellular carcinoma (15)
- Docetaxel for prostate cancer (16)
- Navitoclax in Non-Small-Cell Lung Cancer (17)
- Radiation Therapy for Breast Cancer (18–19)

Mebendazole has been studied in these cell types:

- Ovarian cancer (20)
- Multiple myeloma (21)
- Melanoma (22–23)
- Lung cancer (24)
- Breast cancer (25)
- Brain cancer (26–32)
- Fibrosarcoma (33)
- Squamous cell cancer (34)
- Gastric cancer (35)
- Leukemia (36–38)
- Malignant ascites (39)

Mebendazole pathway interactions are as follows:

- Inactivates BCL-2 (the anti-apoptotic protein)(23)
- Hedgehog inhibitor (Cancer Stem Cell Pathway) (36–37)(43–47)
- Inactivates C-Myc (39)
- Downregulates MDM drug resistance (40)

Mebendazole drug synergies:

- Autophagy inhibitors: chloroquine/ hydroxychloroquine, clarithromycin, thymoquinone, etc.
- Metformin
- Metronomic chemotherapy
- Taxanes of vinca alkaloids microtubule agents
- Albendazole
- Itraconazole
- Cimetidine
- Diclofenac (NSAID)

Mebendazole for Melanoma— Inactivates BCL-2

In 2008, Dr. Nicole Doudican et al. used a high through-put technique to screen 2000 drugs currently approved for human use for anti-cancer activity against virulent melanoma cancer cell lines. They discovered mebendazole as the most promising agent, inducing apoptosis via inactivation of the BCL-2 protein. Many cancers have upregulated BCL-2 to prevent apoptosis and confer "immortality." The new FDA-approved drug venetoclax is a BCL-2 inhibitor approved for hematologic malignancies. Dr. Doudican and colleagues write:

Mebendazole treatment induces apoptosis through the intrinsic and extrinsic pathways in melanoma cells but not in melanocytes ... After treatment with 0.5 µmol/L mebendazole for 14 h, we observed overall **microtubular network disarray** in melanoma, M-14, and SK-Mel-19 cells [melanoma cells], characterized by diffuse staining . (1) (23)

See chapter 20, "Cancer as a Parasitic Disease," for more discussion of mebendazole.

Fenbendazole Microtubule Agent and Glycolysis Inhibitor

The benzimidazole drug family includes mebendazole, albendazole, flubendazole and fenbendazole, all antiparasitic drugs of similar structure. All use microtubule inhibition as the main mechanism of action. A number of very effective chemotherapy drugs (taxanes and vinca alkaloids) also target the microtubule system of the cancer cell. Disrupting microtubule activity blocks the spindle formation needed for cell division and blocks cell division in metaphase (a phase in mitosis), causing cell death (apoptosis).

Joe Tippens's Remarkable Recovery from Lung Cancer

A close cousin of Mebendazole is Fenbendazole (FZ), an antiparasitic veterinary drug, widely used for pets and farm animals, made popular by Joe Tippens, who shared his remarkable story of recovery from metastatic small-cell lung cancer after an old friend, a veterinarian, recommended he take fenbendazole.

Non-Small-Cell Lung Cancer Study in Vitro

Fenbendazole is effective at low micromolar concentrations and is remarkably safe for animals and humans, resulting in relatively mild changes in the microtubule structure of cancer cells. In 2018, Dr. Nilambra Dogra et al. studied the effects of fenbendazole (FZ) on a NSCLC (non-small-cell lung cancer) cell line in vitro and in vivo mouse xenografts and make this favorable conclusion:

> FZ [Fenbendazole] ... is a safe and inexpensive anthelmintic drug possessing an efficient antiproliferative activity.... potent growth-inhibitory activity.... moderate affinity for mammalian tubulin and exerts cytotoxicity to human cancer cells at micromolar concentrations. Simultaneously, it caused mitochondrial translocation of p53 and effectively inhibited glucose uptake, mRNA expression of GLUT transporters as well as HK2 [hexokinase 2]—a key glycolytic enzyme that most cancer cells thrive on. It blocked the growth of human xenografts in nu/nu mice model when mice were fed with the drug orally.... potential therapeutic agent because of its effect on multiple cellular pathways leading to effective elimination of cancer cells. (48)

Treatment of the NSCLC lung cancer cells with 1.0 micromolar FZ for 24 hours resulted in:

> partial alteration of the microtubule network ... the microtubule cage around the nucleus appeared to have lost its intactness when compared with control cells ... relatively mild tubulin depolymerizing activity of FZ as compared to other known microtubule-disrupting agents like **nocodazole** and colchicine... (48)

Fenbendazole GLYCOLYSIS Inhibitor

FZ mimics the structure of glucose and decreases glucose consumption by binding to the enzymatic pocket of HK2, thus impairing the function of hexokinase 2 (HK2). FZ shows augmented anti-cancer effects in combination with GLYCOLYSIS inhibitors DCA (dichloroacetate), and 2DG (2-deoxyglucose). There was "strong synergism by FZ and DCA." See the chapter 5 on DCA for more on this. Dr. Dogra et al. studied oral dosing of fenbendazole to mice bearing lung cancer xenografts over 12 days finding "marked reduction in tumor size and weight" as well as reduced tumor vascularity. (48)

Increased P53 in Nucleus and Mitochondrial Fraction

In addition to its microtubule binding and disruption activities, FZ has a unique ability to induce p53 to a considerably high level, with increased nuclear accumulation and increased P53 protein in the mitochondrial fraction, targeting the VDAC, resulting in activation of apoptosis, mitochondrial cell death pathways. (48–54)

Thymoquinone (black seed oil) also induces mitochondrial apoptosis in cancer cells through the P53 pathway. (55)

Screening for Compounds that Promote P53 Activity

In cancer cell types with a functioning (wild-type) P53 gene, promoting that function is a worthy anti-cancer activity. In 2019, Dr. Zuzana Mrkvová et al. performed a high-throughput screen of 2448 compounds on melanoma cells with functional (wild-type) P53 gene looking for compounds that promote P53 activity. Fenbendazole and albendazole were the best candidates, not only increasing P53-P21 pathway, but also decreasing the MDM2 and MDMx suppressor pathway. (60)

Note: Mdm2 and MdmX are negative regulators of P53, so suppressing them with Fenbendazole restores P53 function.

Mutated P53 Predicts Poor Prognosis

The P53 gene has been coined "the guardian of the genome" because it protects the cell from oncogenic transformation. About half of all cancers have a mutated P53 gene, which predicts poor prognosis with short survival. The mutated P53 cancers are more aggressive, with rapid progression to metastatic disease and resistance to chemotherapy. This is true for all cancer cell types—hematologic cancers, pancreatic, lung, endometrial, ovarian, breast, etc. (56–58)

Making Matters Worse

To make matters worse, the mutant P53 proteins promote oncogenic functions in the cancer cell. The mutant P53 hijacks cell functions to promote cancer cell proliferation. In 2017, Dr. Mantovani reviewed the role of mutated P53 in cancer, writing:

> P53 mutant proteins succeed in subverting a remarkable variety of pathways to promote cancer cell survival, proliferation, invasion, migration, stem cell expansion, chemoresistance, tissue remodeling, and chronic inflammation. (57)

Niclosamide Effective Regardless of P53 Status

P53 protein translocation to the mitochondria is part of the mechanism of cell death for fenbendazole (FZ). One should ask the following question: Does the cancer cell type in question have a functioning P53 gene (wild-type) or a mutant P53? If we are dealing with a mutant P53, since FZ relies on P53 accumulation in the mitochondria to induce apoptosis, this mode of action may not be effective. If the cancer is not responding to the fenbendazole, then one might consider alternate drugs that maintain effect regardless of P53 status. For example, Niclosamide induces apoptosis via mitochondrial ETC (electron transport chain) uncoupling and is effective in P53 mutated cancer cell types, regardless of P53 status.

Screening for Activity against P53 Mutants – a New Paradigm

In 2018, Dr. R. Kumar et al. screened a library of 1600 FDA-approved drugs for compounds that kill P53 deficient ovarian cancer cells and xenografts, finding **Niclosamide** the best candidate at a concentration of only 2 micromolar. The p53 independent mechanism of cancer cell death is "mitochondrial uncoupling." They write:

> We propose a new paradigm for targeting cancers defective in the p53 pathway, by exploiting their vulnerability to **niclosamide-induced mitochondrial uncoupling**. (59)

Fenbendazole for Human Lymphoma Xenografts

In 2008, Dr. Ping Gao et al. studied the effect of fenbendazole in human lymphoma mouse xenografts, finding an "unexpected anti-tumorigenic effect." (61)

Benzimidazoles for Pancreatic Cancer

In 2019, Dr. Rosalba Florio et al. studied the "effects of FDA-approved benzimidazole-based anthelminthics fenbendazole, mebendazole, oxibendazole and parbendazole in PC (pancreatic cancer) cell lines." (62)

Parbendazole was the most potent of the group, with IC50 values (50% inhibitory concentration) in the nanomolar range, inducing "mitotic catastrophe" in the cancer cells. Dr. Floria and colleagues concluded:

> This is the first study providing evidence that parbendazole as a single agent, or in combination with gemcitabine, is a repurposing candidate in the currently dismal PC (pancreatic cancer) therapy. (62)

Fenbendazole is effective in other cell types, including:

- Breast cancer (63)
- Prostate cancer (64)
- Canine glioma (65)

Albendazole is effective in the following cell types:

- Squamous cell cancer (66–67)
- Ehrlich ascites in mice (68)
- Codelivery with nano-silver (69)

Flubendazole is effective in the following:

- Breast cancer stem cells (70–72)
- Melanoma (73)
- Glioma (74)

Oxibendazole is effective for:

- Prostate cancer (75)

Conclusion

The Benzimidazole class of anti-helminthic drugs are microtubule inhibitors with potent anti-cancer activities, as described above. Mebendazole is approved for human use and shows remarkable synergy with autophagy inhibitors such as hydroxychloroquine. Mebendazole inactivates BCL-2, inhibits the Hedgehog cancer stem cell pathway, inactivates c-Myc and downregulates multidrug resistance (MDR). Upregulation of the host immune system is an added bonus. Fenbendazole, a veterinary drug, and albendazole are effective for promoting wild-type P53 with induction of apoptosis. Fenbendazole is also a glycolysis inhibitor. For cancers not responding to fenbendazole because of a mutated P53, niclosamide is an effective alternative. Repurposed use as anti-cancer agents looks very promising for the benzimidazole class of drugs.

References for Chapter 24: Mebendazole and Fenbendazole

1) Pantziarka, Pan et al. "Repurposing Drugs in Oncology (ReDO)—mebendazole as an Anti-Cancer Agent." ecancermedicalscience 8 (2014): 443. PMC. Web. 13 Jan. 2015.

2) Banovic, Pavle, et al. "Drug repurposing: mebendazole as effective antitumor agent. Are we seeing the whole story?" Journal of BU ON.: official journal of the Balkan Union of Oncology 23.6 (2018): 1904-1911.

3) Hamilton, Gerhard, and Barbara Rath. "Repurposing of anthelminthics as anticancer drugs." Oncomedicine 2 (2017): 142-149.

4) Popović, Dušica J., et al. "Application of a widely-used tropical anti-worm agent, mebendazole, in modern oncology." Tropical Journal of Pharmaceutical Research 16.10 (2017): 2555-2562.

5) Jordan, Mary Ann, Douglas Thrower, and Leslie Wilson. "Effects of vinblastine, podophyllotoxin and nocodazole on mitotic spindles. Implications for the role of microtubule dynamics in mitosis." J cell Sci 102.3 (1992): 401-416.

6) Sasaki, Ji-ichiro, et al. "The Anthelmintic Drug Mebendazole Induces Mitotic Arrest and Apoptosis by Depolymerizing Tubulin in Non-Small Cell Lung Cancer Cells." Molecular Cancer Therapeutics 1.13 (2002): 1201-1209.

7) Guerini, Andrea Emanuele, et al. "Mebendazole as a Candidate for Drug Repurposing in Oncology: An Extensive Review of Current Literature." Cancers 11.9 (2019): 1284.

8) Sung, So Jung, et al. "Autophagy Is a Potential Target for Enhancing the Anti-Angiogenic Effect of Mebendazole in Endothelial Cells." Biomolecules & therapeutics 27.1 (2019): 117.

9) Dobrosotskaya, I. Y., et al. "Mebendazole monotherapy and long-term disease control in metastatic adrenocortical carcinoma." Endocrine practice: 17.3 (2011): e59.

10) Martarelli, Daniele, et al. "Mebendazole inhibits growth of human adrenocortical carcinoma cell lines implanted in nude mice." Cancer chemotherapy and pharmacology 61.5 (2008): 809-817.

11) Nygren, Peter, and Rolf Larsson. "Drug repositioning from bench to bedside: Tumour remission by the antihelmintic drug mebendazole in refractory metastatic colon cancer." Acta Oncologica 53.3 (2014): 427-428.

12) He, Licai, et al. "Mebendazole exhibits potent anti-leukemia activity on acute myeloid leukemia." Experimental cell research 369.1 (2018): 61-68

13) Blom, Kristin, et al. "The anticancer effect of mebendazole may be due to M1 monocyte/macrophage activation via ERK1/2 and TLR8-dependent inflammasome activation." Immunopharmacology and immunotoxicology 39.4 (2017): 199-210.

14) Rubin, Jenny, et al. "Mebendazole stimulates CD14+ myeloid cells to enhance T-cell activation and tumour cell killing." Oncotarget 9.56 (2018): 30805.

15) Younis, Nancy S., Amal MH Ghanim, and Sameh Saber. "Mebendazole augments sensitivity to sorafenib by targeting MAPK and BCL-2 signalling in n-nitroso-diethylamine-induced murine hepatocellular carcinoma." Scientific Reports 9.1 (2019): 1-16.

16) Rushworth, Linda K., et al. "Repurposing screen identifies mebendazole as a clinical candidate to synergise with docetaxel for prostate cancer treatment." British Journal of Cancer (2019): 1-11.

17) Lam, Lloyd T., et al. "Antihelminthic benzimidazoles potentiate navitoclax (ABT-263) activity by inducing Noxa-dependent apoptosis in non-small cell lung cancer (NSCLC) cell lines." Cancer cell international 15.1 (2015): 5.

18) Zhang, Le, et al. "Mebendazole Potentiates Radiation Therapy in Triple-Negative Breast Cancer." International Journal of Radiation Oncology* Biology* Physics 103.1 (2019): 195-207.

19) Skibinski, Christine G., Tara Williamson, and Gregory J. Riggins. "Mebendazole and radiation in combination increase survival through anticancer mechanisms in an intracranial rodent model of malignant meningioma." Journal of neuro-oncology 140.3 (2018): 529-538.

20) Elayapillai, Sugantha Priya, et al. "Repurposing mebendazole in combination with PRIMA1MET for ovarian cancer therapy." (2019): 4652-4652.

21) Chen, Xue-han, et al. "Mebendazole elicits potent antimyeloma activity by inhibiting the USP5/c-Maf axis." Acta pharmacologica Sinica 40.12 (2019): 1568-1577.

22) AbdusSamad, Maryam, et al. "Combination therapy with mebendazole, trametinib and metformin

eliminates recalcitrant NRASQ61K melanoma cells." (2016): 2501-2501.

23) Doudican, Nicole, et al. "Mebendazole induces apoptosis via Bcl-2 inactivation in chemoresistant melanoma cells." Molecular Cancer Research 6.8 (2008): 1308-1315.

24) Mukhopadhyay, Tapas, et al. "Mebendazole elicits a potent antitumor effect on human cancer cell lines both in vitro and in vivo." Clinical cancer research 8.9 (2002): 2963-2969.

25) Alam, Syed Mahboob, Farah Asad, and Hina Shams. "Mebendazole Inexplicably Reducing the Breast Cancer Cells Viability Preclinically by Incitement Effects with Methotrexate." RADS Journal of Pharmacy and Pharmaceutical Sciences 6.2 (2018): 101-106.

26) Bai, Ren-Yuan, et al. "Brain penetration and efficacy of different mebendazole polymorphs in a mouse brain tumor model." Clinical Cancer Research 21.15 (2015): 3462-3470.

27) De Witt, Michelle, et al. "Repurposing mebendazole as a replacement for vincristine for the treatment of brain tumors." Molecular Medicine 23.1 (2017): 50.

28) Gamble, Alex, et al. "ATPS-83 Repurposing mebendazole as a replacement for vincristine for the treatment of brain tumors." Neuro-Oncology 17.suppl_5 (2015): v36-v36.

29) Lai, Serene Ruth, et al. "In vitro anti-tubulin effects of mebendazole and fenbendazole on canine glioma cells." Veterinary and comparative oncology 15.4 (2017): 1445-1454.

30) Bai, Ren-Yuan, et al. "Antiparasitic mebendazole shows survival benefit in 2 preclinical models of glioblastoma multiforme." Neuro-oncology 13.9 (2011): 974-982.

31) Riggins, Gregory, Renyaun Bai, and Gary Gallia. "Atnt-21 Preclinical and Initial Phase 1 Experience for Use of Mebendazole as Up Front Therapy for High Grade Glioma." Neuro-Oncology 17.Suppl 5 (2015): v15.

32) Bodhinayake, Imithri, Marc Symons, and John A. Boockvar. "Repurposing mebendazole for the treatment of medulloblastoma." Neurosurgery 76.2 (2015): N15-N16.

33) Popović, Dušica J., et al. "Effect of mebendazole on fibrosarcoma in hamsters." Tropical Journal of Pharmaceutical Research 16.10 (2017): 2445-2451.

34) Zhang, Fugui, et al. "Anthelmintic mebendazole enhances cisplatin's effect on suppressing cell proliferation and promotes differentiation of head and neck squamous cell carcinoma (HNSCC)." Oncotarget 8.8 (2017): 12968.

35) Pinto, Laine Celestino, et al. "The anthelmintic drug mebendazole inhibits growth, migration and invasion in gastric cancer cell model." Toxicology in vitro 29.8 (2015): 2038-2044.

36) Freisleben, Fabian, et al. "Mebendazole Mediates Its Anti-Leukemic Effects By Proteasomal Degradation of GLI Transcription Factors Via Inhibition of HSP70/90-Chaperone Activity in Acute Myeloid Leukemia in a Preclinical and Clinical Setting." (2019): 5050-5050.

37) Freisleben, Fabian, et al. "Mebendazole Exerts Potent Anti-Leukemic Effects By Downregulating Protein Levels of Hedgehog Transcription Factors GLI1 and GLI2." (2018): 5145-5145.

38) Li, Yulin, et al. "Mebendazole for Differentiation Therapy of Acute Myeloid Leukemia Identified by a Lineage Maturation Index." Scientific reports 9.1 (2019): 1-9.

39) Pinto, Laine Celestino, et al. "Mebendazole induces apoptosis via C-MYC inactivation in malignant ascites cell line (AGP01)." Toxicology in Vitro (2019).

40) Mrkvová, Zuzana, et al. "Benzimidazoles Downregulate Mdm2 and MdmX and Activate p53 in MdmX Overexpressing Tumor Cells." Molecules 24.11 (2019): 2152.

43) Larsen, Andrew R., et al. "Repurposing the antihelmintic mebendazole as a hedgehog inhibitor." Molecular cancer therapeutics 14.1 (2015): 3-13.

44) Takebe, Naoko, et al. "Targeting cancer stem cells by inhibiting Wnt, Notch, and Hedgehog pathways." Nature reviews Clinical oncology 8.2 (2011): 97.

45) Trowbridge, Jennifer J., Matthew P. Scott, and Mickie Bhatia. "Hedgehog modulates cell cycle regulators in stem cells to control hematopoietic regeneration." Proceedings of the National Academy of Sciences 103.38 (2006): 14134-14139.

46) Rodova, Mariana, et al. "Sonic hedgehog signaling inhibition provides opportunities for targeted therapy by sulforaphane in regulating pancreatic cancer stem cell self-renewal." PloS one 7.9 (2012).

47) Zhao, Chen, et al. "Hedgehog signalling is essential for maintenance of cancer stem cells in myeloid leukaemia." Nature 458.7239 (2009): 776-779.

48) Dogra, Nilambra, Ashok Kumar, and Tapas Mukhopadhyay. "Fenbendazole acts as a moderate microtubule destabilizing agent and causes cancer cell death by modulating multiple cellular pathways." Scientific reports 8.1 (2018): 11926.

49) Zhao, Yunfeng, et al. "p53 translocation to mitochondria precedes its nuclear translocation and targets mitochondrial oxidative defense protein-manganese superoxide dismutase." Cancer research 65.9 (2005): 3745-3750.

50) Galluzzi, Lorenzo, et al. "Targeting p53 to mitochondria for cancer therapy." Cell cycle 7.13 (2008): 1949-1955.

51) Mihara, Motohiro, et al. "p53 has a direct apoptogenic role at the mitochondria." Molecular cell 11.3 (2003): 577-590.

52) Marchenko, Natalie D., Alexander Zaika, and Ute M. Moll. "Death signal-induced localization of p53 protein to mitochondria a potential role in apoptotic signaling." Journal of Biological Chemistry 275.21 (2000): 16202-16212.

53) Vaseva, Angelina V., et al. "p53 opens the mitochondrial permeability transition pore to trigger necrosis." Cell 149.7 (2012): 1536-1548.

54) Chipuk, Jerry E., et al. "Direct activation of Bax by p53 mediates mitochondrial membrane permeabilization and apoptosis." Science 303.5660 (2004): 1010-1014.

55) Al-Oqail, M. M., et al. "Nigella sativa seed oil suppresses cell proliferation and induces ROS dependent mitochondrial apoptosis through p53 pathway in hepatocellular carcinoma cells." South African journal of botany 112 (2017): 70-78.

56) D'Orazi, Gabriella, and Mara Cirone. "Mutant p53 and cellular stress pathways: a criminal alliance that promotes cancer progression." Cancers 11.5 (2019): 614.

57) Mantovani, Fiamma, Dawid Walerych, and Giannino Del Sal. "Targeting mutant p53 in cancer: a long road to precision therapy." The FEBS journal 284.6 (2017): 837-850.

58) Møller, Michael B., et al. "Disrupted p53 function as predictor of treatment failure and poor prognosis in B-and T-cell non-Hodgkin's lymphoma." Clinical cancer research 5.5 (1999): 1085-1091.

59) Kumar, R., et al. "Mitochondrial uncoupling reveals a novel therapeutic opportunity for p53-defective cancers." Nature Communications 9.1 (2018): 1-13.

60) Mrkvová, Zuzana, et al. "Benzimidazoles Downregulate Mdm2 and MdmX and Activate p53 in MdmX Overexpressing Tumor Cells." Molecules 24.11 (2019): 2152.

61) Gao, Ping, Chi V. Dang, and Julie Watson. "Unexpected antitumorigenic effect of fenbendazole when combined with supplementary vitamins." Journal of the American Association for Laboratory Animal Science 47.6 (2008): 37-40.

62) Florio, Rosalba, et al. "The Benzimidazole-Based Anthelmintic Parbendazole: A Repurposed Drug Candidate That Synergizes with Gemcitabine in Pancreatic Cancer." Cancers 11.12 (2019): 2042.

63) Duan, Qiwen, Yanfeng Liu, and Sara Rockwell. "Fenbendazole as a potential anticancer drug." Anticancer research 33.2 (2013): 355-362.

64) Aycock-Williams, Ari N., et al. "Effects of fenbendazole and vitamin E succinate on the growth and survival of prostate cancer cells." J Cancer Res Exp Oncol 3.9 (2011): 115-121.

65) Lai, Serene Ruth, et al. "In vitro anti-tubulin effects of mebendazole and fenbendazole on canine glioma cells." Veterinary and comparative oncology 15.4 (2017): 1445-1454.

66) Ghasemi, Farhad, et al. "Repurposing Albendazole: new potential as a chemotherapeutic agent with preferential activity against HPV-negative head and neck squamous cell cancer." Oncotarget 8.42 (2017): 71512.

67) Zhang, Qing-Ling, et al. "Antitumor effect of albendazole on cutaneous squamous cell carcinoma (SCC) cells." BioMed Research International 2019 (2019).

68) Castro, L. S. E. P. W., et al. "Albendazole as a promising molecule for tumor control." Redox biology 10 (2016): 90-99.

69) Liang, Jianming, et al. "A novel tumor-targeting treatment strategy uses energy restriction via co-delivery of albendazole and nanosilver." Nano Research 11.9 (2018): 4507-4523.

70) Hou, Zhi-Jie, et al. "Flubendazole, FDA-approved anthelmintic, targets breast cancer stem-like cells." Oncotarget 6.8 (2015): 6326.

71) Oh, Eunhye, et al. "Flubendazole elicits anti-metastatic effects in triple-negative breast cancer via STAT3 inhibition." International journal of cancer 143.8 (2018): 1978-1993.

72) Kim, Yoon-Jae, et al. "Flubendazole overcomes trastuzumab resistance by targeting cancer stem-like properties and HER2 signaling in HER2-positive breast cancer." Cancer Letters 412 (2018): 118-130.

73) Čáňová, K., et al. "Flubendazole induces mitotic catastrophe and apoptosis in melanoma cells." Toxicology in Vitro 46 (2018): 313-322.

74) Zhou, Xumin, et al. "Flubendazole inhibits glioma proliferation by G2/M cell cycle arrest and pro-apoptosis." Cell death discovery 4.1 (2018): 1-10.

75) Chen, Qiaoli, et al. "Oxibendazole inhibits prostate cancer cell growth." Oncology Letters 15.2 (2018): 2218-2226.

Chapter 25

Nicholas Gonzales and the Trophoblastic Theory

I HAD THE PLEASURE OF attending a presentation by the late Nicholas Gonzalez, MD, a keynote speaker at the Boulderfest Conference, July 17–20, 2008, in Denver Colorado. Sadly, Dr. Gonzalez passed away unexpectedly seven years later, July 2015. For many productive years, he practiced integrative oncology in his Manhattan office, treating advanced cancer patients successfully with high-dose pancreatic enzyme capsules taken orally. (1–4)

Dr. Gonzalez's treatment protocol is based on the trophoblastic theory of cancer, originally proposed by Scottish embryologist John Beard (1858–1924) and resurrected by William Donald Kelley, DDS (1926–2005). (5–6)

John Beard and the Trophoblast

John Beard was a Scottish embryologist who used the light microscope to study developmental embryology and cancer histo-pathology. In 1905, Beard was the first to report that trophoblast cells behave in a manner identical to cancer cells, acting invasively and inducing their own blood supply. (7–10)

What are Trophoblasts?

After conception, the developing ovum sends trophoblast cells as finger-like extensions to invade the endometrium, forming the placenta. This layer of trophoblast cells, now called the placenta, induces the maternal blood vessels to grow into the placenta, providing blood flow to the developing fetus. This invasive, infiltrative behavior is very similar to the way cancer cells infiltrate and invade surrounding tissues.

Trophoblasts Produce HCG

These trophoblast cells are known to produce human chorionic gonadotropin (HCG). In fact, production of HCG is the basis for the widely used pregnancy test. If cancer cells and trophoblast cells are similar, one would expect cancer cells to also produce HCG. That is exactly what they do. This was reported in 1995 by Hernan Acevedo, PhD, et al. and published in *Cancer*. Dr. Acevedo and colleagues found that every cancer produces HCG, same as the trophoblast cells of pregnancy. The HCG test is both a pregnancy test and a cancer test. (11–14)

Sharing Same Molecular Circuitry

Since John Beard's time 100 years ago, modern molecular biologists have found even more similarities between trophoblasts and malignant cancer cells. In 2006, Dr. C. Ferretti et al. wrote that both cancer and trophoblast cells share the same molecular circuitry for their proliferative, invasive, and migratory capacities. Both cell types share the following similar pathways:

Proto-Oncogenes: C-Myc, EGFR (endothelial growth factor), PDGF (platelet-derived growth factor), IGF-1 (insulin growth factor).

Proteolytic Enzymes: matrix metalloproteinases (MMPs)

Autocrine and Paracrine Loops: Epidermal growth factor and receptor (EGFR), hepatocyte growth factor and receptor (HGFR), and vascular endothelial growth factor and receptor (VEGFR).

Downregulation of cell adhesion molecule E-cadherin.

Activation of the phosphatidylinositol 3'-kinase **PI3K/AKT axis** as central feature of signaling pathways for proliferative, migratory and invasive processes. (15)

CT Antigens Discovered

Another twist to the story is the recent discovery of a new class of human tumor antigens called cancer/testis (CT) antigens. About 90 genes have been found having messenger RNA expression in both germ cells (testis) and cancer cells and no expression in otherwise normal cells. This is further evidence linking the trophoblast cells, which are in fact germ cells (also called stem cells), with cancer. (16–21)

Recent advances in our understanding of molecular biology have shown that John Beard was quite correct to point out the similarity between placental trophoblast cells and malignant cancer cells. Beard's forgotten predictions in the early 1900s have had an uncanny way of resurfacing. (22)

Pancreatic Enzymes on Day 56

John Beard observed that the trophoblast cells transform from a malignant, invasive cell type into a mature well-behaved cell type. This occurs on Day 56 of gestation, and also coincides with the appearance of enzyme granules (zymogen granules) in the fetal pancreas. Obviously, the developing fetus has no need for pancreatic enzymes, since all nutrition comes from the maternal blood supply. Pancreatic enzymes are needed only after birth when the baby starts feeding. Beard theorized that the appearance of pancreatic enzymes was no accident and that they must have some other function. The most likely explanation, he thought, was that they were responsible for the transformation of behavior of the trophoblast cell from "malignant" to "benign," thereby suggesting the use of digestive enzymes (Trypsin) to control cancer cells. (5)

After this "Eureka Moment", Dr. Nicholas González developed a protocol for treatment of cancer using pancreatic enzymes, finding patient outcomes better than the national average. Other researchers performed preclinical studies confirming the hypothesis, and a number of case reports appeared in the medical literature. (23–34)

In 2003, Dr. Melina Roberts wrote an excellent article in the *Townsend Letter* reviewing the research confirming John Beard's work as well as the value of enzyme treatments for cancer. (35)

John Beard's Work Buried in History Books

About the same time as John Beard's early work, Marie Curie's (1867–1934) work treating cancer with radiation took the spotlight and captured the imagination of the media and the public. Beard's work on the trophoblast theory was dismissed by mainstream medical science and almost forgotten. However, in 1950, the leading biochemist of the time, Ernst Krebs, wrote an important paper supporting the trophoblast theory of cancer. (36)

William Donald Kelley Resurrects John Beard's Work

In the following decade, the 1960s, William Kelly discovered Beard's forgotten papers and resurrected the treatment of cancer with pancreatic enzymes. Kelly had considerable success treating patients with this alternative approach. However, Kelly a dentist, was bitterly opposed by mainstream medicine, and as expected, had difficulties with the authorities. Kelly was convicted of practicing medicine without a license in 1970, and his dental license was suspended in 1976. He died in 2005 at the age of 79.

Nicholas González's Research

In 1981, during Kelly's early years, a medical student at Cornell Medical School by the name of Nicholas Gonzalez was given a summer project to interview Kelly and evaluate Kelly's results using pancreatic enzymes in cancer patients. Gonzalez did a retrospective review of 1300 patients who had been treated over a 20-year period using the Kelley protocol of enzymes, diet, and nutritional support. Gonzalez was so impressed with the data and the superior patient outcomes that this summer project expanded into a book, and he later adopted it as his own life's work. At his Manhattan office, Dr. Gonzalez carried on Kelly's legacy, documenting remarkable success. Selected case reports show dramatic clinical results not possible with conventional cancer treatment. This information is posted on Dr. González's website (www. the gonzalezprotocol.com).

Pilot study of the Enzyme Treatment of Pancreatic Cancer

In 1999, González published a 2-year pilot study of 10 patients with inoperable advanced pancreatic cancer treated with large doses of orally ingested pancreatic enzymes. Results showed 80% survival after 1 year, 45% survival after 2 years and 36% survival after 3 years. (4)

These results are far above the 25% one year, 10% two year, and 6 % three-year survival reported in the National Cancer Data Base for inoperable pancreatic cancer. (25)

Grant for Study Never Completed

Shortly after this, González received a $1.4 million grant from the National Center for Complementary and Alternative Medicine at the National Institutes of Health for further study on enzyme therapy and pancreatic cancer. The study was conducted at Columbia-Presbyterian Medical Center in New York under the supervision of the NCI and with approval from the FDA. The study was never finished and the outcome never published. In his book, *What Went Wrong: the Truth Behind the Clinical Trial of the Enzyme Treatment of Cancer*, Gonzalez reveals how these agencies worked with a common goal of discrediting enzyme therapy under the auspices of what appeared, on the surface, to be a legitimate clinical trial. (24)

The Warburg Effect

Otto Warburg made the important observation that cancer cells share the same metabolic activities as trophoblast cells. They both have high glucose utilization, using the primitive aerobic glycolysis pathway known as the Warburg Effect. They both suppress mitochondrial oxidative phosphorylation and thrive in a low oxygen environment. (37–38)

No Coexistence of Cancer with Circulating Enzymes of Pancreatitis

One last point I am compelled to mention. During my 30-year career as a radiologist, much of my time was spent reading images of metastatic cancer on CAT scans. One thing I noticed was that I never witnessed the presence of metastatic cancer in patients who had pancreatic enzymes circulating freely in the bloodstream from acute or chronic pancreatitis. (Excluded, of course, was focal pancreatitis caused by an obstructed pancreatic duct due to a small pancreatic cancer.) Thus, I had independently confirmed the major tenet of John Beard and Ernst Krebs many years before I even heard of the trophoblastic theory of cancer.

Cancer of Small Bowel Relatively Rare

Most experienced radiologists and surgeons also observe the relative rarity of neoplasm involving the small bowel compared to the relative common appearance (50 times more common) of neoplasm in the colon and the stomach. Ernst Krebs makes this same observation in his landmark 1950 paper on the unified trophoblast theory of cancer, and Krebs suggests that pancreatic enzymes released into the duodenum at the ducts of Wirsung and Santorini are responsible for this 50-times reduction in small-bowel cancer. The age-adjusted death rate for cancer of the colon is 47 times higher than cancer of the small bowel, at 0.4 for small bowel and 18.8 for colon cancer per 100,000 men and women per year. (36)

NIH Grant Proposal to Study Cancer

The National Institute of Health (NIH) has spent literally trillions over four decades on failed cancer research. It is time to take a different approach by allocating NIH funds to study the trophoblast theory of cancer. A widely used technique in molecular biology is the tracer study. The older tracer method involved the use of carbon 14 radio-labeling. The newer method uses insertion of the green fluorescent protein (GFP) into the protein one wishes to study. (39)

Carbon 14 Radio-Labeled Trypsin

The proposed study can be done by using carbon 14 radio-labeling of key amino acids in the pancreatic enzyme trypsin and then feeding these radio-labeled amino acids to the pigs used to harvest the trypsin for later use. The radio-labeled trypsin enzymes can then be administered in an animal model of cancer, looking for the distribution of the radio-label in the sacrificed animals. If there is an effect on the cancer cells, I would expect to find the radio-labeled enzymes at the surface of the cancer cells.

GFP Green Fluorescent Protein

Another more elegant approach would be to genetically modify the pancreatic trypsin enzyme in mice by adding a green fluorescent marker gene (GFP), a common technique used in molecular biology. If pancreatic enzymes control the trophoblast, then the experiments should confirm the presence of the fluorescent marker at the trophoblast cells after day 56 in the developing embryo.

For this study, the green fluorescent gene (GFP) can be inserted into DNA of the animals (usually pigs) used to manufacture the pancreatic enzymes. These labeled enzymes can then be administered to mice pretreated with cancer cells. It would be useful to know the fate of the labeled enzymes in treated vs. control mice. If the enzymes have anti-cancer effects, then one would expect finding the labeled enzymes at the tumor site, taken up by the cancer cells. Further molecular biology studies could investigate intracellular location and mechanism of action. (39-40)

Using the NIH to Find a Cure for Cancer

In 1971, then-President Richard Nixon declared a war on cancer and ramped up funding for NIH research to prove the hypothesis that cancer is a genetic disease caused by viruses. Although the viral theory and genetic theory of cancer do have some elements of truth, this line of research expended massive amounts of money and ended a dismal failure. A new and more promising direction for cancer research would be to investigate the metabolic activities of the trophoblast, which shares so many features in common with cancer cells. These features include the three pillars of cancer cell metabolism (OXPHOS, GLYCOLYSIS and Autophagy) as well as cancer stem cell pathways (Wnt, Hedgehog and Notch).

Further Research on the Enzyme Treatment of Cancer

Further investigation of the enzyme treatment of cancer is also warranted. What is the exact mechanism by which enzymes are effective for treating cancer? I propose a new hypothesis. Perhaps, the orally administered pancreatic enzymes eventually make their way to the tumor micro-environment extracellular space, where they are taken up by macropinocytosis, a form of engulfment by the cancer cell membrane, with the assistance of autophagy/lysosomes to feed the cancer cell's voracious appetite. Once inside the cancer cell, perhaps the enzymes digest the interior organelles, causing cancer cell death. Or perhaps some other mechanism is at work? We await further research to test this hypothesis.

We now have molecular tools that John Beard, a century ago, could only imagine. We await the time when the NIH allocates funding to pursue the trophoblast theory of cancer.

Conclusion

Advances in molecular biology now make the process of validating and expanding on the early work of John Beard, Ernst Krebs, and Otto Warburg fairly straightforward. NIH funding of the costs of such a program would be relatively minimal and the potential gains enormous.

References Chapter 25: Nicholas Gonzales and the Trophoblastic Theory

1) Gonzalez, Nicholas J., and Linda L. Isaacs. "The Gonzalez therapy and cancer: A collection of case reports." Alternative Therapies in Health and Medicine 13.1 (2007): 46.

2) Isaacs, Linda L. "The Gonzalez Best Case Series Presentation to the NCI: 25 Cases, 25 Years Later." Alternative therapies in health and medicine 25.4 (2019): 12-14.

3) Isaacs, Linda L. "An Enzyme-Based Nutritional Protocol in Metastatic Cancer: Case Reports Of A Patient With Colon Cancer And A Patient With Lung Cancer." Alternative therapies in health and medicine 25.4 (2019): 16-19.

4) Gonzales NJ, Isaacs LL. Evaluation of pancreatic proteolytic enzyme treatment of adenocarcinoma of the pancreas, with nutrition and detoxification support. Nutr Cancer 1999; 33(2):117-124.

5) Gonzales NJ, Isaacs LL. The Trophoblast and the Origins of Cancer: One Solution to the Medical Enigma of Our Time. New York, NY: New Spring Press; 2009.

6) Ross, Colin A. "The trophoblast model of cancer." Nutrition and cancer 67.1 (2015): 61-67.

7) Gonzalez, Nicholas James. *One Man Alone: An Investigation of Nutrition, Cancer and William Donald Kelley.* 2010, New Spring Press.

8) Beard J. Embryological aspects and etiology of carcinoma. Lancet 1902; 1:1758.

9) Beard J. *The Enzyme Treatment of Cancer*. London: Chatto & Windus, 1911.

10) Beard, John. "The Action of Trypsin upon the Living Cells of Jensen's Mouse-Tumor." British medical journal 1.2351 (1906): 140.

11) Acevedo HF, et al. Human chorionic gonadotropin-beta subunit gene expression in cultured human fetal and cancer cells of different types and origins. Cancer. 1995 Oct 15;76(8):1467-75.

12) Acevedo HF, et al. Detection of membrane-associated human chorionic gonadotropin and its subunits on human cultured cancer cells of the nervous system. Cancer Detect Prev. 1997; 21(4):295-303.

13) Acevedo HF and Hartsock RJ. Metastatic phenotype correlates with high expression of membrane-associated complete beta-human chorionic gonadotropin in vivo. Cancer. 1996 Dec 1; 78(11):2388-99.

14) Regelson W. Have we found the "definitive cancer biomarker"? The diagnostic and therapeutic implications of human chorionic gonadotropin-beta expression as a key to malignancy. Cancer. 1995; 76:1299-301.

15) Ferretti, C., et al. "Molecular circuits shared by placental and cancer cells, and their implications in the proliferative, invasive and migratory capacities of trophoblasts." Human reproduction update 13.2 (2007): 121-141.

16) Mullen, Catherine A. "Analogies between trophoblastic and malignant cells." American Journal of Reproductive Immunology 39.1 (1998): 41-49.

17) Lala, P. K., et al. "Human placental trophoblast as an in vitro model for tumor progression." Canadian journal of physiology and pharmacology 80.2 (2002): 142-149.

18) Koslowski, Michael, et al. "A placenta-specific gene ectopically activated in many human cancers is essentially involved in malignant cell processes." Cancer research 67.19 (2007): 95

19) Kalejs, Martins, and Jekaterina Erenpreisa. "Cancer/testis antigens and gametogenesis: a review and" brain-storming" session." Cancer cell international 5.1 (2005): 4.

20) Simpson, Andrew JG, et al. "Cancer/testis antigens, gametogenesis and cancer." Nature Reviews Cancer 5.8 (2005): 615.

21) Mahmoud, Abeer M. "Cancer testis antigens as immunogenic and oncogenic targets in breast cancer." Immunotherapy 10.9 (2018): 769-778.

22) Beard, John. "Trypsin and Amylopsin in Malignant Growths." Journal of the American Medical Association 47.6 (1906): 445-445.

23) Gonzalez, N. J. "Nicholas Gonzalez, MD: an enzyme approach to cancer. Interview by Karen Burnett." Alternative therapies in health and medicine 18.6 (2012): 54.

24) Gonzalez, Nicholas J. *What Went Wrong: the truth behind the clinical trial of the enzyme treatment of cancer.* New Spring Press, 2012.

25) Niederhuber, John E., Murray F. Brennan, and Herman R. Menck. "The national cancer data base report on pancreatic cancer." Cancer 76.9 (1995): 1671-1677.

26) Cutfield, A: "Trypsin Treatment in Malignant Disease" Br Med J 5, 525, 1907.

27) Wiggin, FH: "Case of Multiple Fibrosarcoma of The Tongue, With Remarks on the Use of Trypsin and Amylopsin in the Treatment of Malignant Disease" JAMA 47, 2003-08. 1906.

28) Gotze, H, Rotham SS: "Enterohepatic Circulation of Digestive Enzymes as A Conservative Mechanism." (1975) Nature 257, 607–609.

29) Shively, FL: *Multiple Proteolytic Enzyme Therapy Of Cancer.* Dayton, Johnson-Watson, 1969.

30) Little, WL: "A Case of Malignant Tumor, With Treatment." JAMA 50, 1724, 1908.

31) Wald, Martin, et al. "Mixture of trypsin, chymotrypsin and papain reduces formation of metastases and extends survival time of C 57 Bl 6 mice with syngeneic melanoma B16." Cancer chemotherapy and pharmacology 47.1 (2001): S16-S22.

32) Wald M, Olejár T, Poucková P, Zadinová M. Proteinases Reduce Metastatic Dissemination and Increase Survival Time in C57Bl6 Mice with the Lewis Lung Carcinoma. Life Sciences 1998a; 63(17):237-243.

33) Wald M, Olejár T, Poucková P, Zadinová M. The influence of proteinases on in vivo blastic transformation in rat species SD/Ipcv with spontaneous lymphoblastic leukemia. British Journal of Haematology 1998b; 102 (1): 294.

34) Wald M, Poucková P, Hloušková D, Altnerová M, Olejár T. The influence of trypsin, chymotrypsin and papain on the growth of human pancreatic adenocarcinoma transplanted to nu/nu mice. The European Journal of Cancer 1999; 35(4), No. 543:148.

35) Roberts, Melina A. "A Critique of the Kelley Nutritional-Metabolic Cancer Program." Townsend Letter for Doctors and Patients 239 (2003): 76-85.

36) Krebs Jr, Ernst T., and E. T. Krebs. "The Unitarian or Trophoblastic Thesis of Cancer." Medical record (New York: 1934) 163.7 (1950): 149.

37) Warburg O. The Metabolism of Carcinoma Cells. J Cancer Res 1925; 9:148-163.

38) Old, Lloyd J. "Cancer is a Somatic Cell Pregnancy." (2007): 19.

39) Huang, Chaofeng, and Jonathan McConathy. "Radiolabeled amino acids for oncologic imaging." Journal of Nuclear Medicine 54.7 (2013): 1007-1010.

40) Tsien, Roger Y. "The Green Fluorescent Protein." (1998): 509-544.

Chapter 26

Progesterone-Blocking Factor RU 486

Escaping Immune Surveillance

IN PREVIOUS CHAPTERS, WE DISCUSSED cancer stem cells and the failure of chemotherapy to eradicate them. A more successful approach involves using repurposed drugs and supplements to target the cancer stem cell pathways Wnt, Hedgehog, and Notch, and the three pillars of cancer cell metabolism, OXPHOS, GLYCOLYSIS and Autophagy.

Of equal importance are fourth and fifth factors, the cancer cell's escape from immune surveillance, and upregulation of inflammation. The machinery of the cancer cell not only evades destruction by turning off and neutralizing the host immune system, it also hijacks the host inflammatory pathways with a massive cytokine release to feed growth and proliferation. Massive upregulation of inflammation is more completely discussed in chapter 38 on Celecoxib COX 2 Inhibitor.

Evasion of Immune System with PIBF

The previous chapter on cancer as a trophoblastic disease discussed the idea that cancer cells behave similarly to the placental cells of a pregnancy, with similar molecular circuitry. One of these similarities is evasion of the immune system with progesterone-induced blocking factor (PIBF). We now direct our attention to PIBF, a protein secreted by both trophoblast cells and cancer cells to turn off the host immune system and allow the pregnancy or the cancer to grow unimpeded, without interference from the host immune system.

Chemotherapy May Increase Cancer Stem Cells

After chemotherapy, microscopic cancer stem cells will always remain behind, not visible on PET scans. In most cases, as we have discussed, chemotherapy actually increases the number of cancer stem cells. These cancer stem cells re-grow into sizable tumor masses capable of metastasis to remote areas of the body. The new tumors may even be more drug-resistant and aggressive than the original cell type. How can we avoid this scenario?

The Role of the Immune System

You might ask, "Why doesn't the immune system recognize these cancer cells as 'foreign invaders' and kill them as they do other invaders?"

How do the cancer cells evade the immune system? The answer lies in the observation made over a hundred years ago by Scottish embryologist John Beard (1858–1924), who recognized the similarity between embryo implantation and tumor metastasis. See the previous chapter 25 on the trophoblastic theory of cancer.

Both Placenta (Trophoblasts) and Tumors Express PIBF

Invasive cancers induce new blood vessels (angiogenesis) similar to the way the trophoblast cells of the placenta grow into the endometrium during pregnancy, and both are governed by PIBF. Pregnancy lymphocytes secrete PIBF, which modulates the host immune system to allow pregnancy to proceed. Likewise, in cancer cells PIBF suppresses the activity of NK killer cells of the immune system, allowing the cancer cells to evade immune surveillance. Blocking the progesterone receptors on lymphocytes with RU-486 (mifepristone) turns off PIBF production, restoring immune competency. (1–2)

Drs. Julia Szekeres-Bartho and Beata Polgar (2010) write:

> PIBF mRNA and protein are expressed in a variety of malignant tumors. Inhibition of PIBF synthesis increase survival rates of leukemic mice. (1)

Note: PIBF synthesis is inhibited by RU-486 (mifepristone). PIBF mRNA= Progesterone-Induced Blocking Factor Messenger RNA, is used to transmit the code for PIBF to the ribosome, the cellular machinery which actually synthesizes PIBF protein. Detection of mRNA is commonly use in cancer biology as a marker for upregulated pathways.

PIBF Induces More Aggressive Behavior in Cancer, Activating Growth and Proliferation Pathways

In addition to the effect of PIBF on the host immune system, PIBF has a direct action on cancer cells, stimulating tumor invasion by increasing MMP activity, and activating growth and proliferation pathways.

Note: MMP = matrix metallo-proteinase, an enzyme secreted by aggressive cancer cells into the extracellular space to dissolve tissues in preparation for cancer invasion.

In 2013, Dr. Melinda Halasz et al. studied the activity of PIBF in both trophoblast cells and tumor cells, finding that PIBF induces invasive behavior in tumor cells by activation of growth and proliferation pathways. At the same time, quite the opposite happens in trophoblast cells, where PIBF controls invasive behavior by suppressing genes governing invasion:

> In tumor cells PIBF triggered sustained Akt, ERK and late STAT3 activation [gene pathways for invasive behavior] … PIBF binds to the promoters of IL-6, EGF and HB-EGF [cytokines and growth factors]; however, the protein profile of the protein/DNA complex is different in the two cell lines [trophoblasts and tumor cells]. We conclude that in tumor cells PIBF induces proteins which **activate invasion signaling,** while based on our previous data - PIBF might control trophoblast invasion by **suppressing invasive genes.** (2)

Mifepristone (RU-486) and Progesterone Receptor

Discovered in 1982 by the French drug company Roussel-Uclaff, mifepristone (RU-486) is a progesterone receptor blocker known as the "abortion pill," prescribed at abortion clinics to induce abortion and terminate early pregnancy. The steroidal ring chemical structure of mifepristone contains the progesterone backbone with an added moiety, dimethylaminobenzene at the 11th position. (3)

Mifepristone RU-486 Drug is Restricted

Mifepristone may be difficult for the cancer patient to obtain. For political reasons, mifepristone RU-486 is restricted in the U.S. and Europe and may be dispensed only by abortion clinics. For use as a repurposed cancer drug, access to RU-486 can be obtained by filing with the FDA for Investigational New Drug Approval (IND) for compassionate use or by participating in an ongoing clinical trial that already has FDA approval.

Dual Action on Immune System and Cancer Cell

Mifepristone has been repurposed as a form of immunotherapy, an anti-cancer agent blocking progesterone receptors on cell membranes of lymphocytes and preventing PIBF secretion, stripping away the cancer cell's protection from the host immune system. In 2009, Dr. Jerome Check et al. wrote:

> In vitro data has shown that 100% of human leukemia cell lines express mRNA for the PIBF protein. Some leukemia cell lines have been found that actually express the PIBF protein. In fact, **adding progesterone to the culture media upregulated PIBF protein expression and mifepristone inhibited it** ... Thus there is now experimental data to support this hypothesis and a new door to a completely different type of cancer therapy has been opened. (4–5)

Escaping Immune Surveillance

Dr. Check's group writes (2017) that the PIBF protein may hold the key to how cancer cells escape immune surveillance, writing:

Discussion is made about a unique immunomodulatory protein called the progesterone induced blocking factor. The role of this protein, that is unique to rapidly growing cells, may hold a key to how the cancer cells escape immune surveillance. (6)

Mifepristone Anti-Cancer Effects Independent of Progesterone Receptor

Many anti-cancer compounds contain the steroidal ring structure, such as the plant steroidal saponins diosgenin and ginsenosid. The chemist Russell Marker revolutionized modern medicine by utilizing the plant diosgenin steroidal ring for mass production of human steroidal hormones for commercial use. These include cortisone, progesterone, estrogen, testosterone, and ultimately the birth control pill. By the way, diosgenin, like many other plant saponins, has potent anti-cancer stem cell activity. (7–10)

Two other plant anti-cancer agents sharing the steroidal ring mentioned in this book are pterostilbene, and boswellia. Among drugs sharing a steroidal ring are cardiac glycosides (digoxin) and the breast cancer drug, exemestane. As such, mifepristone can be included as another modified steroidal ring molecule with anti-cancer activity. Although mifepristone is a progesterone receptor blocker, the drug has anti-cancer activity of its own, independent of the progesterone receptor.

Dr. Chelsea Tieszen (2011) et al. write:

Contrary to common opinion, growth inhibition of cancer cells by antiprogestin MF [mifepristone] is not dependent upon expression of classical, nuclear PR [progesterone receptor]. (11)

Inhibit Adhesion of Circulating Tumor Cells

In 2015, Dr. Liyuan Wan et al. suggested that the combination of mifepristone together with aspirin, a platelet inhibitor, and the antibiotic doxycycline could prevent metastatic disease. Mifepristone inhibits adhesion of circulating tumor cells (cancer stem cells circulating in the blood stream) to the vascular endothelium, thus preventing implantation of metastatic disease. (12)

Dr. Jianzhong Chen et al. (2014) agree:

Metapristone [the primary metabolite of mifepristone] may have potential for cancer metastatic chemoprevention. (3)

Glioblastoma Model

In 2017, working with a glioblastoma brain cancer cell model, Dr. Gutiérrez-Rodríguez et al. found that PIBF is expressed in astrocytomas (brain cancer), writing:

PIBF promotes proliferation, migration, and invasion of human glioblastoma cells, while RU486 blocked the effect at 10 micromolar. (13)

Much of the work on mifepristone as an anti-cancer agent has been done by Dr. Jerome Check's group at the Cooper Institute for Reproductive Hormonal Disorders. In 2014, Dr. Check published a case report of a 43-year-old male with inoperable glioblastoma, finding a short-term benefit with palliative use of mifepristone. (14)

Leukemia Expresses mRNA for PIBF

Likewise for leukemia cell types, in 2009, Dr. Check et al. found that 100% of human leukemia cell lines express messenger RNA (mRNA) for the PIBF protein, inhibited by the progesterone receptor blocker mifepristone. **Note:** messenger RNA is transcribed by the nuclear DNA, and travels to the ribosome, where it is translated into protein production. (15–16)

Dramatic Regression of CLL Chronic Lymphocytic Leukemia

Emboldened in 2009 by an in vitro mouse model of lymphocytic leukemia showing good response to mifepristone treatment, Dr. Check's group later (2014) treated an elderly female patient with rapidly advancing lymphocytic leukemia who had declined chemotherapy. The patient was given mifepristone 200 mg daily followed by complete remission lasting 12 months. Check et al. theorized that the T cells in the micro-environment secrete PIBF, which allows the tumor to escape immune surveillance. By blocking PIBF production with mifepristone, host-tumor immunity is restored. (17)

Mifepristone Induces Apoptosis in Cancer Cells

As mentioned above, mifepristone has a second anti-cancer mechanism directly inducing apoptosis in cancer cells at appropriate concentrations. In 2013, Dr. Ji Hoon Jang et al. studied the effect of mifepristone on (U937) lymphoma cells, finding reduction in mitochondrial potential, activation of p38 MAPK, and induction of mitochondrial apoptosis. Overexpression of BCL-2 (anti-apoptotic protein) blocked this effect. Induction of apoptosis was also found for breast, lung, and colon cancer cells. (18)

Note: U937 is a myeloid leukaemia cell line consisting of differentiated monocytes derived from the pleura effusion of a 37 year old male with histiocytic lymphoma in 1974 by Drs. Sundström and Nilsson. The cells are typically frozen in liquid nitrogen and distributed for biomedical research. (38)

Melanoma Studies

Similarly, in melanoma studies, mifepristone induced cancer cell apoptosis, seemingly independently of the progesterone receptor. In 2016, Dr. Pandurangan Ramaraj studied mifepristone in a melanoma cell line, finding cell death by apoptosis was NOT mediated through the progesterone receptor. (19)

In 2017, Dr. Ning Zheng et al. found that mifepristone had both antiproliferative and anti-migration effects, suggesting its utility as antimetastatic agent. (20)

Mifepristone for Colon Cancer

In 2009, Dr. Check's group found improvement of quality of life and prolonged survival with mifepristone 200 mg per day in two patients with stage 4 colon cancer with extensive metastatic disease. The metastatic disease did not regress; instead, it appeared to stabilize, the quality of life improved, and the drug was well tolerated. (21)

Lung Cancer

In 2019, Dr. Check et al. reported a 68-year-old female with advanced small-cell lung cancer unresponsive to treatment with chemotherapy and checkpoint inhibitors. Treatment with mifepristone stabilized the disease for one and a half years with good quality of life. (22)

Advanced Cancer Responds to Mifepristone

In 2016, Dr. Check et al. reported on two advanced cancer patients who dramatically improved their long-term survival on mifepristone. The first patient, a "moribund woman with never-treated metastatic lung cancer," responded well to the drug with regression of all lung lesions and remained in remission for over 5 years. The second patient, a male, had bilateral renal carcinoma treated with heminephrectomy (only part of one kidney was surgically removed, with cancer remaining behind) and survived 12 years on the drug. There were no adverse effects from the drug for either patient. (23)

Blocking PIBF with Microtubule Inhibitor Mebendazole

As luck would have it, elimination of PIBF may be accomplished with another drug that is widely available, a microtubule-disrupting agent such as nocodazole, an imidazole similar to mebendazole and fenbendazole. Nocodazole was used in a 2004 study by Dr. Margit Lachmann et al., who found that PIBF is associated with the centrosome, a microtubule spindle structure involved in mitosis cell division. Treatment with the microtubule-disrupting agent, nocodazole, caused the PIBF dots to disappear from the centrosomes.

Note: the centrosome is a microtubule system making up the cell cytoskeleton, also involved in mitosis, cell division.

"PIBF [progesterone-induced blocking factor] is overexpressed in highly proliferating cells and **associated with the centrosom**e," which is involved with the mitotic spindle and its microtubule system. Nocodazole is a microtubule-disrupting agent similar to mebendazole. Dr. Lachman's group writes:

> Treatment with nocodazole [at 5 µg/ml concentration for 4 hr], a microtubule-disrupting agent led to the time-dependent **disappearance of the perinuclear PIBF dots,** which paralleled with the disintegration of the Golgi apparatus. (24)

Dr. Lachmann found that treatment with a microtubule-disrupting drug disturbed production of PIBF, conferring a benefit for the immune system. (24)

Microtubule Agents Benefits for the Immune System

Beneficial effects on the immune system by microtubule-disrupting agents such as nocodazole and mebendazole have been recognized previously.

In 2013, Dr. A. Sevko et al. studied the immune modulating effect of the microtubule agent paclitaxel, showing inhibition of myeloid-derived suppressor cells, with restoration of CD8 T cell-effector (killer T cell) functions in a melanoma model. Is this due to paclitaxel's effect on PIBF, as discussed by Dr. Lachman? This would be a good subject for future NIH funded studies. (25)

Immunomodulation by Microtubule Agents

Dr. Pan Pantziarka et al. (2014) write that mebendazole, like nocodazole and paclitaxel, is a microtubule inhibitor with immunomodulatory effects related to microtubule dynamics. One may speculate this is associated with effects on the PIBF protein at the centrosome. Dr. Pan Pantziarka writes:

> There is also increasing evidence that existing microtubule-disrupting agents used at low or metronomic doses, including the taxanes and vinca alkaloids, exert a positive immunomodulatory action that may help to reverse the immunosuppressive effect of cancer.... We can speculate, mechanistically, that some of this immunomodulatory action is related to microtubule dynamics. Therefore, there may be a similar effect with MBZ [mebendazole] and other benzimidazoles, and this may also be a factor in the anti-cancer effects of these drugs. (26)

Perhaps this immunomodulatory effect of mebendazole and other microtubule-disrupting agents is due to interaction with PIBF, which is highly expressed, and associated with the microtubule structure called the centrosome. We await further studies to confirm or refute this hypothesis.

Mifepristone Disrupts the Cytoskeleton

Others have studied the effect of mifepristone on cancer cells involving disruption of the cytoskeleton with impairment of cancer cell motility and adhesion.

In 2013, Dr. BreeAnn Brandhagen et al. found drastic morphological changes in cancer cells induced by mifepristone, with concentration of tubulin filaments at "neurite-like" extensions. This change in cancer cell morphology included "shrinkage of the cell body with long, thin, neurite-like cellular extensions," that were remarkably similar across four metastatic cancer cell lines. Dr. Brandhagen writes:

> Tubulin, which in untreated and polarized cells usually arranges around the microtubule-organizing center and the Golgi apparatus, was mainly found framing the periphery of the nuclei in control cells; however, **in mifepristone-treated cells, tubulin accumulated mainly in the long-thin neurite-like extensions**. (27)

In 2019, Dr. Sabrina Ritch et al. used fluorescence microscopy to study the effect of mifepristone on cancer cell migration and invasion, finding the alteration in the cancer cell microtubule system. Dr. Ritch observed that mifepristone attenuates the migration, movement, and invasion of cancer cells, preventing metastatic disease. Dr. Ritch also suggested synergy with autophagy inhibitors such as hydroxychloroquine:

> [Mifepristone] alters the morphology of cancer cells in a dose-related manner, and attenuates migration and invasion of cancer cells…. triggers cellular stress and autophagy, making it **useful in combination therapies with proteasome inhibitors and autophagy blockers**. (28)

Meningioma Controlled for 26 Years

In 2020, Dr. Maria Medina-Lopes and Luiz Augusto Casulari reported a women with a large inoperable meningioma controlled for 26 years by mifepristone. (29)

Breast Cancer Studies

A number of studies show the efficacy of mifepristone for breast cancer, suppressing growth, preventing metastatic disease, and suppressing cancer stem cells. (30–33)

Ovarian Cancer in Vitro Studies— Synergy With Chloroquine

In 2017, Dr. Lei Zhang et al. studied mifepristone in an ovarian cancer cell line, showing direct effects on the cancer cells, with triggering of unfolded protein response, increase in "protective autophagy," and induction of apoptosis in combination with lysosomal inhibitors such as chloroquine:

> Moreover, mifepristone increased LC3-II levels [an autophagy marker protein] due to increased autophagic flux. When the autophagic–lysosomal pathway was inhibited with chloroquine, mifepristone was lethal to the cells. (34)

Failure of Clinical Trials of Mifepristone in Ovarian and Endometrial Cancer

Although preclinical studies looked promising, clinical trials of mifepristone in endometrial and ovarian cancer were all considered a failure with poor results. (35–37)

In 2019, Dr. Donata Ponikwicka-Tyszko et al. suggested the reason for failure of the clinical trials was that the beneficial anti-tumor effect of high-doses MF [mifepristone] **could not be achieved** in human cancer tissue, and the low tissue concentrations achieved with the therapeutic doses only promoted the growth of ovarian cancers. (36)

One might speculate that better results could have been obtained with the combination use of mifepristone with an autophagy inhibitor such as chloroquine or hydroxychloroquine, as suggested above by Dr. Zhang in 2017. One might also suggest its use in combination with a third drug such as niclosamide, a mitochondrial uncoupling agent shown to be effective in ovarian cancer. See the two chapters on niclosamide and chloroquine, chapters 23 and 32 respectively.

Conclusion

Despite the failure of clinical trials using mifepristone in endometrial and ovarian cancer, it may serve as an immunomodulating drug for other cancers. The most promising preclinical studies and case reports are in leukemia and lymphoma. Therefore, I would suggest doing clinical trials in leukemia and lymphoma patients, in combination with other agents for inhibition of OXPHOS and GLYCOLYSIS and Autophagy. I would expect improved efficacy of mifepristone when used in such combinations. The protocol here is to use mifepristone as an immune modulator, restore anti-cancer immunity, and use other drugs to inhibit the three pillars of cancer cell metabolism, OXPHOS, GLYCOLYSIS, and Autophagy. We await further studies of the link between mifepristone, PIBF, and other microtubule inhibitors such as mebendazole.

Microtubule agents such as mebendazole have the ability to restore anti-cancer immunity, perhaps related to the link between the cytoskeleton and PIBF as described above. In the event Mifepristone is unavailable or restricted, the use of mebendazole may serve in its place to impair the cancer cells' escape from immune surveillance.

References for 26: Progesterone Blocking Factor RU 486

1) Szekeres-Bartho, Julia, and Beata Polgar. "PIBF: the Double Edged Sword. Pregnancy and Tumor." American Journal of Reproductive Immunology 64.2 (2010): 77-86.

2) Halasz, Melinda, et al. "Progesterone-induced blocking factor differentially regulates trophoblast and tumor invasion by altering matrix metalloproteinase activity." Cellular and molecular life sciences 70.23 (2013): 4617-4630.

3) Chen, Jianzhong, et al. "The unique pharmacological characteristics of mifepristone (RU486): from terminating pregnancy to preventing cancer metastasis." Medicinal research reviews 34.5 (2014): 979-1000.

4) Check, J. H., et al. "Evidence that progesterone receptor antagonists may help in the treatment of a variety of cancers by locally suppressing natural killer cell activity." Clinical and experimental obstetrics & gynecology 34.4 (2007): 207-211.

5) Check, J. H., E. Dix, and L. Sansoucie. "Support for the hypothesis that successful immunotherapy of various cancers can be achieved by inhibiting a progesterone associated immunomodulatory protein." Medical hypotheses 72.1 (2009): 87-90.

6) Check, Jerome H. "The role of progesterone and the progesterone receptor in cancer." Expert Review of Endocrinology & Metabolism 12.3 (2017): 187-197.

7) Escobar-Sánchez, María L., Luis Sánchez-Sánchez, and Jesús Sandoval-Ramírez. "Steroidal saponins

and cell death in cancer." Cell Death—Autophagy, Apoptosis and Necrosis; Ntuli, T., Ed (2015): 331-352.

8) Bhuvanalakshmi, G., et al. "Breast cancer stem-like cells are inhibited by diosgenin, a steroidal saponin, by the attenuation of the Wnt β-catenin signaling via the Wnt antagonist secreted frizzled related protein-4." Frontiers in pharmacology 8 (2017): 124.

9) Raber, Linda. "Steroid industry honored. International historic chemical landmark acclaims success of mexican steroid industry and a US chemist who made it possible." Journal of the Mexican Chemical Society 43.6 (1999): 235-237.

10) Balandrin, Manuel F. "Commercial utilization of plant-derived saponins: an overview of medicinal, pharmaceutical, and industrial applications." Saponins used in traditional and modern medicine. Springer, Boston, MA, 1996. 1-14.

11) Tieszen, Chelsea R., et al. "Antiprogestin mifepristone inhibits the growth of cancer cells of reproductive and non-reproductive origin regardless of progesterone receptor expression." BMC cancer 11.1 (2011): 207.

12) Wan, Liyuan et al. "Aspirin, Lysine, Mifepristone and Doxycycline Combined Can Effectively and Safely Prevent and Treat Cancer Metastasis: Prevent Seeds from Gemmating on Soil." Oncotarget 6.34 (2015): 35157–35172.

13) Gutiérrez-Rodríguez, Araceli, Valeria Hansberg-Pastor, and Ignacio Camacho-Arroyo. "Proliferative and Invasive Effects of Progesterone-Induced Blocking Factor in Human Glioblastoma Cells." BioMed research international 2017 (2017).

14) Check, Jerome H., et al. "Evidence that mifepristone, a progesterone receptor antagonist, can cross the blood brain barrier and provide palliative benefits for glioblastoma multiforme grade IV." Anticancer research 34.5 (2014): 2385-2388.

15) Srivastava, Maya D., et al. "Expression and modulation of progesterone induced blocking factor (PIBF) and innate immune factors in human leukemia cell lines by progesterone and mifepristone." Leukemia & lymphoma 48.8 (2007): 1610-1617.

16) Check, Jerome H., et al. "Mifepristone treatment improves length and quality of survival of mice with

spontaneous leukemia." Anticancer research 29.8 (2009): 2977-2980.

17) Check, Jerome H., et al. "Mifepristone Causing Complete Remission of Rapidly Advancing Leukemia with Measurement of Progesterone-induced Blocking Factor." Anticancer research 34.5 (2014): 2413-2416.

18) Jang, Ji Hoon, et al. "RU486, a glucocorticoid receptor antagonist, induces apoptosis in U937 human lymphoma cells through reduction in mitochondrial membrane potential and activation of p38 MAPK." Oncology reports 30.1 (2013): 506-512.

19) Ramaraj, Pandurangan. "In-vitro inhibition of human melanoma (BLM) cell growth by progesterone receptor antagonist RU-486 (Mifepristone)." Journal of Cancer Therapy 7.13 (2016): 1045-1058.

20) Zheng, Ning, et al. "Metapristone (RU486 derivative) inhibits cell proliferation and migration as melanoma metastatic chemopreventive agent." Biomedicine & Pharmacotherapy 90 (2017): 339-349.

21) Check, Jerome H., et al. "Mifepristone may halt progression of extensively metastatic human adenocarcinoma of the colon-case report." Anticancer research 29.5 (2009): 1611-1613.

22) Check, Jerome H., Diane Check, and Trina Poretta. "Mifepristone Extends Both Length and Quality of Life in a Patient with Advanced Non-small Cell Lung Cancer that Has Progressed Despite Chemotherapy and a Check-point Inhibitor." Anticancer Research 39.4 (2019): 1923-1926.

23) Check, Jerome H., et al. "Long-term high-quality survival with single-agent mifepristone treatment despite advanced cancer." Anticancer Research 36.12 (2016): 6511-6513.

24) Lachmann, Margit, et al. "PIBF (progesterone induced blocking factor) is overexpressed in highly proliferating cells and associated with the centrosome." International journal of cancer 112.1 (2004): 51-60.

25) Sevko A, et al. Antitumor effect of paclitaxel is mediated by inhibition of myeloid-derived suppressor cells and chronic inflammation in the spontaneous melanoma model. J Immunol . 2013;190(5):2464–71.

26) Pantziarka, Pan, et al. "Repurposing Drugs in Oncology (ReDO)—Mebendazole as an Anti-Cancer Agent." ecancermedicalscience 8 (2014).

27) Brandhagen, BreeAnn N., et al. "Cytostasis and morphological changes induced by mifepristone in human metastatic cancer cells involve cytoskeletal filamentous actin reorganization and impairment of cell adhesion dynamics." BMC cancer 13.1 (2013): 35.

28) Ritch, Sabrina J., et al. "Advanced assessment of migration and invasion of cancer cells in response to mifepristone therapy using double fluorescence cytochemical labeling." BMC Cancer 19 (2019).

29) Medina-Lopes, Maria das Dores, and Luiz Augusto Casulari. "Treatment of a Woman with Inoperable Meningioma Using Mifepristone for 26 Years." Case Reports in Neurological Medicine 2020 (2020).

30) Liu, Rong, et al. "Mifepristone Derivative FZU-00,003 Suppresses Triple-negative Breast Cancer Cell Growth partially via miR-153-KLF5 axis." Int J Biol Sci 16.4 (2020): 611-619.

31) Yu, Suhong, et al. "Pharmacoproteomic analysis reveals that metapristone (RU486 metabolite) intervenes E-cadherin and vimentin to realize cancer metastasis chemoprevention." Scientific reports 6 (2016): 22388.

32) Liu, Rong, et al. "Mifepristone suppresses basal triple-negative breast cancer stem cells by down-regulating KLF5 expression." Theranostics 6.4 (2016): 533.

33) Rubin, Ayelen, et al. "Effect of the combined treatment with mifepristone and chemotherapy on breast cancer brain metastases." (2017): 4912-4912.

34) Zhang, Lei, et al. "Mifepristone increases mRNA translation rate, triggers the unfolded protein response, increases autophagic flux, and kills ovarian cancer cells in combination with proteasome or lysosome inhibitors." Molecular oncology 10.7 (2016): 1099-1117.

35) Rocereto, T. F., et al. "A phase II evaluation of mifepristone in the treatment of recurrent or persistent epithelial ovarian, fallopian or primary peritoneal cancer: a gynecologic oncology group study." Gynecologic oncology 116.3 (2010): 332.

36) Ponikwicka-Tyszko, Donata, et al. "Molecular mechanisms underlying mifepristone's agonistic action on ovarian cancer progression." EBioMedicine 47 (2019): 170-183.

37) Ramondetta, Lois M., et al. "Phase 2 trial of mifepristone (RU-486) in advanced or recurrent endometrioid adenocarcinoma or low-grade endometrial stromal sarcoma." Cancer 115.9 (2009): 1867-1874.

38) Sundström, Christer, and Kenneth Nilsson. "Establishment and characterization of a human histiocytic lymphoma cell line (U-937)." International journal of cancer 17.5 (1976): 565-577.

Chapter 27

The Mouse that Killed Cancer

IN 2003, AT WAKE FOREST Medical School in North Carolina, medical students labored tediously for hours on end injecting cancer cells into mice, all of which died promptly after cancer cell injection. Then, one day, the unexpected happened—a mouse survived. This special mouse was renamed "The Mouse That Killed Cancer" and earmarked for further study. As Louis Pasteur once said, "Fortune favors the prepared mind."(1)

Spontaneous Regression of Cancer in the Mouse

These were exciting times, and there were many questions. Why didn't this mouse die of cancer like all the others? How was this mouse able to defeat the injected cancer cells? What kind of immune system protected this mouse?

A Mouse Immune to Cancer

Over the next 3 years, studies showed this strain of mice had an innate immunity to cancer, a genetic trait passed on to the offspring. Their T lymphocytes (T Cells), recognized and killed the cancer cells, just as if cancer were an invading microorganism. These mice were called SR/CR mice, which stands for spontaneous regression/complete resistance to cancer. (2)

Saving Other Mice from Cancer

What about the other wild-type mice with no immunity to cancer who quickly succumb to injected cancer cells? Could these wild-type mice be protected from cancer by transferring the immune system from a SR/CR mouse? What if we infused the T Cells, the immune cells from a SR/CR mouse, into a plain mouse? More experiments showed that, yes, protection from the injected cancer cells could be transferred to plain mice after transfusion with T cells from SR/CR mice. (3–4)

Tumor Cell Equilibrium with the Immune System

In 2007, Dr. Catherine Koebel et al. studied a mouse model of chemical carcinogenesis, finding that the immune system of a mouse is capable of controlling cancer growth for long periods of time, a process called "Equilibrium":

> In addition to destroying tumour cells and sculpting tumour immunogenicity, the immune system of a naive mouse can also restrain cancer growth for extended time periods. (5)

Eventually, the tumor spontaneously "escapes" from immune surveillance and goes wild, spreading throughout the body.

Human Mice—Spontaneous Regression of Cancer

What about us humans? Can we be like the mice? Do we have similar immunity to cancer? Are some of us humans "immune" from cancer? The answer is yes—this is called "tumor immune surveillance," first described over 100 years ago. The immune system destroys cancer cells before they can cause harm. Drs. Jeremy Swann and Mark Smyth (2007) write:

> The idea that the immune system, which so effectively protects the host from microbial pathogens, might also recognize and destroy tumor cells was first discussed over a century ago … tumor immune surveillance, whereby the immune system identifies cancerous and/or precancerous cells and **eliminates them before they can cause harm.** (6)

Malignant Melanoma Immune Surveillance.

Perhaps tumor immune surveillance is best illustrated in humans in malignant melanoma, which undergoes spontaneous regression in about 25%–50% of cases. (7-9)

In 2017, Dr. Arielle Gray et al. studied 14 melanomas of the skin, finding, on microscopic evaluation of the biopsy sample, a unique subset of lymphocytes associated with cancer regression:

> A unique subset of T lymphocytes found in areas of regression can be histologically distinguished from tumor-infiltrating T lymphocytes [TIL] found in areas of tumor progression. We call this unique subset of T lymphocytes **regression associated T lymphocytes** [RATs]. (7)

Cancer-Cell Killing Ability in Healthy Humans

In 2011, Dr. Michael Blanks et al. studied freshly isolated human leukocytes (white cells) from 22 cancer cases and 25 healthy controls and was able to detect innate cancer-cell killing activity in the healthy patients' white cells similar to the cancer resistant SR/CR mice. Cell-killing ability was lower in the cancer patients. (10)

Transferring Anti-Cancer Immunity in Humans

Remember the mouse experiments that protected the mouse from cancer by infusing the T Cells from an SR/CR mouse into a plain mouse? This can be done in humans, protecting us from cancer the same way mice are protected.

In 2017, Dr. Dipnarine Maharaj studied eleven patients with advanced end-stage solid tumors refractory to further conventional treatment. White cells were collected by leukapheresis from young, healthy donors and then infused in to the cancer patients. Of the eleven patients so treated, three patients with metastatic ovarian, colon, and breast cancer later died within 90 days of treatment and had post mortem tissue available for histology revealing extensive tumor necrosis and leukocyte (neutrophils) infiltration:

> Post mortem examination of all three patients showed similar diffuse histological evidence of tumor necrosis … in about 80% of tumor in Patients 1 and 2 and 40–50% in Patient 3, which appeared to be treatment related … Evidence of leukocyte [neutrophil] infiltration was seen in all cases.…

minimal side effects related to this novel immunotherapy. (11)

Stimulating Neutrophils with Neupogen

In 2011, Dr. Juan Carlos Souto et al. suggested that intense, sustained neutrophilia (increased neutrophils – leukocytes or white cells) induced by the Neupogen drug (granulocyte colony-stimulating factor) creates an inflammatory response around the tumor and could represent an effective anti-cancer treatment for solid tumors. (12)

The Power of the Immune System in Cancer Treatment

The above discussion highlights the importance in cancer surveillance of the immune system, which prevents cancer from growing in our bodies. "Immune evasion" is a requirement for cancer to persist in our bodies. (13–18)

Escape from Immune Surveillance

The concept of escape from immune surveillance was an old one originally proposed in 1909 by Paul Ehrlich. (19) This idea is nicely summarized by Dr. Miao in 2019: "Our bodies are equipped with powerful immune surveillance to clear cancerous cells as they emerge." (20)

Cancer Stem Cells Evade Immune Surveillance

In 2019, Dr. Yuxuan Miao used squamous cell cancer to study how cancer stem cells evade the immune system, finding that cancer stem cells acquire the CD80 surface protein, which directly blocks cytotoxic T cells from killing the cancer cells. (20)

Likewise in 2019, Mr. Chiara Marchiori et al. studied colon cancer preneoplastic lesions finding that CD80 surface protein plays a "major role in orchestrating immune surveillance " Indeed, soluble CD80 was patented in 2019 as a therapy to reverse immune suppression in cancer patients. (21–22)

In 2018, Dr. Judith Agudo et al. studied cycling and quiescent stem cells, finding that stem cells are routinely eliminated by activated T cells. However, quiescent stem cells in hair follicles or muscle were resistant to the cytotoxic effect of T cells by using their immune-evasion machinery. (24)

Cancer Stem Cells and Immune Evasion

In 2019, Dr. Alex Miranda et al. studied 21 sold cancers, finding "stemness" to be associated with anti-cancer immunity. **Note:** stemness is defined as having features of stem cells.

The cancer stem cells had the most effective immune evasion. Dr. Miranda writes:

> Thus, **stemness** is not only a fundamental process in cancer progression but may represent a unifying mechanism linking antigenicity, intratumoral heterogeneity, and **immune suppression across cancers.** (25)

Quiescent cancer stem cells "fly under the radar," so to speak, by virtue of their ability to escape from immune surveillance. (26–27)

Escape from Immune Surveillance—Fourth Pillar

For this reason, I propose "Escape from Immune Surveillance" of equal important to the first three pillars of cancer cell metabolism, a "fourth pillar" for our *Cracking Cancer Toolkit*. Remember, the first three pillars are concerned with blocking metabolic pathways inside the cancer cell—OXPHOS, GLYCOLYSIS and Autophagy. This fourth pillar is concerned with restoring the host immune response to the cancer, roughly described as "immunotherapy," having a long history in medicine.

The Father of Immunotherapy— Coley's Toxins

The recognized father of immunotherapy is a New York orthopedic surgeon by the name of William Coley (1890–1936). In 1891, Dr. Coley performed a forearm amputation for osteosarcoma (bone cancer) of the hand in a young lady who succumbed to metastatic disease only a few months after the amputation. This dismal outcome made an impact and motivated Dr. Coley to review the hospital records of the previous 90 cases, revealing the only surviving patient experienced complete tumor regression after contracting erysipelas, a streptococcus infection of the skin. Dr. Coley then hypothesized that injecting similar bacterial toxins into patients could stimulate the immune system to reject the tumor. The injected concoction was labeled "Coley's Toxins," consisting of heat-killed Streptococcus pyogenes and Serratia marcescens (two bacterial strains). In total, Dr. Coley injected more than 1,000 patients and published 150 papers. After enjoying considerable success with many tumor regressions from 1893 to 1960, enthusiasm for Coley's toxins waned after the introduction of chemotherapy and radiation. In 1963, the FDA deemed Coley's Toxins an investigational new drug, essentially banning its use outside of a clinical trial. (28–33)

In 1909, Paul Ehrlich was the first to propose the idea of "immune surveillance," a term later coined in 1957 by Lewis Thomas and Sir Frank Macfarlane Burnet. This is the idea that cancer cells arise in the body and are removed by the immune system on a routine basis. (28)

Immune Surveillance

Lending validity to the concept of "immune surveillance"' are both animal and human studies. Patients with dysfunctional immune systems have higher incidence of cancer. In 2018, Dr. Mayor studied patient registries of patients with primary immunodeficiency syndrome, finding a 10-fold increase in lymphoma in males. (32)

Similarly, patients on immunosuppressive drugs for organ transplants had higher incidence of neoplasm. (28)

In 2011, Drs. Robert Schreiber et al. proposed the concept of the three stages of "cancer immunoediting." In the first stage, elimination, tumor cells are completely eliminated by the immune system. In the second stage, equilibrium, the tumor cells persist in a quiescent state. In the third stage, escape, tumor cells evade the immune system altogether, proliferating rapidly into large masses that spread to distant organs. (33)

In 2020, Dr. Carlson reviewed immunotherapy, writing:

> Thus, the fundamental goal of cancer immunotherapy is to overcome the years to decades of immunoediting to generate anti-tumor immunity that is sufficient to completely eliminate the patient's cancer and cure their disease. (28)

The Invention of Checkpoint Inhibitors

The next great milestone in the history of immunotherapy came with the invention of checkpoint inhibitors, antibody treatments that block the suppression of T lymphocytes, restoring anti-cancer immunity. The first agent to be FDA-approved in 2011, Ipilimumab, is an anti–CTLA-4 monoclonal antibody approved for metastatic melanoma. The second agent, a PD-1 Antibody, nivolumab, was approved in 2014. In 2016, anti-PD-L1 mAb (monoclonal antibodies) pembrolizumab and atezolizumab were FDA-approved. The checkpoint inhibitors were proven efficacious; however, there remains a population of non-responders, either failing to respond to initial treatment or acquiring resistance with relapse after initial response. (34–37)

Note: CTLA = cytotoxic T-lymphocyte-associated protein, PD-L1 = Programmed Death Ligand-1

In the following chapters, we will discuss strategies in *Cracking Cancer Toolkit* to enhance the efficacy of checkpoint inhibitor immune-therapy.

The Miracle of CAR T cell Therapy

Immunotherapy research reached its crowning achievement with the introduction of CAR T cell therapy for CD19+ B-cell hematologic malignancies (leukemias and lymphomas).

(**Note:** CAR T cell = Chimeric Antigen Receptor T Cell).

CAR T cell therapy involves harvesting the patient's own T cells with a leukapheresis machine. The T cells are sent to a lab where they are genetically engineered to express antibodies to the CD19 surface protein marker exclusively present on normal and malignant B cells. The anti-CD-19 antibodies are embedded on the outer membrane of the T Cells, facilitating attachment to malignant B cells, thus overcoming immune evasion, killing the cancer cells.

The modified T cells are allowed to expand (multiply) and then re-infused into the patient as a treatment for B-cell lymphoma or leukemia. Patients routinely receive a short course of lympho-depleting chemotherapy prior to reinfusion of the T cells. If all goes well, the CAR T cells attack and destroy the patient's malignant B cells, leading to long-term durable remission. The patient's normal B cells are also destroyed, leading to profound B-Cell depletion, which by the way is beneficial in lupus and other auto-immune diseases. The treatment is not without adverse effects—among the most common are cytokine storm, CNS toxicity, and cytopenias. Durable remissions have been reported. However, up to 40% of patients relapse with CD19 negative disease, called "CD19 escape."

Future CAR T constructs are planned with co-targeting of multiple surface markers CD19/20/22 to avoid this type of relapse. A major criticism of CAR T is cost. The treatment is very expensive. Another criticism is lack of efficacy in solid tumors. Co-treatment with CAR T and Ibrutinib, a tyrosine kinase inhibitor (TKI) drug routinely used in lymphoma, shows considerable synergy, enhancing T cell expansion and persistence. (38–44)

Strategies for Restoring Host Immune Surveillance

The next chapters discuss strategies to enhance immune surveillance and restore the host immune system.

Cimetidine is one such off-patent repurposed drug that is capable of upregulating the host immune system. Another is AHCC mushroom extracts, also called beta glucans. We will discuss additional immune enhancing strategies such as optimizing vitamin D levels, vitamin C, vitamin A, iodine, selenium, thyroid hormone, probiotics, etc. Working in combination, these strategies can have powerful benefits for the cancer patient in restoring anti-cancer immunity.

References for Chapter 27: The Mouse that Killed Cancer

1) Cui, Zheng, et al. "Spontaneous regression of advanced cancer: identification of a unique genetically determined, age-dependent trait in mice." Proceedings of the National Academy of Sciences 100.11 (2003): 6682-6687.

2) Hicks, Amy M., et al. "Effector mechanisms of the anti-cancer immune responses of macrophages in SR/CR mice." Cancer Immunity Archive 6.1 (2006): 11.

3) Hicks, Amy M., et al. "Transferable anticancer innate immunity in spontaneous regression/complete resistance mice." Proceedings of the National Academy of Sciences 103.20 (2006): 7753-7758.

4) Stehle, John R., et al. "Impact of sex, MHC, and age of recipients on the therapeutic effect of transferred leukocytes from cancer-resistant SR/CR mice." BMC cancer 9.1 (2009): 328.

5) Koebel, Catherine M., et al. "Adaptive immunity maintains occult cancer in an equilibrium state." Nature 450.7171 (2007): 903-907.

6) Swann, Jeremy B., and Mark J. Smyth. "Immune surveillance of tumors." The Journal of Clinical Investigation 117.5 (2007): 1137-1146.

7) Gray, Arielle, et al. "The microenvironment in primary cutaneous melanoma with associated spontaneous tumor regression: evaluation for T-regulatory cells and the presence of an immunosuppressive microenvironment." Melanoma research 27.2 (2017): 104-109.

8) Cervinkova, Monika, Petra Kucerova, and Jana Cizkova. "Spontaneous regression of malignant melanoma-is it based on the interplay between host immune system and melanoma antigens?" Anti-cancer drugs 28.8 (2017): 819-830.

9) Kappauf, Herbert, and Gregor Esser. "Metachronous spontaneous remission of melanoma lung metastasis and mediastinal lymph node metastases." Oncology research and treatment 41.3 (2018): 135-138.

10) Blanks, Michael J., et al. "Novel innate cancer killing activity in humans." Cancer cell international 11.1 (2011): 26.

11) Maharaj, Dipnarine, et al. "Young donor white blood cell immunotherapy induces extensive tumor necrosis in advanced-stage solid tumors." Heliyon 3.10 (2017): e00438.

12) Souto, Juan Carlos, Luis Vila, and Antonio Bru. "Polymorphonuclear neutrophils and cancer: intense and sustained neutrophilia as a treatment against solid tumors." Medicinal research reviews 31.3 (2011): 311-363.

13) Muenst, S., et al. "The immune system and cancer evasion strategies: therapeutic concepts." Journal of internal medicine 279.6 (2016): 541-562.

14) Rao, Samhita, Karim Gharib, and Arnold Han. "Cancer immunosurveillance by T cells." International review of cell and molecular biology. Vol. 342. Academic Press, 2019. 149-173.

15) Baker, Mairead, et al. "Spontaneous regression of Merkel cell carcinoma is driven by adaptive immune activation and clonal T cell expansion." (2018): 4676-4676.

16) Shatola, Ashley, et al. "Spontaneous Regression of Non-small Cell Lung Cancer: A Case Report and Literature Review." Cureus 12.1 (2020).

17) Chin, Ken Min, Chung Yip Chan, and Ser Yee Lee. "Spontaneous regression of pancreatic cancer: A case report and literature review." International journal of surgery case reports 42 (2018): 55-59.

18) Cserni, Gábor, et al. "Spontaneous pathological complete regression of high-grade triple-negative breast cancer with axillary metastasis." Polish Journal of Pathology 70.2 (2019): 139-143.

19) Ribatti, Domenico. "The concept of immune surveillance against tumors: The first theories." Oncotarget 8.4 (2017): 7175.

20) Miao, Yuxuan, et al. "Adaptive immune resistance emerges from tumor-initiating stem cells." Cell 177.5 (2019): 1172-1186.

21) Marchiori, Chiara, et al. "Epithelial CD80 promotes immune surveillance of colonic preneoplastic lesions and its expression is increased by oxidative stress through STAT3 in colon cancer cells." Journal of Experimental & Clinical Cancer Research 38.1 (2019): 1-14.

22) Ostrand-Rosenberg, Suzanne. "Soluble CD80 as a therapeutic to reverse immune suppression in cancer patients." U.S. Patent No. 10,377,810. 13 Aug. 2019.

24) Agudo, Judith, et al. "Quiescent tissue stem cells evade immune surveillance." Immunity 48.2 (2018): 271-285.

25) Miranda, Alex, et al. "Cancer stemness, intratumoral heterogeneity, and immune response across cancers." Proceedings of the National Academy of Sciences 116.18 (2019): 9020-9029.

26) Boyd, Ashleigh S., and Neil P. Rodrigues. "Stem Cells Cycle toward Immune Surveillance." Immunity 48.2 (2018): 187-190.

27) Bird, Lucy. "Leukaemic Stem Cells Go Under the Radar." Nature Reviews Immunology 19.9 (2019): 533-533.

28) Carlson, Robert D., John C. Flickinger, and Adam E. Snook. "Talkin' Toxins: From Coley's to Modern Cancer Immunotherapy." Toxins 12.4 (2020): 241.

29) Coley, W. "Contribution to the knowledge of sarcoma." Am Surg 14 (1891): 190.

30) Coley, William B. "The Treatment of Inoperable Sarcoma with the Mixed Toxins of Erysipelas and Bacillus Prodigiosus: Immediate and Final Results, One Hundred and Forty Cases." Journal of the American Medical Association 31.9 (1898): 456-465.

31) Coley, William B. "The treatment of inoperable sarcoma by bacterial toxins (the mixed toxins of the Streptococcus erysipelas and the Bacillus prodigiosus)." Proceedings of the Royal Society of Medicine 3.Surg_Sect (1910): 1-48.

32) Mayor, Paul C., et al. "Cancer in primary immunodeficiency diseases: cancer incidence in the United States Immune Deficiency Network Registry." Journal of Allergy and Clinical Immunology 141.3 (2018): 1028-1035.

33) Schreiber, Robert D., Lloyd J. Old, and Mark J. Smyth. "Cancer immunoediting: integrating immunity's roles in cancer suppression and promotion." Science 331.6024 (2011): 1565-1570.

34) Nikolaou, Michail, et al. "Immunotherapy of Cancer: Developments and Reference Points, an Unorthodox Approach." Integrative Cancer Therapies 18 (2019): 1 –10.

35) Joshi, Kroopa, et al. "The "Achilles' Heel" of Cancer and its implications for the development of novel immunotherapeutic strategies." Cold Spring Harbor Perspectives in Medicine 8.1 (2018): a027086.

36) Trapani, Joseph A., and Phillip K. Darcy. "Immunotherapy of cancer." Australian Family Physician 46.4 (2017): 194.

37) Fuereder, Thorsten. "The adolescence of cancer immunotherapy: from a difficult childhood to a pillar of modern anticancer therapy." (2018): 82-83.

38) Feins, Steven, et al. "An introduction to chimeric antigen receptor (CAR) T-cell immunotherapy for human cancer." American journal of hematology 94.S1 (2019): S3-S9.

39) Sermer, David, and Renier Brentjens. "CAR T-cell therapy: Full speed ahead." Hematological oncology 37 (2019): 95-100.

40) Santomasso, Bianca, et al. "The other side of CAR T-cell therapy: cytokine release syndrome, neurologic toxicity, and financial burden." American Society of Clinical Oncology Educational Book 39 (2019): 433-444.

41) Fousek, Kristen, et al. "CAR T-cells that target acute B-lineage leukemia irrespective of CD19 expression." Leukemia (2020): 1-15.

42) Kansal, Rita, et al. "Sustained B cell depletion by CD19-targeted CAR T cells is a highly effective treatment for murine lupus." Science translational medicine 11.482 (2019): eaav1648.

43) Shah, Nirav, et al. "Multi targeted CAR-T cell therapies for B-cell malignancies." Frontiers in oncology 9 (2019): 146.

44) Sun, L., et al. "Synergistic effect of ibrutinib and CD19 CAR-T cells on Raji cells in vivo and in vitro." (2020).

Chapter 28

Cimetidine

Overcoming Cancer Cell Immune Evasion—Complete Remission of Lymphoma with Cimetidine

THE FIRST PATIENT, A 73-YEAR-OLD man presented to the hospital with upper abdominal pain and weight loss. Upper endoscopy of the stomach revealed a large ulcerated mass. Endoscopic biopsy confirmed the mass was a malignant lymphoma. To treat the gastric ulcer, the patient was started on cimetidine, 900 mg daily, until surgery could be performed 14 weeks later. At surgery, an antral ulcer was found. However, the lymphoma had disappeared, solely with cimetidine treatment. (1)

A second patient, an 84-year-old man presented to the hospital with chest pain. Upper endoscopy of the stomach revealed multiple areas of ulceration and narrowing of the lumen. Gastric biopsy revealed malignant lymphoma, and the patient was started on cimetidine, 1200 mg daily, and ranitidine, 150 mg daily. Five weeks later at surgery, the lymphoma had gone into a durable complete remission. (1)

The remarkable anti-cancer benefits of cimetidine have been reported by many others. (2–6) Inhibition of suppressor cell function (myeloid-derived suppressor cells) involved in tumor immune evasion is thought to be the mechanism of action. (7–10)

Cimetidine Antacid Drug

FDA-approved in 1979 as histamine receptor blocker (H2 receptor), cimetidine (Tagamet®) was originally marketed as an antacid drug for treatment of gastric hyperacidity, gastritis, and ulcer. Cimetidine inhibits gastric acid secretion by binding to the H2 receptors in parietal cells in the gastric wall. In its day, cimetidine was a top-selling drug and today is still available over the counter. For the most part, cimetidine has been replaced by the newer proton pump inhibitor antacids (PPI drugs). Doctors using cimetidine observed remarkable cancer regressions that seemingly involved the drug's ability to stimulate host immune cell expansion and reverse immune tumor evasion.

Remarkable Cancer Regression in Melanoma

In 1983, Dr. P. Flodgren et al. studied the combined use of cimetidine and interferon in 20 melanoma patients, finding remarkable tumor regression in 6 of the 20 patients associated with marked lymphocyte infiltration at the tumor site. Dr. Flodgren writes:

> Five out of eight patients with metastases confined to skin and subcutaneous tissue had complete tumour regressions, while one patient with skin and lung metastases achieved an extensive partial regression of the skin tumour and a complete roentgenological regression of the lung metastasis. Three additional patients attained a stable

disease status for prolonged periods of time. Histopathological examinations confirmed disappearance and/or degeneration of melanoma cells and demonstrated a marked lymphocyte infiltration in tumour sites of the patients with objective tumour regression. (11)

Cimetidine in Mouse Xenograft Models

In 1985, Dr. Yoshihiro Kikuchi et al. studied ovarian cancer engrafted into nude mice, finding that mice given cimetidine had decreased the tumor volume to one third that of control mice at 36 days. The spleen cells (immune cells) of the cimetidine-treated mice had the capacity to lyse tumor cells at day 14, while the control mice did not. (12)

In 1981, Dr. Gifford studied cimetidine in a mouse lymphoma xenograft model, finding an improved survival rate (56%) for cimetidine-treated mice, compared to controls (10%) at 30 days. (13–14)

Cimetidine – Reversing Immunosuppression of Histamine

In 2019 Dr. Abdollah Jafarzadeh reviewed the Immunomodulatory properties of cimetidine, finding reversal of histamine induced immunosuppression and stimulation of immune cell "effector functions," writing that by binding to histamine receptor 2 (H2R),

Cimetidine, as an H2R antagonist, reverses the histamine-mediated immunosuppression, as it has powerful stimulatory effects on the effector functions of neutrophils, monocytes, macrophages, DCs, NK cells, NKT cells, Th1-, Th2-, Th17-, and CD8+ cytotoxic T cells..... The therapeutic potentials of cimetidine as an immunomodulatory agent [extends to] a number of human diseases such as cancers, viral warts, allergic disorders, burns, etc. (15)

Cimetidine Induced IL-18 Production in Monocytes

In 2006, the research breakthrough was made by Dr. Hideo Kohka Takahashi et al., who found that cimetidine induces IL-18 production in monocytes. Interleukin-18 (IL-18) is an immunostimulatory cytokine with anti-tumor activity. (16)

In 2013, Dr. Michael Robertson et al. conducted a study in 19 patients using recombinant IL-18 combined with Rituximab for NHL (non-Hodgkin's lymphoma). Rituximab is an anti-CD20 antibody routinely used for B-cell lymphoma. Of 19 patients in the study, there were 2 complete and 3 partial tumor responses. (17)

CAR T Cells Engineered to Secrete IL-18

The use of IL-18 in next-generation CAR T cells highlights its importance in cancer therapy. (18–20) **Note:** CAR T cells are Chimeric Antigen Receptor T Cells.

Three studies investigate CAR T cells bio-engineered to secrete IL-18. In 2017, Dr. Biliang Hu et al. used a melanoma mouse model to study CAR T Cells bio-engineered to secrete IL-18, finding "augmented anti-tumor immunity."

Dr. Hu and colleagues write:

In an intact mouse tumor model, CD19-IL-18 CAR T cells induced deeper B-cell aplasia, significantly enhanced CAR T cell proliferation, and effectively augmented anti-tumor effects in mice with B16F10 melanoma. In other words, the IL-18 made the CAR T cells much more effective for killing the tumor cells.(20)

Another CAR T melanoma study in mice in 2018 by Dr. André Kunert et al. was summarized as follows:

> Transfer of T cells expressing a melanoma specific-TCR [T cell receptor] and inducible iIL-18 [into mice] was without side effects, enhanced the presence of therapeutic CD8+ T cells within tumors, reduced tumor burden and prolonged survival…. treatment with T cells engineered with a TCR and iIL18 T cells is safe and able to skew the tumor micro-environment in favor of an improved anti-tumor T cell response. (19)

Note: iIL-12 is inducible IL-12. One might speculate on a similar benefit with cimetidine for CAR-T therapy, since cimetidine indices IL-18. This would be a good topic for further study with NIH funding.

A third study in 2018 by Drs. Markus Chmielewski, and Hinrich Abken showed the "release of IL-18 by CAR T cells promotes Th1 effector functions and recruitment of innate immune cells resulting in enhanced eradication of solid tumors."(18)

Immunomodulatory Effects of IL-18—A 56-Fold Expansion of Anti-Tumor NK Killer Cells

Now that we have your attention, let's explore the cell biology mechanisms of IL-18.

In 2018, Dr. Hiroaki Senju studied the effect of IL-18 and IL-12 on expansion of human natural killer (NK) Cells. These are the immune cells that kill cancer cells in the body. When IL-12, followed by IL-18 was added to the NK-cell suspension, by Day 4, NK cells proliferated vigorously, and by Day 10, there was a 56-fold expansion of NK cells. "IL-18 promoted the expansion of NK cells. "(21)

IL-12/IL-18 Preactivated Donor NK cells

In 2018, Dr. Yuan Song et al. studied IL-12/IL-18 preactivated donor NK cells in a murine model of B-cell lymphoma, finding enhancement of the graft vs. lymphoma effect. **Note:** graft vs. lymphoma effect is a term used for the anti-lymphoma immune response of transplanted bone marrow stem cells. Dr. Song et al. found:

> IL-12/18 preactivated NK cells mediated stronger GVL [Graft vs. Lymphoma] effect than control NK cells mainly due to their elevated activation/cytotoxicity and sustained proliferative potential. The IL-12/18 preactivated NK cells mitigate aGVHD [Acute Graft vs. Host Disease] despite the severity of the disease. IL-12/18-preactivated donor NK-cell infusion may be an effective and safe adoptive therapy after allo-HSCT [Allogeneic Hematopoietic Stem Cell Transplant]. (22)

In 2017, Drs. Esmailbeig and Abbas Ghaderi reported on IL-18 cytokine as a regulator of anti-tumor immunity with the activation of cytotoxic T cells (CTLs) and NK cells. Dr. Esmailbeig writes about the IL-18 cytokine:

> This cytokine synergistically with IL-12 contributes to Th1 differentiation and, therefore, is important in host defense mechanisms against intracellular bacteria, viruses, and fungi…. IL-18 in combination with IL-12 can activate cytotoxic T cells

[CTLs], as well as natural killer (NK) cells, to produce IFN-γ and, therefore, may contribute to tumor immunity (23)

2014 Review

In 2014, Dr. Pan Pantziarka et al. reviewed the anti-cancer effects of cimetidine, and identification four mechanisms.

1) Antiproliferative: Oral cimetidine blocks histamine stimulated growth of colon cancer cells in a mouse model.

2) Immunomodulatory

Histamine is associated with an immunosuppressive tumour micro-environment [TME], including increased regulatory T cell [T-reg] activity, reduced antigen-presenting activity of dendritic cells [DC], reduced NK-cell activity and increased myeloid-derived suppressor cell [MDSC] activity.... histamine binding to the H2 receptor is associated with suppression of IL-12 and stimulation of IL-10 secretion and is implicated with a shift in Th1/Th2 balance toward Th2-dominance of the immune response. This effect was reversed by CIM [Cimetidine] in human PBMC [peripheral blood monocytes] ... MDSCs [myeloid-derived suppressor cells] express H1–H3 receptors, and there is in vitro and in vivo evidence that blockade of H1 [using the H1RA cetirizine] or H2 [using CIM], can reverse the immunosuppressive action of these cells ... An increase in NK activity compared to non-CIM-treated controls has also been noted in cardiopulmonary bypass surgery. (24)

3) Effects on cell adhesion: By downregulating and inhibiting tumor cell adhesion, CIM prevents metastatic spread of tumor cells.

In a nude mouse model, CIM dose-dependently reduced the incidence of HT-29 liver metastases, suppressing it completely at the highest dose (200 mg/kg/day). The effect on cell adhesion was mediated by the interaction between tumour sialyl Lewis antigens and E-selectin expressed on the endothelium. (24)

4) Anti-Angiogenic Action

Production of VEGF which leads to angiogenesis (new vessels) is mediated by histamine. The upregulation of VEGF (vascular endothelial growth factor) and PDGF (platelet-derived growth factor) induced by histamine is reversed by cimetidine. This blocks the growth of tumor micro-vascularity needed to support the enlarging tumor mass. (24)

Many of these same points were made by Dr. Martina Kubecova et al. in a 2011 "Review of Cimetidine as an Anti-Cancer Drug," and by Dr. Florence LeFranc et al. in 2006. (25–26)

Cimetidine for Cutaneous Warts (HPV)— Enhancing Cell-Mediated Immunity

In 2018, Dr. Bibhuti Das et al. found cimetidine effective in restoring immune response and clearing refractory HPV induced cutaneous warts in children who were immuno-suppressed after heart transplants. Seven of eight patients had complete resolution of their warts after 3–6 months of cimetidine. Dr. Das's group found that cimetidine enhances cell-mediated immunity, writing:

Cimetidine is postulated to act as an immunomodulatory agent at high doses by inhibiting suppressor T cell function. The paradigm between T-helper 2 cells

[Th-2], and Th1 cells predominance is reflected in the level of cytokines that are released. Cimetidine activates Th1 cells to produce interleukin-2 [IL-2], IL-12, tumor necrosis factor alpha [TNF-α], and interferon gamma [IFN-γ] and their expression correlates with improvement in cellular immunity and wart remission... Patients who received cimetidine were shown to exhibit **enhanced cell-mediated immunity,** restoration of sensitivity following development of acquired tolerance, and increased response of lymphocytes to mitogen stimulation. (27)

Cimetidine for Viral Disease— Activating Th1 Cells

In 2003, Drs. Tsuyoshi Mitsuishi et al. studied cimetidine for viral warts, finding enhanced IL-2 and IFN-gamma expression in punch biopsy specimens of the warts after cimetidine treatment. Dr. Mitsuishi writes:

> Cimetidine activates Th1 cells to produce IL-2 and IFN-c and that their expression correlates with wart remission. (28)

Cimetidine for Shingles Herpes Zoster

Herpes Zoster (Shingles) is a reactivated chickenpox virus that involves the trunk and can be quite painful. Cimetidine has also been suggested for herpes zoster for reduction in pain and speeding healing. (29–33)

Cimetidine for Herpes Simplex

Orofacial herpes breakouts and genital herpes can be quite annoying. Cimetidine has been studied and shows considerable efficacy against herpes simplex, reducing blister time and speeding healing. (34–37)

Combined Use of Cimetidine with Mebendazole

In 1987, Dr. Bekhti reported that treatment of hepatic echinococcal cyst (hyatid parasitic disease) with mebendazole (1.5 grams three times a day) was enhanced with cimetidine, which increased the serum concentration of mebendazole (1200 mg/day x 30 days), resulting in complete resolution of the previously unresponsive liver cysts.(38)

Cimetidine for Painful Bladder Syndrome (IC Interstitial Cystitis)

Interstitial Cystitis/Painful Bladder syndrome in women is a poorly understood medical condition. The etiology and treatment have not been determined. One medical hypothesis is that occult infection accompanied by a defect or suppression of the immune system causes the condition. If this is true, then upregulating the immune system with a drug such as cimetidine might help. Indeed, a number of studies suggest cimetidine provides symptom relief in women with interstitial cystitis/ painful bladder. (39–41)

Adverse Side Effects of Cimetidine CIM

Dr. Pan Pantziarka et al. (2014) summarize the adverse effects of cimetidine. The Cytochrome P-450 enzyme system in the liver is inhibited by cimetidine, so interactions with other drugs may increase their exposure, as in the case of mebendazole:

> CIM has low toxicity, with the most common side effects being headache, dizziness, diarrhea, and rash. Rare side effects include

gynecomastia, reversible impotence (particularly reported in patients receiving very high doses) ... Rarely, CIM has also been associated with reversible leukopenia and thrombocytopenia, effects that may be particularly important to watch for in cancer patients who may be undergoing chemotherapy.... CIM is an inhibitor of cytochrome P450, through multiple [CYP] enzymes. (24) (42–43)

Prolonged suppression of gastric acid production with cimetidine (or PPI's) may produce malabsorption of vitamin B12 and iron. (44)

Conclusion

Cimetidine as an antihistamine and immuno-modulatory drug has a significant role as anti-cancer agent. Cimetidine's ability to reverse tumor-induced immunity and restore host cancer-killing cellular immunity is remarkable. The drug's antiviral activity for warts and herpes viruses is due, again, to its remarkable upregulation of the immune system.

References for Chapter 28: Cimetidine

1) Strauchen, James A., et al. "Spontaneous regression of gastric lymphoma." Cancer 60.8 (1987): 1872-1875.

2) Ankerst, Jaro, et al. "Complete remission in a patient with acute myelogenous leukemia treated with leukocyte α-interferon and cimetidine." Cancer Immunology, Immunotherapy 17.1 (1984): 69-71.

3) Inhorn, L., et al. "High-dose cimetidine for the treatment of metastatic renal cell carcinoma. A Hoosier Oncology Group study." American journal of clinical oncology 15.2 (1992): 157-159.

4) Pedersen, Lise, Carsten Rose, and Eyvind Langvad. "Combined treatment of advanced malignant melanoma with coumarin and cimetidine." Cancer Immunology, Immunotherapy 24.2 (1987): 178-179.

5) Burtin, Claude, et al. "Clinical improvement in advanced cancer disease after treatment combining histamine and H2-antihistaminics (ranitidine or cimetidine)." European Journal of Cancer and Clinical Oncology 24.2 (1988): 161-167.

6) Lefranc, Florence, et al. "Cimetidine, an unexpected anti-tumor agent, and its potential for the treatment of glioblastoma." International journal of oncology 28.5 (2006): 1021-1030.

7) Zheng, Yisheng, et al. "Cimetidine suppresses lung tumor growth in mice through proapoptosis of myeloid-derived suppressor cells." Molecular immunology 54.1 (2013): 74-83.

8) Kumar, Ashir, and Ronald P. Cleveland. "Immunoregulatory effects of cimetidine: inhibition of suppressor cell effector function in vivo." Immunopharmacology and immunotoxicology 10.3 (1988): 327-332.

9) Jin, Zaiwang, et al. "Inhibition of suppressor cell function by cimetidine in a murine model." Clinical immunology and immunopathology 38.3 (1986): 350-356.

10) Sahasrabudhe, Deepak M., et al. "Inhibition of suppressor T lymphocytes (Ts) by cimetidine." The Journal of Immunology 138.9 (1987): 2760-2763.

11) Flodgren, P., et al. "Metastatic malignant melanoma: Regression induced by combined treatment with interferon [HuIFN-α (Le)] and cimetidine." International journal of cancer 32.6 (1983): 657-665.

12) Kikuchi, Yoshihiro, et al. "Effects of cimetidine on tumor growth and immune function in nude mice bearing human ovarian carcinoma." Journal of the National Cancer Institute 74.2 (1985): 495-498.

13) Gifford, R. R., Bruce V. Voss, and Ronald M. Ferguson. "Cimetidine protection against lethal tumor challenge in mice." Surgery 90.2 (1981): 344-351.

14) Gifford, RobertR M., RonaldM Ferguson, and BruceV Voss. "Cimetidine reduction of tumour formation in mice." The Lancet 317.8221 (1981): 638-640.

15) Jafarzadeh, Abdollah, et al. "Immunomodulatory properties of cimetidine: Its therapeutic potentials for

treatment of immune-related diseases." International immunopharmacology 70 (2019): 156-166.

16) Takahashi, Hideo Kohka, et al. "Cimetidine induces interleukin-18 production through H2-agonist activity in monocytes." Molecular pharmacology 70.2 (2006): 450-453.

17) Robertson, Michael J., et al. "A dose-escalation study of recombinant human interleukin-18 in combination with rituximab in patients with non-Hodgkin's lymphoma." Journal of immunotherapy 36.6 (2013): 331.

18) Chmielewski, Markus, and Hinrich Abken. "TRUCKs with IL-18 payload: Toward shaping the immune landscape for a more efficacious CAR T-cell therapy of solid cancer." Advances in Cell and Gene Therapy 1.1 (2018): e7.

19) Kunert, Andre, et al. "Intra-tumoral production of IL18, but not IL12, by TCR-engineered T cells is non-toxic and counteracts immune evasion of solid tumors." Oncoimmunology 7.1 (2018): e1378842.

20) Hu, Biliang, et al. "Augmentation of antitumor immunity by human and mouse CAR T cells secreting IL-18." Cell reports 20.13 (2017): 3025-3033.

21) Senju, Hiroaki, et al. "Effect of IL-18 on the Expansion and Phenotype of Human Natural Killer Cells: Application to Cancer Immunotherapy." International journal of biological sciences 14.3 (2018): 331.

22) Song, Yuan, et al. "IL-12/IL-18-preactivated donor NK cells enhance GVL effects and mitigate GvHD after allogeneic hematopoietic stem cell transplantation." European journal of immunology 48.4 (2018): 670-682.

23) Esmailbeig, Maryam, and Abbas Ghaderi. "Interleukin-18: a regulator of cancer and autoimmune diseases." European cytokine network 28.4 (2017): 127-140.

24) Pantziarka, Pan, et al. "Repurposing drugs in oncology (ReDO)—cimetidine as an anti-cancer agent." (2014).

25) Kubecova, Martina, et al. "Cimetidine: An anticancer drug?" European Journal of Pharmaceutical Sciences 42.5 (2011): 439-444.

26) Lefranc, Florence, et al. "Cimetidine, an unexpected anti-tumor agent, and its potential for the treatment of glioblastoma." International journal of oncology 28.5 (2006): 1021-1030.

27) Das, Bibhuti, et al. "Cimetidine: a safe treatment option for cutaneous warts in pediatric heart transplant recipients." Medical Sciences 6.2 (2018): 30.

28) Mitsuishi, Tsuyoshi, I. I. D. A. Kazumi, and Seiji Kawana. "Cimetidine treatment for viral warts enhances IL-2 and IFN-γ expression but not IL-18 expression in lesional skin." European Journal of Dermatology 13.5 (2003): 445-448.

29) Kapińska-Mrowiecka, M., and G. Turowski. "Efficacy of cimetidine in treatment of Herpes zoster in the first 5 days from the moment of disease manifestation." Polski tygodnik lekarski 51.23-26 (1996): 338-339.

30) Komlos, Luise, et al. "In vitro cell-mediated immune reactions in herpes zoster patients treated with cimetidine." Asian Pacific journal of allergy and immunology 12 (1994): 51-51.

31) Miller, Ariel, et al. "Cimetidine as an immunomodulator in the treatment of herpes zoster." Journal of neuroimmunology 22.1 (1989): 69-76.

32) Levy, D. W., A. K. Banerjee, and Helen P. Glenny. "Cimetidine in the treatment of herpes zoster." Journal of the Royal College of Physicians of London 19.2 (1985): 96.

33) Hayne, S. T., and J. B. Mercer. "Herpes zoster: treatment with cimetidine." Canadian Medical Association Journal 129.12 (1983): 1284.

34) Cohen, Philip R., and Razelle Kurzrock. "Herpes simplex virus infections and cimetidine therapy." Journal of the American Academy of Dermatology 19.4 (1988): 762-763.

35) Kurzrock, R., M. Auber, and G. M. Mavligit. "Cimetidine therapy of herpes simplex virus infections in immunocompromised patients." Clinical and experimental dermatology 12.5 (1987): 326-331.

36) Levy, D. W., and W. Levin. "Cimetidine in the treatment of herpes virus infections." South African medical journal 58.3 (1980): 112-116.

37) Wakefield, Denis. "Cimetidine in recurrent genital herpes simplex infection." Annals of internal medicine 101.6 (1984): 882-882.

38) Bekhti, A., and J. Pirotte. "Cimetidine increases serum mebendazole concentrations. Implications for treatment of hepatic hydatid cysts." British journal of clinical pharmacology 24.3 (1987): 390-392.

39) Thilagarajah, R., R. O'N. Witherow, and M. M. Walker. "Oral cimetidine gives effective symptom relief in painful bladder disease: a prospective, randomized, double-blind placebo-controlled trial." BJU international 87.3 (2001): 207-212.

40) Seshadri, Pieter, Laurel Emerson, and Alvaro Morales. "Cimetidine in the treatment of interstitial cystitis." Urology 44.4 (1994): 614-616.

41) Dasgupta, P., et al. "Cimetidine in painful bladder syndrome: a histopathological study." BJU international 88.3 (2001): 183-186.

42) Richter, Joel E., et al. "Cimetidine and hematologic suppression." Digestive diseases and sciences 25.12 (1980): 960-963.

43) Carloss, Harry W., et. Al. "Cimetidine-Induced Granulocytopenia." Annals of internal medicine 93.1 (1980): 57-58.

44) Aymard, Jean-Pierre, et al. "Haematological adverse effects of histamine H 2-receptor antagonists." Medical toxicology and adverse drug experience 3.6 (1988): 430-448.

Chapter 29

AHCC (Beta Glucans) Immune Strategies

IN THIS CHAPTER, WE DISCUSS a number of strategies to enhance the immune system, restoring the anti-cancer immunity we all naturally possess. As mentioned in previous chapters, cancer stem cells have the ability to evade immune surveillance, hijacking immune suppressive pathways pre-existing in our cell physiology. This is not surprising, as illustrated in the following two examples.

Maternal-Fetal Tolerance

The first example was discussed in chapter 25 on cancer as a trophoblastic disease. In order for a pregnancy to proceed, the trophoblast must disable the mother's immune system. Otherwise, the developing embryo, which is 50% genetically different from the mother, would be rejected, much like a rejected organ transplant. (1–2)

We discussed PIBF, which helps to "switch off" the mother's immune system. Perhaps increased number of T-reg cells (regulatory T cells) play a role in the immune tolerance of pregnancy. In 2020, Dr. Nada R. Al-Khunaizi et al. lament that the exact mechanism of "maternal-fetal tolerance" is still a mystery to medical science, writing:

> Fetal antigens are allogeneic [foreign] to the mother's immune system and should theoretically elicit an immune response. The fact that this does not occur and that

the fetus thrives for so long in the mother without undergoing rejection by her immune system is a scientific mystery. (3)

How Our Bodies Prevent Auto-Immune Disease

The second illustrative example is our current state of knowledge concerning auto-immune disease and why healthy people's immune systems do not attack their own bodies. This process, called "self-tolerance," is thought to be controlled by a subset of T lymphocytes called T-reg cells (regulatory T cells), and the balance between suppressor regulatory T-reg cells and T-helper (Th17) cells.(3–6) Our bodies already have pre-existing pathways and mechanisms for "turning off" the immune system, all of which can be hijacked by the opportunistic cancer cell, virus, or parasite. (7)

Cancer Stem Cell Crosstalk with T-Regulatory Cells

In 2019, Dr. A. Dutta et al. achieved a new insight in the mechanism of how cancer cells evade immune surveillance. Dr. Dutta studied breast cancer stem cells and breast tumor tissues, finding that the breast cancer stem cells actually generated their own immunosuppressive T-reg cells. This was done by secretion of exosomes (small vesicles related to macropinocytosis) into the micro-environment. The exosomes contain the FOXP3 protein, which binds to a receptor on the T cell, which then converts the T cell into an immunosuppressive T-reg cell. Thus, Dr. Dutta and colleagues linked together immune evasion of cancer stem cells to the lysosmal/autophagy pathway.

Note: T cells are thymus-derived lymphocytes, associated with cell-mediated immunity. B cells are bone-marrow-derived lymphocytes associated with antibody mediated immunity.

Dr. Dutta et al. write:

Collectively our data demonstrates that bCSC [breast cancer stem cell]-shed exosomal FOXP3 [protein] plays an important role in procreation of T-reg cells within the tumor micro-environment thus leading to tumor-induced immune suppression. (8–9)

Indeed, autophagy is the common pathway for endo/exosomal vesicular trafficking, which provides the cancer cell with the ability to secrete various proteins, enzymes and bioactive substances to achieve an immunosuppressive micro-environment. (10–12)

One might speculate that inhibiting the release of these exosomes and autophagosomes from the cancer cell would play a role in reducing the numbers of suppressive T-reg cells and restore anti-tumor immunity in the micro-environment. This can be done with various autophagy/lysosomal agents discussed in this book, such as mefloquine, chloroquine, hydroxychloroquine, loratadine, thymoquinone, PPI inhibitors etc. See the chapters 31-35 on autophagy inhibitors for more on this topic.

Autophagy Inhibitors Target Regulatory T Cells

In 2018, Dr. Elise Jacquin and Lionel Apetoh studied the role of autophagy inhibition in restoring anti-tumor immunity in the micro-environment, suggesting use of the autophagy inhibitor hydroxychloroquine to "restrain T-reg functions," which then may enhance checkpoint inhibitor immunotherapy. They write:

The role for autophagy inhibition in **restraining T-reg cell functions** and promoting TH9 cell differentiation evidenced in recent studies opens new therapeutic perspectives regarding the combination of autophagy inhibitors with anti-cancer immunotherapies [checkpoint inhibitors]. Recent cancer clinical trials have suggested that the clinically approved autophagy inhibitor **hydroxychloroquine** may be considered for cancer therapy … (13–14)

Cancer Stem Cells, Immune Evasion, Wnt Pathway

Recent studies, in 2019 and 2020, by Drs. Amol Suryawanshi, M. Feng et al. reveal a link between the Wnt pathway (a cancer stem cell pathway), and T-reg cells. Inhibiting the Wnt pathway serves to downregulate the T-reg cells and enhances immunotherapy with checkpoint inhibitors. (15–16)

In earlier chapter 10 on nontoxic natural substances to eradicate cancer stem cells, we discussed a number of agents to inhibit cancer stem cells via the Wnt pathway. As it turns out, these also regulate the "immunosuppressive tumor micro-environment." A few are resveratrol (pterostilbene), curcumin, EGCG (from green tea) and quercetin. (17–19)

As mentioned previously, OXPHOS inhibitors are also Wnt pathway inhibitors and cancer stem cell agents. So, in the above discussion, we have connected the inhibition of two metabolic pathways, OXPHOS and Autophagy, as beneficial for the reduction of T-reg cells and for restoring anti-cancer immunity. I might remind the reader that microtubule agents such as mebendazole are also enormously useful for restoring anti-cancer immunity, as discussed in chapter 24.

Beta Glucans for Immune Stimulation

In addition to the over-the-counter drug cimetidine, another useful anti-cancer strategy involves upregulating the immune system with dietary beta glucans, a group of plant polysaccharides (sugars) found in edible mushrooms, baker's yeast, and cereals in the diet since ancient times. Mushrooms used for beta glucan extraction include reishi, maitake, and shiitake.

Note: The chemical name of Beta glucans is: (1–3) (1–6) beta-d-glucans.

Beta Glucans are PAMPs

Although the exact mechanism is still in dispute, one popular theory is that beta glucans represent pathogen associated molecular patterns (PAMPs). These are molecules in the cell wall of pathogenic yeasts and bacteria that "strongly contribute to microorganism recognition and clearance." In other words, the beta glucans have molecular structures that "mimic" pathogenic organisms recognized by our immune system, which then stimulate an immune response. Remember the discussion of

Coley's toxins in the previous chapter 27? Since the FDA has rendered Coley's toxins unavailable, beta glucans may serve the same purpose of stimulating the immune system to reject the cancer cells.

In 2020, Dr. Manuela Del Cornò, Sandra Gessani, and Lucia Conti studied the role of beta glucans in controlling cancer, writing:

> In vitro studies have shown that Beta-Glucans from yeasts, mushrooms or cereals are able to enhance the responsiveness or function of human primary immune cells, eliciting potent immune responses ... the immune stimulating effects of Beta Glucans can be elicited in a wide variety of species, including earthworms, insects, shrimp, birds, mammals and humans. (19–24)

AHCC Active Hexose Correlate Compound

AHCC, containing both beta and alpha glucans, is a widely used food supplement in Japan and China originally formulated in 1989 by Amino Up Chemical Co., Ltd., and Dr. Toshihiko Okamoto, School of Pharmaceutical Sciences, University of Tokyo. (25–26)

AHCC Enhances Tumor Immune Surveillance

In 2006, Dr. Yunfei Gao studied AHCC (alpha and beta glucans) in a mouse xenograft model of melanoma and lymphoma, finding delayed tumor development associated with activation of increased anti-tumor immune cells, CD4 and CD8 T Cells, and natural killer (NK cells, writing:

AHCC [Active Hexose Correlate Compound Beta Glucan] can **enhance tumor immune surveillance** through regulating both innate and adaptive immune responses. (33)

Case Report: Dramatic Response to AHCC in Prostate Cancer

In 2009, Dr. Jeffrey Turner published a case report of a 66-year-old male with castration-resistant prostate cancer (CR-PC). The patient initially presented to the hospital with a two-month history of left hip pain and 12-pound weight loss. MRI imaging showed blastic metastatic disease of the lumbar spine. (Blastic means the lesions are "white" on X-ray and CAT scan, meaning dense calcified lesions typical for prostate cancer).

The initial PSA was quite elevated at 2,000. (Normal is less than 4.0) Biopsy showed prostate cancer and treatment with androgen blockade with leuprolide and bicalutamide produced an initial decline in PSA to 993 ng/ml/, and 4 months later further declined to 2.5 (normal). Unfortunately, the remission was temporary, with gradually increasing PSA reaching 30.0 about 8 months later. About 10 months later, androgen blockade had been withdrawn, and the PSA had risen to 69.3. About this time, after withdrawal of all medical treatment, the patient began self-treatment with AHCC mushroom supplement, and the PSA after one month on the mushroom extract had dropped to 3.34 and later to 1.5 ng/ml. The patient's metastatic bone disease remained stable on repeat imaging, and ambulation improved with alleviation of bone pain. (35)

Benefits of Beta Glucans as listed by Dr. Del Cornò in 2020: (19)

- Reduces allergy symptoms
- Safe with lack of toxicity in Phase II clinical trials
- Attenuates chemotherapy-induced leukopenia
- Decreases myeloid-derived suppressor cells (MDSC)
- Reduces chemotherapy-associated side effects on loss of appetite, alopecia, fatigue
- Stimulates hematopoiesis
- Useful as adjunct with checkpoint inhibitor immunotherapy or conventional chemotherapy
- Increases natural killer (NK) cell activity
- Simulates both cellular and humoral immunity
- Promotes T-helper response (TH17)

Beta glucans benefits in various cancer cell lines:

- Breast cancer, stem cells (27–28)
- AML (acute myeloid leukemia) (29)
- Hepatoma (30–32)
- Lymphoma (33)
- Melanoma (33–34)
- Prostate cancer (35)
- Pancreatic cancer, synergy with gemcitabine (36–37)
- Ovarian cancer on chemotherapy (38)
- Non-small-cell lung cancer (40)
- Gastric and colon cancer (41–42)
- Ovarian and peritoneal cancer with platinum chemo (45)

- Alleviation of toxicity of chemotherapy (43–50)

Combinations of AHCC and Wasabi in Breast and Pancreatic Cell Lines— Clinical Trial Under Way (51)

Note: Wasabi= allyl isothiocyanate (6-HITC), found in mustard, horseradish, and wasabi.

A clinical trial is under way evaluating the combination of beta glucans with checkpoint inhibitor drugs in melanoma or triple-negative breast cancer patients. (Clinical Trial NCT02981303, completion date, Nov 2021). (52)

Combining Beta Glucans with Adoptive T Cell Therapies

In 2018, Dr. Priscilla de Graff et al. proposed using beta glucans derived from bacteria, fungi, yeast, and cereal in combination with adoptive T Cell therapies. Such therapies include:

- Infusion of autologous tumor-specific T cells
- Infusion of CAR T cells (genetically engineered T cells)
- Infusion of immune checkpoint inhibitor antibodies

Dr. de Graff et al. write:

> When tested in mouse cancer models, β-glucans result in better control of tumor growth and shift the TME [tumor micro-environment] toward a T cell-sensitive environment. Along these lines, we advocate that intake of β-glucans provides an accessible and immune-potentiating adjuvant when combined with adoptive T cell treatments of cancer. (53–54)

Beta Glucans Inhibits STAT3 Signaling

In 2018, Dr. Jin Young Choi et al. studied AHCC in an ovarian cancer cell model, finding reduced viability of cancer cells through inhibition of STAT3 signaling. As we will see below, inhibition of STAT3 signaling is an enormously useful anti-cancer target. Dr. Choi and colleagues write:

> AHCC treatment … suppressed the expression of cyclin D1, Bcl-2, Mcl-1, survivin, and VEGF, which are STAT3-regulated gene products that are associated with cell proliferation or apoptosis. These results suggest that AHCC has an antiproliferative effect on ovarian cancer cell lines, **via STAT3 phosphorylation.** (38)

Note: STAT3 = signal transducer and activator of transcription 3.

What is STAT3?

In 2018, Dr. Yu Wang et al. reviewed the role of STAT3 in tumor progression, explaining the dual role of STAT3, both triggering oncogene expression in the cancer cells as well as promoting immunosuppression in the micro-environment. In cancer progression, STAT3 is activated both in the cancer cells as well the immune cells (T lymphocytes), creating immunosuppressive effects in the micro-environment. Dr. Wang et al. write:

> STAT3 is activated both in tumor cells and tumor-infiltrated immune cells. Activated STAT3 persistently triggers tumor progression through direct regulation of oncogenic gene expression. Apart from its oncogenic role in regulating gene expression in tumor cells, STAT3 also paves the way for human

cancer growth through immunosuppression. Activated STAT3 in immune cells results in inhibition of immune mediators and promotion of immunosuppressive factors. Therefore, STAT3 modulates the interaction between tumor cells and host immunity. Accumulating evidence suggests that targeting STAT3 may enhance anti-cancer immune responses and rescue the suppressed immunologic micro-environment in tumors. Taken together, STAT3 has emerged as a promising target in cancer immunotherapy. (39)

Beta Glucans for Eradication of HPV and Prevention of Cervical Cancer

Human papilloma virus (HPV) is a common, sexually transmitted disease that causes dysplastic changes in the female cervix, considered to be precancerous lesions, due to the E6 oncoprotein. HPV-16 and 18 are considered "high risk" strains. Ninety percent of HPV infections are cleared by the patient's immune system. However, due to the virus's ability to downregulate the host immune system, HPV cervical infection may persist on serial PAP smears, which may ultimately clear in most cases or, unfortunately in a minority of cases, progress from dysplasia to cervical cancer over a number of years. Conventional gynecology treatments involve cone biopsy, loop curettage, and laser ablation of the cervical epithelium. Beta glucans can play a role here in upregulating the immune system, allowing the invigorated immune system to clear the HPV infection. Combination use of beta glucans with pterostilbene and curcumin may provide more robust efficacy. (55–64)

Beta Glucans in Athletes and Healthy Adults

A number of studies using athletes and healthy adults confirmed the safety and efficacy of beta glucans as a "functional food." Typically, studies show upregulation of the circulating NK immune cells compared to the placebo treated group, and promotion of T-helper response (TH17). (65–69)

Similar enhancement of NK-cell activity was found in cancer patients and aged mice. (70–73)

Beta Glucans Antiviral Effects

A number of studies challenging mice with a lethal dose of influenza virus found beta glucans to dramatically reduce mortality via upregulation of the immune system. Efficacy against other viruses such as West Nile and Herpes Simplex was also found. (74–77)

Drs. Shoko Nogusa et al. (2009) write:

dietary glucan can significantly reduce the effects of influenza infection. Lower mortality and overall effects of infection are most probably affected by stimulation of both cellular and humoral responses leading to the lower viral load in many organs. These results suggest that consumption of dietary glucan might be potentially useful as a complementary or alternative approach to treatment of influenza infection. (74)

Beta Glucans for Lyme Disease

Lyme disease, affecting an estimated 300,000 people in the U.S. annually, is a parasitic spirochete (Borrelia burgdorferi) transmitted by ticks. The disease is prevalent in the Northeast United States and commonly treated with antibiotics such as doxycycline, with poor results. Due to the stealth nature of the organism, which can hide intracellularly and evade the immune system, persistent disease is common after antibiotic treatment. "Lyme post-treatment syndrome" may be associated with fatigue, flu-like symptoms, headache, arthritis, myocarditis, neurologic changes, facial palsies, etc.

AHCC for Lyme Study

In 2019, Dr. John Salerno of New York studied the effect of beta glucans (AHCC) in 12 patients with Lyme disease, finding resolution or improvement in flu-like symptoms and other manifestations of the disease. Patients were treated with 3 grams of AHCC daily for 8 weeks. All patients reported improvement in one or more symptoms of Lyme disease and laboratory studies showed reduction in inflammatory markers, sedimentation rate, and interleukin 8 (IL-8) inflammatory cytokine.

Dr. John Salerno et al. speculate that post-treatment Lyme disease syndrome (PLDS) is caused by a dysfunctional immune system, a "post-infectious auto-immune response." In this scenario, prolonged treatment with conventional antibiotics is fruitless, and efforts should be directed toward restoring functionality of the immune system. Other studies have found long-term persistence of the Lyme organism in various body tissues within antibiotic resistance biofilms that provoke an inflammatory response. (78–82)

Integrative Protocol for the Lyme Patient

In 2011, Dr. Barbara Siminovich-Blok and Michelle Hessberger proposed a complementary/integrative protocol for the Lyme patients to complement conventional antibiotics and hopefully prevent chronic disease. This protocol includes immune modulation with beta glucans among a long list of other agents. (83)

Cimetidine for Lyme Disease

Like beta glucans, cimetidine is another agent with immunomodulatory effects. In 2019, Dr. Justin Shemenski proposed the addition of cimetidine to conventional antibiotics for initial treatment of Lyme disease to obtain better results and prevent post-treatment chronic Lyme disease, writing:

> The author proposes a novel theory that CIM [cimetidine] therapy during early Bb [Borrelia burgdorferi] infection may promote a more appropriate immune response and increase the utility of antibiotic therapy during early stage Lyme disease, thus improving clinical outcomes of the disease. (84)

See chapter 28 on cimetidine as an immunomodulating agent for more on this topic.

Repurposing Statin Drugs as Anti-Microbials

In 2016, Dr. Tricia Van Laar et al. suggested repurposing statin drugs as anti-microbials, observing that statin drugs inhibit the mevalonate pathway that is present in the Lyme (B. burgdorferi) organism, showing efficacy in a mouse model of Lyme disease. (85–86)

Case Report: Beta Glucans for Cholangiocarcinoma

A 59-year-old female presented to the hospital with obstructive jaundice from cancer of the bile ducts (cholangiocarcinoma). In spite of initial treatment with radiation and chemotherapy (gemcitabin+ cisplatin), the patient quickly developed metastatic disease of lung, liver, and brain. The tumor was found to possess a BRAF mutation, indicating sensitivity to mitogen-activated extracellular signal regulation kinase (MEK) inhibitors. Using this information, the patient was then started on new treatment with a MEK inhibitor (trametinib) and a BRAF inhibitor (dabrafenib) as well as a beta glucan in the form of BioBran/ MGN-3, rice bran arabinoxylan concentrate, 3 grams a day for four months. This combination treatment resulted in rapid remission in metastatic disease and a dramatic drop in cancer markers CEA and CA19–9. This case illustrates the basic premise of this book, that combination therapies are the most powerful and most likely to succeed.

> a combination of protein kinase signaling pathway inhibitors [Tyrosine Kinase Inhibitors] and natural immunomodulators [Beta Glucans] may open new perspectives in the tumor therapy. This case report may support this hypothesis ... Pathogenic Associated Molecular Pattern molecules [PAMPs such as Beta Glucans] are the best candidates for this combination of targeting therapy with immunomodulation.... the best evidence based and standardized immunodulators without any side effects are ... food supplements. (87–88)

Like other beta glucan products, rice bran arabinoxylan concentrate studies show upregulation of NK-cell activity and enhancement of cytotoxic CD8+ T cells without adverse side effects. (89–96)

Case Report: Beta Glucans for Glioblastoma

In 2016, Dr. John Berg declared a "paradigm shift" in glioblastoma treatment, proposing a combination of repurposed drugs and supplements. This includes both cimetidine and beta glucans, two of the immunomodulatory agents we have already discussed. Also included in his drug cocktail is fenofibrate, discussed in chapter 37. (98)

As you have surmised by now, I am in agreement with Dr. Berg's opinion that a combination of targeted repurposed drugs is the key to a successful outcome. This approach was advocated by Ben Williams, who describes how he survived glioblastoma using repurposed drugs in his 2002 book, *Surviving Terminal Cancer*. (97)

Conclusion

Earlier in this book, we discussed inducing cancer cell apoptosis by inhibiting the "three pillars of cancer cell metabolism," OXPHOS, GLYCOLYSIS and Autophagy. The fourth pillar, restoration of the immune system, is of equal if not greater importance. This can be accomplished with the combined use of cimetidine and beta glucans as suggested by Dr. Berg. In the next chapter, we will discuss additional immune enhancing strategies. (97–98)

References for Chapter 29:
AHCC Immune Strategies

1) Cadili, Ali. "Why the mother's immune system does not reject her fetus." Archives of Medical Science 4.3 (2008): 229.

2) Liu, Jia, et al. "Human placental trophoblast cells contribute to maternal–fetal tolerance through expressing IL-35 and mediating iT R 35 conversion." Nature communications 10.1 (2019): 1-10.

3) Al-Khunaizi, Nada R., Khaled S. Tabbara, and Eman M. Farid. "Is there a Role for HLA-G in the Induction of Regulatory T cells during the Maintenance of a Healthy Pregnancy?." American Journal of Reproductive Immunology (2020): e13259.

4) Alissafi, Themis, et al. "Tregs restrain dendritic cell autophagy to ameliorate autoimmunity." The Journal of clinical investigation 127.7 (2017): 2789-2804.

5) Göschl, Lisa, Clemens Scheinecker, and Michael Bonelli. "Treg cells in autoimmunity: from identification to Treg-based therapies." Seminars in Immunopathology. Vol. 41. No. 3. Springer Berlin Heidelberg, 2019.

6) Knochelmann, Hannah M., et al. "When worlds collide: Th17 and Treg cells in cancer and autoimmunity." Cellular & molecular immunology 15.5 (2018): 458-469.

7) Joosten, Simone A., and Tom HM Ottenhoff. "Human CD4 and CD8 regulatory T cells in infectious diseases and vaccination." Human immunology 69.11 (2008): 760-770.

8) Dutta, A., et al. "338P A new insight into tumour immune-evasion: Crosstalk between cancer stem cells and T regulatory cells." Annals of Oncology 30.Supplement_9 (2019): mdz438-020.

9) Wee, Ian, et al. "Role of tumor-derived exosomes in cancer metastasis." Biochimica et Biophysica Acta (BBA)-Reviews on Cancer 1871.1 (2019): 12-19.

10) Papandreou, Margarita-Elena, and Nektarios Tavernarakis. "Autophagy and the endo/exosomal pathways in health and disease." Biotechnology journal 12.1 (2017): 1600175.

11) Wen, Zhi-Fa, et al. "Tumor cell-released autophagosomes (TRAPs) promote immunosuppression through induction of M2-like macrophages with increased expression of PD-L1." Journal for immunotherapy of cancer 6.1 (2018): 1-16.

12) Chen, Yong-Qiang, et al. "Tumor-released autophagosomes induces CD4+ T cell-mediated immunosuppression via a TLR2–IL-6 cascade." Journal for immunotherapy of cancer 7.1 (2019): 178.

13) Jacquin, Elise, and Lionel Apetoh. "Cell-intrinsic roles for autophagy in modulating CD4 T cell functions." Frontiers in immunology 9 (2018): 1023.

14) Schabowsky, Rich-Henry, et al. "Targeting CD4+ CD25+ FoxP3+ regulatory T-cells for the augmentation of cancer immunotherapy." Current opinion in investigational drugs (London, England: 2000) 8.12 (2007): 1002-1008.

15) Suryawanshi, Amol, et al. "Wnt signaling cascade in dendritic cells and regulation of anti-tumor immunity." Frontiers in immunology 11 (2020).

16) Feng, M., et al. "Pharmacological inhibition of β-catenin/BCL9 interaction overcomes resistance to immune checkpoint blockades by modulating Treg cells." Science advances 5.5 (2019): eaau5240.

17) Wang, Yizhi, et al. "The roles of curcumin in regulating the tumor immunosuppressive microenvironment." Oncology Letters 19.4 (2020): 3059.

18) Moody, Rhiane, et al. "Natural Compounds with Potential to Modulate Cancer Therapies and Self-Reactive Immune Cells." Cancers 12.3 (2020): 673.

19) Del Cornò, Manuela, Sandra Gessani, and Lucia Conti. "Shaping the Innate Immune Response by Dietary Glucans: Any Role in the Control of Cancer?." Cancers 12.1 (2020): 155.

20) Vetvicka, V., and J. Vetvickova. "β-Glucan–Is the Current Research Relevant." Int Clin Pathol J 4.2 (2017): 00089.

21) Vetvicka, Vaclav, and Jana Vetvickova. "Immune-enhancing effects of Maitake (Grifola frondosa) and Shiitake (Lentinula edodes) extracts." Annals of translational medicine 2.2 (2014).

22) Vetvicka, Vaclav, and Jana Vetvickova. "Comparison of immunological effects of commercially available β-glucans." Appl Sci Rep 1.2 (2014): 1-7.

23) Vetvicka, V., and J. Vetvickova. "Comparison of immunological effects of commercially available β-glucans: Part III." Int. Clin. Pathol. J 2.4 (2016): 78-83.

24) Vetvicka, Vaclav, et al. "Beta glucan: Supplement or drug? From laboratory to clinical trials." Molecules 24.7 (2019): 1251.

25) Nishizawa, Takashi, Koji Wakame, and Hiroshi Okawa. "αGlucan (AHCC Compound Liquid derived from Basidiomycetes) Contributes to Macrophage Activation More than βGlucan."

26) Ulbricht, Catherine, et al. "An evidence-based systematic review of active hexose correlated compound (AHCC) by the Natural Standard Research Collaboration." Journal of dietary supplements 10.3 (2013): 264-308.

27) Graham, Émilie A., et al. "MicroRNA signature in the chemoprevention of functionally-enriched stem and progenitor pools (FESPP) by active hexose correlated compound (AHCC)." Cancer biology & therapy 18.10 (2017): 765-774.

28) Matsushita, Kazuhiro, et al. "Combination therapy of active hexose correlated compound plus UFT significantly reduces the metastasis of rat mammary adenocarcinoma." Anti-cancer drugs 9.4 (1998): 343-350.

29) Fatehchand, Kavin, et al. "Active hexose-correlated compound enhances extrinsic-pathway-mediated apoptosis of Acute Myeloid Leukemic cells." PloS one 12.7 (2017).

30) Matsui, Yoichi, et al. "Improved prognosis of postoperative hepatocellular carcinoma patients when treated with functional foods: a prospective cohort study." Journal of Hepatology 37.1 (2002): 78-86.

31) Cowawintaweewat, Suwanna, et al. "Prognostic improvement of patients with advanced liver cancer after active hexose correlated compound (AHCC) treatment." Asian Pacific journal of allergy and immunology 24.1 (2006): 33.

32) Cao, Zhiyun, et al. "Active hexose correlated compound potentiates the antitumor effects of low-dose 5-fluorouracil through modulation of immune function in hepatoma 22 tumor-bearing mice." Nutrition research and practice 9.2 (2015): 129-136.

33) Gao, Yunfei, et al. "Active hexose correlated compound enhances tumor surveillance through regulating both innate and adaptive immune responses." Cancer Immunology, Immunotherapy 55.10 (2006): 1258-1266.

34) Ignacio, Rosa Mistica, et al. "Therapeutic effect of Active Hexose-Correlated Compound (AHCC) combined with CpG-ODN (oligodeoxynucleotide) in B16 melanoma murine model." Cytokine 76.2 (2015): 131-137.

35) Turner, Jeffrey, and Uzair Chaudhary. "Dramatic prostate-specific antigen response with activated hemicellulose compound in metastatic castration-resistant prostate cancer." Anti-cancer drugs 20.3 (2009): 215-216.

36) Suenaga, Shigeyuki, et al. "Active hexose-correlated compound down-regulates HSP27 of pancreatic cancer cells, and helps the cytotoxic effect of gemcitabine." Anticancer research 34.1 (2014): 141-146.

37) Tokunaga, Masayuki, et al. "Active hexose-correlated compound down-regulates heat shock factor 1, a transcription factor for HSP27, in gemcitabine-resistant human pancreatic cancer cells." Anticancer research 35.11 (2015): 6063-6067.

38) Choi, Jin Young, et al. "Active hexose correlated compound (AHCC) inhibits the proliferation of ovarian cancer cells by suppressing signal transducer and activator of transcription 3 (STAT3) activation." Nutrition and cancer 70.1 (2018): 109-115.

39) Wang, Yu, et al. "The role of STAT3 in leading the crosstalk between human cancers and the immune system." Cancer letters 415 (2018): 117-128.

40) Ishizuka, Reiki, et al. "Personalized cancer therapy for stage IV non-small cell lung cancer: combined use of active hexose correlated compound and genistein concentrated polysaccharide." Personalized Medicine Universe 1.1 (2012): 39-44.

41) Kawaguchi, Yusai. "Improved survival of patients with gastric cancer or colon cancer when treated with active hexose correlated compound (AHCC): effect of AHCC on digestive system cancer." Nat Med J 1.1 (2009): 1-6.

42) Hazama, Shoichi, et al. "Efficacy of orally administered superfine dispersed lentinan (β-1, 3-glucan) for the treatment of advanced colorectal cancer." Anticancer Research 29.7 (2009): 2611-2617.

43) Sun, Buxiang, et al. "The effect of active hexose correlated compound in modulating cytosine arabinoside-induced hair loss, and 6-mercaptopurine-and methotrexate-induced liver injury in rodents." Cancer epidemiology 33.3-4 (2009): 293-299.

44) Ito, Toshinori, et al. "Reduction of adverse effects by a mushroom product, active hexose correlated compound (AHCC) in patients with advanced cancer during chemotherapy—the significance of the levels of HHV-6 DNA in saliva as a surrogate biomarker during chemotherapy." Nutrition and cancer 66.3 (2014): 377-382.

45) Suknikhom, Wineeya, Ruangsak Lertkhachonsuk, and Tarinee Manchana. "The effects of Active Hexose Correlated Compound (AHCC) on levels of CD4+ and CD8+ in patients with epithelial ovarian cancer or peritoneal cancer receiving platinum based chemotherapy." Asian Pacific journal of cancer prevention: APJCP 18.3 (2017): 633.

46) deleted

47) Shigama, Kota, et al. "Alleviating effect of active hexose correlated compound (AHCC) for anticancer drug-induced side effects in non-tumor-bearing mice." Journal of experimental therapeutics & oncology 8.1 (2009).

48) Yanagimoto, Hiroaki, et al. "Alleviating effect of active hexose correlated compound (AHCC) on chemotherapy-related adverse events in patients with unresectable pancreatic ductal adenocarcinoma." Nutrition and cancer 68.2 (2016): 234-240.

49) Nakamoto, Daisuke, et al. "Active hexose correlated compound (AHCC) alleviates gemcitabine-induced hematological toxicity in non-tumor-bearing mice." International Journal of Clinical Medicine 3.05 (2012): 361.

50) Hirose, Aya, et al. "The influence of active hexose correlated compound (AHCC) on cisplatin-evoked chemotherapeutic and side effects in tumor-bearing mice." Toxicology and applied pharmacology 222.2 (2007): 152-158.

51) Corradetti, Bruna, et al. "Bioactive Immunomodulatory Compounds: A Novel Combinatorial Strategy for Integrated Medicine in Oncology? BAIC Exposure in Cancer Cells." Integrative cancer therapies 18 (2019): 1534735419866908.

52) Iglesias, Jose Luis, et al. "A multicenter, open-label, phase II study of PGG beta-glucan and pembrolizumab in patients (pts) with advanced melanoma (MEL) following progression on treatment with checkpoint inhibitors (CPI) or triple negative breast cancer (TNBC) failing front-line chemotherapy for metastatic disease." (2017): TPS3105-TPS3105.

53) de Graaff, Priscilla, et al. "Consumption of β-glucans to spice up T cell treatment of tumors: A review." Expert opinion on biological therapy 18.10 (2018): 1023-1040.

54) Houot, Roch, et al. "T-cell–based immunotherapy: adoptive cell transfer and checkpoint inhibition." Cancer immunology research 3.10 (2015): 1115-1122.

55) Song, Dan, et al. "Effect of human papillomavirus infection on the immune system and its role in the course of cervical cancer." Oncology letters 10.2 (2015): 600-606.

56) Chatterjee, Kaushiki, et al. "Dietary polyphenols, resveratrol and pterostilbene exhibit antitumor activity on an HPV E6-positive cervical cancer model An in vitro and in vivo analysis." Frontiers in oncology 9 (2019): 352.

57) Westrich, Joseph A., Cody J. Warren, and Dohun Pyeon. "Evasion of host immune defenses by human papillomavirus." Virus research 231 (2017): 21-33.

58) Piersma, Sytse J. "Immunosuppressive tumor microenvironment in cervical cancer patients." Cancer Microenvironment 4.3 (2011): 361-375.

59) Smith, Judith Ann, et al. "Phase II randomized, double-blind, placebo-controlled evaluation of ahcc for the eradication of HPV infections in women with HPV positive pap smears." Gynecologic Oncology 154 (2019): 39.

60) Smith, Judith Ann, et al. "From Bench to Bedside: Evaluation of AHCC supplementation to modulate the host immunity to eradicate high-risk human papillomavirus infections." Frontiers in Oncology 9 (2019): 173.

61) Smith, J. A., et al. "In vitro and in vivo evaluation of active hexose correlated compound (AHCC) for the eradication of HPV." Gynecologic Oncology 133 (2014): 189.

62) Smith, Judith A., et al. "Abstract B79: Evaluation of active hexose correlated compound (AHCC) for the prevention or delay of tumor growth in human cervical cancer xenograft model." (2011): B79-B79.

63) Basu, Partha, et al. "Clearance of cervical human papillomavirus infection by topical application of curcumin and curcumin containing polyherbal cream: a phase II randomized controlled study." Asian Pac J Cancer Prev 14.10 (2013): 5753-5759.

64) Mishra, Alok, and Bhudev C. Das. "Curcumin as an anti-human papillomavirus and anti-cancer compound." Future Oncology 11.18 (2015): 2487-2490.

65) Yin, Zhinan, Hajime Fujii, and Thomas Walshe. "Effects of active hexose correlated compound on frequency of CD4+ and CD8+ T cells producing interferon-γ and/or tumor necrosis factor−α in healthy adults." Human immunology 71.12 (2010): 1187-1190.

66) Mallard, Brody, et al. "Synergistic immuno-modulatory activity in human macrophages of a medicinal mushroom formulation consisting of Reishi, Shiitake and Maitake." PloS one 14.11 (2019): e0224740-e0224740.

67) Spierings, Egilius LH, et al. "A Phase I study of the safety of the nutritional supplement, active hexose correlated compound, AHCC, in healthy volunteers." Journal of nutritional science and vitaminology 53.6 (2007): 536-539.

68) Bergendiova, Katarina, Elena Tibenska, and Juraj Majtan. "Pleuran (β-glucan from Pleurotus ostreatus) supplementation, cellular immune response and respiratory tract infections in athletes." European journal of applied physiology 111.9 (2011): 2033-2040.

69) Lee, Won-Woo, et al. "Active Hexose Correlated Compound promotes T helper (Th) 17 and 1 cell responses via inducing IL-1β production from monocytes in humans." Cellular immunology 275.1-2 (2012): 19-23.

70) Ghoneum, Mamdooh, et al. "Enhancement of NK cell Activity in Cancer Patient by Active Hemicellulose Compound (AHCC)." Proceedings of the Adjuvant Nutrition in Cancer Treatment Symposium (Tulsa, OK. 1992.

71) Ghoneum, Mamdooh. "NK-immunomodulation by active hemicellulose compound AHCC in 17 cancer patients." Abstract of 2nd Meeting Society of Natural Immunity, Taormina, Italy. 1994.

72) deleted

73) Ghoneum, M., et al. "Active hemicellulose compound (AHCC) enhances NK cell activity of aged mice in vivo." FASEB J 6 (1992): A1213.

74) Nogusa, Shoko, Jeffrey Gerbino, and Barry W. Ritz. "Low-dose supplementation with active hexose correlated compound improves the immune response to acute influenza infection in C57BL/6 mice." Nutrition Research 29.2 (2009): 139-143.

75) Vetvicka, Vaclav, and Jana Vetvickova. "Glucan supplementation enhances the immune response against an influenza challenge in mice." Annals of translational medicine 3.2 (2015).

76) Wang, Shuhui, et al. "Oral administration of active hexose correlated compound enhances host resistance to West Nile encephalitis in mice." The Journal of nutrition 139.3 (2009): 598-602.

77) Urbancikova, Ingrid, et al. "Efficacy of Pleuran (β-Glucan from Pleurotus ostreatus) in the Management of Herpes Simplex Virus Type 1 Infection." Evidence-Based Complementary and Alternative Medicine 2020 (2020).

78) Salerno, John, et al. "A Pilot Open-Label Study Assessing the Effects of AHCC Supplementation on Lyme Disease Patients." Bioactive Compounds in Health and Disease 2.11 (2019): 221-229.

79) Vetvicka, Vaclav, et al. "Beta glucan: Supplement or drug? From laboratory to clinical trials." Molecules 24.7 (2019): 1251.

80) Vaclav, Vetvicka, and Vetvickova Jana. "Glucan supplementation ameliorates some health problems related to the development of Lyme disease." World Journal of Pathology 8.2 (2019).

81) Shaw, Gina. "Prolonged Antibiotics Do Not Improve Neurocognitive Outcomes in Persistent Lyme Disease." Neurology Today 19.5 (2019): 27-31.

82) Sapi, Eva, et al. "The long-term persistence of Borrelia burgdorferi antigens and DNA in the tissues of a patient with Lyme disease." Antibiotics 8.4 (2019): 183.

83) Siminovich-Blok, Barbara, and Michelle Hessberger. "Designing and Implementing a Novel CAM Protocol Using Laboratory Analysis and Supplementation to Reduce Morbidity Outcomes in the Treatment of Lyme Disease." (2011).

84) Shemenski, Justin. "Cimetidine as a novel adjunctive treatment for early stage Lyme disease." Medical hypotheses 128 (2019): 94-100.

85) Van Laar, Tricia A., et al. "Statins reduce spirochetal burden and modulate immune responses in the C3H/HeN mouse model of Lyme disease." Microbes and infection 18.6 (2016): 430-435.

86) Rana, Ritika, Ruchika Sharma, and Anoop Kumar. "Repurposing of Existing Statin Drugs for Treatment of Microbial Infections: How Much Promising?." Infectious Disorders-Drug Targets (Formerly Current Drug Targets-Infectious Disorders) 19.3 (2019): 224-237.

87) Hajto, Tibor. "Can a standardized plant immunomodulator (rice bran arabinoxylan concentrate/MGN-3) increase the effects of MEK and BRAF inhibitors with clinical benefit? Case report of a patient with carcinoma in biliary duct." Res Rew Insight 1.3 (2017): 1-4.

88) Solit, David B., et al. "BRAF mutation predicts sensitivity to MEK inhibition." Nature 439.7074 (2006): 358-362.

89) Ooi, Soo Liang, et al. "Evidence-based review of BioBran/MGN-3 arabinoxylan compound as a complementary therapy for conventional cancer treatment." Integrative cancer therapies 17.2 (2018): 165-178.

90) Ghoneum, M. "From Bench to Bedside: The Growing Use of Arabinoxylan Rice Bran (MGN-3/ImunoBran) in." Cancer Immunotherapy. Austin Immunol 1.2 (2016): 1006.

91) Elsaid, Ahmed F., Magda Shaheen, and Mamdooh Ghoneum. "Biobran/MGN-3, an arabinoxylan rice bran, enhances NK cell activity in geriatric subjects: A randomized, double-blind, placebo-controlled clinical trial." Experimental and therapeutic medicine 15.3 (2018): 2313-2320.

92) El-Din, Nariman K. Badr, et al. "Biobran/MGN-3, arabinoxylan from rice bran, sensitizes breast adenocarcinoma tumor cells to paclitaxol in mice." (2015): 5312-5312.

93) Cholujova, Dana, et al. "MGN-3 arabinoxylan rice bran modulates innate immunity in multiple myeloma patients." Cancer Immunology, Immunotherapy 62.3 (2013): 437-445.

94) Pérez-Martínez, Antonio, et al. "Arabinoxylan rice bran (MGN-3/Biobran) enhances natural killer cell–mediated cytotoxicity against neuroblastoma in vitro and in vivo." Cytotherapy 17.5 (2015): 601-612.

95) Ghoneum, Mamdooh, et al. "Arabinoxylan rice bran (MGN-3/Biobran) provides protection against whole-body γ-irradiation in mice via restoration of hematopoietic tissues." Journal of radiation Research 54.3 (2013): 419-429.

96) Ghoneum, M., and S. Agrawal. "MGN-3/Biobran enhances generation of cytotoxic CD8+ T cells via upregulation of DEC-205 expression on dendritic cells." International journal of immunopathology and pharmacology 27.4 (2014): 523-530.

97) Williams, Ben A. Surviving" Terminal" Cancer: Clinical Trials, Drug Cocktails and Other Treatments Your Oncologist Won't Tell You About. Fairview Press, 2002.

98) Berg, John. "A Paradigm Shift in Glioblastoma Treatment and Research: A Multi-mechanistic, Multi-agent Approach to Target Glioblastoma Multiforme." Journal of Advanced Medical Sciences and Applied Technologies 2.4 (2016): 323-326.

Chapter 30

Thyroid, Iodine, Vitamin D, Probiotics

Thyroid Hormone, the Immune System, and Cancer

THE GREATEST AMERICAN ENDOCRINOLOGIST, BRODA Barnes, MD (1906–1988), was an astute clinician who observed that people with hypothyroidism, a low thyroid condition, have reduced immunity to infection. (1) Unfortunately, the mainstream endocrinologists of his time rejected Dr. Barnes's teachings. Recent studies using hypothyroid mice show that Dr. Barnes was right all along.

Hypothyroid Mice Unable to Survive Infection

In 2014, Dr. Cristiana Perrotta of Milan, Italy, et al. studied the ability of hypothyroid mice to survive an infectious insult, finding that T3 thyroid hormone protected mice against gram-negative endotoxemia. The hypothyroid mice challenged with gram-negative bacteria lipopolysaccharide (LPS) had 90% mortality after 96 hours. However, when the hypothyroid mice were injected with T3 (thyroid hormone) for five days before gram-negative endotoxemia, they were now protected from death with 70 % survival. This is an impressive demonstration of the importance of thyroid hormone for boosting our immune system and protecting us from infectious disease. (2)

Stress-Induced Model of Lymphoma— Thyroid Hormone Protective

If thyroid hormone enhances our immune system and protects us from infectious disease, one might predict thyroid hormone confers a similar protection from cancer, restoring immune surveillance.

To answer this question, in 2009, Dr. Luciana Frick et al. studied a mouse model of stress-induced lymphoma model. The mice were subjected to chronic stress by restraining them in a narrow confinement tube. The chronically restrained mice exhibited impaired T-cell mediated immunity and enhanced progression of lymphoma. (3–4)

In addition, treatment of the mice with thyroid hormone (thyroxine, T4) enhanced their immune systems, reversed the impaired T cell immunity, and inhibited the lymphoma cell proliferation. Dr. Frick's group concluded:

> These results show that thyroid hormones are regulators of tumor evolution, acting through the modulation of T cell-mediated immunity affected by chronic stress.… experimental hypothyroidism leads to a general depression of the immune system. (3)

Experimental hypothyroidism leads to a "general depression of the immune system," reducing resistance to infection as well as reducing immune surveillance for cancer. (5–12)

Thyroid Hormone (T3) Potentiates Anti-Tumor Immunity

Indeed, Dr. V. A. Alamino et al. (2016) write:

> T3 thyroid hormone reinvigorates dendritic cells [immune cells] and potentiates anti-tumor immunity. (13–14)

In 2019, Dr. Eilon Krashin et al. reviewed the effect of thyroid hormones in cancer, finding that:

> hypothyroidism creates an immunosuppressive milieu that allows for immune tolerance toward metastasizing tumor cells. (15)

Thyroid as Growth Promotor for Cancer Cells

The idea of enhancing immune surveillance by giving thyroid hormone to all cancer patients is an attractive one. However, things are not so simple, as thyroid hormone can be regarded as a growth factor for the cancer cell. It seems that many cancer types have overexpressed thyroid hormone receptors which stimulate growth. Dr. Krashin's group writes:

> The thyroid hormones are increasingly acknowledged for their tumor-promoting effects..... This is highly relevant, specifically in the context of the discovery of the T4 receptor site upon the $\alpha v \beta 3$ integrin, which is overexpressed in many tumor cells. (15)

In 2019, Dr. Soeren Latteyer et al. studied the effect of thyroid hormone thyroxine (T4) in a mouse model of Lewis lung cancer, finding tumor growth slowed by hypothyroidism, and accelerated tumor growth with the addition of thyroid hormone (T4). Surprisingly, only T4, thyroxine, but not T3, promoted tumor growth, which was abrogated by blocking the T4 receptor with Tetrac.

> We conclude that T4 promotes lung cancer growth in this orthotopic mouse model.... These data suggest that such effects of levothyroxine [T4 thyroid hormone] may need to be considered in cancer patients on T4 substitution. (16)

In 2019, Dr. Yi-Ru Chen et al. found that thyroid hormone induces PD-L1 (programmed death ligand) expression in cancer cells, which inhibits tumor-specific T cells, creating an immunosuppressive environment and allowing cancer proliferation (17).

Here we have contradictory effects of thyroid hormone for the cancer patient. On the one hand, there is beneficial upregulation of the immune system. One the other hand, thyroid hormone, specifically T4, acts as cancer growth promotor and assists in creating an immunosuppressive micro-environment.

Medically Induced Hypothyroidism as Cancer Treatment

If thyroid hormone (T4) aggravates tumor growth, then perhaps inducing a hypothyroid state would be beneficial for slowing tumor growth. This is exactly what was found in 2013 by Dr. Osnat Ashur-Fabian et al., who treated a high-grade optic glioma patient with medically induced hypothyroidism with methimazole, a thyroid blocking drug, and thyroid hormone replacement with T3 (Liothyronine). This blocks T4 while providing T3. The treatment was considered beneficial with prolonged patient survival. (18)

Encouraged by Dr. Ashur-Fabian's group's success in 2015, Dr. Aleck Hercbergs et al. went on to treat 23 patients with various end-stage cancers. Only 20% were expected to survive beyond one year based on survival tables; however, 83% of patients survived beyond one year, indicating considerable benefit in prolonging survival. Dr. Hercbergs et al. write that

> compassionate medical induction of hypo-thyroxinemia should be considered for patients with advanced cancers to whom other avenues of treatment are closed. (19)

The above contradictory studies on the use of thyroid hormone in cancer patients explains the reluctance of conventional oncology to prescribe thyroid hormones to the cancer patient. Will the practice of medically induced hypothyroidism with T3 replacement be vindicated and proven effective as a cancer treatment? Or will it be relegated to the dustbin of history as just another failed experiment? Only time will tell.

Next, we look at the dietary supplement iodine for enhancement of anti-tumor immunity.

Iodine for Fibrocystic Breast Disease

As an interventional radiologist for 30 years, part of my job was to read mammograms and perform the breast biopsies and needle-aspiration procedures. Women with fibrocystic breast disease typically had multiple scattered cysts and nodules throughout the breast tissue visible on mammograms and ultrasound. Many of these women returned to the department every year for repeated ultrasound guided needle aspirations and biopsy procedures. After the procedure, they would always corner me in the reading room and ask, "Doctor, what can I do to make these cysts and nodules in my breast go away?" And, for 30 years I would throw up my hands and say, "We just don't know."

After I retired from radiology and returned to clinical medicine in 2004, I attended medical meetings and listened to David Brownstein, MD, and George Flechas, MD, speaking about the health benefits of iodine supplementation.

Iodine is the answer to fibrocystic breast disease. Iodine is the answer for breast cancer prevention. Iodine is the answer I should have been giving to all the women over the years I worked in the hospital X-ray department. But I didn't, so I am making up for it now. We routinely test for iodine level, and give iodine supplements to every woman in my clinic. I consider this extremely important. (20–22)

Iodine Deficiency and Breast Cancer

Iodine deficiency is a risk factor for breast cancer. Iodine levels in young women have been declining since the mid-1970s. Could this be the link with increasing breast cancer? Dr. Jay Rappaport says yes. In 2017, Dr. Jay Rappaport proposed a link between dietary iodine deficiency and increasing incidence of breast cancer:

> Dietary iodine insufficiency represents a plausible explanation for the increasing incidence of breast cancer in young women with distant metastasis. In view of the established reduction in iodine levels in US women of childbearing age since the mid-70s, this group would be most vulnerable to increased breast cancer risk.... iodine testing and management may be consid-

ered as a potentially important aspect for clinical practice. (23)

The Gerson Therapy Incorporated Iodine

Iodine supplementation is included in the Gerson Therapy, a diet-based anti-cancer therapy developed by Max Gerson, MD, in the early 1900s, initially devised to relieve his migraines, and later as a treatment for tuberculosis and type II diabetes.

Initally, Dr Gerson insisted his diet was not a cancer treatment. However, when a cancer patient insisted on trying his protocol, he reluctantly agreed and was pleasantly surprised to find considerable benefit. The Gerson therapy involves detoxification and immune enhancing strategies and incorporates Lugol's solution, a widely available form of iodine, as well as potassium, B vitamins, pancreatic enzymes, and coffee enemas. By the way, Dr. Max Gerson also routinely used natural desiccated thyroid in his protocol, as discussed above in the section on thyroid and the immune system. (24)

Molecular Iodine as Treatment for Breast Cancer

Dr. Gerson had no way of knowing that medical research would eventually show he was quite correct to use iodine for cancer patients. Over the years, a number of studies have accumulated evidence that molecular iodine is effective treatment for breast cancer. The mechanism of action (MOA) involves activation of peroxisome proliferator-activated receptors (PPAR) and production of iodolactones, which mediate apoptotic effects. (25–29)

Molecular Iodine Effective Form

A drop of the 2% iodine Lugol's solution contains 1 mg of molecular iodine (I2) and 2 mg of potassium iodide (I-). An iodine supplement called Iodoral® is available for people who prefer Lugol's iodine in tablet form. The tablet avoids annoying yellow stains on clothing from accidental spills of the liquid product. (30–31)

The anti-cancer effects of iodine are thought to be related to the type of iodine used, with molecular iodine (I2) and not iodide (I-) considered the effective anti-cancer agent, via increasing expression of PPAR-gamma (peroxisome proliferator-activated receptor gamma), which in turn induces cancer cell apoptosis. (33)

Activation of the PPAR nuclear receptor family requires a vitamin A cofactor such as ATRA. In 2020, Dr. Irasema Mendeita found that molecular iodine (which activates PPAR-gamma) augmented the anticancer activity of ATRA in a neuroblastoma model. Similarly, fenofibrate activates PPAR by forming a heterodimer with the retinoid X receptor (RXR). See chapter 37 on Fenofibrate for more. (32)

Clinical Study: Iodine as Adjuvant for Breast Cancer

Iodine treatment has a dual anti-cancer effect. It has a direct anti-cancer effect by inducing apoptosis of the cancer cells, and secondarily, iodine "activates the anti-tumor immune response." In 2019, Dr. Aura Morena-Vega et al. studied the use of molecular iodine in thirty breast cancer patients, either alone or as adjuvant with chemotherapy, in two groups—

early and advanced. In the early group, thirty women were treated with either 5 mg per day of molecular iodine (I2) or placebo for 7 to 35 days before surgery. For the advanced group, all patients received chemotherapy (5-fluorouracil/epirubicin/cyclophosphamide or taxotere/epirubicin (FEC/TE) and were randomized to receive either molecular iodine 5 mg/day or placebo before and 170 days after surgery. Five-year disease-free survival was significantly higher for patients treated with molecular iodine (I2) before and after surgery compared to placebo—82 per cent vs. 46 per cent. Examination of histology of tissue samples showed Iodine treated patients had "activation of the anti-tumoral immune response."

Dr. Moreno-Vega et al. write:

> I2 supplementation showed a significant attenuation of the [chemotherapy] side effects and an absence of tumor chemoresistance ... I2-treated tumors exhibit less invasive potential, and significant increases in apoptosis, estrogen receptor expression, and immune cell infiltration.... Transcriptomic analysis indicated activation of the antitumoral immune response. (34)

Iodine in Breast Cancer Animal Xenograft Studies

In 2019, further studies by Dr. Irasema Mendieta et al. using human breast cancer cell lines in vitro and in vivo animal xenografts confirm Dr. Morena's conclusions, finding that supplementation with I2 reduced the ability to implant tumor cells into immunosuppressed mice and reduced the proliferation rate and invasive capacity of the cancer cells. Various cancer markers such as CD44 and vascular endothelial growth factor (VEGF) were reduced by iodine, and PPAR-gamma was increased. In the mouse xenograft model, evidence of immune enhancement was seen with increased levels of circulating immune cells (leukocytes) and increased intra-tumor infiltration of CD8+ lymphocytes (anti-tumor lymphocytes).

Dr. Mendieta proposes iodine supplementation as a possible adjuvant in breast cancer therapy, writing:

> I2 [Iodine] decreases the invasive potential of a triple-negative basal cancer cell line, and under in vivo conditions the oral supplement of this halogen [iodine] activates the anti-tumor immune response, preventing progression of xenografts from laminal and basal mammary cancer cells. These effects allow us to propose iodine supplementation as a possible adjuvant in breast cancer therapy. (35)

Iodine for Other Cancer Cell Types

In 2016, Dr. Harald Rösner et al. studied iodine as an anti-cancer agent, finding considerable efficacy in breast cancer and seven other malignant cancer cell lines, including:

- Breast cancer, melanoma, lung cancer (35–37)
- Cervical cancer (38)
- Prostate cancer (39)
- Colon cancer (40)
- Canine mammary cancer (41)

In 2018, Dr. Xóchitl Zambrano-Estrada et al. studied canine mammary cancer using the combination of Iodine and chemotherapy, writing:

> The [combination Doxorubicin chemotherapy plus iodine] mDOX+I2 scheme

improves the therapeutic outcome, diminishes the invasive capacity, attenuates the adverse events and increases disease-free survival. These data led us to propose mDOX+I2 as an effective treatment for canine mammary cancer. (41)

Iodine Adverse Effects

Extremely large quantities of iodine are routinely prescribed in the form of SSKI for COPD (chronic obstructive lung disease) and amiodarone for cardiac arrhythmias. These are well tolerated for the most part with a few adverse events reported, such as metallic taste, headache, GI upset, and skin rash thought to be related to dermo-bromism.

Iodine is contra-indicated in a few relatively rare thyroid conditions, such as toxic multinodular goiter and autonomous thyroid nodule, in which case the administration of iodine supplements, such as iodized salt, may induce hyperthyroidism which can be fatal in some cases. These are all good reasons to be under the care of a competent health care professional who can monitor the patient during such treatment. The use of high-dose iodine supplementation during pregnancy may influence fetal thyroid function, so caution is advised. (42–48)

In addition to iodine, a typical breast cancer prevention program includes supplementation with DIM (di-indole-methane) and calcium-D-glucarate, while avoiding xeno-estrogens in food and plastics. It is also useful to test for selenium and vitamin D3 and supplement if found low. (163-165) (169)

In conclusion, molecular iodine (I2) is a useful anti-cancer agent with the dual effects of upregulating host immune surveillance and directly inducing apoptosis in cancer cells. Iodine supplements are widely available over the counter without a prescription. Because of the rare yet serious adverse side effects of iodine supplementation, it is advisable to seek the assistance of a competent health care provider for iodine testing and monitoring.

Next, we discuss vitamin D as an immune modulator and anti-cancer agent.

Vitamin D as Immune Modulator

It has been suggested that vitamin D is not really a vitamin but is actually a steroid hormone that works as an immune modulator synergistic with vitamin A to prevent auto-immune disease and cancer. Indeed, the chemical structure of vitamin D (Calcitriol) is that of a "seco-steroid," which bears a striking resemblance to the steroid ring of hormones. (49–64)

Vitamin D deficiency is a risk factor predisposing the patient to cancer and auto-immune diseases, such as multiple sclerosis. In 2016, Dr. Yingyu Ma reviewed the anti-cancer effects of vitamin D, which include

- Induction of cell cycle arrest
- Induction of apoptosis
- Induction of differentiation
- Suppression of inflammation
- Suppression of angiogenesis
- Suppression of invasion
- Suppression of metastasis
- Potentiates effects of chemotherapy

Dr. Yingyu Ma et al. write:

Preclinical studies show that 1,25D3, the active metabolite of vitamin D, and its analogs have anti-tumor effects in vitro and in vivo through multiple mechanisms including the induction of cell cycle arrest, apoptosis, differentiation and the suppression of inflammation, angiogenesis, invasion, and metastasis. 1,25D3 also potentiates the effect of chemotherapeutic agents and other agents in the combination treatment. (65)

Low Vitamin D in Cancer Patients

Unfortunately, when tested, many cancer patients are vitamin D deficient, a state commonly ignored yet easily corrected with administration of vitamin D supplements. (66–70)

Antiviral Effects of Vitamin D

The immune modulating effects of vitamin D are illustrated by its antiviral effects against herpes simplex, herpes zoster, human papilloma virus (HPV), hepatitis C virus, and respiratory viruses such as influenza, RSV, and corona virus. (71–83)

Preventing Auto-immune Disease

Vitamin D's immune modulating effects are also demonstrated by the ability of vitamin D to prevent various auto-immune diseases, such as multiple sclerosis and rheumatoid arthritis, (84–88)

Vitamin D in Combination Therapies

In 2018, Dr. Stephen Bigelsen proposed vitamin D (paricalcitol form) to upregulate cytotoxic T lymphocytes in combination with repurposed anti-cancer drugs such as hydroxychloroquine, intravenous vitamin C, statins, metformin, curcumin and aspirin for treatment of pancreatic cancer, discussed elsewhere in this book. (89–91)

Probiotics for the Cancer Patient

Once, while visiting a cancer patient on the chemotherapy ward, I had a conversation with the attending oncologist, who stepped into the room while on rounds. I nonchalantly asked him if probiotics were OK for the cancer patient to take. He deflected the question and instead suggested I ask the gastroenterologists, since this was not his area of expertise.

I didn't have the heart to point out to the oncologist that all his patients are getting a probiotic drink with every meal tray. Apparently, the dietary department had decided without consulting him that all the cancer patients should be taking probiotics. Exactly what did the dietary department know that the oncologist did not know?

The Microbiome and Anti-Cancer Immunity

As illustrated by the above story, the subject of probiotics (and the microbiome) has been largely ignored by oncologists. We all carry in our gut three to five pounds of "friendly bacteria", also called the "microbiome," containing a trillion organisms (bacteria, viruses and fungi) representing a vast amount of genetic material, 100-fold larger than the human genome. When we ingest probiotics, we are ingesting friendly bacteria that colonize our gut, and become part of our microbiome. A number of examples illustrate the importance of the microbiome for the cancer patient. (92)

Microbiome and Checkpoint Immunotherapy

The introduction of immunotherapy, in the form of checkpoint inhibitor drugs such as anti–CTLA-4 and anti-PD-1 antibody drugs, have revolutionized oncology by activating T Cells and restoring the patient's own anti-cancer immune response. Unfortunately, response rates are disappointing and in need improvement. According to Drs. Fyza Shaikh et al. (2019), "only a minority of patients respond to the available immunotherapy drugs."(93)

Oncologists were surprised when researchers discovered that the response rate of checkpoint inhibitor immunotherapy depends largely on the status of the microbiome.

In 2012, Dr. Ivaylo Ivanov and Kenya Honda studied the influence of friendly bacteria, the "gut microbiome," on the efficacy of checkpoint inhibitor drugs in patients with melanoma, non-small-cell lung cancer and renal cell carcinoma, finding that recent antibiotic use (within 30–60 days) was associated with shorter overall survival (OS) and shorter progression-free survival (PFS). The antibiotics kill off the friendly bacteria of the microbiome.

Dr. Ivanov et al. write:

> The recent discovery of the microbiome's impact on the efficacy of checkpoint inhibitors and the subsequent work to elucidate the immunological mechanisms driving these effects have revolutionized microbiome research in oncology. (94)

Baseline Microbiome Determines Efficacy

In 2017, Dr. Nathalie Chaput et al. studied use of the checkpoint inhibitor drug ipilimumab, targeting CTLA-4 in 26 melanoma patients. However, prior to treatment, Dr. Chaput studied the microbiomes with 16s ribosomal RNA sequencing, a new microbiology tool for identifying bacterial species. Dr. Chaput's team found that the species of bacteria in the microbiome determined the response to immunotherapy, writing:

> Ipilimumab led to a higher inducible T cell Costimulator induction on CD4+ T cells and to a higher increase in serum CD25 in patients who belonged to Faecalibacterium-driven cluster A... Baseline gut microbiota enriched with Faecalibacterium and other Firmicutes is associated with beneficial clinical response to ipilimumab and more frequent occurrence of ipilimumab-induced colitis. (95–97)

Note: Faecalibacterium and Firmicutes are species of friendly bacteria found in the microbiome, found to augment immunotherapy.

Year of the Breakthrough of the Microbiota

In 2018, Dr. Kroemer considers 2017 the year of the "breakthrough of the microbiota" for cancer immunotherapy, writing:

> In 2017, epidemiological studies in humans and experiments in mouse models showed that the intestinal microbiota determines the effectiveness of anti-cancer immunotherapies. (98–100)

Selecting the Correct Bacterial Strain

Drs. Jiwan Sidhu and Dina Alkandari (2020) provide an overview of all previous research on probiotics in cancer prevention and therapy, emphasizing that one must select the correct bacterial strain (species) intended to produce the desired immunostimulatory, cholesterol-lowering, anti-obesity, anti-anxiety, antidiabetic, anti-inflammatory, anticarcinogenic, and antidepressant results. This desired beneficial strain of probiotic can now be bio-engineered with new precision technology called CRISPR. Drs. Sidhu and Alkandari write:

> Now, with the development of the CRISPR system [Clustered Regularly Interspaced Short Palindromic Repeats], a system for precision genetic engineering, the production of designer Lactobacilli such as Streptococcus thermophilus has become much easier to establish their immunostimulatory functions in dairy products. (101)

Cancer Hijacks Inflammatory Pathways

As we discuss elsewhere in this book, cancers will commonly upregulate inflammatory pathways (with pro-inflammatory cytokines such as IL-6) to feed rapid growth and invasive behavior. Treatments that downregulate IL-6 and other inflammatory cytokines are enormously useful. Certain probiotic strains have been found to do exactly this, upregulating anti-inflammatory cytokines and downregulating pro- inflammatory cytokines. (101)

Reasonable to Think

Other strains of probiotics enhance the immune system and improve efficacy of chemotherapy and immunotherapy drugs, as reviewed by Dr. Luciana Marinelli et al. (2017), who write:

> It is **reasonable to think** that cocktails of beneficial bacteria together with an ad hoc diet or food supplements may be used as novel anti-cancer adjuvant agents in future therapeutic regimens. (102)

High-Dose Antibiotics for Febrile Neutropenia

As we discussed in the Introduction and Chapter 1, high-dose intra-venous antibiotics are commonly given to cancer patients after chemotherapy in order to treat the resulting "febrile neutropenia" caused by bone marrow suppression and toxicity to the gut (with loss of mucosal barrier and "leaky gut"). The more intensive chemotherapy regimens such as hyper-CVAD are notorious for prolonged bone marrow toxicity and febrile neutropenia. (103)

Untreated febrile neutropenia rapidly leads to septic shock and a very high mortality rate. The antibiotic drug of choice is Zosyn® (Piperacillin and Tazobactam), as recommended by the National Institute of Health (NIH). These antibiotics essentially kill off all the friendly bacteria in the gut, creating a state called "dysbiosis," with severely reduced diversity, which, as we have seen above, is associated with poor outcomes after immunotherapy with checkpoint inhibitors. In addition, this disruption of the microbiome by high-dose antibiotics is associated with increased risk of clostridia difficile enterocolitis (C.Diff) and increased mortality after allogeneic stem cell transplantation, both of which are remedied by the judicious use of high-dose probiotics. C. Diff enterocolitis tends to be recurrent, an event which carries a high mortality rate. High dose probiotics prevent initital C. Diff infection, and reduces recurrence rate. High dose probiotics also reduces mortality for patients undergoing Allogeneic Bone Marrow Transplant, commonly done for hematologic malignancies. Thus, high dose probiotics have been shown enormously useful for the cancer patient. (104–112)

Kefir: A Probiotic Food with Anti-Cancer Effects

One of the more promising probiotic foods, originating from Tibet, is kefir, consisting of a yeast and bacteria combination. Kefir is a fermented milk product that can be made at home by adding widely available kefir grains to milk and allowing the mixture to ferment overnight.

In 2002, Dr. Je-Ruei Liu et al. studied the anti-tumor effect of milk kefir in mouse xenografts inoculated with human sarcoma cells, finding 64% tumor inhibition compared to controls in mice fed the kefir. Other in vitro and in vivo studies show efficacy in colorectal cancer, malignant T lymphocytes, breast cancer, and lung carcinoma. (113–114)

Dr. Mohammadreza Sharifi et al. (2017), write:

> Kefir is one of the best therapeutic natural ingredients, applying its anti-cancer effect through different cellular and molecular pathways. Kefir is likely to be recognized for effective treatment of malignancies and as an anti-cancer agent in the near future. (114)

Gut Bacteria as Drug Factories

As we have seen in previous chapters, many drug discoveries come from the bacterial world—for example, the antiparasitic drug ivermectin, a repurposed anti-cancer drug derived from a single Japanese soil sample bacterium. Likewise, the gut microbiome can be considered a production factory for anti-cancer molecules, proteins, and peptides. (115–116)

Clostridium Butyricum Probiotic

Another example is butyrate, a short-chain fatty acid (SCFA) that has anti-cancer activity as an HDAC inhibitor (histone deacetylase inhibitor) providing synergy with artemisinin. To increase butyrate levels, one may ingest butyrate itself, or else the widely available butyrate-producing clostridium butyricum probiotic that manufactures butyrate in the gut. (117–123)

Conclusion

Iodine and Vitamin D supplementation for the cancer patient seems like a "no brainer" with considerable benefits. When levels are measured and followed, this is a very low risk anti-cancer strategy wih no adverse side effects. Both Iodine and Vitamin D enhances anti-cancer immunity, and have direct anti-cancer effects as well. Vitamin D prevents autoimmune disease.

The science of the microbiome and its interaction with the immune system is still in its infancy. Even at this early stage, it is clear that maintaining a robust and diverse microbiome has enormous benefits for the cancer patient, including improving the efficacy of immune checkpoint inhibitors, prevention of C. diff enterocolitis, reduction in mortality from allogeneic bone marrow transplant, modulating or upregulating the immune system, and production of anti-cancer molecules and substances directly by the gut microbiome. The use of high-dose probiotics in the cancer patient is another "no brainer." Over the next decade, it is highly likely that more precise, targeted probiotic cocktails will be discovered with even more potent anti-cancer activity. (124–131)

Although this concludes our discussion of immune enhancing strategies for the *Cracking Cancer Toolkit*, the reader should be aware that this list is by no means complete. I must apologize, due to time and space considerations, we have not fully discussed immune enhancing benefits of selenium, zinc, vitamin C, vitamin A, chlorella (microalgae), colostrum, modified citrus pectin, and many others. (132–167)

References for Chapter 30: Thyroid, Iodine, Vitamin D, Probiotics

1) Galton, Lawrence, and Broda Otto Barnes. Hypothyroidism: The unsuspected illness. Crowell, 1976.

2) Perrotta, Cristiana, et al. "The thyroid hormone triiodothyronine controls macrophage maturation and functions: protective role during inflammation." The American journal of pathology 184.1 (2014): 230-247.

3) Frick, Luciana Romina, et al. "Involvement of thyroid hormones in the alterations of T-cell immunity and tumor progression induced by chronic stress." Biological psychiatry 65.11 (2009): 935-942.

4) Frick, L. R., et al. "Chronic restraint stress impairs T-cell immunity and promotes tumor progression in mice." Stress 12.2 (2009): 134-143.

5) De Vito, Paolo, et al. "Thyroid hormones as modulators of immune activities at the cellular level." Thyroid 21.8 (2011): 879-890.

6) Alamino, V. A., et al. "The thyroid hormone triiodothyronine reinvigorates dendritic cells and potentiates anti-tumor immunity." OncoImmunology 5.1 (2016): e1064579.

7) Hodkinson, Clare F., et al. "Preliminary evidence of immune function modulation by thyroid hormones in healthy men and women aged 55–70 years." Journal of Endocrinology 202.1 (2009): 55-63.

10) Schoenfeld, Philip S., et al. "Suppression of cell-mediated immunity in hypothyroidism." Southern medical journal 88.3 (1995): 347-349.

11) del Mar Montesinos, María, and Claudia Pellizas. "Thyroid hormone action on innate immunity." Frontiers in endocrinology 10 (2019).

12) Hodkinson, Clare F., et al. "Preliminary evidence of immune function modulation by thyroid hormones in healthy men and women aged 55-70 years." Journal of endocrinology 202.1 (2009): 55.

13) Alamino, Vanina A., et al. "Antitumor responses stimulated by dendritic cells are improved by triiodothyronine binding to the thyroid hormone receptor β." Cancer research 75.7 (2015): 1265-1274.

14) Alamino, V. A., et al. "The thyroid hormone triiodothyronine reinvigorates dendritic cells and potentiates anti-tumor immunity." Oncoimmunology 5.1 (2016): e1064579.

15) Krashin, Eilon, et al. "Thyroid hormones and cancer: A comprehensive review of preclinical and clinical studies." Frontiers in endocrinology 10 (2019): 59.

16) Latteyer, Soeren, et al. "Thyroxine promotes lung cancer growth in an orthotopic mouse model." Endocrine-related cancer 1.aop (2019).

17) Chen, Yi-Ru, et al. "Thyroid hormone, PD-L1, and cancer." Journal of Cancer Research and Practice 6.4 (2019): 162.

18) Ashur-Fabian, Osnat, et al. "Long-term response in high-grade optic glioma treated with medically induced hypothyroidism and carboplatin: a case report and review of the literature." Anti-cancer drugs 24.3 (2013): 315-323.

19) Hercbergs, Aleck, et al. "Medically induced euthyroid hypothyroxinemia may extend survival in compassionate need cancer patients: an observational study." The oncologist 20.1 (2015): 72.

20) Ghent, W. R., et al. "Iodine replacement in fibrocystic disease of the breast." Canadian journal of surgery. Journal canadien de chirurgie 36.5 (1993): 453-460.

21) Kessler, Jack H. "The effect of supraphysiologic levels of iodine on patients with cyclic mastalgia." The breast journal 10.4 (2004): 328-336.

22) Mansel, Robert E., et al. "A Randomized Controlled Multicenter Trial of an Investigational Liquid Nutritional Formula in Women with Cyclic Breast Pain Associated with Fibrocystic Breast Changes." Journal of Women's Health 27.3 (2018): 333-340.

23) Rappaport, Jay. "Changes in dietary iodine explains increasing incidence of breast Cancer with distant involvement in young women." Journal of Cancer 8.2 (2017): 174.

24) Gerson Therapy, by Charlotte Gerson and Morton Walker, DPM (2001) NY: Kensington Publishing Corp. ISBN 1-57566-628-6 (Trade paperback, 371 pages, plus appendixes and index.)

25) Aceves, Carmen, et al. "Antineoplastic effect of iodine in mammary cancer: participation of 6-iodo-lactone (6-IL) and peroxisome proliferator-activated receptors (PPAR)." Molecular Cancer 8.1 (2009): 33.

26) Arroyo-Helguera, O., et al. "Signaling pathways involved in the antiproliferative effect of molecular iodine in normal and tumoral breast cells: evidence that 6-iodolactone mediates apoptotic effects." Endocrine-related cancer 15.4 (2008): 1003-1011.

27) Nava-Villalba, Mario, and Carmen Aceves. "6-Iodolactone, key mediator of antitumoral properties of iodine." Prostaglandins & other lipid mediators 112 (2014): 27-33.

28) Nava-Villalba, Mario, et al. "Activation of peroxisome proliferator-activated receptor gamma is crucial for antitumoral effects of 6-iodolactone." Molecular cancer 14.1 (2015): 168.

29) Xu, Zack, et al. "Elucidating the mechanism of action of molecular iodine on breast cancer cells." (2017): 2243-2243.

30) Abraham, Guy E. "Serum inorganic iodide levels following ingestion of a tablet form of Lugol solution: Evidence for an enterohepatic circulation of iodine." The Original Internist 11.3 (2004): 29-34.

31) Brownstein, David. "Clinical experience with inorganic, non-radioactive iodine/iodide." The Original Internist 12.3 (2005): 105-108.

32) Mendieta, Irasema, et al. "Molecular iodine synergized and sensitized neuroblastoma cells to antineoplastic effect of ATRA." Endocrine-Related Cancer 1.aop (2020).

33) De la Vieja, Antonio, and Pilar Santisteban. "Role of iodide metabolism in physiology and cancer." Endocrine-related cancer 25.4 (2018): R225-R245.

34) Moreno-Vega, Aura, et al. "Adjuvant Effect of Molecular Iodine in Conventional Chemotherapy for Breast Cancer. Randomized Pilot Study." Nutrients 11.7 (2019): 1623.

35) Mendieta, Irasema, et al. "Molecular iodine exerts antineoplastic effects by diminishing proliferation and invasive potential and activating the immune response in mammary cancer xenografts." BMC cancer 19.1 (2019): 261.

36) Rösner, Harald, et al. "Antiproliferative/cytotoxic effects of molecular iodine, povidone-iodine and Lugol's solution in different human carcinoma cell lines." Oncology letters 12.3 (2016): 2159-2162.

37) Elio Torremante, Pompilio, and Harald Rosner. "Antiproliferative effects of molecular iodine in cancers." Current Chemical Biology 5.3 (2011): 168-176.

38) Bigoni-Ordóñez, Gabriele Davide, et al. "Molecular iodine inhibits the expression of stemness markers on cancer stem-like cells of established cell lines derived from cervical cancer." BMC cancer 18.1 (2018): 928.

39) Aranda, Nuri, et al. "Uptake and antitumoral effects of iodine and 6-iodolactone in differentiated and undifferentiated human prostate cancer cell lines." The Prostate 73.1 (2013): 31-41.

40) Thomasz, Lisa, et al. "6 Iodo-δ-lactone: A derivative of arachidonic acid with antitumor effects in HT-29 colon cancer cells." Prostaglandins, Leukotrienes and Essential Fatty Acids 88.4 (2013): 273-280.

41) Zambrano-Estrada, Xóchitl, et al. "Molecular iodine/doxorubicin neoadjuvant treatment impair invasive capacity and attenuate side effect in canine mammary cancer." BMC veterinary research 14.1 (2018): 87.

42) Goyal, Itivrita, Manu Raj Pandey, and Rajeev Sharma. "Hypothyroidism and Goiter in a Young Male with Suspected Iodine Deficiency Followed by Thyrotoxicosis after Iodine Supplementation." AACE Clinical Case Reports 6.1 (2020): e19-e22.

43) Bülow Pedersen, Inge, et al. "Increase in incidence of hyperthyroidism predominantly occurs in young people after iodine fortification of salt in Denmark."

The Journal of Clinical Endocrinology & Metabolism 91.10 (2006): 3830-3834.

44) Delange, F., B. De Benoist, and D. Alnwick. "Risks of iodine-induced hyperthyroidism after correction of iodine deficiency by iodized salt." Thyroid 9.6 (1999): 545-556.

45) Connolly, R. J., G. I. Vidor, and J. C. Stewart. "Increase in thyrotoxicosis in endemic goitre area after iodation of bread." The Lancet 295.7645 (1970): 500-502.

46) Kohn, Lawrence A. "The Midwestern American" epidemic" of iodine-induced hyperthyroidism in the 1920s." Bulletin of the New York Academy of Medicine 52.7 (1976): 770.

47) Livadas, D. P., et al. "The toxic effects of small iodine supplements in patients with autonomous thyroid nodules." Clinical endocrinology 7.2 (1977): 121-127.

48) Connolly, Kara J., et al. "Congenital hypothyroidism caused by excess prenatal maternal iodine ingestion." The Journal of pediatrics 161.4 (2012): 760-762.

49) Sassi, Francesca, Cristina Tamone, and Patrizia D'Amelio. "Vitamin D: nutrient, hormone, and immunomodulator." Nutrients 10.11 (2018): 1656.

50) Monastra, G., et al. "Vitamin D: a steroid hormone with progesterone-like activity." Eur Rev Med Pharmacol Sci 22.8 (2018): 2502-2512.

51) Verstuyf, Annemieke, et al. "Vitamin D: a pleiotropic hormone." Kidney international 78.2 (2010): 140-145.

52) Wimalawansa, S. J. "Biology of Vitamin D." J Steroids Horm Sci 10.1 (2019).

53) Grant, William B. "A review of the evidence supporting the vitamin D-cancer prevention hypothesis in 2017." Anticancer research 38.2 (2018): 1121-1136.

54) Grant, W. B., and M. Moukayed. "Vitamin D3 from Ultraviolet-B Exposure or Oral Intake in Relation to Cancer Incidence and Mortality." Current nutrition reports (2019).

55) Dovnik, Andraž, and Nina Fokter Dovnik. "Vitamin D and Ovarian Cancer: Systematic Review of the Literature with a Focus on Molecular Mechanisms." Cells 9.2 (2020): 335.

56) Srivastava, Amit Kumar, et al. "Depleting ovarian cancer stem cells with calcitriol." Oncotarget 9.18 (2018): 14481.

57) Barreto, Savio G., and Rachel E. Neale. "Vitamin D and pancreatic cancer." Cancer letters 368.1 (2015): 1-6.

58) Iqbal, Sarah, and Imrana Naseem. "Pancreatic cancer control: is vitamin D the answer?" European Journal of Cancer Prevention 25.3 (2016): 188-195.

59) Gilzad-Kohan, Hamed, Shabnam Sani, and Mehdi Boroujerdi. "Calcitriol reverses induced expression of efflux proteins and potentiates cytotoxic activity of gemcitabine in capan-2 pancreatic cancer cells." Journal of Pharmacy & Pharmaceutical Sciences 20 (2017): 295-304.

60) Trump, Donald L. "Calcitriol and cancer therapy: A missed opportunity." Bone reports 9 (2018): 110-119.

61) García-Quiroz, Janice, et al. "Synergistic Antitumorigenic Activity of Calcitriol with Curcumin or Resveratrol is Mediated by Angiogenesis Inhibition in Triple Negative Breast Cancer Xenografts." Cancers 11.11 (2019): 1739.

62) Huang, Zixian, et al. "Vitamin D promotes the cisplatin sensitivity of oral squamous cell carcinoma by inhibiting LCN2-modulated NF-κB pathway activation through RPS3." Cell Death & Disease 10.12 (2019): 1-14.

63) Wicks, Sheila, et al. "Combinations of vitamins A, D2 and D3 have synergistic effects in gastric and colon cancer cells." Functional Foods in Health and Disease 9.12 (2019): 749-771.

64) Griffin, Niamh, and Maura Dowling. "Vitamin D supplementation and clinical outcomes in cancer survivorship." British Journal of Nursing 27.19 (2018): 1121-1128.

65) Ma, Yingyu, Candace S. Johnson, and Donald L. Trump. "Mechanistic insights of vitamin D anticancer effects." Vitamins & Hormones. Vol. 100. Academic Press, 2016. 395-431.

66) Seyedalipour, Fatere, et al. "High prevalence of vitamin D deficiency in newly diagnosed acute myeloid leukemia patients and its adverse outcome." International journal of hematology-oncology and stem cell research 11.3 (2017): 209.

67) Acevedo, Francisco, et al. "High prevalence of vitamin D deficiency in women with breast cancer: The first Chilean study." The Breast 29 (2016): 39-43.

68) Crew, Katherine D., et al. "High prevalence of vitamin D deficiency despite supplementation in premenopausal women with breast cancer undergoing adjuvant chemotherapy." Journal of Clinical Oncology 27.13 (2009): 2151.

69) Napoli, Nicola, et al. "High prevalence of low vitamin D and musculoskeletal complaints in women with breast cancer." The breast journal 16.6 (2010): 609-616.

70) Tangpricha, Vin, et al. "Prevalence of vitamin D deficiency in patients attending an outpatient cancer care clinic in Boston." Endocrine Practice 10.3 (2004): 292.

71) Kumar, Archit, et al. "25-Hydroxyvitamin D3 and 1, 25 dihydroxyvitamin D3 as an antiviral and immunomodulator against herpes simplex virus-1 infection in HeLa cells." Viral immunology 31.8 (2018): 589-593.

72) Zdrenghea, Mihnea T., et al. "Vitamin D modulation of innate immune responses to respiratory viral infections." Reviews in medical virology 27.1 (2017): e1909.

73) Tanner, Alex, and Stephen Allen. "The Case for Vitamin D Supplementation to Improve Protection against Respiratory Tract Infections." Current Respiratory Medicine Reviews 14.3 (2018): 128-134.

74) Martineau, Adrian R., et al. "Vitamin D supplementation to prevent acute respiratory infections: individual participant data meta-analysis." Health Technol Assess (2019).

75) McCartney, D. M., and D. G. Byrne. "Optimisation of Vitamin D Status for Enhanced Immuno-protection Against Covid-19." Irish Medical Journal 113.4 (2020): 58-58.

76) Teymoori-Rad, Majid, et al. "The interplay between vitamin D and viral infections." Reviews in medical virology 29.2 (2019): e2032.

77) Telcian, Aurica G., et al. "Vitamin D increases the antiviral activity of bronchial epithelial cells in vitro." Antiviral research 137 (2017): 93-101.

78) Hansdottir, Sif, et al. "Vitamin D decreases respiratory syncytial virus induction of NF-κB–linked chemokines and cytokines in airway epithelium while maintaining the antiviral state." The journal of immunology 184.2 (2010): 965-974.

79) Gal-Tanamy, Meital, et al. "Vitamin D: an innate antiviral agent suppressing hepatitis C virus in human hepatocytes." Hepatology 54.5 (2011): 1570-1579.

80) Ozgu, Emre, et al. "Could 25-OH vitamin D deficiency be a reason for HPV infection persistence in cervical premalignant lesions." J. Exp. Ther. Oncol 11 (2016): 177-180.

81) Chao, Chia-Ter, et al. "Serum vitamin D levels are positively associated with varicella zoster immunity in chronic dialysis patients." Scientific reports 4.1 (2014): 1-8.

82) Chao, Chia-Ter, et al. "Vitamin D is closely linked to the clinical courses of herpes zoster: From pathogenesis to complications." Medical hypotheses 85.4 (2015): 452-457.

83) Grant, William B., et al. "Evidence that vitamin D supplementation could reduce risk of influenza and COVID-19 infections and deaths." Nutrients 12.4 (2020): 988.

84) Yamamoto, Erin, and Trine N. Jørgensen. "Immunological effects of vitamin D and their relations to autoimmunity." Journal of autoimmunity (2019).

85) Murdaca, Giuseppe, et al. "Emerging role of vitamin D in autoimmune diseases: an update on evidence and therapeutic implications." Autoimmunity reviews (2019): 102350.

86) Harrison, Stephanie R., et al. "Vitamin D, autoimmune disease and rheumatoid arthritis." Calcified tissue international (2019): 1-18.

87) Biström, Martin, et al. "High serum concentration of vitamin D may protect against multiple sclerosis." Multiple Sclerosis Journal–Experimental, Translational and Clinical 5.4 (2019): 2055217319892291.

88) Manousaki, Despoina, and J. Brent Richards. "Vitamin D deficiency is an etiological factor for MS–Yes." Multiple Sclerosis Journal 25.5 (2019): 637-639.

89) Marcinkowska, Ewa, Graham R. Wallace, and Geoffrey Brown. "The use of 1α, 25-dihydroxyvitamin

D3 as an anticancer agent." International journal of molecular sciences 17.5 (2016): 729.

90) Sarkar, Surojit, et al. "Role of vitamin D in cytotoxic T lymphocyte immunity to pathogens and cancer." Critical reviews in clinical laboratory sciences 53.2 (2016): 132-145.

91) Bigelsen, Stephen. "Evidence-based complementary treatment of pancreatic cancer: a review of adjunct therapies including paricalcitol, hydroxychloroquine, intravenous vitamin C, statins, metformin, curcumin, and aspirin." Cancer management and research 10 (2018): 2003.

92) Nuti, Marianna, et al. "The microbiota impact: bacteria shaping immunity, disease and response to therapy." Science 359 (2018): 91-7.

93) Shaikh, Fyza Y., Joell J. Gills, and Cynthia L. Sears. "Impact of the microbiome on checkpoint inhibitor treatment in patients with non-small cell lung cancer and melanoma." EBioMedicine (2019).

94) Ivanov, Ivaylo I., and Kenya Honda. "Intestinal commensal microbes as immune modulators." Cell host & microbe 12.4 (2012): 496-508.

95) Chaput, Nathalie, et al. "Baseline gut microbiota predicts clinical response and colitis in metastatic melanoma patients treated with ipilimumab." Annals of Oncology 28.6 (2017): 1368-1379.

96) Routy, Bertrand, et al. "Gut microbiome influences efficacy of PD-1–based immunotherapy against epithelial tumors." Science 359.6371 (2018): 91-97.

97) Matson, Vyara, et al. "The commensal microbiome is associated with anti–PD-1 efficacy in metastatic melanoma patients." Science 359.6371 (2018): 104-108.

98) Kroemer, Guido, and Laurence Zitvogel. "Cancer immunotherapy in 2017: The breakthrough of the microbiota." Nature Reviews Immunology 18.2 (2018): 87.

99) Tinsley, Nadina, et al. "Cumulative antibiotic use significantly decreases efficacy of checkpoint inhibitors in patients with advanced cancer." The oncologist 25.1 (2020): 55.

100) Sivan, Ayelet, et al. "Commensal Bifidobacterium promotes antitumor immunity and facilitates anti–PD-L1 efficacy." Science 350.6264 (2015): 1084-1089.

101) Sidhu, Jiwan S., and Dina Alkandari. "Overview of probiotics in cancer prevention and therapy." Functional Foods in Cancer Prevention and Therapy. Academic Press, 2020. 261-282.

102) Marinelli, Luciana, Gian Carlo Tenore, and Ettore Novellino. "Probiotic species in the modulation of the anticancer immune response." Seminars in cancer biology. Vol. 46. Academic Press, 2017.

103) Gill, Saar, et al. "Prolonged haematological toxicity from the hyper-CVAD regimen: manifestations, frequency, and natural history in a cohort of 125 consecutive patients." Annals of Hematology 87.9 (2008): 727-734.

104) Taur, Ying, et al. "The effects of intestinal tract bacterial diversity on mortality following allogeneic hematopoietic stem cell transplantation." Blood 124.7 (2014): 1174-1182.

105) Shono, Yusuke, et al. "Increased GVHD-related mortality with broad-spectrum antibiotic use after allogeneic hematopoietic stem cell transplantation in human patients and mice." Science translational medicine 8.339 (2016): 339ra71-339ra71.

106) Bilinski, Jaroslaw, et al. "Impact of gut colonization by antibiotic-resistant bacteria on the outcomes of allogeneic hematopoietic stem cell transplantation: a retrospective, single-center study." Biology of Blood and Marrow Transplantation 22.6 (2016): 1087-1093.

107) Andermann, T. M., A. Rezvani, and A. S. Bhatt. "Microbiota Manipulation With Prebiotics and Probiotics in Patients Undergoing Stem Cell Transplantation." Current hematologic malignancy reports 11.1 (2016): 19.

108) Holler, Ernst, et al. "Metagenomic analysis of the stool microbiome in patients receiving allogeneic stem cell transplantation: loss of diversity is associated with use of systemic antibiotics and more pronounced in gastrointestinal graft-versus-host disease." Biology of Blood and Marrow Transplantation 20.5 (2014): 640-645.

109) Mercadante, Ana CT, et al. "Oral Combined Therapy with Probiotics and Alloantigen Induces B Cell–Dependent Long-Lasting Specific Tolerance." The Journal of Immunology 192.4 (2014): 1928-1937.

110) Gerbitz, Armin, et al. "Probiotic effects on experimental graft-versus-host disease: let them eat yogurt." Blood 103.11 (2004): 4365-4367.

111) Tung, Jennifer M., Lisa R. Dolovich, and Christine H. Lee. "Prevention of Clostridium difficile infection with Saccharomyces boulardii: a systematic review." Canadian Journal of Gastroenterology and Hepatology 23.12 (2009): 817-821.

112) Hickson, Mary. "Probiotics in the prevention of antibiotic-associated diarrhoea and Clostridium difficile infection." Therapeutic advances in gastroenterology 4.3 (2011): 185-197.

113) Liu, Je-Ruei, et al. "Antitumor activity of milk kefir and soy milk kefir in tumor-bearing mice." Nutrition and cancer 44.2 (2002): 183-187.

114) Sharifi, Mohammadreza, et al. "Kefir: a powerful probiotics with anticancer properties." Medical Oncology 34.11 (2017): 183.

115) Karpiński, Tomasz M., and Artur Adamczak. "Anticancer activity of bacterial proteins and peptides." Pharmaceutics 10.2 (2018): 54.

116) Rodrigues, Gisele, et al. "Bacterial proteinaceous compounds with multiple activities toward cancers and microbial infection." Frontiers in microbiology 10 (2019).

117) Singh, Narendra P., and Henry C. Lai. "Synergistic cytotoxicity of artemisinin and sodium butyrate on human cancer cells." Anticancer research 25.6B (2005): 4325-4331.

118) Han, Anna, et al. "Butyrate regulates its own metabolic fate as an HDAC inhibitor in colorectal cancer cells." The FASEB Journal 31.1_supplement (2017): 300-2.

119) Semaan, Josiane, et al. "Comparative effect of sodium butyrate and sodium propionate on proliferation, cell cycle and apoptosis in human breast cancer cells MCF-7." Breast Cancer (2020): 1-10.

120) Yagi, Akira, Megumi Hasegawa, and Hiroyuki Abe. "Beneficial Roles of Histone Deacetylase Inhibitor Butyrate to Multiple Myeloma, Acute Leukemia and Acute Myeloid Leukemia." Journal of Gastroenterology and Hepatology Research 9.2 (2020): 3107-3112.

121) Cao, Mingming, et al. "Butyrate inhibits the proliferation and induces the apoptosis of colorectal cancer HCT116 cells via the deactivation of mTOR/S6K1 signaling mediated partly by SIRT1 downregulation." Molecular medicine reports 19.5 (2019): 3941-3947.

122) Chen, Danfeng, et al. "Clostridium butyricum, a butyrate-producing probiotic, inhibits intestinal tumor development through modulating Wnt signaling and gut microbiota." Cancer Letters 469 (2020): 456-467.

123) Scharlau, Daniel, et al. "Mechanisms of primary cancer prevention by butyrate and other products formed during gut flora-mediated fermentation of dietary fibre." Mutation Research/Reviews in Mutation Research 682.1 (2009): 39-53.

124) Zhang, Chen-xing, Hui-yu Wang, and Tong-xin Chen. "Interactions between Intestinal Microflora/Probiotics and the Immune System." BioMed Research International 2019 (2019).

125) Helmink, Beth A., et al. "The microbiome, cancer, and cancer therapy." Nature medicine 25.3 (2019): 377-388.

126) Zhang, Ziying, et al. "Demystifying the manipulation of host immunity, metabolism, and extraintestinal tumors by the gut microbiome." Signal transduction and targeted therapy 4.1 (2019): 1-34.

127) Galdeano, Carolina Maldonado, et al. "Beneficial effects of probiotic consumption on the immune system." Annals of Nutrition and Metabolism 74.2 (2019): 115-124.

128) Mendoza, Luis. "Potential effect of probiotics in the treatment of breast cancer." Oncology reviews 13.2 (2019).

129) Shi, Linlin, et al. "Combination Therapy of TGF-β Blockade and Commensal-derived Probiotics Provides Enhanced Antitumor Immune Response and Tumor Suppression." Theranostics 9.14 (2019): 4115.

130) Utz, Virginia Emilce Mendez, Gabriela Perdigón, and Alejandra de Moreno de LeBlanc. "Oral administration of milk fermented by Lactobacillus casei CRL431 was able to decrease metastasis from breast cancer in a murine model by modulating immune response locally in the lungs." Journal of functional foods 54 (2019): 263-270.

131) Maghsood, Faezeh, et al. "Anti-proliferative and Anti-metastatic Potential of High Molecular Weight Secretory Molecules from Probiotic Lactobacillus Reuteri Cell-Free Supernatant Against Human Colon Cancer Stem-Like Cells (HT29-ShE)." International Journal of Peptide Research and Therapeutics (2020): 1-13.

132) Kuršvietienė, Lolita, et al. "Selenium Anticancer Properties and Impact on Cellular Redox Status." Antioxidants 9.1 (2020): 80.

133) Cui, Jinling, et al. "Inorganic Selenium Induces Nonapoptotic Programmed Cell Death in PC-3 Prostate Cancer Cells Associated with Inhibition of Glycolysis." Journal of Agricultural and Food Chemistry 67.38 (2019): 10637-10645.

134) Wintergerst, Eva S., Silvia Maggini, and Dietrich H. Hornig. "Immune-enhancing role of vitamin C and zinc and effect on clinical conditions." Annals of Nutrition and Metabolism 50.2 (2006): 85-94.

135) Heuser, Gunnar, and Aristo Vojdani. "Enhancement of natural killer cell activity and T and B cell function by buffered vitamin C in patients exposed to toxic chemicals: the role of protein kinase-C." Immunopharmacology and immunotoxicology 19.3 (1997): 291-312.

136) Carr, Anitra C., and Silvia Maggini. "Vitamin C and immune function." Nutrients 9.11 (2017): 1211.

137) Jafari, Davood, et al. "Vitamin C and the Immune System." Nutrition and Immunity. Springer, Cham, 2019. 81-102.

138) Kashiouris, Markos G., et al. "The emerging role of vitamin C as a treatment for sepsis." Nutrients 12.2 (2020): 292.

139) Xi, Dan. "Vitamin C in Cancer Therapeutics and Metastasis." Journal of orthopedic research and therapy 10.1 (2019).

140) Semba, Richard D. "The role of vitamin A and related retinoids in immune function." Nutrition reviews 56.1 (1998): S38-S48.

141) Dennert, Gunther. "Retinoids and the immune system: immunostimulation by vitamin A." The retinoids. Academic Press, 1984. 373-390.

142) Montrone, Michele, et al. "Retinoids as critical modulators of immune functions: new therapeutic perspectives for old compounds." Endocrine, Metabolic & Immune Disorders-Drug Targets (Formerly Current Drug Targets-Immune, Endocrine & Metabolic Disorders) 9.2 (2009): 113-131.

143) Cao, Xin. "Retinoids Induced Cancer Stem Cell Differentiation and Apoptosis for Cancer Therapies." Molecular and Cellular Therapies (2019): 1-8.

144) Tripathi, Surya Kant, et al. "The potential of retinoids for combination therapy of lung cancer: Updates and future directions." Pharmacological research 147 (2019): 104331.

145) Ishiguro, Susumu, et al. "Cell Wall Membrane Fraction of Chlorella sorokiniana Enhances Host Antitumor Immunity and Inhibits Colon Carcinoma Growth in Mice." Integrative Cancer Therapies 19 (2020): 1534735419900555.

146) El-Hack, Mohamed E. Abd, et al. "Microalgae in modern cancer therapy: Current knowledge." Biomedicine & Pharmacotherapy 111 (2019): 42-50.

147) Kunte, Mugdha, and Krutika Desai. "The protein extract of chlorella minutissima inhibits the expression of MMP-1, MMP-2 and MMP-9 in cancer cells through upregulation of TIMP-3 and down regulation of c-Jun." Cell Journal (Yakhteh) 20.2 (2018): 211.

148) Martínez Andrade, Kevin A., et al. "Marine microalgae with anti-cancer properties." Marine drugs 16.5 (2018): 165.

149) Cheng, Dai, et al. "Dietary Chlorella vulgaris ameliorates altered immunomodulatory functions in cyclophosphamide-induced immunosuppressive mice." Nutrients 9.7 (2017): 708.

150) Lin, Ping-Yi, et al. "Chlorella sorokiniana induces mitochondrial-mediated apoptosis in human non-small cell lung cancer cells and inhibits xenograft tumor growth in vivo." BMC complementary and alternative medicine 17.1 (2017): 88.

151) Kubatka, Peter, et al. "Antineoplastic effects of Chlorella pyrenoidosa in the breast cancer model." Nutrition 31.4 (2015): 560-569.

152) Tanaka, Kuniaki, et al. "A novel glycoprotein obtained from Chlorella vulgaris strain CK22

shows antimetastatic immunopotentiation." Cancer Immunology, Immunotherapy 45.6 (1998): 313-320.

153) Vermeil, C., and O. Morin. "Experimental role of the unicellular algae Prototheca and Chlorella (Chlorellaceae) in anti-cancer immunogenesis (murine BP8 sarcoma)." Comptes rendus des seances de la Societe de biologie et de ses filiales 170.3 (1976): 646-649.

154) do Carmo França-Botelho, Aline. "Beneficial Components of Colostrum for Cancer Patients: A Mini-review Focused on Oxidative Aspects and Properties of Colostrinin." Asian Oncology Research Journal (2019): 1-6.

155) Samuel, Monisha, et al. "Bovine milk-derived exosomes from colostrum are enriched with proteins implicated in immune response and growth." Scientific reports 7.1 (2017): 1-10.

156) Agarwal, Prashant, and Ritika Gupta. "A Review on Anticancer Property of Colostrum." Research and Reviews Journal of Medical and Health Sciences 5.4 (2016).

157) Farziyan, Mohammad Ali, Fatemeh Moradian, and Ali Reza Rafiei. "Anticancer effect of bovine lactoferrin on human esophagus cancer cell line." Research in Molecular Medicine 4.1 (2016): 18-23.

158) Xu, Mei Ling, et al. "The effect of dietary bovine colostrum on respiratory syncytial virus infection and immune responses following the infection in the mouse." Journal of Microbiology 53.9 (2015): 661-666.

159) Wong, Eric B., et al. "Bovine colostrum enhances natural killer cell activity and immune response in a mouse model of influenza infection and mediates intestinal immunity through toll-like receptors 2 and 4." Nutrition research 34.4 (2014): 318-325.

160) Uchida, Kenji, et al. "Augmentation of cellular immunity and protection against influenza virus infection by bovine late colostrum in mice." Nutrition 28.4 (2012): 442-446.

161) LI, Li, et al. "Effect of Bovine Colostrum Powder on Immune Function in Cancer Patients: A Randomized Controlled Study." Acta Nutrimenta Sinica 6 (2005).

162) Rona, Zoltan P. "Bovine colostrum emerges as immune system modulator." American Journal of Natural Medicine 3 (1998): 19-23.

163) Short, Sarah P., and Christopher S. Williams. "Selenoproteins in tumorigenesis and cancer progression." Advances in cancer research. Vol. 136. Academic Press, 2017. 49-83.

164) Sanmartín, Carmen, et al. "Selenium compounds, apoptosis and other types of cell death: an overview for cancer therapy." International journal of molecular sciences 13.8 (2012): 9649-9672.

165) Misra, Sougat, et al. "Redox-active selenium compounds—From toxicity and cell death to cancer treatment." Nutrients 7.5 (2015): 3536-3556.

166) Merheb, Rihab, Roula M. Abdel-Massih, and Marc C. Karam. "Immunomodulatory effect of natural and modified Citrus pectin on cytokine levels in the spleen of BALB/c mice." International journal of biological macromolecules 121 (2019): 1-5.

167) Eliaz, Isaac, and Avraham Raz. "Pleiotropic Effects of Modified Citrus Pectin." Nutrients 11.11 (2019): 2619.

168) Dach, Jeffrey. Natural Medicine 101: How to Win the Medical Information War and Take Control of Your Health. BookSurge Publishing. (2009)

169) Thomson, Cynthia A., Emily Ho, and Meghan B. Strom. "Chemopreventive properties of 3, 3'-diindolylmethane in breast cancer: evidence from experimental and human studies." Nutrition reviews 74.7 (2016): 432-443.

Chapter 31

Mefloquine Autophagy Inhibitor

Antimalaria Drug Mefloquine

CHAPTER 11 ON REPURPOSED DRUGS discussed the antimalarial drug mefloquine as a good candidate targeting cancer stem cells (CSCs). In addition, mefloquine has been safely used for malaria treatment in combination with doxycycline, atovaquone, and most commonly, artemisinin (or a derivative). The combination of artemisinin (or derivative) with mefloquine is well tolerated and has been extensively studied, with many published papers in the medical literature. Synergy of this combination for cancer treatment has been found, as we discuss below. (1–6)

Mefloquine for Travelers

Mefloquine is currently recommended for malaria prophylaxis in travelers. Dosage is usually one 250 mg tablet per week for a few weeks prior to the trip. (7)

Mefloquine single doses as high as 1,000 mg have been effective for malaria falciparum and found to be safe. For example, in 1983, Dr. T. Harinasuta et al. ran a phase II randomized clinical trial of mefloquine for treatment of malaria in 147 adult males using single oral doses of 500 mg, 750 mg, and 1,000 mg, finding cure rates of 92.5, 95, and 100 per cent respectively. Regarding the adverse side effects observed, Dr. Harinasuta writes that they were mild and transient:

The side effects, which were transient and generally mild, included nausea, vomiting, and diarrhea. No significant changes were noted in hematological or biochemical parameters in any of the three groups. Sinus bradycardia, which started 4–7 days after drug administration and lasted for a few weeks, was seen in 10 patients. It was symptomless and needed no treatment. Acute brain syndrome was observed in one patient on day 21 after receiving a 1000-mg dose of mefloquine. (7)

Although single-dose mefloquine is generally considered safe for short-term use, neuropsychiatric adverse side effects have been described with long-term use. The combination use of mefloquine and artemisinin is associated with reactive astrocyte formation and glial degeneration in the hippocampus of mice, a troubling indication of brain toxicity. (8–13)

Dr. G. Dow et al. (2006) write:

Mefloquine has also been associated with neurological sequelae, including anxiety, panic attacks, suicidal ideation, nightmares, sleep disturbances, dizziness, tremor, headache, mood changes, and fatigue. These effects generally occur more frequently at the treatment dose, even in the absence of malaria, than at the prophylaxis dose…. the continued use of mefloquine will remain controversial given its association with neurological effects in some individuals … mefloquine induces dose- and concentration-related neurological effects in rats that may have clinical relevance and could result in permanent damage to the central nervous system. (8)

Neuropsychiatric Adverse Effects

The possible neuropsychiatric adverse effects induced by mefloquine, such as psychosis and violence, are not to be taken lightly. No doubt, these side effects damper enthusiasm for the use of the drug. However, limited use of the drug at the lower, prophylactic dosage might be acceptable for the cancer patient. In 2018, Dr. Philip Fischer declared mefloquine "still safe and effective" for malaria chemo-prophylaxis. (14)

Regardless of the potential adverse effects, we will next examine the role of mefloquine as an anti-cancer drug, hoping to learn more about autophagy and lysosomes in cancer biology.

Mefloquin: Lysosomal Agent Autophagy Inhibitor

As mentioned above, all three commonly used antimalaria drugs—mefloquine, chloroquine and hydroxychloroquine are autophagy inhibitors. After administration, the drugs are trapped and accumulate in lysosomes, causing an increase in pH, thus changing the normal acidic lysosome to alkaline. The drugs also prevent fusion of the lysosome to the autophagosome in the late stage of autophagy.

Autophagy Inhibitors Interrupt Macropinocytosis

All Autophagy inhibitors, including antimalaria drugs, interrupt lysosome functions at the outer cell membrane, a location associated with malignant cancer behavior. These activities are called "antegrade lysosome trafficking," in which lysosomes migrate to the cell membrane where they release acid and digestive enzymes into the extracellular matrix in preparation for invasion of cancer into the tissues. Once tissues in the extracellular space are digested by the enzymes, the free proteins, fats, and sugars can be engulfed by the folds in the cancer cell membrane in a process called "macropinocytosis," providing building blocks and nutrition for the cancer cell's voracious appetite for growth and replication. (15–22)

Mefloquine Most Potent

In 2012, Dr. Natasha Sharma et al. studied the effect of mefloquine on breast cancer cells in vitro, finding mefloquine the most potent of the three antimalarial drugs, causing expansion and disruption of lysosomes. (23)

Artemisinin/Mefloquin Anti-Cancer Synergy

Since considerable synergy for malaria treatment can be found with the artesunate/mefloquine combination, one might expect synergy for anti-cancer treatment, as well. This was found to be the case in 2013, by Dr. Sukhai's group in Toronto, working with a leukemia cell line in vitro and in vivo. After screening a list of on- and off-patent drugs for anti-leukemic activity, Dr. Mahadeo Sukhai's group found ivermectin to be most active, and mefloquine second most active. Dr. Sukhai determined that mefloquine accumulates in lysosomes of cancer cells and disrupts the lysosome outer membrane, causing release of lysosomal acid and enzymes (called cathepsins) into the cytosol (the fluid contents of the cell), triggering cell death. Dr. Sukhai et al. write:

> Unregulated release of lysosomal hydrolases and proteases into the cytosol triggers caspase-independent cell death. (24)

Once mefloquine was identified as the second most active anti-cancer drug for leukemia, Dr. Sukhai's group screened 500 drugs for synergy with mefloquine. The drugs showing the best synergy were artemisinin and artesunate derivatives, which also disrupt lysosomes by generating ROS in the lysosome. This is caused by a "Fenton Reaction." The oxygen in the peroxide bridge of the artesunate molecule reacts with iron in the lysosomes, which release ROS, which damages and disrupts the lysosome membrane, releasing free iron into the cytosol, as described by Dr. Hamacher-Brady in 2011. (25)

Next, Dr. Sukhia's group used haploinsufficiency profiling (HIP), a genomics platform, to elucidate the mechanism of mefloquine's anti-leukemic activity. This testing indicated that mefloquine specifically targets lysosomal functions. This was previously demonstrated in 1992 by Dr. Hans Glaumann et al. who studied the effect of mefloquine on mouse hepatic (liver) lysosomes after a single drug administration, finding the mefloquine was trapped and accumulated in the lysosomes, which appeared to expand. The effect lasted for 7 days after a single drug administration. This explains the weekly 250 mg mefloquine tablet for travelers.

Dr. Glaumann et al. write:

Expansion of intra-hepatic lysosomes starting at 24 hours after administration, and lasting for 7 days in mice. The lysosomes later harbored multi-lamellar bodies which disappeared after 7–10 days. (26)

Lysosomal Disruption from Mefloquine

Dr. Sukhai's group then studied the effect of Mefloquine on isolated lysosomes taken from cell samples from Leukemia patients, finding that mefloquine disrupted lysosomes with the release of lysosomal contents (enzymes, cathepsins B and L). Moreover, there were no similar effects on mitochondria, which were spared. The lysosomal disrupting effect of mefloquine effects were selective for (AML) leukemia cells, which showed abundant lysosomal enzyme contents (cathepsin B) which had been released into the cytoplasm. Normal hematopoietic cells were unaffected, with intact lysosomes and no release of cathepsin B (lysosomal contents) into the cytoplasm. (24)

Leukemia Cell have Upregulated, Larger Lysosomes

Targeting the lysosome of the cancer cell has been suggested by various authors as an "Achilles heel" to be exploited. When stressed by starvation, hypoxia, or anti-cancer drug treatment, many cancers switch into "survival mode" by activating "protective autophagy," in which lysosomes migrate centrally in the cell and cluster around the cell nucleus (perinuclear clustering). One might envision this process as a two-way railroad system made up of the cell's microtubules system for back and forth migration of lysosomes from periphery (antegrade trafficking) to central (perinuclear clustering-protective autophagy).

The movement of lysosomes from central to peripheral location in the cancer cell is associated with aggressive cancer behavior. This scenario is described nicely by Drs. Flora Guerra and Ceclia Buccioi (2019), who studied RAB7, a protein closely associated with endosomal and lysosomal functions in prostate cancer cells.

Dr. Guerra et al. write:

> It is known that in human prostate cancer DU-145 cells the intracellular localization of lysosomes generally closer to the cell surface determines the secretion of proteases favoring cell invasion ... Instead, perinuclear localization of lysosomes is a common feature of less invasive cells, which do not usually secrete large amounts of acid hydrolases. The movement of lysosomes in the cells are guaranteed by microtubules and actin filaments utilizing molecular motor protein such as dynein, kinesin, and/or myosin family members. (27)

In the scenario of "protective autophagy" with perinuclear clustering of lysosomes, the cancer cell becomes more susceptible to apoptosis from lysosomal targeting drugs, which push the cancer cell closer to a cliff called the "apoptotic threshold," as discussed below by Drs. Kenneth Tompkins et al. and Shengfu Piao et al. (28–29)

Leukemia Has Larger Lysosomes

Dr. Sukhai reported that Leukemia cells have lysosomes two to three times larger than those of normal cells and have upregulated the genes responsible for lysosome biogenesis with overexpressed messenger RNA coding for the cathepsin enzymes inside lysosomes. This was also true for LIC (leukemia-initiating stem cells). Dr. Mahadevo Sukahi's group then did in vivo xenograft studies in mice with implanted leukemia cells, again showing mefloquine effective at reducing tumor size and weight with little or no toxicity to the mouse. (24)

Mefloquin Effective for Various Cancer Cells Types

For gastric cancer, mefloquine potently inhibits proliferation and induces apoptosis in vitro and in vivo at low concentrations (EC50 = 0.5–0.7 micromolar). Mefloquine has synergy with the chemotherapy drug paclitaxel and downregulates the PI3K/Akt/mTOR pathway. (30) It is effective for the following cancer cell types:

- Breast cancer (23)
- Prostate cancer (31–32)
- Cervical cancer (33)
- CLL chronic lymphocytic leukemia (34)
- Esophageal squamous cell cancer (induction of mitophagy - mitochondrial autophagy) (35)
- Neuroblastoma (36)
- Colorectal cancer (37) (inhibits NF-kB)
- Liver cancer (38) (targets Wnt/β-Catenin)
- Acute myeloid leukemia (AML) (24) (39)
- Enhancement of chemotherapy in MDR drug resistance (40–41) (inhibits p-glycoprotein)
- Glioblastoma (42) (inhibits ATP synthase)

- Blast-phase chronic leukemia—synergy with tyrosine kinase inhibitors (43–44)

Mefloquin is a CSC agent (45–47)

Mefloquin Synergy with Tyrosine Kinase Inhibitors in Leukemia

In 2019, Dr. Hui Lam Yi et al. studied combining mefloquine with tyrosine kinase inhibitor drugs (TKIs, imatinib, dasatinib and ponatinib) in chronic myelogenous leukemia (CML) cell lines, in vitro. Dr. Yi et al. found that the antimalarial agent mefloquine augments the efficacy of TKIs in CML cell lines and primary CML cells in vitro, including those with the T315I mutation. This effect is selective, sparing normal cells. (43)

Dr. Yi's group write that mefloquine preferentially targets CSCs (we will later discuss the link between autophagy inhibition and CD34+ leukemia CSCs):

> Mefloquine preferentially targets CML [chronic myelogenous leukemia stem cells] CD34+ stem/progenitor cells and augments the efficacy of BCR-ABL1 TKIs [B-Cell receptor tyrosine kinase drugs] by inducing lysosomal dysfunction. (43)

Mefloquin Eliminates Colon Cancer Stem Cells

In 2019, Dr. Mitsunobu Takeda et al. studied a colon cancer mouse xenograft model, finding that disruption of lysosomal activity with mefloquine is the key to eliminating CSCs. Specifically, inhibition of the endolysosomal RAB5/7 proteins with mefloquine eliminated colorectal CSCs. Of the three antimalarial autophagy inhibitors, mefloquine was more effective at lower serum concentration than chloroquine and hydroxychloroquine.

Cancer Stem Cells Express Lower ROS Levels

Dr. Takeda's lab knew that CSCs have upregulated their metabolism and upregulated defenses against ROS (i.e., they are able to eliminate ROS). This confers drug resistance and protects the CSC from the toxic effects of chemotherapy and radiation. Dr. Takeda's lab screened colon cancer cells for a surface antigen marker for lower ROS levels, identifying the lysosomal-associated membrane protein 1 (LAMP1). This is the main protein of the endosome/lysosome pathway and identifies these cells as CSCs with lower ROS levels, compared to non-stem cells. The bold goal of Dr. Takeda's group is to develop a curative therapy for colon cancer based on the CSC concept, writing:

> We aimed to clarify the role of the endosome/lysosome pathway in the maintenance of colorectal CSCs and to identify key regulators of the endosome/lysosome pathway that potentially become a target for the development of curative colorectal cancer treatment based on the CSC concept. (45)

Dr. Takeda et al. made a number of findings during their study:

- Autolysosome-activated cells are tumor-initiating and long-term dye-retaining cells.
- Long-term dye-retaining ability also revealed cell dormancy or slow growth as unique characteristics of stem cells and CSCs.

- LysoTracker labeling and LAMP1 expression were moderately down-regulated by CQ (chloroquine) or HQ (hydroxychloroquine) treatment but almost completely suppressed by MQ (mefloquine) treatment.

- Autolysosome-activated cells are tumor-initiating (CSCs) and long-term dye-retaining cells (dormant).

- MQ (Mefloquine) treatment completely suppressed LAMP1 and LAMP2 expression.

- Chemotherapy **increased** CSC fraction (84%). MQ **decreased** it (9.4%).

- The combination of mefloquine with chemotherapy dramatically decreased CSC population (0.1%).

- Mefloquine treatment in cancer xenografts decreased LAMP protein and CSC markers, and inhibited lysosomal activity by targeting RAB 5 and RAB7 proteins.

- In mouse xenografts, the combination of MQ with chemotherapy "drastically reduced" tumor volume compared to single-agent use.

- Treatment with MQ alone or MQ with chemotherapy was safe with no adverse effects.

Dr. Takeda's group write:

We expect that mefloquine may induce depletion of CSCs and, due to a synergistic effect, demolish the cancer hierarchy, including cancer precursor cells, when given in combination with cytotoxic anti-cancer drugs ... Accordingly, we suggest that mefloquine is a promising candidate for colon CSC-targeting therapy. (45)

Mefloquine Targets the RAB7 Protein

One of Dr. Takeda's group's findings, above, was that mefloquine targets the RAB 7 protein (Ras-related in brain 7), the key protein regulating endosomal/ lysosomal trafficking and perinuclear clustering.

Drs. Flora Guerra and Bucci (2019) reviewed the role of the RAB7 protein, writing:

The RAB [Ras-related in brain] protein family ... regulates ... vesicular trafficking events.... ubiquitously expressed, mainly localized to late endosomes and with a pivotal role in endocytic trafficking. Indeed, RAB7A regulates maturation of early endosome into late endosome, transport from early endosomes to late endosome and lysosomes, clustering and fusion of late endosomes and lysosomes in perinuclear region and lysosomal biogenesis ... In addition of these functions.... RAB7A has many other cellular roles, being involved in autophagy, apoptosis, phagocytosis, in retromer regulation, mitophagy, and lipophagy as well as in cytoskeleton organization ... (27)

RAB7 Protein and Cancer Progression

In addition, RAB7 is an oncogenic protein with various functions in cancer progression. According to Drs. Flora Guerra and Cecilia Bucci in 2019,

RAB7A determines the acquisition of invasion and metastasis features [by the cancer cell] via the following activities:

Induction of actin cytoskeleton organization.

Internalization and recycling of MT-1-MMP [Matrix Metallo-Proteinase Enzyme] to allow digestion and degradation of the extracellular matrix.

Interaction with mTOR to decrease number of mitochondria, induce MDSC [myeloid-derived suppressor cells], and T cell suppression to allow cancer evasion of the host immune system.

Induction of Akt-mediated survival signaling, resisting apoptosis, evading growth suppressors, and sustained proliferation signaling. (27) [end quote]

Autophagy as a Major Metabolic Pathway

Now we can easily understand why we have included Autophagy as one of the "three pillars of cancer cell metabolism," the other two being, OXPHOS and GLYCOLYSIS. In addition, as we see above, autophagy/lysosomal function is a major component of CSC maintenance. Here we have expanded the concept of "Autophagy" to broadly include all other functions of the endosome/lysosomal system in the cancer cell.

Autophagy/Lysosomes are Metabolic Players

Dr. L. Martinez-Carreres et al. (2017) write:

Many investigations have proved that lysosomes are not only degradative organelles but also participate in metabolism of the entire cell at different levels, and their modifications can promote or repress cell proliferation.

In this beautifully written passage, Dr. Martinez-Carreres et al. aptly describe how cell starvation (hypoxia or stress) induces lysosomal perinuclear clustering, while nutrient replenishment induces the opposite, antegrade lysosomal trafficking to the cell membrane:

[Cancer cell] starvation increases pH, causing lysosomes to cluster near the microtubule-organizing center (MTOC), facilitating autophagosome–lysosome fusion…. Conversely, nutrient replenishment restores basal pH, inducing lysosomal scattering, which brings lysosomal mTORC1 to the cell periphery and stimulates its activity by increasing its coupling to the gradient of signaling molecules emanating from the plasma membrane. (46)

Anti-Cancer Stem Cell Activity in AML

In 2012, Dr. Eleftherios Sachlos et al. screened a library of 590 compounds for anti-CSC activity in AML by inducing differentiation of hematopoietic CSCs, while not affecting normal cells. Mefloquine was one of two candidate drugs showing LC50 values below the 10 micromolar threshold. This is certainly consistent with Dr. Takeda's study above. Surprisingly, Dr. Sachlos's group's top candidate drug was thioridazine, an FDA-approved antipsychotic dopamine receptor antagonist of the phenothiazine group. (**Note**: LC50=lethal dose causing 50% cell death)(47)

Clotrimazole Synergy with Mefloquin

Although artesunate/mefloquine combination showed the highest synergy against leukemia cells, Dr. Sukhai et al. also found the antifungal drug clotrimazole had good anti-cancer synergy when used in combination with mefloquine. However, clotrimazole is not available as an oral drug, being limited to topical use only. (24)

Mefloquine for AML Cancer Stem Cells

Dr. Sukhai's group's AML (acute myelogenous leukemia) study showed that mefloquine was equally effective for leukemia CSCs both in vitro and in vivo mouse xenografts. Leukemia stem cells have "overexpressed" genes for lysosomes, and indeed, have larger and more numerous lysosomes. They wrote:

> Leukemia-initiating cells [stem cells] overexpressed lysosomal biogenesis genes. These results demonstrate that **lysosomal disruption preferentially targets AML cells and AML progenitor cells,** providing a rationale for testing lysosomal disruption as a novel therapeutic strategy for AML. (24)

Mefloquine Patents

Mefloquin is patented as a treatment for cancer, specifically in combination with tyrosine kinase inhibitor drugs in CML. (48–50)

Mefloquine Anti-Cancer Blood Levels

In 2013, Dr. Kun-Huang Yan et al. studied mefloquine (MQ) in a prostate cancer cell model, finding that mefloquine had highly selective anti-cancer activities. Although prostate cancer cells were sensitive to the cytotoxic effects of MQ at 10 micromolar, other normal cells such as fibroblasts were unaffected. Dr. Yan's group noted that mefloquine blood levels in the 2.1–23 micromolar range are typically found with antimalaria therapy, while blood levels in the 3–4 micromolar range are found with malaria prophylaxis for travelers. This can be compared to the 4–10 micromolar range found effective for cancer treatment in Dr. Sukhai's in vitro leukemia cell study. (24) (32)

Mefloquine Retinal Toxicity and Neurotoxicity

Caution is advised before using mefloquine as well as other quinolone drugs, such as chloroquine and hydroxychloroquine. Although originally marketed as safe for malaria prophylaxis, recent studies show an alarming incidence of neurologic toxicity, which may be "clinically occult, and in some cases, irreversible." (7–13)

A possible mechanism of mefloquin toxicity was elucidated by Dr. Anthony Mawson in 2013, suggesting a retinoid (vitamin A) toxicity hypothesis. (13)

Mefloquin Inhibition of Drug Efflux Pumps

In 2018, Drs. G. Mereddy and C. T. Ronayne reviewed mefloquine (MQ) as a repurposed anti-cancer agent for glioblastoma, writing this very enthusiastic summary:

> MQ showed potent inhibition of Glioblastoma cells at low 10 micromolar concentration. MQ inhibits autophagy at the stage of autophagosome formation in … BCa [Breast Cancer] cells. MQ potently inhibited cell proliferation and induced apoptosis against several human gastric cancer cell lines with IC50 values ranging from 0.5–0.7 μM.… MQ **potently inhibits drug efflux pumps** that are often upregulated in drug-resistant cancer cells. By inhibiting these pumps, MQ chemo-sensitized resistant cells to standard chemotherapeutic agents … Although long-term

usage of MQ has psychiatric and neurological side effects in some patients, **its utility may be justified in late-stage cancer patients with limited treatment options** … MQ has pleiotropic effects on cancer cells that include inhibition of autophagy, lysosomal disruption, inhibition of various signaling pathways, and inhibition of Pgp pumps [drug resistance pumps].… **MQ's ready and inexpensive availability and long-standing record of clinical use qualify this drug for repurposing for anti-cancer applications.** (50)

Conclusion

Autophagy inhibition is one of the three pillars of cancer cell metabolism, and inclusion of an autophagy inhibitor is considered essential for a successful repurposed drug program. Although more potent as an anti-cancer agent, mefloquine's associated toxicities have made hydroxychloroquine (Plaquenil®) a safer choice for autophagy inhibitor (see the following chapter). Alternate autophagy inhibitors such as propranolol, clarithromycin, and pyrvinium might be considered, as these agents are both OXPHOS and Autophagy inhibitors that synergize with GLYCOLYSIS inhibitors such as DCA. Safer alternate autophagy inhibitors with a less toxic profile include loratadine (Claritin®), PPI inhibitors, and thymoquinone. There appears to be a link between autophagy and CSCs, making the addition of autophagy inhibitor essential for CSC eradication. As always, work closely with a knowledgeable physician when contemplating such a repurposed drug program.

References for Chapter 31: Mefloquine Autophagy Inhibitor

1) Agomo, P. U., and Lagos Yaba. "Efficacy and safety of Artesunate+ Mefloquine (Artequin 8) in the Treatment of Uncomplicated Falciparum malaria in Ijede Community, Ikorodu LGA, Lagos State, Nigeria" J. Med. Sci 7.5 (2007): 816-824.

2) Krudsood, S., et al. "Artesunate and mefloquine given simultaneously for three days via a prepacked blister is equally effective and tolerated as a standard sequential treatment of uncomplicated acute Plasmodium falciparum malaria: randomized, double-blind study in Thailand." The American journal of tropical medicine and hygiene 67.5 (2002): 465-472.

3) Reuter, Stephanie E., et al. "Population pharmacokinetics of orally administered mefloquine in healthy volunteers and patients with uncomplicated Plasmodium falciparum malaria." Journal of Antimicrobial Chemotherapy (2014): dku430.

4) Krudsood, S., et al. "New fixed-dose artesunate-mefloquine formulation against multidrug-resistant Plasmodium falciparum in adults: a comparative phase IIb safety and pharmacokinetic study with standard-dose nonfixed artesunate plus mefloquine." Antimicrobial agents and chemotherapy 54.9 (2010): 3730-3737.

5) Marquino, Wilmer, et al. "Efficacy of mefloquine and a mefloquine-artesunate combination therapy for the treatment of uncomplicated Plasmodium falciparum malaria in the Amazon Basin of Peru." The American journal of tropical medicine and hygiene 68.5 (2003): 608-612.

6) Wang, W., W. Yang, and S. T. Micha. "Efficacy of dihydroartemisinin-mefloquine on acute uncomplicated falciparum malaria." Chinese medical journal 114.6 (2001): 612-613.

7) Harinasuta, T., Danai Bunnag, and W. H. Wernsdorfer. "A phase II clinical trial of mefloquine in patients with chloroquine-resistant falciparum malaria in Thailand." Bulletin of the World Health Organization 61.2 (1983): 299.

8) Dow, G., et al. "Mefloquine induces dose-related neurological effects in a rat model." Antimicrobial agents and chemotherapy 50.3 (2006): 1045-1053.

9) Nevin, Remington L. "A serious nightmare: psychiatric and neurologic adverse reactions to mefloquine are serious adverse reactions." Pharmacology research & perspectives 5.4 (2017): e00328.

10) Lee, Sue J., et al. "Adverse effects of mefloquine for the treatment of uncomplicated malaria in Thailand: A pooled analysis of 19,850 individual patients." PloS one 12.2 (2017): e0168780.

11) Ekanem, Theresa, et al. "Combination therapy antimalarial drugs mefloquine and artequin induce reactive astrocyte formation on the hippocampus of rats." BMC Proceedings. Vol. 2. No. S1. BioMed Central, 2008.

12) Udoh, Nsikan-Abasi B., et al. "Hippocampal Glial Degenerative Potentials of Mefloquine and Artequin in Adult Wistar Rats." International Journal of Brain Science 2014 (2014).

13) Mawson, Anthony. "Mefloquine use, psychosis, and violence: a retinoid toxicity hypothesis." Medical Science Monitor Basic Research 19 (2013): 579-583.

14) Fischer, Philip R. "Mefloquine: Still Effective and Still Safe for Malaria Chemoprophylaxis." Infectious Disease Alert 37.6 (2018).

15) Nujić, Krunoslav, et al. "Impairment of lysosomal functions by azithromycin and chloroquine contributes to anti-inflammatory phenotype." Cellular immunology 279.1 (2012): 78-86.

16) Tietz, Pamela S., Kiyoshi Yamazaki, and Nicholas F. Larusso. "Time-dependent effects of chloroquine on pH of hepatocyte lysosomes." Biochemical pharmacology 40.6 (1990): 1419-1421.

17) Gonzalez-Noriega, Alfonso, et al. "Chloroquine inhibits lysosomal enzyme pinocytosis and enhances lysosomal enzyme secretion by impairing receptor recycling." The Journal of cell biology 85.3 (1980): 839-852.

18) Krogstad, Donald J., and Paul H. Schlesinger. "The basis of antimalarial action: non-weak base effects of chloroquine on acid vesicle pH." The American journal of tropical medicine and hygiene 36.2 (1987): 213-220.

19) Browning, David J. "Pharmacology of chloroquine and hydroxychloroquine." Hydroxychloroquine and chloroquine retinopathy. Springer, New York, NY, 2014. 35-63.

20) Florey, Oliver, and Michael Overholtzer. "Macropinocytosis and autophagy crosstalk in nutrient scavenging." Philosophical Transactions of the Royal Society B 374.1765 (2019): 20180154.

21) Yoshida, Sei, et al. "Macropinocytosis, mTORC1 and cellular growth control." Cellular and Molecular Life Sciences 75.7 (2018): 1227-1239.

22) Jayashankar, Vaishali, and Aimee L. Edinger. "Macropinocytosis confers resistance to therapies targeting cancer anabolism." Nature Communications 11.1 (2020): 1-15.

23) Sharma, Natasha, et al. "Inhibition of autophagy and induction of breast cancer cell death by mefloquine, an antimalarial agent." Cancer Letters 326.2 (2012): 143-154.

24) Sukhai, Mahadeo A., et al. "Lysosomal disruption preferentially targets acute myeloid leukemia cells and progenitors." The Journal of clinical investigation 123.1 (2013): 315-328.

25) Hamacher-Brady, Anne, et al. "Artesunate activates mitochondrial apoptosis in breast cancer cells via iron-catalyzed lysosomal reactive oxygen species production." Journal of Biological Chemistry 286.8 (2011): 6587-6601.

26) Glaumann, Hans, Anne-Marie Motakefi, and Helena Jansson. "Intracellular distribution and effect of the antimalarial drug mefloquine on lysosomes of rat liver." Liver 12.4 (1992): 183-190.

27) Guerra, Flora, and Cecilia Bucci. "Role of the RAB7 Protein in Tumor Progression and Cisplatin Chemoresistance." Cancers 11.8 (2019): 1096.

28) Tompkins, Kenneth D., and Andrew Thorburn. "Focus: Death: Regulation of Apoptosis by Autophagy to Enhance Cancer Therapy." The Yale Journal of Biology and Medicine 92.4 (2019): 707.

29) Piao, Shengfu, and Ravi K. Amaravadi. "Targeting the lysosome in cancer." Annals of the New York Academy of Sciences 1371.1 (2016): 45.

30) Liu, Yanwei, et al. "Mefloquine effectively targets gastric cancer cells through phosphatase-dependent inhibition of PI3K/Akt/mTOR signaling pathway." Biochemical and biophysical research communications 470.2 (2016): 350-355.

31) Yan, Kun-Huang, et al. "Mefloquine induces cell death in prostate cancer cells and provides a potential novel treatment strategy in vivo." Oncology letters 5.5 (2013): 1567-1571.

32) Yan, Kun-Huang, et al. "Mefloquine exerts anticancer activity in prostate cancer cells via ROS-mediated modulation of Akt, ERK, JNK and AMPK signaling." Oncology letters 5.5 (2013): 1541-1545.

33) Li, Hui, et al. "Therapeutic effects of antibiotic drug mefloquine against cervical cancer through impairing mitochondrial function and inhibiting mTOR pathway." Canadian journal of physiology and pharmacology 95.1 (2017): 43-50.

34) Das, Subhadip, et al. "Antimalarial drugs trigger lysosome-mediated cell death in chronic lymphocytic leukemia (CLL) cells." Leukemia research 70 (2018): 79-86.

35) Xie, Yifei, et al. "Mefloquine Inhibited Esophageal Squamous Cells Carcinoma Proliferation by Induction of Mitochondrial Autophagy." Available at SSRN 3429885 (2019).

36) Kumar, Abhishek, Debasish Kumar Ghosh, and Akash Ranjan. "Mefloquine binding to human acyl-CoA binding protein leads to redox stress mediated apoptotic death of human neuroblastoma cells." NeuroToxicology (2020).

37) Xu, Xin, et al. "Antimalarial drug mefloquine inhibits nuclear factor kappa B signaling and induces apoptosis in colorectal cancer cells." Cancer science 109.4 (2018): 1220-1229.

38) Li, Yu-Hui, et al. "Mefloquine targets β-catenin pathway and thus can play a role in the treatment of liver cancer." Microbial pathogenesis 118 (2018): 357-360.

39) Phan, Jessica L., et al. "The Evaluation of Mefloquine Drug Repurposing on Acute Myeloid Leukemia." (2018).

40) Fujita, R., et al. "Enhancement of doxorubicin activity in multidrug-resistant cells by mefloquine." Methods and findings in experimental and clinical pharmacology 22.5 (2000): 281-284.

41) Kim, Ju-Hwa, et al. "Co-treatment with the anti-malarial drugs mefloquine and primaquine highly sensitizes drug-resistant cancer cells by increasing P-gp inhibition." Biochemical and biophysical research communications 441.3 (2013): 655-660.

42) Sharma, Natasha, et al. "Reduced glucose uptake and inhibition of ATP synthase by mefloquine results in death of glioblastoma multiforme." (2013): 1853-1853.

43) Yi, Hui Lam, et al. "Lysosome Inhibition by Mefloquine Preferentially Enhances the Cytotoxic Effects of Tyrosine Kinase Inhibitors in Blast Phase Chronic Myeloid Leukemia." Translational oncology 12.9 (2019): 1221-1228.

44) Xiang, Wei, et al. "Mefloquine enhances the cytotoxic effects of tyrosine kinase inhibitors in blast phase chronic myeloid leukaemia by lysosome membrane disruption." (2017): 1050-1050.

45) Takeda, Mitsunobu, et al. "Disruption of endolysosomal rab5/7 efficiently eliminates colorectal cancer stem cells." Cancer research 79.7 (2019): 1426-1437.

46) Martinez-Carreres, L., A. Nasrallah, and L. Fajas. "Cancer: Linking Powerhouses to Suicidal Bags." Frontiers in Oncology 7 (2017).

47) Sachlos, Eleftherios, et al. "Identification of drugs including a dopamine receptor antagonist that selectively target cancer stem cells." Cell 149.6 (2012): 1284-1297.

48) Carson, Dennis, Lorenzo Leoni, and Howard Cottam. "Treatment of Cancer with Mefloquine, its purified enantiomers, and mefloquine analogs." U.S. Patent Application No. 10/509,693.

49) Muller, Edgar, and Max Scheiwe. "Pharmaceutical combination of artesunate and mefloquine for therapy of malaria." U.S. Patent Application No. 10/504,651.

50) Mereddy, G. R., and C. T. Ronayne. "Repurposing Antimalarial Drug Mefloquine for Cancer Treatment." Transl Med (Sunnyvale) 8.199 (2018): 2161-1025.

Chapter 32

Autophagy Inhibitors Part 2:
Chloroquine and Hydroxychloroquine

ALTHOUGH MEFLOQUINE IS A SUPERB anti-cancer stem cell (CSC) drug, discussed in the previous chapter, concerns about neurotoxicity have cooled initial enthusiasm for its use as a repurposed anti-cancer drug. Attention has been redirected to safer versions of the quinolone family of antimalaria drugs, chloroquine and hydroxychloroquine. Although safer, they are less potent as anti-cancer drugs when compared to mefloquine.

Chloroquine Antimalaria Drug from Cinchona Tree

Chloroquine, originally derived from the bark of the cinchona tree, was synthesized in 1934 and FDA-approved in 1949. Hydroxychloroquine (Plaquenil®) was FDA-approved in 1955. Both are used for prevention and treatment of malaria, serving as autophagy inhibitors, with accumulation of the drug in lysosomes, raising the pH (more alkaline, less acid) and preventing fusion of lysosomes with autophagosomes. (1)

Inhibiting Macropinocytosis

In addition, autophagy inhibitor drugs such as chloroquine and hydroxychloroquine inhibit macropinocytosis, a process utilized by cancer cells to promote tumor invasion involving the engulfment of fluids and nutrients from the extracellular matrix into the cancer cell to provide nutrition. The reverse is also true: The extrusion of acid and digestive proteins from the cancer cell into the extracellular matrix serves to dissolve tissues to aid tumor invasion. (2)

What is Macropinocytosis?

Remember those old biology class movies of single-celled amoeba parasites engulfing their food with pseudopod extensions? Human and mammalian cells do the same thing. It's called macropinocytosis, originally observed in the 1930s by Warren Lewis viewing macrophages, tumor cells, and amoebas under the microscope. (2–6)

In 2019, Dr. Jason King and Robert Jay write on the origins and evolution of macropinocytosis:

> In macropinocytosis, cells take up…. droplets of medium into internal vesicles. These vesicles are acidified and fused to lysosomes, their contents digested and useful compounds extracted…. Macropinocytosis … is described in both metazoa and amoebae, but not in plants or fungi. Its evolutionary origin goes back to at least the common ancestor of the amoebozoa … The primary function of macropinocytosis in amoebae and some cancer cells is feeding … [and] has been adapted in immune cells for antigen presentation. Macro-pinocytic cups are large, actin-driven processes, closely related to phagocytic cups and pseudopods. (4)

Note: Actin is a scaffolding protein of the cytoskeleton, the cell's microtubule system.

Invadopedia and Matrix Degradation

Cancer cells can use macropinocytosis to take in nutrients from outside the cell, and the endosome/lysosome can also be used by the cancer cell to extrude various substances out to the extracellular space. In a process visually similar to the way an amoeba sends out pseudopods, the cancer cell sends out "invadopedia" or "podosomes" to degrade the extracellular matrix. In a process called exocytosis, acidic lysosomal contents (cathepsin B) and digestive proteins such as matrix metallo-proteinase (MMP) are extruded by the cancer cell to the extracellular matrix to dissolve tissues and promote tumor invasion. So, when we are talking about autophagy inhibitors, we are speaking in broad terms, which include the inhibition of these other lysosomal functions—namely, the use of endosomes/lysosomes to obtain nutrition from the micro-environment and the use of lysosomes to degrade the extracellular matrix, promoting tumor invasion. (7–9)

Autophagy Inhibition and Apoptotic Threshold

The role of autophagy inhibition in cancer treatment was discussed in 2019 by Drs. Kenneth D. Tompkins and Andrew Thorburn. They propose that autophagy inhibition affects the "threshold for apoptosis" (programmed cell death), with implications for all of cancer therapy. Here is their bold statement:

We propose that … autophagy inhibition is affecting something much more fundamental –- **the apoptotic threshold**, which as we described above, ultimately determines whether all cells, normal or cancer, die or not and explains the fundamental basis for why cancer therapy is possible at all. (10)

The idea is a simple one. Dormant CSCs resist anti-cancer drugs by going into a hibernation mode called "protective autophagy." This is analogous to how mammals downregulate their metabolism by "hibernating" during winter months when food is scarce, surviving on their fat stores until spring. The cancer cells hibernate until some later time when they are triggered to reactivate and become aggressive.

In addition, protective autophagy prevents apoptosis. Adding an autophagy inhibitor such as chloroquine blocks "protective autophagy" and alters the apoptotic threshold, resensitizing the cancer cell to any form of treatment, chemotherapy, repurposed drug, or nontoxic natural substance.

Providing the Extra "Apoptotic Push": It Doesn't Matter What the Other Drug Is!!

Drs. Tompkins and Thorburn go on to write:

Autophagy inhibition works with many different kinds of anti-cancer agent – **it doesn't matter what the other drug is** so long as it is capable of providing **an extra pro-apoptotic push** in that cancer cell. (10)

Their article has a vivid illustration of this process—a graphic of a cancer cell falling off a cliff when the apoptotic threshold is reached.

Pancreatic Cancer—Autophagy Inhibitor Combination

In 2019, Dr. Conan Kinsey et al. illustrated this point nicely by adding an autophagy inhibitor to pancreatic cancer cells, thereby pushing them over the "apoptotic threshold." Dr. Kinsey's group studied a pancreatic cancer cell line in a mouse xenograft model, finding that activation of the K-RAS/RAF/MEK/ERK signaling pathway was key to cancer cell proliferation. Paradoxically, inhibiting this key pathway with a MEK inhibitor, the FDA-approved drug, trametinib (trade name Mekinist), provided no clinical benefit for pancreatic cancer patients. The reason for this is that the pancreatic cancer cells go into "protective autophagy" mode, making them resistant to the cytotoxic effects of the drug. Dr. Kinsey et al. then added the autophagy inhibitor hydroxychloroquine (HCQ) to the MEK inhibitor drug in the mouse xenograft model, finding the combination was now dramatically effective. They then tried the experiment with other cancers—melanoma and colorectal cancer—showing, similarly, very effective response in the xenograft model with this combination of drugs. (11)

Dr. Kinsey Patient Case Report on Pancreatic Cancer

Emboldened by successful xenograft studies, Dr. Kinsey and his colleagues then treated an 81-year-old refractory pancreatic cancer patient in the clinic with the combination of hydroxychloroquine (600 mg twice daily) along with the MEK inhibitor (2mg of trametinib), finding a remarkable 50% regression of tumor size, resolution of debilitating pain, and dramatic reduction in the CA19–9 tumor marker, with no toxicity. Monthly ophthalmologic exams and weekly electrocardiograms were conducted showing no evidence of ocular or cardiac toxicity.

Superior to Traditional Cytotoxic Chemotherapy

Dr. Kinsey et al. write that this autophagy inhibitor combination is "likely to be superior to traditional cytotoxic chemotherapy":

> Since both trametinib and hydroxychloroquine are orally administered, FDA-approved drugs…. these observations were translated to the clinic for a single, heavily pretreated PDA [pancreatic ductal adenocarcinoma] patient. Remarkably, the T/HCQ [trametinib/hydroxychloroquine] combination resulted in substantial reduction in this patient's overall tumor burden, CA19–9 tumor marker, and resolution of debilitating cancer pain. Moreover, the safety and tolerability of **the T/HCQ combination is likely to be superior to traditional cytotoxic chemotherapy** for PDA patients. (11)

Autophagy Clinical Trials a Failure for Pancreatic Cancer

As mentioned above, preclinical studies in pancreatic cancer using chloroquine and hydroxychloroquine as autophagy inhibitors in vitro and in vivo mouse xenograft studies have been encouraging. However, human clinical trials such as the 2020 study by Dr. Herbert Zeh et al. have been disappointing. (13)

In 2020, Dr. Maria New and Sharon Tooze write:

Despite the promising data in PDAC [pancreatic ductal cancer] cell lines and mouse xenografts showing that autophagy inhibition reduces cell proliferation and tumor size and prolongs mouse survival, clinical outcomes in [human] autophagy inhibitor trials have not seen an improvement on standard-of-care treatment. (12)

In searching for a reason for the failure of clinical trials of autophagy inhibitors in pancreatic cancer, Drs. New and Tooze suggest the problem could be insufficient levels of autophagy inhibition, which could be monitored with the LC3-II marker in human peripheral lymphocytes after hydroxychloroquine (HCQ) treatment.

Drs. New and Tooze make another comment that is in agreement with a basic point made throughout this book: Because of the metabolic plasticity of the CSC, the inhibition of only one metabolic pathway is insufficient to achieve clinical success. Drug combinations to inhibit multiple pathways are needed. In this book, I propose simultaneous inhibition of all three major metabolic pathways (OXPHOS, GLYCOLYSIS and Autophagy) to achieve "synthetic lethality" and long-term remission.

They write:

It is important to ensure that autophagy in tumors is adequately inhibited. It might be that autophagy inhibition alone is insufficient to affect pancreatic tumor growth, and in this case **combination treatments** will likely be explored to elicit a therapeutic response. (12)

Combination Therapy for Stage 4 Pancreatic Cancer: Hydroxychloroquine, Vitamin D3, and Chemotherapy

One such case report of successful use of "combination therapy" is that of Stephen Bigelson, MD. In July 2016, Dr. Bigelson was treated at Weill-Cornell Medical Center for metastatic pancreatic cancer with peritoneal spread and a massively elevated CA19–9 marker of 11,575.

Dr. Bigelson knew chemotherapy alone carried a dismal prognosis. This prompted him to perform a medical literature search looking for combination therapies in addition to the conventional chemotherapy drugs gemcitabine and capecitabine. Dr. Bigelson was also treated with the combination of intravenous paricalcitol (Zemplar®), a vitamin D3 analog (25 mcg three times a week), and the autophagy inhibitor, hydroxychloroquine (600 mg twice a day).

Dr. Bigelson's research paid off with a "complete response" to treatment. As of 2018, he was cancer free with a CA19–9 cancer marker of only 15 U/ml. (down from 11,575), and a follow-up CAT scan showing "no evidence of disease" (NED). Based on large-scale studies, the chances for such a favorable outcome is 1 in 340 or about 0.3 per cent. Dr. Bigelson also references the repurposed use of intravenous vitamin C, statins, metformin, curcumin and aspirin as anti-cancer agents, all discussed elsewhere in this book. (14–15)

The Role of Vitamin D in Cancer Treatment

Paricalcitol is a synthetic version of vitamin D3, considered safer and without the adverse effects of hypercalcemia. Vitamin D analogs in pancreatic cancer have a number of benefits. One is the reduction in the protective layer of stromal cells surrounding the cancer mass, cloaking and protecting the mass from cytotoxic drug treatment. The stromal cells (also called stellate cells) have upregulated vitamin D receptors, and treatment with vitamin D analogs inactivates stromal cell production.

Vitamin D also upregulates the cell cycle inhibitor proteins p21 and p27. Vitamin D blocks the Wnt pathway, suppressing β-catenin mediated gene transcription and reducing inflammatory signaling. Vitamin D also inhibits the mTOR pathway, a major pathway for cancer cell growth and proliferation. Vitamin D also acts as an immunomodulator, increasing anti-tumor T cell penetration into the tumor 10–100 fold. Vitamin D is synergistic with vitamin A and Metformin. Vitamin D is discussed in more detail in Chapter 30. (16–28)

Screening for Synthetic Lethality

In 2014, Dr. V. Bhattacharjee et al. ran a "synthetic lethal screen" on a genome-wide siRNA library looking for gemcitabine sensitizers, finding the vitamin D receptor (VDR) as a top candidate. **Note:** Gemcitabine is the conventional chemotherapy for pancreatic cancer, which stalls DNA replication in cancer cells. The added treatment with paricalcitol depletes the VDRs (Vitamin D receptors) in cancer cells, reducing capacity for repair of chemotherapy-induced DNA damage.

Dr. Bhattacharjee and colleagues write:

Gemcitabine sensitivity was shown to be VDR dependent in multiple PCa [pancreatic cancer] cell lines in clonogenic survival assays ... Thus, inhibition of VDR in PCa cells provides a new way to enhance the efficacy of genotoxic drugs.... We believe that gemcitabine sensitization of VDR-depleted cells is due to their reduced capacity to repair damaged DNA. (18)

In 2010, Dr. Wei-dong Yu et al. studied the effect of calcitriol (the active metabolite of vitamin D) on a pancreatic cancer xenograft model, finding synergy with gemcitabine with "significant reduction in tumor volume compared to single agent" treatment in the xenograft model. Dr. Yu and colleagues write:

Calcitriol causes antiproliferative effects through multiple mechanisms, including the induction of cell cycle arrest, apoptosis and differentiation in vitro and in vivo in a variety of cancer cell types including prostate, breast, colon, skin and leukemic cells. (19)

Autophagy Upregulated in Pancreatic Cancer

Numerous studies over the years have shown upregulated autophagy in pancreatic cancer and inhibition of autophagy has been shown to be beneficial in preclinical studies. (29–36)

In 2011, Dr. Shenghong Yang et al. studied autophagy inhibitors (such as chloroquine) in pancreatic cancer finding robust tumor regression and prolonged survival in mouse xenograft studies, writing:

Inhibition of autophagy by genetic means or chloroquine treatment leads to **robust tumor regression and prolonged survival** in pancreatic cancer xenografts and genetic mouse models. These results suggest autophagy is actually required for tumorigenic growth of pancreatic cancers de novo, and drugs that inactivate this process may have a unique clinical utility in treating pancreatic cancers and other malignancies with a similar dependence on autophagy. As chloroquine and its derivatives are potent inhibitors of autophagy and have been used safely in human patients for decades for a variety of purposes, these results are immediately translatable to the treatment of pancreatic cancer patients, and provide a much needed, novel vantage point of attack. (30)

Pancreatic Cancer Stem Cells Increased Autophagy

In 2012, Dr. Vanessa Rausch et al. studied autophagy in pancreatic cancer cells, finding that hypoxia and starvation in the micro-environment enhanced the survival of CSCs, which had higher levels of Autophagy compared to non-CSCs. Autophagy inhibition reduced the migratory capacity and tumorigenicity of the CSCs and primed them for apoptosis. Dr. Rausch et al. write:

> Our data suggest that enhanced autophagy levels may enable survival of CSC under H/S [hypoxia/starvation]. Interference with autophagy-activating or -inhibiting drugs disturbs the fine-tuned physiological balance of enhanced autophagy in CSC and switches survival signaling to suicide [apoptosis]. (36)

Autophagy Inhibitor Combination in Lymphoma Model

In 2007, Dr. Ravi Amaravadi et al. studied a c-Myc-induced model of lymphoma in genetically modified mice. **Note:** c-Myc is an oncogene (see the Glossary). This type of lymphoma lacks a nuclear P53 gene, which makes it resistant to apoptosis. The lymphoma cells were genetically modified to give them back a P53 gene, which had been re-engineered to activate when a drug, tamoxifen, is administered to the mice. As expected, the c-Myc lymphoma cells resisted treatment with cytotoxic chemotherapy in these mice. However, when the P53 gene in the lymphoma was activated by the administration of tamoxifen, the lymphoma promptly regressed for a short time but then recurred because of induction of "protective autophagy." Addition of autophagy inhibition (i.e., by adding chloroquine) enhanced the ability of either P53 or the chemotherapy drug to induce lymphoma cell death (apoptosis) and prolong the remission. Dr. Amaravadi and colleagues write:

> Activation of p53 was associated with the rapid appearance of apoptotic cells [dead cancer cells] and the induction of autophagy in surviving cells. Inhibition of autophagy with either chloroquine or ATG5 shRNA [short hairpin RNA] enhanced the ability of either p53 activation or alkylating drug therapy to induce tumor cell death. These studies provide evidence that autophagy serves as a survival pathway in tumor cells treated with apoptosis activators and a rationale for the use of autophagy inhibitors such as chloroquine in combination with therapies designed to induce apoptosis in human cancers. (37)

In 2008, Dr. Kirsteen Maclean et al. studied a transgenic mouse model of human Burkitt lymphoma, finding that intermittent chloroquine treatment activates P53 dependent cell death, thus preventing development of lymphoma. This suggests intermittent autophagy inhibition could be used as part of a maintenance program to prevent recurrence or relapse of cancer. Dr. Maclean's group writes:

> Thus chloroquine induces lysosomal stress and provokes a p53-dependent cell death that does not require caspase-mediated apoptosis. These findings specifically demonstrate that intermittent chloroquine use effectively prevents cancer in mouse models of 2 genetically distinct human cancer syndromes, Burkitt lymphoma and ataxia telangiectasia, suggesting that agents targeting lysosome-mediated degradation may be effective in cancer prevention. (87)

Inhibiting Autophagy and Hedgehog in B-cell Lymphoma

In 2016, Dr. Jiajun Fan et al. studied B-cell lymphoma in vitro (B-NHL Raji cells) finding that treatment with vismodegib, an inhibitor of the Hedgehog signaling pathway, induced apoptosis and stimulated "protective autophagy." Simultaneous treatment with an autophagy inhibitor was synergistic. (38–40)

In 2012, Dr. Laia Rosich et al. studied the mTOR inhibitor everolimus in vitro with a B-cell lymphoma line (mantle cell lymphoma), a cell type with activated the mTOR pathway. Resistant lymphoma cells showed a high level of autophagy.

Accordingly, selective triple knockdown of the autophagy genes ATG7, ATG5 and ATG3, and pretreatment with the autophagy inhibitor hydroxychloroquine, efficiently overcame the resistance to Akt/mTOR inhibitors, leading to the activation of the mitochondrial apoptotic pathway.... These results suggest that autophagy induction protects MCL cells from Akt/mTOR targeting and counteracting autophagy may represent an attractive strategy for sensitizing MCL cells to everolimus-based therapy. (41)

Triple-Negative Breast Cancer Cell Model: Combining OXPHOS and Autophagy Inhibition

In 2019, Dr. Etna Abad et al. studied in vitro and in vivo mouse xenografts of a triple-negative breast cancer cell line, using a combination of antibiotic to target mitochondrial ribosomes, along with an autophagy inhibitor. Dr. Abad's group first created in their lab parent CSCs, as well as chemotherapy resistant cancer cells, finding the latter had increased mitochondrial metabolic activity and higher metastatic ability compared to the parent cancer cells. They theorized that an antibiotic to induce mitochondrial dysfunction would inhibit OXPHOS and suppress cancer growth. The antibiotic selected was linezolid, which inhibits mitochondrial ribosomal protein production, similar to the mechanism of doxycycline and clarithromycin. The authors found the antibiotic increased reactive oxygen species (ROS) and activated "protective autophagy." The authors then added the autophagy inhibitor hydroxychloroquine, finding this combination reduced metastatic capacity and delayed tumor growth for both CSCs and drug-resistant cancer cells. One might speculate that Dr. Abad's results would have been even better if a glycolysis Inhibitor (DCA) had been added, targeting all three major metabolic pathways. Dr. Abad et al. write:

> we propose that antibiotics serving as MDF-inducers [MDF= mitochondrial dysfunction] can suppress cancer cell proliferation and decrease tumor growth. In combination with autophagy blockers, such drugs can be repurposed as part of the multitarget anti-cancer therapy. (42)

Preventing the Switch from Dormant to Aggressive

In 2018, Dr. Laura Vera-Ramirez et al. studied autophagy inhibition in "dormant" breast cancer using in vitro and in vivo mouse xenograft models. "Dormant" breast cancer cells are synonymous with the CSC phenotype. As we discussed in previous chapters, CSCs have metabolic plasticity and can switch back and forth from a dormant to an aggressive proliferative state. Autophagy inhibition prevented the "wake-up" of dormant breast CSCs, preventing the switch from the dormant to the proliferative state. Dr. Vera-Ramirez et al. write:

> Autophagy inhibition effectively reduced the metastatic burden in the lungs of transplanted mice and it was proposed that autophagy is required for the switch from dormancy to tumor cell growth, as autophagy inhibition specifically depleted dormant cells from tumors, leaving the proliferative tumor cells intact ... Inhibition

of autophagy may therefore be a potential mechanism to eliminate dormant tumour cells and prevent recurrence of BC [breast cancer]. (43)

Glioblastoma Case Report Autophagy Inhibitor Combination

In 2014, Dr. Jean Levy et al. published a case report of autophagy inhibition in a patient with brainstem ganglioglioma successfully treated with vemurafenib (inhibitor of BRAF kinase) and vinblastine (vinca alkaloid microtubule inhibitor) for one year, until tumor recurrence refractory to further drug or radiation treatment. Quite dramatically, the patient enjoyed a sudden improvement when chloroquine was added to the vemurafenib drug. Dr. Levy et al. write:

> The patient had rapid improvement in the neurologic deficits accompanied by decreased inflammatory signal and stabilization of intracranial CNS [central nervous system] lesions. For a period of time, this patient had to stop taking vemurafenib but remained on CQ [chloroquine]. This too led to increased tumor growth and disease progression. Most importantly, when she was again treated with the combination of vemurafenib plus CQ, her tumor regressed, neurological deficits were again reduced and continued tumor control was maintained for more than two years ... autophagy inhibition with CQ is not only capable of making an active drug better, it can actually overcome the acquired resistance that occurs when a kinase inhibitor stops working. (44–46)

Chloroquine for Glioblastoma Clinical Study: Dr. Sotelo

As of 2019, there were 21 clinical trials evaluating chloroquine for cancer treatment, and 66 for hydroxychloroquine. Perhaps the most promising outcome so far is the 2006 randomized clinical trial by Dr. Julio Sotelo et al. in Mexico, adding oral chloroquine (150 mg/day) to conventional treatment (chemo-radiation) in thirty glioblastoma patients over 12 months. Conventional chemotherapy with temozolomide was given. (47–48) The hydroxychloroquine treated group had two patients still in remission at 24 months, while the control group had no patients surviving past 22 months. Median survival for the chloroquine-treated group was double that of the control patients. Dr. Sotelo and his colleagues write:

> Median survival after surgery was 24 months for chloroquine-treated patients and 11 months for controls. (47–49)

I thought this was very impressive.

Autophagy Inhibition and Cancer Stem Cells

In 2019, Drs. Alexandra Smith and Kay F. Macleod made the bold statement that autophagy is required for CSC maintenance, and confers the ability of CSCs to remain dormant for years:

> Autophagy has emerged over the past several years as a requirement for the maintenance of stemness in both normal tissue stem cells and CSCs. (50)

In 2019, Dr. Francesca Nazio et al. similarly write that autophagy and mitophagy (autophagy involving mitochondria) are key mechanisms for CSCs. (51)

The autophagy inhibitor, chloroquine has been identified as a CSC targeting agent for breast cancer, glioblastoma, chronic myeloid leukemia, and pancreatic cancer. (52–53) In combination with metformin, chloroquine eliminates CSCs in pre malignant lesions. (54)

Chloroquine Targets Cancer Stem Cells and Decreases Ability to Metastasize

In 2016, Dr. Diana Liang et al. studied the effect of chloroquine on triple-negative CSCs in vitro and in vivo xenografts, finding that:

> CQ [chloroquine] effectively targets CSCs via autophagy inhibition, mitochondrial structural damage, and impairment of double-stranded DNA break repair.... CQ effectively diminishes the TNBC [triple negative breast cancer] cells' ability to metastasize in vitro and in a TNBC xenograft model (55)

Numerous studies have revealed the connection between autophagy and CSC maintenance and function; cancer drug chemoresistance, recurrence, and ability to metastasize; and the conversion of non-stem cells to CSCs. (56–66)

Important!! Autophagy Inhibitors must be part of any long-term maintenance program after complete remission to target the dormant CSCs!

CQ or HQ has been studied in the following cancer cell lines:

- Gastric CA in combination with cisplatin (67–68)

- Lung cancer (69–70)
- Acute myelogenous leukemia (71–72)
- Endometrial cancer (resveratrol plus chloroquine) (73–75)
- GI stromal tumors (76)
- Hypopharyngeal and nasopharyngeal cancer (77–78)
- Oral squamous cell cancer (79)
- Glioblastoma with temozolomide (80–81)
- Bladder cancer (82)
- Osteosarcoma (mg63) (83)
- Melanoma (84)
- Advanced solid tumors (85)
- Pancreatic cancer (86)
- Lymphoma (87)(37)(40–41)
- Leukemia (40)

Chloroquine Synergy with Sulforaphane

In 2013, Dr. Vyas reported sulforaphane and chloroquine had synergistic effects in prostate cancer chemoprevention. (88)

Autophagy Inhibition for Viral Disease

Some viruses require uptake into cells via macropinocytosis and replicate within the acidic lysosomes. Lysosomal agents such as chloroquine, hydroxychloroquine and azithromycin alter lysosomal pH, and impair lysosomal function, thus preventing viral replication. These drugs have been repurposed as antiviral agents. Another mechanism of action is that CQ and HCQ act as "zinc ionophores",

meaning they facilitate zinc transport into cells, concentrating zinc in lysosomes, the site of viral replication. It has been known that zinc is a potent antiviral agent by inhibiting RNA polymerase, thus preventing viral replication. A number of clinical studies have shown efficacy of the combination of zinc with hydroxychloroquine (or chloroquine) and azithromycin for coronavirus specifically; efficacy for other RNA viruses might be expected. Other zinc ionophores mentioned are quercetin, epigallocatechin gallate (EGCG), and thymoquinone (89–95) (117–123).

Adverse Effects of Chloroquine and Hydroxychloroquine

Dosage for chloroquine ranges between 100 and 500 mg per day. Dosage for hydroxychloroquine is commonly in the range of 400 mg per day, although dosage as high as 2 grams daily have been used. (96–97)

Hydroxychloroquine (Plaquenil®) is considered safer and less toxic than chloroquine or mefloquine and has been used off-label for decades for various rheumatologic conditions such as systemic lupus erythematosus and connective tissue diseases. About 5 million prescriptions for hydroxychloroquine were written annually from 2011 to 2017. (98) The drug is considered safe when used as a single agent. However, combined use with other mitochondrial toxins may aggravate or increase toxicity.

Toxicity May be Amplified when Used with other Mitochondrial Toxins, Such as OXPHOS Inhibitors

Although the mechanism of action of CQ and HQ involves autophagy and lysosomes, the net sum of their effects results in mitochondrial toxicity. These toxic effects on the mitochondria may be amplified when used in combination with other mitochondrial toxins such as most OXPHOS inhibitors, statins, beta blockers, doxycycline, clarithromycin, niclosamide, pyrvinium, etc. Caution is advised when used in such combinations, as toxicity may limit such use.

Important: Extreme caution is advised when using multiple repurposed drugs that are mitochondrial toxins. Careful clinical and laboratory monitoring for adverse effects is warranted. Pulsed or intermittent use may decrease exposure and reduce toxicity.

The side effects of chloroquine are usually minimal at low doses, while many more toxic effects, such as visual disturbances, gastrointestinal upset, electrocardiographic changes, headache, and pruritus occur at higher doses. Two deaths associated with hydroxychloroquine recorded in the medical literature were middle-aged females with long-standing history of systemic lupus, taking 400 mg of hydroxychloroquine for more than 10 years. Both died of acute heart failure. (100)

Side effects include:

- Mitochondrial dysfunction (toxicity) (102)
- Myopathy (99–100)
- Cardiotoxicity, prolonged QT interval on EKG (100–103)
- Retinopathy (100)(104–106)
- Neuropathy (103)

Other Autophagy Inhibitors—Propranolol

In 2018, Dr. Laura Brohée et al. studied prostate cancer cells in vitro and in vivo, using a combination treatment of glycolysis inhibitor (2DG) and autophagy inhibitor (propranolol), finding that:

> the blockage by propranolol of the autophagy flux induced by 2DG resulted in a strong accumulation of LC3-II and p62 [autophagy marker proteins] and in a massive accumulation of autophagic vesicles … due to autophagy blockade. The propranolol + 2DG treatment efficiently prevents prostate cancer cell proliferation, induces cell apoptosis, alters mitochondrial morphology, inhibits mitochondrial bioenergetics and aggravates ER [endoplasmic reticulum] stress in vitro and also suppresses tumor growth in vivo. (107)

Note: Propranolol serves as both an OXPHOS and an autophagy Inhibitor, so combining propranolol with a GLYCOLYSIS inhibitor such as 2 DG or DCA targets all "three pillars of cancer cell metabolism."

- OXPHOS
- GLYCOLYSIS
- Autophagy

Conclusion

Autophagy inhibition is of equal importance to the other two major metabolic pathways in the cancer cell, OXPHOS and GLYCOLYSIS, all three representing the "three pillars of cancer cell metabolism." Inclusion of autophagy inhibition is essential for initial treatment of the cancer patient and later for a maintenance program for the cancer survivor in remission.

Although mefloquine has more potency as an anti-cancer and anti-CSC agent, the associated retinal, neuropsychiatric and mitochondrial toxicity has made hydroxychloroquine (Plaquenil®) a safer choice as an autophagy inhibitor. Alternate autophagy inhibitors include propranolol, clarithromycin (azithromycin), and pyrvinium; these agents are both OXPHOS and autophagy inhibitors that synergize with GLYCOLYSIS inhibitors such as dichloroacetate (DCA). Alternate autophagy inhibitors with less toxic profile include loratadine (Claritin®), proton pump (PPI) inhibitors, and thymoquinone. Autophagy inhibition is key for eradication of CSCs. As always, work closely with a knowledgeable physician who can assist in laboratory testing and monitor for drug toxicity. (108–116)

References for Chapter 32: Autophagy Inhibitors Part Two Chloroquine and Hydroxychloroquine

1) Verbaanderd, Ciska, et al. "Repurposing Drugs in Oncology (ReDO)—chloroquine and hydroxychloroquine as anti-cancer agents." ecancermedicalscience 11 (2017).

2) Ha, Kevin D., Scott M. Bidlingmaier, and Bin Liu. "Macropinocytosis exploitation by cancers and cancer therapeutics." Frontiers in physiology 7 (2016): 381.

3) Yoshida, Sei, et al. "Macropinocytosis, mTORC1 and cellular growth control." Cellular and Molecular Life Sciences 75.7 (2018): 1227-1239.

4) King, Jason S., and Robert R. Kay. "The origins and evolution of macropinocytosis." Philosophical Transactions of the Royal Society B 374.1765 (2019): 20180158.

5) Meza, Isaura, and Margaret Clarke. "Dynamics of endocytic traffic of Entamoeba histolytica revealed by confocal microscopy and flow cytometry." Cell motility and the cytoskeleton 59.4 (2004): 215-226.

6) Godbold, G. D., and B. J. Mann. "Involvement of the actin cytoskeleton and p21rho-family GTPases in the pathogenesis of the human protozoan parasite Entamoeba histolytica." Brazilian journal of medical and biological research 31.8 (1998): 1049-1058.

7) Tu, Chun, et al. "Lysosomal cathepsin B participates in the podosome-mediated extracellular matrix degradation and invasion via secreted lysosomes in v-Src fibroblasts." Cancer research 68.22 (2008): 9147-9156.

8) Poincloux, Renaud, Floria Lizárraga, and Philippe Chavrier. "Matrix invasion by tumour cells: a focus on MT1-MMP trafficking to invadopodia." Journal of cell science 122.17 (2009): 3015-3024.

9) Frittoli, Emanuela, et al. "Secretory and endo/exocytic trafficking in invadopodia formation: the MT1-MMP paradigm." European journal of cell biology 90.2-3 (2011): 108-114.

10) Tompkins, Kenneth D., and Andrew Thorburn. "Focus: Death: Regulation of Apoptosis by Autophagy to Enhance Cancer Therapy." The Yale Journal of Biology and Medicine 92.4 (2019): 707.

11) Kinsey, Conan G., et al. "Protective autophagy elicited by RAF→ MEK→ ERK inhibition suggests a treatment strategy for RAS-driven cancers." Nature medicine 25.4 (2019): 620-627.

12) New, Maria, and Sharon Tooze. "The Role of Autophagy in Pancreatic Cancer—Recent Advances." Biology 9.1 (2020): 7.

13) Zeh, Herbert, et al. "A randomized phase II preoperative study of autophagy inhibition with high-dose hydroxychloroquine and gemcitabine/nab-paclitaxel in pancreatic cancer patients." Clinical Cancer Research (2020).

14) Bigelsen, Stephen. "AB091. P063. Case report: stage 4 pancreatic cancer to remission using paricalcitol and hydroxychloroquine in addition to traditional chemotherapy." Annals of Pancreatic Cancer (2018).

15) Bigelsen, Stephen. "Evidence-based complementary treatment of pancreatic cancer: a review of adjunct therapies including paricalcitol, hydroxychloroquine, intravenous vitamin C, statins, metformin, curcumin, and aspirin." Cancer Management and Research 10 (2018): 2003.

16) Sherman, Mara H., et al. "Vitamin D receptor-mediated stromal reprogramming suppresses pancreatitis and enhances pancreatic cancer therapy." Cell 159.1 (2014): 80-93.

17) Schwartz, Gary G., et al. "19-nor-1α, 25-Dihydroxyvitamin D2 (Paricalcitol) inhibits the proliferation of human pancreatic cancer cells in vitro and in vivo." Cancer biology & therapy 7.3 (2008): 430-436.

18) Bhattacharjee, V., Y. Zhou, and T. J. Yen. "A synthetic lethal screen identifies the Vitamin D receptor as a novel gemcitabine sensitizer in pancreatic cancer cells." Cell cycle 13.24 (2014): 3839-3856.

19) Yu, Wei-Dong, et al. "Calcitriol enhances gemcitabine antitumor activity in vitro and in vivo by promoting apoptosis in a human pancreatic carcinoma model system." Cell cycle 9.15 (2010): 3094-3101.

20) Javadinia, Seyed Alireza, et al. "Therapeutic potential of targeting the Wnt/β-catenin pathway in the treatment of pancreatic cancer." Journal of cellular biochemistry 120.5 (2019): 6833-6840.

21) He, Weichun, et al. "Blockade of Wnt/β-catenin signaling by paricalcitol ameliorates proteinuria and kidney injury." Journal of the American Society of Nephrology 22.1 (2011): 90-103.

22) Guo, Li-Shu, et al. "Synergistic antitumor activity of vitamin D3 combined with metformin in human breast carcinoma MDA-MB-231 cells involves m-TOR related signaling pathways." Die Pharmazie-An International Journal of Pharmaceutical Sciences 70.2 (2015): 117-122.

23) Abu el Maaty, Mohamed A., et al. "Differences in p53 status significantly influence the cellular response and cell survival to 1, 25-dihydroxyvitamin D3-metformin cotreatment in colorectal cancer cells." Molecular carcinogenesis 56.11 (2017): 2486-2498.

24) Halder, Sunil K., et al. "Paricalcitol, a vitamin D receptor activator, inhibits tumor formation in a murine model of uterine fibroids." Reproductive sciences 21.9 (2014): 1108-1119.

25) Han, Jing, et al. "Antitumor effects and mechanisms of 1, 25 (OH) 2D3 in the Pfeiffer diffuse large B lymphoma cell line." Molecular medicine reports 20.6 (2019): 5064-5074.

26) Wicks, Sheila, et al. "Combinations of vitamins A, D2 and D3 have synergistic effects in gastric and colon cancer cells." Functional Foods in Health and Disease 9.12 (2019): 749-771.

27) Von Essen, Marina Rode, et al. "Vitamin D controls T cell antigen receptor signaling and activation of human T cells." Nature immunology 11.4 (2010): 344-349.

28) Alagbala, Adebusola A., et al. "Antitumor effects of two less-calcemic vitamin D analogs (Paricalcitol and QW-1624F2-2) in squamous cell carcinoma cells." Oncology 70.6 (2006): 483-492.

29) Bryant, Kirsten L., and Channing J. Der. "Blocking autophagy to starve pancreatic cancer." Nature Reviews Molecular Cell Biology 20.5 (2019): 265-265.

30) Yang, Shenghong, et al. "Pancreatic cancers require autophagy for tumor growth." Genes & development 25.7 (2011): 717-729.

31) New, Maria, et al. "Molecular pathways controlling autophagy in pancreatic cancer." Frontiers in oncology 7 (2017): 28.

32) Boone, Brian A., Herbert J. Zeh III, and Nathan Bahary. "Autophagy inhibition in pancreatic adenocarcinoma." Clinical colorectal cancer 17.1 (2018): 25-31.

33) Yang, Annan, et al. "Autophagy sustains pancreatic cancer growth through both cell-autonomous and nonautonomous mechanisms." Cancer discovery 8.3 (2018): 276-287.

34) Endo, Sho, et al. "Autophagy is required for activation of pancreatic stellate cells, associated with pancreatic cancer progression and promotes growth of pancreatic tumors in mice." Gastroenterology 152.6 (2017): 1492-1506.

35) Sousa, Cristovão M., et al. "Pancreatic stellate cells support tumour metabolism through autophagic alanine secretion." Nature 536.7617 (2016): 479-483.

36) Rausch, Vanessa, et al. "Autophagy mediates survival of pancreatic tumour-initiating cells in a hypoxic microenvironment." The Journal of pathology 227.3 (2012): 325-335.

37) Amaravadi, Ravi K., et al. "Autophagy inhibition enhances therapy-induced apoptosis in a Myc-induced model of lymphoma." The Journal of clinical investigation 117.2 (2007): 326-336.

38) Fan, Jiajun, et al. "A novel therapeutic approach against B-cell non-Hodgkin's lymphoma through co-inhibition of Hedgehog signaling pathway and autophagy." Tumor Biology 37.6 (2016): 7305-7314.

39) Zeng, Xian, and Dianwen Ju. "Hedgehog signaling pathway and autophagy in cancer." International journal of molecular sciences 19.8 (2018): 2279.

40) Djavaheri-Mergny, Mojgan, et al. "Therapeutic modulation of autophagy in leukaemia and lymphoma." Cells 8.2 (2019): 103.

41) Rosich, Laia, et al. "Counteracting autophagy overcomes resistance to everolimus in mantle cell lymphoma." Clinical cancer research 18.19 (2012): 5278-5289.

42) Abad, Etna, et al. "Common metabolic pathways implicated in resistance to chemotherapy point to a key mitochondrial role in breast cancer." Molecular & Cellular Proteomics 18.2 (2019): 231-244.

43) Vera-Ramirez, Laura, et al. "Autophagy promotes the survival of dormant breast cancer cells and metastatic tumour recurrence." Nature communications 9.1 (2018): 1-12.

44) Levy, Jean M. Mulcahy, et al. "Autophagy inhibition improves chemosensitivity in BRAFV600E brain tumors." Cancer Discovery 4.7 (2014): 773-780.

45) Levy, Jean M. Mulcahy, et al. "Autophagy inhibition overcomes multiple mechanisms of resistance to BRAF inhibition in brain tumors." Elife 6 (2017): e19671.

46) Levy, Jean M. Mulcahy, Christina G. Towers, and Andrew Thorburn. "Targeting autophagy in cancer." Nature Reviews Cancer 17.9 (2017): 528.

47) Sotelo, Julio, Eduardo Briceno, and Miguel Angel López-González. "Adding chloroquine to conventional treatment for glioblastoma multiforme: a randomized, double-blind, placebo-controlled trial." Annals of internal medicine 144.5 (2006): 337-343.

48) Weyerhäuser, Patrick, Sven R. Kantelhardt, and Ella L. Kim. "Re-purposing chloroquine for glioblastoma: potential merits and confounding variables." Frontiers in oncology 8 (2018): 335.

49) Pérez-Hernández, Marta, et al. "Targeting autophagy for cancer treatment and Tumor chemosensitization." Cancers 11.10 (2019): 1599.

50) Smith, Alexandra G., and Kay F. Macleod. "Autophagy, cancer stem cells and drug resistance." The Journal of pathology 247.5 (2019): 708-718.

51) Nazio, Francesca, et al. "Autophagy and cancer stem cells: molecular mechanisms and therapeutic applications." Cell Death & Differentiation 26.4 (2019): 690-702.

52) Choi, Dong Soon, et al. "Chloroquine eliminates cancer stem cells through deregulation of Jak2 and DNMT1." Stem cells 32.9 (2014): 2309-2323.

53) Balic, Anamaria, et al. "Chloroquine targets pancreatic cancer stem cells via inhibition of CXCR4 and hedgehog signaling." Molecular cancer therapeutics 13.7 (2014): 1758-1771.

54) Vazquez-Martin, Alejandro, et al. "Repositioning chloroquine and metformin to eliminate cancer stem cell traits in pre-malignant lesions." Drug Resistance Updates 14.4-5 (2011): 212-223

55) Liang, Diana H., et al. "The autophagy inhibitor chloroquine targets cancer stem cells in triple negative breast cancer by inducing mitochondrial damage and impairing DNA break repair." Cancer letters 376.2 (2016): 249-258

56) Vitale, Ilio, et al. "Role of autophagy in the maintenance and function of cancer stem cells." International Journal of Developmental Biology 59.1-2-3 (2015): 95-108.

57) Lei, Yuanyuan, et al. "Targeting autophagy in cancer stem cells as an anticancer therapy." Cancer letters 393 (2017): 33-39.

58) Maycotte, Paola, et al. "Autophagy supports breast cancer stem cell maintenance by regulating IL6 secretion." Molecular cancer research 13.4 (2015): 651-658.

59) Narter, Fehmi. "Re: Autophagy in Cancer Stem Cells: A Potential Link Between Chemoresistance, Recurrence and Metastasis." Journal of Urological Surgery 3.2 (2016): 57.

60) Han, Yanyan, et al. "Role of autophagy in breast cancer and breast cancer stem cells." International journal of oncology 52.4 (2018): 1057-1070.

61) Guan, Jun-Lin, et al. "Autophagy in stem cells." Autophagy 9.6 (2013): 1-20.

62) Bousquet, Guilhem, et al. "Targeting autophagic cancer stem-cells to reverse chemoresistance in human triple negative breast cancer." Oncotarget 8.21 (2017): 35205.

63) Cufí, Sílvia, et al. "Autophagy positively regulates the CD44+ CD24-/low breast cancer stem-like phenotype." Cell cycle 10.22 (2011): 3871-3885.

64) Zhu, Haitao, et al. "Role of the Hypoxia-inducible factor-1 alpha induced autophagy in the conversion of non-stem pancreatic cancer cells into CD133+ pancreatic cancer stem-like cells." Cancer cell international 13.1 (2013): 119.

65) Kawaguchi-Ihara, Noriko, et al. "Chloroquine Inhibits Self-Renewal of Blast Progenitors Synergistically With Phytochemicals or Nonsteroidal Anti-inflammatory Drugs in Hematological Malignant Cell Lines." Anticancer research 39.1 (2019): 87-98.

66) Pascolo, Steve. "Time to use a dose of chloroquine as an adjuvant to anti-cancer chemotherapies." European journal of pharmacology 771 (2016): 139-144.

67) Zhang, Hui-Qing, et al. "Antitumor activity of chloroquine in combination with Cisplatin in human gastric cancer xenografts." Asian Pac J Cancer Prev 16.9 (2015): 3907-3912.

68) Kim, Mi-Young, et al. "Combination Therapy with a PI3K/mTOR Dual Inhibitor and Chloroquine Enhances Synergistic Apoptotic Cell Death in Epstein–Barr Virus-Infected Gastric Cancer Cells." Molecules and cells 42.6 (2019): 448.

69) Liu, Likun, et al. "Chloroquine inhibits cell growth in human A549 lung cancer cells by blocking autophagy and inducing mitochondrial-mediated apoptosis." Oncology reports 39.6 (2018): 2807-2816.

70) Datta, Satabdi, et al. "Autophagy inhibition with chloroquine reverts paclitaxel resistance and attenuates metastatic potential in human nonsmall lung adenocarcinoma A549 cells via ROS mediated modulation of β-catenin pathway." Apoptosis 24.5-6 (2019): 414-433.

71) Mukhopadhyay, Arunima, et al. "Hydroxychloroquine for chronic myeloid leukemia: complete cure on the horizon?." Expert review of hematology 4.4 (2011): 369-371.

72) Kim, Yundeok, et al. "Induction of cytosine arabinoside-resistant human myeloid leukemia cell death through autophagy regulation by hydroxychloroquine." Biomedicine & Pharmacotherapy 73 (2015): 87-96.

73) Nuñez-Olvera, Stephanie I., et al. "Autophagy Machinery as a Promising Therapeutic Target in Endometrial Cancer." Frontiers in Oncology 9 (2019).

74) Fukuda, Tomohiko, et al. "The anti-malarial chloroquine suppresses proliferation and overcomes cisplatin resistance of endometrial cancer cells via autophagy inhibition." Gynecologic oncology 137.3 (2015): 538-545.

75) Fukuda, Tomohiko, et al. "Autophagy inhibition augments resveratrol-induced apoptosis in Ishikawa endometrial cancer cells." Oncology letters 12.4 (2016): 2560-2566.

76) Gupta, Anu, et al. "Autophagy inhibition and antimalarials promote cell death in gastrointestinal stromal tumor (GIST)." Proceedings of the National Academy of Sciences 107.32 (2010): 14333-14338.

77) Zhao, Xing-guo, et al. "Chloroquine-enhanced efficacy of cisplatin in the treatment of hypopharyngeal carcinoma in xenograft mice." PLoS One 10.4 (2015).

78) Aga, Tomomi, et al. "Inhibition of autophagy by chloroquine makes chemotherapy in nasopharyngeal carcinoma more efficient." Auris Nasus Larynx 46.3 (2019): 443-450.

79) Jia, Lihua, et al. "In vitro and in vivo antitumor effects of chloroquine on oral squamous cell carcinoma." Molecular medicine reports 16.5 (2017): 5779-5786.

80) Liu, Lin-qing, et al. "Hydroxychloroquine potentiates the anti-cancer effect of bevacizumab on

glioblastoma via the inhibition of autophagy." Biomedicine & Pharmacotherapy 118 (2019): 109339.

81) Yan, Yuanliang, et al. "Targeting autophagy to sensitive glioma to temozolomide treatment." Journal of experimental & clinical cancer research 35.1 (2016): 23.

82) Wang, Feng, et al. "Chloroquine enhances the radiosensitivity of bladder cancer cells by inhibiting autophagy and activating apoptosis." Cellular Physiology and Biochemistry 45.1 (2018): 54-66.

83) Ishibashi, Yoichi, et al. "Chloroquine Enhances Rapamycin-induced Apoptosis in MG63 Cells." Anticancer research 39.2 (2019): 649-654.

84) Egger, Michael E., et al. "Inhibition of autophagy with chloroquine is effective in melanoma." journal of surgical research 184.1 (2013): 274-281.

85) Abdel Karim, Nagla Fawzy, et al. "Phase I trial of chloroquine (CQ)/hydroxychloroquine (HCQ) in combination with carboplatin-gemcitabine (CG) in patients with advanced solid tumors." (2019): 3027-3027.

86) Frieboes, Hermann B., et al. "Chloroquine-Mediated Cell Death in Metastatic Pancreatic Adenocarcinoma Through Inhibition of Autophagy." JOP. Journal of the Pancreas 15.2 (2014): 189-197.

87) Maclean, Kirsteen H., et al. "Targeting lysosomal degradation induces p53-dependent cell death and prevents cancer in mouse models of lymphomagenesis." The Journal of clinical investigation 118.1 (2008): 79-88.

88) Vyas, Avani R., et al. "Augmentation of D, L-sulforaphane-mediated prostate cancer chemoprevention by pharmacologic inhibition of autophagy using chloroquine in a transgenic mouse model." Cancer Research 73.8 Supplement (2013): 3695-3695.

89) Carlucci, Philip, et al. "Hydroxychloroquine and azithromycin plus zinc vs hydroxychloroquine and azithromycin alone: outcomes in hospitalized COVID-19 patients." medRxiv (2020).

90) Nujić, Krunoslav, et al. "Impairment of lysosomal functions by azithromycin and chloroquine contributes to anti-inflammatory phenotype." Cellular immunology 279.1 (2012): 78-86.

91) Gautret, Philippe, et al. "Hydroxychloroquine and azithromycin as a treatment of COVID-19: results of an open-label non-randomized clinical trial." International Journal of Antimicrobial Agents (2020): 105949.

92) Liu, Jia, et al. "Hydroxychloroquine, a less toxic derivative of chloroquine, is effective in inhibiting SARS-CoV-2 infection in vitro." Cell Discovery 6.1 (2020): 1-4.

93) Savarino, Adrea, et al. "Effects of chloroquine on viral infections: an old drug against today's diseases." The Lancet infectious diseases 3.11 (2003): 722-727.

94) Gao, Jianjun, Zhenxue Tian, and Xu Yang. "Breakthrough: Chloroquine phosphate has shown apparent efficacy in treatment of COVID-19 associated pneumonia in clinical studies." Bioscience trends (2020).

95) Kono, Masakazu, et al. "Inhibition of human coronavirus 229E infection in human epithelial lung cells (L132) by chloroquine: involvement of p38 MAPK and ERK." Antiviral research 77.2 (2008): 150-152.

96) Yao, Xueting, et al. "In vitro antiviral activity and projection of optimized dosing design of hydroxychloroquine for the treatment of severe acute respiratory syndrome coronavirus 2 (SARS-CoV-2)." Clinical Infectious Diseases (2020).

97) Kimura, Tomonori, et al. "Chloroquine in cancer therapy: a double-edged sword of autophagy." Cancer research 73.1 (2013): 3-7.

98) Schrezenmeier, Eva, and Thomas Dörner. "Mechanisms of action of hydroxychloroquine and chloroquine: implications for rheumatology." Nature Reviews Rheumatology (2020): 1-12.

99) Macdonald, Ronald D., and Andrew G. Engel. "Experimental chloroquine myopathy." Journal of Neuropathology & Experimental Neurology 29.3 (1970): 479-499.

100) Joyce, Emer, Aurelie Fabre, and Niall Mahon. "Hydroxychloroquine cardiotoxicity presenting as a rapidly evolving biventricular cardiomyopathy: key diagnostic features and literature review." European Heart Journal: Acute Cardiovascular Care 2.1 (2013): 77-83.

101) Tselios, Konstantinos, et al. "Antimalarial-induced cardiomyopathy in systemic lupus erythematosus: as

rare as considered?." The Journal of rheumatology 46.4 (2019): 391-396.

102) Chaanine, Antoine H., et al. "High-dose chloroquine is metabolically cardiotoxic by inducing lysosomes and mitochondria dysfunction in a rat model of pressure overload hypertrophy." Physiological reports 3.7 (2015): e12413.

103) Roos, J. M., M. C. Aubry, and W. D. Edwards. "Chloroquine cardiotoxicity: clinicopathologic features in three patients and comparison with three patients with Fabry disease." Cardiovascular pathology: the official journal of the Society for Cardiovascular Pathology 11.5 (2002): 277.

104) Rosenthal, A. R., et al. "Chloroquine retinopathy in the rhesus monkey." Investigative ophthalmology & visual science 17.12 (1978): 1158-1175.

105) Leung, Loh-Shan B., et al. "Rapid onset of retinal toxicity from high-dose hydroxychloroquine given for cancer therapy." American journal of ophthalmology 160.4 (2015): 799-805.

106) Marmor, Michael F., et al. "Recommendations on screening for chloroquine and hydroxychloroquine retinopathy (2016 revision)." Ophthalmology 123.6 (2016): 1386-1394.

107) Brohée, Laura, et al. "Propranolol sensitizes prostate cancer cells to glucose metabolism inhibition and prevents cancer progression." Scientific reports 8.1 (2018): 1-14.

108) Solitro, A. R., and J. P. MacKeigan. "Leaving the lysosome behind: novel developments in autophagy inhibition." Future medicinal chemistry 8.1 (2016): 73.

109) Shi, Ting-Ting, et al. "Research progress of hydroxychloroquine and autophagy inhibitors on cancer." Cancer chemotherapy and pharmacology 79.2 (2017): 287-294.

110) Poillet-Perez, Laura, and Eileen White. "Role of tumor and host autophagy in cancer metabolism." Genes & development 33.11-12 (2019): 610-619.

111) Du, Fang-Yu, et al. "Targeting cancer stem cells in drug discovery: Current state and future perspectives." World journal of stem cells 11.7 (2019): 398.

112) El Hout, Mouradi, et al. "Crosstalk between autophagy and metabolic regulation of cancer stem cells." Molecular Cancer 19.1 (2020): 27.

113) Baradaran Eftekhari, Reza, Niloufar Maghsoudnia, and Farid Abedin Dorkoosh. "Chloroquine: A brand-new scenario for an old drug." (2020).

114) Gewirtz, David A. "The Switch between Protective and Nonprotective Autophagy; Implications for Autophagy Inhibition as a Therapeutic Strategy in Cancer." Biology 9.1 (2020): 12.

115) Varisli, Lokman, Osman Cen, and Spiros Vlahopoulos. "Dissecting pharmacological effects of Chloroquine in cancer treatment: interference with inflammatory signaling pathways." Immunology (2019).

116) Xu, Ran, et al. "The clinical value of using chloroquine or hydroxychloroquine as autophagy inhibitors in the treatment of cancers: A systematic review and meta-analysis." Medicine 97.46 (2018).

Chapter 33

Autophagy Inhibitors Part 3:
Clarithromycin, Propranolol, Pyrvinium, Thymoquinone, PPI's, loratadine (Claritin®), Dipyridamole, Niclosamide

Clarithromycin

MACROLIDE ANTIBIOTICS SUCH AS AZITHRO-MYCIN and clarithromycin are OXPHOS inhibitors that work by blocking the large ribosome in the mitochondria of the cancer cell. In addition, they also serve as potent autophagy inhibitors acting on lysosomes, providing synergy with tyrosine kinase inhibitors, and are useful as antiviral agents. For more, see chapter 35 on clarithromycin. (1–12)

Propranolol

In 2018, Dr. Laura Brohée et al. studied prostate cancer cells in vitro and in vivo, using the combination of glycolysis inhibitor (2DG) and autophagy inhibitor (propranolol), and found the following:

> The blockage by propranolol of the autophagy flux induced by 2DG resulted in a strong accumulation of LC3-II and p62 [lysosomal proteins] and in a massive accumulation of autophagic vesicles ... due to autophagy blockade. The propranolol + 2DG treatment efficiently prevents prostate cancer cell proliferation, induces cell apoptosis, alters mitochondrial morphology, inhibits mitochondrial bioenergetics and aggravates ER [Endoplasmic Reticulum] stress in vitro and also suppresses tumor growth in vivo. (13)

Note: Propranolol serves as dual OXPHOS inhibitor and autophagy inhibitor. Combining propranolol with a glycolysis inhibitor such as 2 DG (or DCA) targets all "three pillars of cancer cell metabolism."

- OXPHOS
- Glycolysis
- Autophagy

Propranolol may be a chloroquine-like autophagy inhibitor. For more, see chapter 6 on propranolol. (14–15)

Pyrvinium Autophagy Inhibitor

Pyrvinium is an antiparasitic drug, a repurposed anti-cancer drug, an OXPHOS inhibitor that accumulates in mitochondria, a potent inhibitor of the Wnt pathway, and a cancer stem cell (CSC) agent.

In 2013, Dr. Longfei Deng et al. studied the antiparasitic drug pyrvinium as an autophagy inhibitor in a cervical cancer model in vitro and in vivo (HeLa cells). Dr. Deng's group first stimulated autophagy in the cancer cells with the use of 2 DG, a glycolysis inhibitor that activates autophagy. In cancer cells with upregulated autophagy induced by 2DG, the application of pyrvinium-induced potent anti-cancer activity in vivo inhibited autophagosome formation and reduced transcription of autophagy-associated genes.

Pyrvinium Inhibits Autophagy Genes

Cancer cells are "addicted" to autophagy, especially when stimulated with glycolysis inhibitors (2DG) or other anti-cancer drugs that induce "protective autophagy." In 2013, Dr. Deng et al. studied the antiparasitic drug pyrvinium, demonstrating inhibition of autophagy both in vitro and in vivo by "transcriptional inhibition of autophagy genes." They write that the mechanism of action is:

> transcriptional inhibition of autophagy genes. Moreover, the combination of pyrvinium with autophagy stimuli improves its toxicity against cancer cells.... in vivo studies show that the combination therapy of pyrvinium with the anti-cancer and autophagy stimulus agent, 2-deoxy-glucose (2-DG), is significantly more effective in inhibiting tumor growth than pyrvinium or 2-DG alone.... we identify pyrvinium as a potent small molecule inhibitor of autophagy with an IC50 of 50 nanoMolar. (16)

For more, see chapter 12 on Pyrvinium.

Thymoquinone Autophagy Inhibitor

In 2013, Dr. Ira Racoma et al. studied the effect of thymoquinone (TQ) in a glioblastoma cell model, finding induction of apoptosis in a caspase-independent manner (meaning the mechanism was related to lysosomal disruption and not mitochondrial apoptosis):

> Exposure to TQ caused an increase in the recruitment and accumulation of the microtubule-associated protein light chain 3-II (LC3-II). TQ also caused an accumulation of the LC3-associated protein p62, confirming the inhibition of autophagy.... our results describe a novel mechanism of action for

TQ as an autophagy inhibitor selectively targeting glioblastoma cells. (17)

Thymoquinone was also found to induce autophagic cell death in squamous cell carcinoma and colon cancer cell models. (18–19) The obvious advantage of using thymoquinone as an alternate to chloroquine and hydroxychloroquine is the avoidance of retinal, cardiac and neurologic toxicity. For more on this topic, see the chapter 34 on thymoquinone.

Proton Pump Inhibitors (PPI) as Lysosomal/Autophagy Inhibitors

As we have discussed in the preceding chapters, cancer cells have upregulated autophagy as a major metabolic pathway for obtaining nutrition; for aggressive, invasive behavior; and for maintaining CSCs. Autophagy depends on acidification of the lysosome. This is accomplished by a molecular proton pump called the "V-ATPase," representing yet another "Achilles heel" in the cancer cell. Blocking the V-ATPase proton pump raises the lysosomal pH from acid to alkaline, rendering lysosomes and autophagy dysfunctional. We are fortunate proton pump inhibitor anti-acid drugs are widely available, over the counter for heartburn and hyper-acidity. Routinely used proton pump inhibitor (PPI) drugs are Dexlansoprazole (Dexilant), Esomeprazole (Nexium), Lansoprazole (Prevacid), Pantoprazole (Protonix), Omeprazole (Prilosec), Rabeprazole (AcipHex), etc. About 100 million prescriptions for PPI drugs were written in 2017, according to the Medical Expenditure Panel Survey (MEPS). (22-23)

Increased Lysosomal Activity in Cancer

In 2016, Dr. Laura Stransky et al. reviewed the function of V-ATPase in cancer, commenting that cancer cells typically have increased lysosomal activity. Inhibition of V-ATPase (with a PPI drug) blocks autophagy flux, and inhibits Wnt and Notch signaling (CSC pathways):

> Lysosomes undergo a variety of changes during carcinogenesis. Cancer cells often display enhanced lysosomal biogenesis, lysosomal protease activity, and lysosomal trafficking towards the leading edge [ante-grade trafficking] … Enhanced V-ATPase expression in cancer cells allows lysosomes to participate in processes critical to carcinogenesis … **Thus inhibition of the V-ATPase blocks autophagic flux** … proton pump inhibitors such as omeprazole are commonly used in the clinic and have been shown to reduce V-ATPase activity … Wnt signaling requires V-ATPase function for proper trafficking and activation … Like Wnt, Notch signaling relies on the V-ATPase for proper trafficking and activation. (20)

ATPase Controls Cancer Stem Cell Pathways

Another revelation provided by Dr. Stransky is that the CSC pathways, Wnt and Notch, are dependent on the V-ATPase function, writing:

> Wnt and Notch signaling requires V-ATPase function for proper trafficking and activation. (20)

This means that blocking V-ATPase also blocks CSC pathways. (42)

Important: Wnt and Notch Pathways are CSC pathways that require V-ATPase for proper functioning. This is highly significant!!! Blocking V-ATPase with PPIs eradicates CSCs!!

Aberrant Location of ATPase on Cell Membrane

In 2018, Dr. Bradleigh Whitton et al. noted that the aberrant location of the V-ATPase molecular acid pump on the cancer cell membrane plays an important role in degrading the extracellular matrix and promoting cancer invasion.

> Increased cancer cell invasive activity is frequently associated with aberrant V-ATPase plasma membrane localization suggesting that increased acidification of the extracellular space plays an important role … V-ATPase can increase the activity of extracellular proteases, such as cathepsins and matrix metalloproteinases [enzymes], via both increased protease secretion and decreased extracellular pH which enhances activity of these enzymes…. Once activated, these proteases increase extracellular matrix degradation and facilitate migration of cancer cells…. PPI's such as omeprazole and esomeprazole, also inhibit V-ATPase and can increase sensitivity to chemotherapeutics in vitro and in vivo. (21)

Benefits of Targeting Lysosomes

In 2016, Dr. Jessie Yanxiang Guo and Eileen White commented that blocking V-ATPase function in lysosomes has the added advantage of inhibiting macropinocytosis, which is upregulated in cancers with the K-Ras oncogene mutation, a survival mechanism for pancreatic cancer. Dr. Jessie Yanxiang Guo writes:

> Targeting lysosomes has the added advantage of not only blocking intracellular protein scavenging by autophagy but also blocking extracellular protein scavenging by macropinocytosis. Macropinocytosis and lysosomal degradation of albumin [and

presumably other extracellular proteins] is an important survival mechanism for K-Ras–driven pancreatic cancer. (24)

Note: K-Ras is an oncogene which upregulates autophagy and micropinocytosis.

Because of their widespread clinical use and relative safety, repurposing proton pump inhibitor drugs as anti-cancer agents has been suggested by a number of authors. (22–26)

PPIs for B-Cell Lymphoma

In 2007, Dr. Angelo Yanxiang studied PPI treatment in a pre-B acute lymphoblastic leukemia cell line finding use of PPI drug increased sensitivity to the chemotherapy agent, vinblastine. Next, the cells showed typical changes in the lysosomes with increased pH and rupture of lysosomal membranes. This was followed by induction of mitochondrial apoptosis. This cell-death process could be halted by the anti-oxidant N-Acetyl cysteine (NAC), a vitamin available at the health food store. In vivo studies in immune deficient mice confirmed inhibition of tumor growth with PPI treatment. Read Dr. Milito's play-by-play description of apoptosis in a leukemia cell model with a PPI drug:

> The effect of PPI was mediated by a very early production of reactive oxygen species [ROS] that preceded alkalinization of lysosomal pH, lysosomal membrane permeabilization, and cytosol acidification, suggesting an early destabilization of the acidic vesicular compartment. Lysosomal alterations were followed by mitochondrial membrane depolarization, release of cytochrome c, chromatin condensation, and caspase activation [mitochondrial apoptosis]. (27)

Like other autophagy inhibitors such as clarithromycin, azithromycin, and hydroxychloroquine, PPIs also enhance sensitivity of cancer cells to tyrosine kinase inhibitor drugs, as described in 2018 by Drs. Merve Ergül and Mustafa Ergül, who found PPIs enhanced the chemo-sensitivity of chronic myelogenous leukemia to imatinib (Gleevec®). (28)

Eradicating Cancer Stem Cells with PPIs: Embryonal Rhabdomyosarcoma in Children

Embryonal rhabdomyosarcoma (ER), the most frequent soft tissue sarcoma of children, is notoriously difficult to treat, responding briefly to chemotherapy after which relapse is common, thought to be caused by residual CSCs. In 2014, Dr. Manuela Salerno et al. studied ER CSCs, which had higher invasive ability and more chemo resistance compared to native ER cancer cells. This was thought to be related to higher V-ATPase activity in CSCs. Inhibition of lysosomal acidification with PPI drugs "significantly enhanced doxorubicin (chemotherapy) toxicity":

> Unexpectedly, lysosomal targeting also blocked cell growth and reduced the invasive potential of rhabdomyosarcoma CSC, even at very low doses of omeprazole [10 and 50 microMolar µM, respectively]. (29)

PPIs Enhance Activity of Chemotherapy Docetaxel

In 2015, Dr. Q. Tan et al. note that thirty clinical trials with autophagy inhibitors chloroquine and hydroxychloroquine have not been entirely fulfilling due to the difficulty in achieving the high micromolar concentrations needed to completely inhibit autophagy. They write that "new and safer inhibitors of autophagy are worthy of investigation." (30)

One such new agent is a second-generation chloroquine analog (Lys05), 5–10 times more potent than the original version of chloroquine when used against leukemia stem cells. In 2019, Dr. Baquero studied this new drug (Lys05), and found it effective in eradicating CSCs in CML (chronic myelogenous leukemia) when combined with TKI drug (tyrosine kinase inhibitor). Another answer to the quest for more potent autophagy inhibitors could be the PPI V-ATPase inhibitor drugs. (31)

In Vivo Studies PPI Drugs Enhance Chemotherapy

In 2015, Dr. Tan et al. studied the PPI drug pantoprazole, added to the chemotherapy agent docetaxol, against three cancer cell lines (breast, prostate, and epidermoid skin cancer) as mouse xenografts, finding dramatic enhancement of docetaxol activity by the PPI drug. **Note:** docetaxol is a taxane microtubule agent. This was further studied and found to be due to autophagy inhibition by the PPI drug. Similar to many other chemotherapy drugs, docetaxol upregulates "protective autophagy" which promotes survival in cancer cells. Inhibition of "protective autophagy" with a PPI drug is confirmed by finding increased protein markers LC3-II and p62. Dr. Tan and colleagues write:

> Our results suggest that pantoprazole inhibits autophagy by raising lysosomal pH and/or by inhibiting fusion of autophagosomes with lysosomes, leading to the accumulation of autophagosomes…. pantoprazole increased the accumulation

of both LC3-II and p62. (30–32)

The Pandora Trial

Dr. Tan's mouse xenograft results were so promising in prostate cancer that his group then initiated a phase II clinical trial of a PPI drug combined with docetaxol for prostate cancer. Identifier: NCT01748500; the PANDORA Trial in Toronto. Unfortunately, in 2019 Dr. Aaron Hansen et al. reported disappointing results. The drug combination did not work and most of the patients died.

> The PANDORA trial has demonstrated that the combination of high-dose pantoprazole with docetaxel is tolerable, but the clinical activity was not sufficient to warrant further testing. (33)

Regarding the failure of the PANDORA study, in 2020, Drs. Alan Lombard and Allen Gao write:

> It appears that targeting autophagy may prove beneficial in combating taxane resistance, but it should be noted that recent results of the PANDORA trial failed to show that autophagy inhibition using pantoprazole meaningfully enhanced docetaxel treatment. (34)

Why Did the Pandora Trial Fail?

My assessment of the Pandora trial failure is that there were two important factors. First, the PPI drug was given intravenously every 3 weeks. This is a mistake; it should be given daily, orally, the same as prescribed to the general population. Indeed, the attraction of a PPI drug as autophagy inhibitor is the ease of using it orally and the fact that millions of users have taken the drug as oral tablet for months and years. Why the authors decided to use the drug intravenously every 21 days is a mystery to me and an obvious mistake. Second, the trial did not use the proper combination of drugs to target all three metabolic pathways. Although autophagy was addressed, the other two pathways, OXPHOS and GLYCOLYSIS were ignored.

Dr. Lombard Assesses Reason for Failure

In 2020, Dr. Lombard et al. suggested targeting additional metabolic pathways with a FASN inhibitor (orlistat, Xenical). Instead of using orlistat, why not use fenofibrate, also a FASN and OXPHOS inhibitor? Fenofibrate may serve in place of orlistat, as discussed in the chapter 37. In addition, fenofibrate is known to enhance prostate cancer sensitivity to docetaxol, as described by Dr. Marcin Luty et al. in 2019. (34–35)

Devising a More Robust Protocol for Prostate Cancer

A more robust drug combination program for prostate cancer would include:

- DCA (plus poly-MVA) or diclofenac- glycolysis inhibitor.
- Daily oral PPI drug such as pantoprazole as autophagy inhibitor. A second lysosomal agent, loratadine 10 mg/day might also be added.
- Fenofibrate OXPHOS inhibitor, 400 mg per day with evening meal.
- Propranolol OXPHOS and autophagy inhibitor (80 mg per day) or niclosamide (dual OXPHOS/autophagy inhibitor)
- Sulforaphane (broccoli extract) depletes glutathione and is synergistic with autophagy inhibitors, eradicates

CSCs. Sulforaphane was discussed in the chapter 10 on natural substances targeting CSCs.

- Other supplements such as melatonin, thymoquinone, curcumin, boswellia, pterostilbene, iodine, poly-MVA (alpha lipoic and thiamine) etc.

This protocol could be studied with and without the docetaxol chemotherapy agent. The above combination would be worthy of study with NIH funding, as it is more likely to succeed in clinical trials, assuming no problems arise with added toxicities.

PPIs Enhance Chemotherapy for Ovarian Cancer

Autophagy inhibition with a PPI drug was found to overcome drug resistance and enhance the effect of the chemotherapy agent paclitaxel for ovarian cancer by Dr. Yoo-Young Lee et al. in 2015 and Cisplatin by Dr. Arpita Kulshrestha et al. in 2019. (36–37)

PPIs studied in other cancers:

- B-cell lymphoblastic leukemia (27)
- Pancreatic cancer (38–39)
- Breast cancer (40)
- Head-and-neck squamous cell cancer (41)
- Gastric CSCs (42)
- Melanoma (43)
- Multiple myeloma (44)
- Gastric cancer (45–47)

Results of PPIs in Clinical Trials

As described by Dr. Elisabetta Iessi et al. in 2018, a number of clinical trials showing adjuvant PPI use increases efficacy of chemotherapy in osteosarcoma and metastatic breast cancer, metastatic colorectal cancer and other solid tumors. PPI use increased survival in head-and-neck squamous cell carcinoma.

Animal studies show PPI treatment reverses chemoresistance in refractory tumors such as lymphoma, melanoma, and squamous carcinoma, and increases efficacy of chemotherapy. Dr. Iessi and colleague writes:

> All these studies provided the first clinical evidence that **PPIs pretreatment could be easily included into the standard protocols in clinical oncology with a clear benefit for patients** having the less favorable prognostic factors. Indeed, pretreatment with PPIs, by inhibiting proton pumps, induced a decrease of the protonation of extracellular tumor environment, in turn allowing the chemotherapeutics to be fully effective, improving the effectiveness of either chemical and biological drugs against cancer. Thus, tumor alkalinization could improve the outcome of patients by counteracting tumor chemoresistance. (54–55)

PPI's Adverse Side Effects

Adverse effects of PPI drugs associated with long-term use are related to the marked suppression of stomach acid, a gastric juice required for digestion and absorption of protein and key vitamins and minerals such as calcium, iron, and B12. These deficiencies may lead to pathologic fractures, iron deficiency anemia, and megaloblastic anemia. In addition, gastric acid acts as a barrier to pathogenic microbes. Removing this acid barrier with a PPI drug increases the risk for community acquired pneumonia (CAP) and clostridia difficile enterocolitis. (48–50)

Summary

To summarize, proton pump inhibitors are useful agents for inhibition of V-ATPase, the molecular proton pump in lysosomes; they thus serve as autophagy inhibitors, restore drug sensitivity for chemotherapy resistant cell types, and target CSCs. In addition, PPI's have more extensive anti-cancer effects related to their ability to dysregulate pH and electrolyte balance in the cancer cell. The use of PPIs in combination with OXPHOS and GLYCOLYSIS inhibitor is advised for targeting all "three pillars of cancer cell metabolism." (51–53)

Loratadine and Cationic Amphiphilic Antihistamines (CAD)

Antihistamines such as diphenhydramine (Benadryl) have been household names ever since I can remember, used for allergy symptoms of runny nose and itchy eyes since they were first introduced in 1947, and widely used with a high level of safety. Here in Florida, we open a Benadryl capsule and mix it with skin lotion and apply it to mosquito bites for prompt relief of the "histamine wheal." Other uses for Benadryl include treatment for the tremor of Parkinson's disease, extra-pyramidal symptoms caused by antipsychotic drugs (involuntary movements called tardive dyskinesia), and as a sleep aid for insomnia.

Accumulates in Lysosomes 1,000 Fold

A less sedating version of Benadryl, loratadine, a second-generation antihistamine, was FDA-approved in 1993 and off-patent in 2002 when it became available over the counter.

Loratadine acts by blocking the H1 histamine receptor.

Loratadine is a cationic amphiphilic drug (CAD), which enters the acidic lysosome, where once protonated, it is trapped and accumulates a thousand fold. As one can imagine, this interrupts lysosomal function, and serves as an autophagy inhibitor. (56)

In 2016, Dr. Anne-Marie Ellegaard et al. studied CAD drugs in non-small-cell lung cancer (NSCLC) and suggested repurposing loratadine as an anti-cancer drug. Dr. Ellegaard's group writes that cancer progression depends on upregulated lysosomal activity, which makes the cancer cell lysosomes more fragile and easier targets for inducing "lysosomal cell death" with a CAD drug:

> Cancer progression to metastatic disease depends on the activation of the lysosomal compartment, which is manifested by increased lysosomal biogenesis and acidification. Besides being tumor-promoting, these lysosomal changes associate with reduced lysosomal membrane stability. This frailty of cancer cell lysosomes can be targeted by several cationic amphiphilic drugs (CADs) that accumulate in the acidic lysosomes and induce lysosomal damage preferentially in cancer cells. (56)

Next, Dr. Ellegaard's group screened a library of 72 CAD drugs for activity against NSCLC (non-small cell lung cancer), finding two antihistamines among the top 5 hits. By the way, the antimalarial mefloquine, showed up prominently in the list. See chapter 31 on mefloquine for more on this topic.

Further study of the antihistamine group showed that loratadine induced lysosomal cell death in lung cancer cells at IC50 concentration of (60.1–85.6 micromolar). Because these concentrations are somewhat high, and cannot be achieved with standard oral dosage (10 mg daily), Dr. Ellegaard's group suggested the real value of loratadine is in combination therapy with microtubule-based chemotherapy, with enhancement of cytotoxic effects.

Next, Dr. Ellegaard's group performed a cohort study, examining Denmark's nationwide registries for CAD antihistamine use over 6 months (3 months before and 3 months after a cancer diagnosis) between 1995 and 2011. The use of loratadine

> was associated with significantly reduced all-cause mortality among patients with non-localized NSCLC or any non-localized cancer when compared with use of non-CAD antihistamines. (56)

In patients on loratadine also receiving chemotherapy, the hazard ratio (HR) was 0.64; without chemotherapy, it was 0.81. Other cancer cell types showed similar benefits. Further laboratory studies confirmed the ability of CADs to synergize with chemotherapy and overcome drug resistance. Dr. Ellegaard's group concluded:

> CAD Antihistamines Destabilize Lysosomal Membranes.

> CAD Antihistamines and Chemotherapy Synergize to Induce Apoptotic and Lysosomal Cell Death.

> Use of cationic amphiphilic antihistamines is associated with reduced mortality among patients with non-localized cancer.

Clinically relevant concentrations of cationic amphiphilic antihistamines sensitize cancer cells to chemotherapy.

Clinically relevant concentrations of cationic amphiphilic antihistamines revert multidrug resistance. (56)

Loratadine/ Sulforaphane Combination

Perhaps loratadine efficacy in lung cancer and other solid cancers would have been more effective if combined with sulforaphane, as reported by Dr. Desai, who studied this combination in a pancreatic cell model, finding a 40-fold reduction in IC (inhibitory concentration) compared to using either alone. (57)

Sulforaphane is an OXPHOS inhibitor, depletes prostate cancer cells of glutathione, and is synergistic with autophagy inhibitors, as discussed in chapter 10 on Natural Supplements Targeting Cancer Stem Cells.

Loratadine for AML – Dual Lysosome/ Mitochondrial Targeting

As discussed in chapter 31, leukemia cells are much more sensitive to lysosomal agents because they have larger and more active lysosomes. It is possible to transform perfectly normal white blood cells into leukemia cells in the laboratory using MLL fusion genes, commonly used in transgenic mouse model for MLL-AF9-driven leukemia. **Note:** MLL = mixed lineage leukemia gene. (58)

Reversing the Gene Signature

In 2019, Dr. Josep Cornet-Masana et al. did in-silico screening of a connectivity map database, searching for drugs to revert the gene signature in MLL-AF9 leukemia cells and found a group of antihistamines (CADs) that "reversed the transformation gene signature." When studied in vitro and in vivo mouse xenografts, these antihistamines selectively killed leukemia cells, while sparing normal cells, with EC 50 in the low micromolar range (10 micromolar). The effect was independent of the H1 histamine receptor and instead involved simultaneous "dual targeting" with mitochondrial and lysosomal disruption. Note that in these leukemia studies, loratadine (CADs) was much more effective than in the lung cancer studies by Dr. Ellegaard's group, which required higher concentrations of the drug to be effective.

Vitamin E Prevents the Cytotoxic Effect

Dr. Cornet-Masana et al. found that vitamin E (alpha-tocopherol) protects lysosomal membranes and strongly prevented cytotoxicity induced by loratadine. For this reason, avoiding concurrent vitamin E use with lysosomal/ autophagy inhibitors is advised.

Dr. Cornet-Masana et al. conclude:

A group of antihistamines possessing cationic amphiphilic structure [CADs, loratadine] selectively eradicate AML [acute myelogenous leukemia] cells independently of histamine receptors by targeting both lysosomes and mitochondria, known to be altered and more fragile in AML compared to their healthy counterpart. This dual mechanism is based on physicochemical properties of drugs and emerges as a novel therapeutic approach for AML eradication. (59–60)

In agreement with these conclusions was a 2019 study by Dr. Chanas LaRue using antihistamines combined with ibrutinib (a tyrosine kinase inhibitor) to induce synergistic cancer cell death in B-Cell lymphoma and leukemia. (61)

CADs for Glioblastoma

In 2019, Dr. Vadim Le Joncour et al. studied the beneficial effect of clemastine (CAD) for glioblastoma, writing that CAD drugs should be included as adjuvant therapy to the standard of care. Clemastine is an antihistamine similar to loratadine:

> Bearing in mind the chemo-resistant nature of infiltrating gliomas and the poor delivery of conventional drugs due to the BBB [Blood Brain Barrier], the repurposing of antihistamines and other CADs to trigger the LMP [lysosome membrane permeability] in invasive neoplasms should be considered as an adjuvant therapy to the standard of care, i.e. the surgical resection of the primary tumour and conventional radio- and chemotherapies. (62)

More Cohort Studies

Additional cohort studies have been done for melanoma, ovarian cancer, and breast cancer, finding that loratadine users have improved survival. Melanoma patients using loratadine had striking reduction in mortality with HR of 0.50 (hazard ratio reduced by half). (63–66)

Other cancer cell types studied with loratadine:

- Chronic B-Cell leukemia (CLL) synergy with ibrutinib (67)
- Hepatoma in combination with cisplatin (68)

Loratadine Drug Interactions

Drugs that inhibit the CYP3A4 enzyme system in the liver, such as itraconazole, ketoconazole, clarithromycin, cimetidine, and grapefruit lead to increased plasma levels of loratadine.

Loratadine Relieves Bone Pain from G-CSFs

Studies suggest loratadine relieves bone pain associated with granulocyte colony-stimulating factor (G-CSFs), commonly used in cancer patients after chemotherapy to increase the white blood cell count. (69)

Adverse Side Effects of Loratadine

Unlike earlier antihistamines, which cause sedation, loratadine is a "non-sedating" antihistamine, without adverse CNS or cardiovascular effects. (70–71) Loratadine may aggravate muscle pain induced by statin drugs. (72)

Summary

In summary, the widely used, over-the-counter allergy pill, loratadine, accumulates in and causes dysfunction in lysosomes. Loratidine is a promising repurposed anti-cancer drug, especially for hematologic cancers which appear to be more sensitive to lysosomal inhibition. Synergy with Tyrosine Kinase Inhibitors and Chemotherapy agents makes the drug useful as adjunctive therapy.

Dipyridamole as Autophagy Inhibitor

The old antiplatelet drug dipyridamole is discussed in chapter 40, and should be mentioned here as another autophagy inhibitor, as reported by Dr. Marcos P. Thomé et al. (2018) in a prostate cancer cell model. Thomé found that treatment of cancer cells resulted in an increased number of autophagosomes and autolysosomes, indicating blockage of autophagic flux, thought to be secondary to increased intracellular cAMP (cyclic AMP).(73-74)

Antiviral Effects of Dipyridamole

Anti-cancer effects of Dipyridamole are thought related to inhibition of lysosomeal activity, the site for viral replication. A numer of studies show inhibition of EBV (Epstein Barr virus), Herpes Simplex, RSV (respiratory syncytial virus), rhinovirus, vaccinia virus, and COVID-19. An added bonus in COVID (coronavirus) patients is the anti-platelet effect of dipyridamole which prevents the intravascular clot formation known to occur in late stage of disease. (75-86)

Antiviral Effects of Niclosamide

As discussed previously, many viruses are dependent on acidic vesicular pH for replication. Niclosamide and other agents that alter lysosomal pH and cause lysosomal dysfunction may serve as broad spectrum antivirals, similar to hydroxychloroquine, azithromycin, loratadine, and PPIs. Niclosamide's ability to target lysosomes confers broad antiviral efficacy against influenza, dengue and SARS-Cov-2, MERS-CoV, and adenovirus, rhinovirus etc. For more on Niclosamide, see chapter 23.

Dr. Andreas Jurgeit (2012) studied antiviral effects of niclosamide finding mode of action distinct from chloroquine and hydroxychloroquine. Dr. Jurgeit suggested synergy with combination of Niclosamide with V-ATPase inhibitors (such as PPI drugs), writing:

Niclosamide neutralizes acidic membrane-bounded compartments. Niclosamide did not affect the vacuolar ATPase but acted as a protonophore, both in vesicles isolated from cells, and protein-free liposome assays. It blocked

rhinovirus infections synergistically with the proton ATPase inhibitor bafilomycin A1. Niclosamide targets endosomes by a mode of action distinct from that of endosomal pH neutralizing agents, such as chloroquine, which accumulates in acidic endosomes. (89-94)

High Thru-Put Screening for Anti-Viral Activity

As we have seen above, many repurposed drugs serve as autophagy inhibitors by accumulating in lysosomes, neutralizing lysosomal pH, and inhibiting lysosomal function. Not only is this a valid anti-cancer strategy, this is also an effective anti-viral strategy, owing to the fact that viruses use endosomal/exosomal/lysosomal machinery to enter cells. The lysosome is the site for viral replication, and as "platform for virus particle maturation and release". (96-98)

In 2020, Dr. Frank Touret at al. screened the Prestwick Library of 1,520 approved and off-patent drugs, using a SARS-CoV-2 infection cell-based assay, finding 90 drugs with antiviral activity. Not surprisingly, the top candidates are lysosomal/autophagy inhibitor drugs, azithromycin and hydroxychloroquine/chloroquine, already discussed above. PPI drugs such as omeprazole followed closely behind, next on the list. Dr. Touret writes:

Omeprazole [PPI drug] is specifically of interest because it is massively used and well tolerated. It has been demonstrated to increase the pH of endosomial/golgian pathway either by inhibiting ATPase proton pump, or by buffering the pH. We can thus expect that such endosomial pH modification would limit the processing of the Spike protein [of the COVID virus] by endosomal proteases and, in turn, block the virus entry mediated by membrane fusion process. (95)

Conclusion

Lysosomal/autophagy activity has emerged not only as a major pillar of cancer cell metabolism but also as a major mechanism for cancer invasion and aggressive behavior via antegrade lysosomal trafficking, with extrusion of acid and enzymes into the micro-environment to facilitate tumor invasion. In addition, lysosomal/autophagy plays a key role involved in CSC maintenance, dormancy, and activation. Autophagy inhibitors serve as CSC agents and work in synergy with OXPHOS and GLYCOLYSIS inhibitors. Although currently ignored by the mainstream oncologist, autophagy inhibition occupies a prominent role in our *Cracking Cancer Toolkit* as one of the "three pillars of cancer cell metabolism." Surprisingly, many of these lysosomal drugs repurposed as anti-cancer autophagy inhibitors, also have potent anti-viral effects, since viral replication depends on acidic lysosomes. (95-98)

References for Chapter 33: Autophagy Inhibitors Part Three

1) Petroni, Giulia, et al. "Clarithromycin inhibits autophagy in colorectal cancer by regulating the hERG1 potassium channel interaction with PI3K." Cell Death & Disease 11.3 (2020): 1-18.

2) Kang, Minyong, et al. "Concurrent autophagy inhibition overcomes the resistance of epidermal growth factor receptor tyrosine kinase inhibitors in human bladder cancer cells." International journal of molecular sciences 18.2 (2017): 321.

3) Mukai, Shuntaro, et al. "Macrolides sensitize EGFR-TKI-induced non-apoptotic cell death via blocking autophagy flux in pancreatic cancer cell lines." International journal of oncology 48.1 (2016): 45-54.

4) Sugita, Shohei, et al. "EGFR-independent autophagy induction with gefitinib and enhancement of its cytotoxic effect by targeting autophagy with clarithromycin in non-small cell lung cancer cells." Biochemical and biophysical research communications 461.1 (2015): 28-34.

5) Schafranek, Lisa, et al. "Clarithromycin enhances dasatinib-induced cell death in chronic myeloid leukemia cells, by inhibition of late stage autophagy." Leukemia & lymphoma 54.1 (2013): 198-201.

6) Carella, Angelo Michele, et al. "Clarithromycin potentiates tyrosine kinase inhibitor treatment in patients with resistant chronic myeloid leukemia." Leukemia & lymphoma 53.7 (2012): 1409-1411.

7) Carella, A. M., et al. "Inhibition of autophagy with clarithromycin: a new strategy to enhance sensitivity of CML stem cells to tyrosine kinase inhibitors." Leukemia supplements 1.2 (2012): S49-S50.

8) Altman, Jessica K., and Leonidas C. Platanias. "A new purpose for an old drug: inhibiting autophagy with clarithromycin." Leukemia & lymphoma 53.7 (2012): 1255.

9) Van Nuffel, An MT, et al. "Repurposing Drugs in Oncology (ReDO)—clarithromycin as an anti-cancer agent." ecancermedicalscience 9 (2015).

10) Nakamura, Miki, et al. "Clarithromycin attenuates autophagy in myeloma cells." International journal of oncology 37.4 (2010): 815-820.

11) Asada, Masanori, et al. "Macrolide antibiotics inhibit respiratory syncytial virus infection in human airway epithelial cells." Antiviral research 83.2 (2009): 191-200.

12) Damle, Bharat, et al. "Clinical Pharmacology Perspectives on the Antiviral Activity of Azithromycin and Use in COVID-19." Clinical Pharmacology & Therapeutics (2020).

13) Brohée, Laura, et al. "Propranolol sensitizes prostate cancer cells to glucose metabolism inhibition and prevents cancer progression." Scientific reports 8.1 (2018): 1-14.

14) Li, Yuan, et al. "A cell-based quantitative high-throughput image screening identified novel autophagy modulators." Pharmacological research 110 (2016): 35-49.

15) Wu, Haiwei, et al. "Enhanced Efficacy of Propranolol Therapy for Infantile Hemangiomas based on a Mesoporous Silica Nanoplatform through Mediating Autophagy Dysfunction." Acta Biomaterialia (2020).

16) Deng, Longfei, et al. "Pyrvinium targets autophagy addiction to promote cancer cell death." Cell death & disease 4.5 (2013): e614-e614.

17) Racoma, Ira O., et al. "Thymoquinone inhibits autophagy and induces cathepsin-mediated, caspase-independent cell death in glioblastoma cells." PLoS One 8.9 (2013).

18) Chu, Shu-Chen, et al. "Thymoquinone induces cell death in human squamous carcinoma cells via caspase activation-dependent apoptosis and LC3-II activation-dependent autophagy." PloS one 9.7 (2014).

19) Chen, Ming-Cheng, et al. "Thymoquinone induces caspase-independent, autophagic cell death in CPT-11-resistant lovo colon cancer via mitochondrial dysfunction and activation of JNK and p38." Journal of agricultural and food chemistry 63.5 (2015): 1540-1546.

20) Stransky, Laura, Kristina Cotter, and Michael Forgac. "The function of V-ATPases in cancer." Physiological reviews 96.3 (2016): 1071-1091.

21) Whitton, Bradleigh, et al. "Vacuolar ATPase as a potential therapeutic target and mediator of treatment resistance in cancer." Cancer medicine 7.8 (2018): 3800-3811.

22) Spugnini, Enrico Pierluigi, and Stefano Fais. "Drug repurposing for anticancer therapies. A lesson from proton pump inhibitors." Expert Opinion on Therapeutic Patents just-accepted (2020).

23) Lu, Zhen-Ning, Bing Tian, and Xiu-Li Guo. "Repositioning of proton pump inhibitors in cancer therapy." Cancer chemotherapy and pharmacology 80.5 (2017): 925-937.

24) Guo, Jessie Yanxiang, and Eileen White. "Autophagy, metabolism, and cancer." Cold Spring Harbor symposia on quantitative biology. Vol. 81. Cold Spring Harbor Laboratory Press, 2016.

25) Meo-Evoli, Nathalie, et al. "V-ATPase: a master effector of E2F1-mediated lysosomal trafficking, mTORC1 activation and autophagy." Oncotarget 6.29 (2015): 28057.

26) Fako, Valerie E., et al. "Repositioning proton pump inhibitors as anticancer drugs by targeting the thioesterase domain of human fatty acid synthase." Journal of medicinal chemistry 58.2 (2015): 778-784.

27) De Milito, Angelo, et al. "Proton pump inhibitors induce apoptosis of human B-cell tumors through a caspase-independent mechanism involving reactive oxygen species." Cancer research 67.11 (2007): 5408-5417.

28) Ergül, Merve, and Mustafa Ergül. "Protein pump inhibitors esomeprazole and pantoprazole increase the chemosensitivity of CML cells against imatinib." Cumhuriyet Medical Journal 40.4 (2018): 351-355.

29) Salerno, Manuela, et al. "Impairment of lysosomal activity as a therapeutic modality targeting cancer stem cells of embryonal rhabdomyosarcoma cell line RD." PloS one 9.10 (2014).

30) Tan, Q., et al. "Effect of pantoprazole to enhance activity of docetaxel against human tumour xenografts by inhibiting autophagy." British journal of cancer 112.5 (2015): 832-840.

31) Baquero, Pablo, et al. "Targeting quiescent leukemic stem cells using second generation autophagy inhibitors." Leukemia 33.4 (2019): 981-994.

32) Tan, Qian, et al. "Up-regulation of autophagy is a mechanism of resistance to chemotherapy and can be inhibited by pantoprazole to increase drug sensitivity." Cancer chemotherapy and pharmacology 79.5 (2017): 959-969.

33) Hansen, Aaron R., et al. "Pantoprazole Affecting Docetaxel Resistance Pathways via Autophagy (PANDORA): Phase II Trial of High Dose Pantoprazole (Autophagy Inhibitor) with Docetaxel in Metastatic Castration-Resistant Prostate Cancer (mCRPC)." The Oncologist 24.9 (2019): 1188-1194.

34) Lombard, Alan P., and Allen C. Gao. "Resistance Mechanisms to Taxanes and PARP Inhibitors in Advanced Prostate Cancer." Current Opinion in Endocrine and Metabolic Research (2020).

35) Luty, Marcin, et al. "Fenofibrate Augments the Sensitivity of Drug-Resistant Prostate Cancer Cells to Docetaxel." Cancers 11.1 (2019): 77.

36) Lee, Yoo-Young, et al. "Proton pump inhibitors enhance the effects of cytotoxic agents in chemoresistant epithelial ovarian carcinoma." Oncotarget 6.33 (2015): 35040.

37) Kulshrestha, Arpita, et al. "Targeting V-ATPase Isoform Restores Cisplatin Activity in Resistant Ovarian Cancer: Inhibition of Autophagy, Endosome Function, and ERK/MEK Pathway." Journal of oncology 2019 (2019).

38) Tozzi, Marco, et al. "Proton Pump Inhibitors Reduce Pancreatic Adenocarcinoma Progression by Selectively Targeting H+, K+-ATPases in Pancreatic Cancer and Stellate Cells." Cancers 12.3 (2020): 640.

39) Udelnow, Andrej, et al. "Omeprazole inhibits proliferation and modulates autophagy in pancreatic cancer cells." PloS one 6.5 (2011).

40) Wang, Chao. "Utilization of Proton Pump Inhibitors in Combination Regimen for Breast Cancer Treatment by Targeting Fatty Acid Synthase." (2019).

41) Papagerakis, Silvana, et al. "Proton pump inhibitors and histamine 2 blockers are associated with improved overall survival in patients with head and neck squamous carcinoma." Cancer Prevention Research 7.12 (2014): 1258-1269.

42) Feng, Shuitu, et al. "Proton pump inhibitor pantoprazole inhibits the proliferation, self-renewal and chemoresistance of gastric cancer stem cells via the EMT/β-catenin pathways." Oncology reports 36.6 (2016): 3207-3214.

43) De Milito, Angelo, et al. "pH-dependent antitumor activity of proton pump inhibitors against human melanoma is mediated by inhibition of tumor acidity." International journal of cancer 127.1 (2010): 207-219.

44) Canitano, Andrea, et al. "Proton pump inhibitors induce a caspase-independent antitumor effect against human multiple myeloma." Cancer letters 376.2 (2016): 278-283.

45) Zhang, Bin, et al. "Proton pump inhibitor pantoprazole inhibits gastric cancer metastasis via suppression of telomerase reverse transcriptase gene expression." Cancer letters 452 (2019): 23-30.

46) Zhang, Bin, et al. "Proton pump inhibitor pantoprazole abrogates adriamycin-resistant gastric cancer cell invasiveness via suppression of Akt/GSK-β/β-catenin signaling and epithelial–mesenchymal transition." Cancer letters 356.2 (2015): 704-712.

47) Huang, Shuling, et al. "Proton pump inhibitor selectively suppresses proliferation and restores the chemosensitivity of gastric cancer cells by inhibiting STAT3 signaling pathway." International immunopharmacology 17.3 (2013): 585-592.

48) Elias, Evan, and Laura E. Targownik. "The clinician's guide to proton pump inhibitor related adverse events." Drugs 79.7 (2019): 715-731.

49) Schoenfeld, Adam Jacob, and Deborah Grady. "Adverse effects associated with proton pump inhibitors." JAMA internal medicine 176.2 (2016): 172-174.

50) Abraham, Neena S. "Proton pump inhibitors: potential adverse effects." Current opinion in gastroenterology 28.6 (2012): 615-620.

51) Cao, Yu, et al. "The proton pump inhibitor pantoprazole disrupts protein degradation systems and sensitizes cancer cells to death under various stresses." Cell death & disease 9.6 (2018): 1-19.

52) Spugnini, Enrico Pierluigi, and Stefano Fais. "Drug repurposing for anticancer therapies. A lesson from proton pump inhibitors." Expert Opinion on Therapeutic Patents just-accepted (2020).

53) Alfarouk, Khalid O., et al. "The Interplay of Dysregulated pH and Electrolyte Imbalance in Cancer." Cancers 12.4 (2020): 898.

54) Iessi, Elisabetta, et al. "Rethinking the combination of proton exchanger inhibitors in cancer therapy." Metabolites 8.1 (2018): 2.

55) Papagerakis, Silvana, et al. "Proton pump inhibitors and histamine 2 blockers are associated with improved overall survival in patients with head and neck squamous carcinoma." Cancer Prevention Research 7.12 (2014): 1258-1269.

56) Ellegaard, Anne-Marie, et al. "Repurposing cationic amphiphilic antihistamines for cancer treatment." EBioMedicine 9 (2016): 130-139.

57) Desai, Preshita, et al. "Loratadine self-microemulsifying drug delivery systems (SMEDDS) in combination with sulforaphane for the synergistic chemoprevention of pancreatic cancer." Drug delivery and translational research 9.3 (2019): 641-651.

58) Winters, Amanda C., and Kathrin M. Bernt. "MLL-rearranged leukemias—an update on science and clinical approaches." Frontiers in pediatrics 5 (2017): 4.

59) Cornet-Masana, Josep M., et al. "Dual lysosomal-mitochondrial targeting by antihistamines to eradicate leukaemic cells." EBioMedicine 47 (2019): 221-234.

60) Winter, Stuart S. "The emergence of antihistamines as unexpected allies in our fight against acute myeloid leukaemia." EBioMedicine 48 (2019): 7-8

61) Chanas-LaRue, Aaron P. Antihistamines Induce Synergistic Cell Death When Combined with Ibrutinib in Malignant B Cell Lines and Primary Chronic Lymphocytic Leukemia Cells. Dissertation. University of Manitoba, 2019.

62) Le Joncour, Vadim, et al. "Vulnerability of invasive glioblastoma cells to lysosomal membrane destabilization." EMBO molecular medicine 11.6 (2019).

63) Fritz, Ildikó, et al. "Desloratadine and loratadine use associated with improved melanoma survival." Allergy (2020).

64) Verdoodt, Freija, et al. "Antihistamines and ovarian cancer survival: nationwide cohort study and in vitro cell viability assay." JNCI: Journal of the National Cancer Institute (2019).

65) Olsson, Håkan Lars, Ildiko Fritz, and Philippe Wagner. "Abstract P5-06-07: Desloratadine and loratadine increase breast cancer survival." (2020): P5-06.

66) Bens, Annet, et al. "The role of H1 antihistamines in contralateral breast cancer: a Danish nationwide cohort study." British Journal of Cancer (2020): 1-7.

67) Chanas-LaRue, Aaron P., James B. Johnston, and Spencer B. Gibson. "Antihistamines as synergists with targeted therapies in chronic lymphocytic leukemia." (2018): 3976-3976.

68) Adly, Nouran. "Evaluation of cytotoxic potential of loratadine and the combination of loratadine and cisplatin on hepatocellular carcinoma cell lines." (2017).

69) Duggan, Caitriona, et al. "Oral loratadine in the management of G-CSF-induced bone pain: a pilot study." British Journal of Nursing 28.4 (2019): S4-S11.

70) Hey, J. A., et al. "Loratadine Produces Antihistamine Activity without Adverse CNS, ECG or Cardiovascular Effects in Guinea Pigs." International archives of allergy and immunology 107.1-3 (1995): 418-419.

71) Kay, G. G., and A. G. Harris. "Loratadine: a non-sedating antihistamine. Review of its effects on cognition, psychomotor performance, mood and sedation." Clinical & Experimental Allergy 29 (1999): 147-150.

72) Leung, Yat Hei, Jacques Turgeon, and Veronique Michaud. "Study of statin-and loratadine-induced muscle pain mechanisms using human skeletal muscle cells." Pharmaceutics 9.4 (2017): 42.

73) Thomé, Marcos P., et al. "Dipyridamole impairs autophagic flux and exerts antiproliferative activity on prostate cancer cells." Experimental cell research 382.1 (2019): 111456.

74) El-Sisi, Alaa E., et al. "Enhanced anticancer activity of combined treatment of imatinib and dipyridamole in solid Ehrlich carcinoma-bearing mice." Naunyn-Schmiedeberg's Archives of Pharmacology (2020): 1-17.

75) Thomé, Marcos P., et al. "Dipyridamole as a new drug to prevent Epstein-Barr virus reactivation." Antiviral Research 172 (2019): 104615.

76) Hay, Kathleen A., Andrew Gaydos, and Richard B. Tenser. "Inhibition of herpes simplex virus reactivation by dipyridamole in a mouse model." Journal of medical virology 50.2 (1996): 198-203.

77) Jiarun, Zheng, Tang Meiyu, and Yu Yanhua. "Study on Anti Herpes Simplex Virus Activity of Dipyridamole in Vitro." Chinese Journal of Dermatology 4 (1998): 12.

78) Tonew, M., E. Tonew, and R. Mentel. "The antiviral activity of dipyridamole." Acta virologica 21.2 (1977): 146-150.

79) Kozhukharova, M. S., et al. "Evaluation of dipyridamole efficacy as an agent for preventing acute

respiratory viral diseases." Voprosy virusologii 32.3 (1987): 294-297.

80) Jiahua, Pan, Lou Wanling, and Chen Lanjü. "An experimental study on treatment of respiratory syncytial virus pneumonia in mice with dipyridamole." Chinexe Journal of Pediatrics 6 (1998).

81) Oehring, H., and J. Schmidt. "The antiviral action of dipyridamole on rhinoviruses." Zeitschrift fur Attgemeine Mikrobiologie, Morphologic, Physiologic, Genetik und Okologie der Microorganismen 24.6 (1978): 447-449.

82) Korbecki, M., et al. "Dipyridamole as an inhibitor of vaccinia virus replication." Molekuliarnaia genetika, mikrobiologiia i virusologiia 1 (1985): 29-32.

83) Liu, Xiaoyan, et al. "Potential therapeutic effects of dipyridamole in the severely ill patients with COVID-19." Acta Pharmaceutica Sinica B (2020).

84) Li, Zhe, et al. "FEP-based screening prompts drug repositioning against COVID-19." bioRxiv (2020).

85) Liu, Xiaoyan, et al. "Therapeutic effects of dipyridamole on COVID-19 patients with coagulation dysfunction." medRxiv (2020).

86) Rogosnitzky, Moshe, Esther Berkowitz, and Alejandro R. Jadad. "Delivering Benefits at Speed through Real-World Repurposing of Off-Patent Drugs: The COVID-19 Pandemic as a Case in Point." JMIR Public Health and Surveillance 6.2 (2020): e19199.

87) Gao, Ying, et al. "Niclosamide blocks autophagy via lysosomal dysfunction (663.18)." The FASEB Journal 28.1_supplement (2014): 663-18.

88) Circu, Magdalena L., et al. "A novel high content imaging-based screen identifies the anti-helminthic niclosamide as an inhibitor of lysosome anterograde trafficking and prostate cancer cell invasion." PloS one 11.1 (2016).

89) Jurgeit, Andreas, et al. "Niclosamide is a proton carrier and targets acidic endosomes with broad antiviral effects." PLoS pathogens 8.10 (2012).

90) Xu, Jimin, et al. "Broad spectrum antiviral agent niclosamide and its therapeutic potential." ACS infectious diseases (2020).

91) Kao, Jo-Chi, et al. "The antiparasitic drug niclosamide inhibits dengue virus infection by interfering with endosomal acidification independent of mTOR." PLoS neglected tropical diseases 12.8 (2018): e0006715.

92) Gassen, Nils C., et al. "Analysis of SARS-CoV-2-controlled autophagy reveals spermidine, MK-2206, and niclosamide as putative antiviral therapeutics." bioRxiv (2020).

93) Pindiprolu, Sai Kiran SS, and Sai Harshini Pindiprolu. "Plausible mechanisms of Niclosamide as an antiviral agent against COVID-19." Medical Hypotheses (2020): 109765.

94) Pindiprolu, Sai Harshini, and Sai Kiran SS Pindiprolu. "CD133 receptor mediated delivery of STAT3 inhibitor for simultaneous elimination of cancer cells and cancer stem cells in oral squamous cell carcinoma." Medical hypotheses 129 (2019): 109241.

95) Touret, Franck, et al. "In vitro screening of a FDA approved chemical library reveals potential inhibitors of SARS-CoV-2 replication." Scientific reports 10.1 (2020): 1-8.

96) Spence, Jennifer S., et al. "IFITM3 directly engages and shuttles incoming virus particles to lysosomes." Nature chemical biology 15.3 (2019): 259-268.

97) Seggewiß, Nicole, Dajana Paulmann, and Andreas Dotzauer. "Lysosomes serve as a platform for hepatitis A virus particle maturation and nonlytic release." Archives of virology 161.1 (2016): 43-52.

98) Ballout, Rami A., et al. "The lysosome: A potential juncture between SARS-CoV-2 infectivity and Niemann-Pick disease type C, with therapeutic implications." The FASEB Journal (2020).

Chapter 34

Thymoquinone as Natural Autophagy Inhibitor

USED AS A FOOD SPICE in India and the Middle East, black cumin (nigella sativa) contains the active ingredient, thymoquinone (TQ), used since ancient times for its anti-inflammatory, antimicrobial, analgesic, anti-cancer, anti-diabetic, anti-hypertensive, bronchodilator, immunomodulatory, hepato-protective, and anti-oxidant effects.

Egyptian Pharaohs

Black cumin seeds were found in the pyramid tomb of Egyptian Pharaoh Tutankhamen, and references to medicinal use of black cumin seeds can be found in the oldest religious and medical texts. While TQ has anti-cancer activity, there is negligible toxicity to normal cells. TQ anti-cancer mechanisms involve inhibition of proliferation, induction of apoptosis, cell cycle interruption, generation of reactive oxygen species (ROS), prevention of angiogenesis (new blood vessels), and prevention of metastatic spread.(1–7)

Thymoquinone Potent Anti-Inflammatory Agent- Blocks NF-kB Activation

Thymoquinone has potent anti-inflammatory effects by preventing activation of nuclear factor kappa B (NF-kB), the master controller of inflammation. Studies in cholangiocarcinoma, B-cell lymphoma, and colon cancer show inactivation of the NF-kB pathway with induction of apoptosis. Anti-inflammatory effects include attenuation of cis-platinum chemotherapy toxicity, protection from testicular and hepatic injury from diabetes, lead, cadmium and methotrexate chemotherapy. Protective anti-inflammatory effects were found in rheumatoid arthritis and osteoarthritis. (8–10)(87–98) Thymoquinone has antiviral and antimicrobial effects. (99–103)

Thymoquinone Mechanisms of Action (MOA)

- **Inactivates NF-kB** and inhibits its downstream signaling (COX-2, 5-LOX, TNF, Cyclin D1) (8–10)
- Reverses DNA hyper methylation by inhibiting DNMT1.(11)
- Inhibitor of late-stage autophagy. (12–14)
- Suppresses HIF-1 mediated GLYCOLYSIS.(15–22)

Thymoquinone for Leukemia. TQ Reverses DNA Hypermethylation

In 2017, Dr. Jiuxia Pang et al. studied the anti-cancer effects of thymoquinone using acute myeloid leukemia (AML) cells, finding potent inhibition of cell proliferation and growth in both the in vitro and in vivo mouse xenograft models.

DNA hypermethylation caused by over-expression of DNA methyltransferase 1 (DNMT1) is commonly observed in leukemia cells. Thymoquinone (TQ) binds to the DNMT1 catalytic pocket, and suppresses DNMT1 methylation activity thus reversing DNA hyper-methylation. This is done at a low concentration of 30 nanomolar. Thus, thymoquinone, induces "global DNA hypo methylation." In addition, blocking the NF-kB pathway is the "central mediator of TQ anti-cancer actions."(11)

Curcumin and berberine also inhibit DNMT.

Thymoquinone Modulates Epigenetic Machinery

Controlling DNA methylation is one facet of thymoquinone's ability to "modulate epigenetic machinery" of the cancer cell.

In 2019, Dr. M. Khan wrote:

Thymoquinone can modulate epigenetic machinery, like modifying histone acetyla-tion and deacetylation, DNA methylation and demethylation, which are among the major epigenetic changes that can contrib-ute to carcinogenesis. Moreover, thymo-quinone can alter the genetic expression of various non-coding RNAs, such as miRNA and lncRNA, which are the key parts of cellular epigenetics. (7)

Thymoquinone as Late-Stage Autophagy Inhibitor

In 2013, Dr. Ira Racoma et al. studied TQ in a glioblastoma cell model, finding that cell death (apoptosis) was due to inhibition of later stage autophagy. The mechanism was caspase-independent, meaning independent of mitochondrial apoptosis. Dr. Racoma sug-gested a similarity between thymoquinone and chloroquine as two autophagy inhibitors ben-eficial for glioblastoma, causing accumulation of LC3-II and p62 protein, the two markers for autophagy inhibition:

TQ induces lysosome membrane perme-abilization … result(ing) in a leakage of cathepsin B (lysosomal enzymes) into the cytosol, which mediates caspase-indepen-dent cell death … Exposure to TQ caused an increase in the recruitment and accumu-lation of the microtubule-associated pro-tein light chain 3-II (LC3-II). TQ also caused an accumulation of the LC3-associated protein p62, confirming the inhibition of autophagy. (12)

Note: LC3 and p62 are markers for autophagy inhibition. In addition, thymoquinone caused lysosomal membranes to become "permeable," releasing lysosomal enzymes, cathepsins, into the cytosol, an event which triggers cell death.

Master Regulator Hypoxia-Inducible Factor-1 (HIF-1)

Cancer cells have upregulated the genes for hypoxia-inducible factor-1 (HIF-1) responsi-ble for cell survival, proliferation, angiogenesis, metastasis, and the metabolic derangements found in cancer cells. Tissue hypoxia activates HIF, which then activates the hypoxia response element (HRE) gene promoter. This results in activation of mTOR, and MAPK (mitogen-acti-vated protein kinase), all of which orchestrates the Warburg Effect, with expression of hexoki-nase II relocated to the VDAC, upregulation of GLYCOLYSIS, and downregulation of OXPHOS. In other words, HIF-1 is a "master regulator" of cancer progression, and inhibition of HIF-1 is a valid anti-cancer target. (15–22)

Thymoquinone Suppresses HIF-1 (Hypoxia-Inducible Factor)

Hypoxia Inducing Factor (HIF-1) is a key growth stimulator in cancer cells. Hypoxic conditions in the micro-environment activate HIF-1α activation, which then induces transcriptional reprogramming of the cancer cell to switch metabolism toward GLYCOLYSIS (Warburg Effect) and "switch on" angiogenesis and invasiveness. Blocking HIF-1 activity is a valid anti-cancer strategy.

In 2019, Dr. Yoon-Mi Lee et al. screened a library of 502 natural compounds for HIF-1 inhibition, finding thymoquinone (TQ) the lead candidate. A few other natural substances identified are: curcumin, quercetin, resveratrol, and EGCG epigallocatechin as HIF-1α inhibitors.

Dr. Lee's group then studied the anti-cancer effects of TQ on a renal cell cancer line, writing that TQ rapidly degrades HIF-1 protein and kills hypoxic renal cancer cells:

> TQ causes rapid degradation of HIF-1α by inhibiting interaction between HIF-1α and HSP90 ... TQ suppressed HIF-1α protein levels, which significantly downregulated the hypoxia-induced tumor-promoting HIF-1α target genes ... TQ Suppresses Glycolysis [the Warburg Effect] in Hypoxic Renal Cancer Cells, ... TQ-mediated suppression of angiogenesis via HIF-mediated VEGF expression. (22)

Thymoquinone Inhibits HIF Stimulated Glycolysis

TQ reduced HIF-1 protein levels by increasing its degradation, and TQ suppressed downstream genes affected by HIF-1. TQ downregulates nuclear factor-κB (NF-κB) and signal transducer and activator of transcription 3 (STAT-3). In addition, GLYCOLYSIS was inhibited with altered glucose, lactate, and ATP levels. Dr. Lee et al. write:

> In cancer, hypoxic condition is a common occurrence due to increased oxygen consumption resulting from rapidly growing cells, thus leading to HIF-1α activation. HIF-1α exacerbates tumor growth upon oxygen and nutrient deprivation through transcriptional reprogramming of angiogenesis, anaerobic glycolysis [Warburg Effect], and invasiveness. HIF-1α is associated with high incidence of cancer, poor prognosis, and resistance to chemotherapy or radiotherapy in cancer patients. Thus, extensive studies have demonstrated that targeting HIF-1α could be a promising anti-cancer therapeutic strategy.... Overall, our finding suggested that TQ, as an HIF-1α inhibitor, is a potential natural compound involved in clearance of hypoxic renal cancer cells. (22)

TQ Synergy with Chemotherapy for Glioblastoma

Autophagy Inhibitor

In 2016, Dr. Monao Pazhouhi et al. showed that TQ synergistically potentiates the cytotoxicity of the chemotherapy drug temozolomide in a glioblastoma cell line through inhibition of autophagy. (13–14)

Most chemotherapy drugs induce protective autophagy, conferring drug resistance and cell survival. In most cases, the addition of an autophagy inhibitor will overcome the drug resistance and make the chemotherapy more effective.

TQ induces Apoptosis and Autophagic Cell Death

In 2014, Dr. Shu-Chen Chu et al. studied squamous cell carcinoma cells in vitro and in vivo, finding thymoquinone treatment had two distinct anti-cancer activities. Firstly, induction of autophagy with accumulation of autophagosomes, and secondly, induction of apoptosis. Accumulation of autophagosomes indicates inhibition of late stage autophagy.

> TQ induced cell death in SASVO3 [squamous cell cancer] cells via two distinct antineoplastic activities that can induce apoptosis and autophagy. [Firstly] TQ induced autophagosome accumulation, resulting in autophagic cell death and…. [Secondly] caspase-9 activation-dependent apoptosis…. (23)

Accumulation of Autophagosomes

Similar upregulation of autophagy with accumulation of autophagosomes was seen in 2018 by Dr. Yujiao Zhang et al. in a renal cell cancer model treated with TQ. In this model, inhibition of autophagy with 3-methyladenine (3-MA) attenuated the anti-cancer effects of TQ. Treatment with TQ caused AMPK activation and downregulated mTOR, which stimulated autophagy. TQ significantly inhibited renal cell cancer growth and metastasis in an in vivo mouse xenograft model, via inhibition of EMT (epithelial to mesenchymal transition). In this model, TQ stimulated early stage autophagy. However, late-stage autophagy was blocked, as indicated by accumulation of autophagosomes with good inhibition of metastasis. (24)

Combinations Provide Synergy

In 2019, Dr. M. Aumeeruddy et al. found synergy of thymoquinone with combined use of sulforaphane and piperine (black pepper). (25)

In 2017, Dr. Omar Alobaedi et al. found synergy of TQ with resveratrol. One might expect similar synergy with pterostilbene. (26)

Immune System Activation by TQ

In 2018, Dr. Lena Odeh et al. found synergy of TQ with melatonin in a breast cancer mouse xenograft model. In addition, there was a beneficial effect on the immune system with activation of T-helper-1 anti-cancer immune response. (27)

Similarly, in 2018, Dr. Santosh Singh found that TQ enhanced anti-cancer NK-cell (killer cells) activity in a lung cancer model. (28)

Combined Use of Thymoquinone with Artemisinin

The use of combined artemisinin and thymoquinone in a hybrid compound was explored in 2018 by Drs. Gruber and Froehlich in a colon cancer model, finding 20-fold increased activity compared to parent compounds and even greater potency than the chemotherapy drug 5FU. (29–30)

TQ Effective for Cancer Stem Cells

In 2019, Dr. Benardina Ndreshkjana et al. studied the combination of TQ with the chemotherapy drug 5FU (5 flouro-uracil), finding the combination simultaneously inhibited the "Wnt /ß-Catenin and PI3K/AKT signaling pathways" and was highly effective against CD133+ CSCs. (31)

TQ Effective Independent of P53 Status

Thymoquinone triggers P53-mediated mitochondrial apoptosis in breast and colon cancer cell lines that do have a functioning P53 gene. However, about half of cancers have a mutated P53 gene. Surprisingly, thymoquinone induces apoptosis in cancer cell lines lacking a functioning p53. *This is remarkable!*

TQ Upregulates the Functioning P53 Gene

In 2010, Dr. André Wirries et al. studied TQ derivatives in a p53-competent colorectal and hepatoma cell line, finding induction of apoptosis via a P53 dependent mechanism, writing:

> We developed further TQ derivatives ... investigated for ... activity in HCT116 colon cancer cells and the human hepatoma cell line HepG2. Dependent on p53 status, these new molecules induced a cytostatic effect at low concentrations by the upregulation of p21.... (32)

In 2016, Dr. Mehdi Nikbakht Dastjerdi et al. studied TQ in a MCF-7 breast cancer cell line, finding induction of apoptosis associated with dramatic upregulation of the P53 gene. (33)

In 2017, Dr. Belkis Atasever Arslan et al.

studied TQ in a lymphoma cell line, finding induction of P53 mediated apoptosis. (34)

P53 Null Cancer Models

In 2005, Dr. Mohamed El-Mahdy et al. studied the anti-cancer effects of thymoquinone in a P53-null leukemia cell model (having no functioning P53 gene), finding induction of apoptosis in the leukemia cells without a functioning P53 gene by activating caspase 8, a part of the extrinsic apoptotic signaling pathway. (35)

In 2007, Dr. Martin Roepke et al. studied TQ in a P53-null osteosarcoma line, finding induction of apoptosis in spite of loss of function of the P53 gene. Dr. Roepke's group write that TQ could be useful for cancers that have a loss of P53:

> TQ induces p53-independent apoptosis in human osteosarcoma cells. As the loss of p53 function is frequently observed in osteosarcoma patients, our data suggest the potential clinical usefulness of TQ for the treatment of these malignancies. (36)

Important: Thymoquinone is effective in P53 mutated cancer cell lines. Efficacy is independent of P53 status.

Notch Signaling -Cancer Stem Cell Activity

TQ suppresses notch signaling, indicating anti-CSC activity. (37–38)

TQ Effective for Cancer Cell Lines

TQ has been studied and found effective in these cancer cell lines:

- Hepatocellular carcinoma (37–38)
- B-cell lymphoma (10)(34)

- Colorectal cancer (31–32)(39)(45)
- Melanoma (40–41)
- Acute lymphoblastic leukemia (42–44)
- Leukemia (45–46)(11)
- Hepatocellular cancer (37–38)(46–47)
- Osteosarcoma (36)
- Breast cancer (25–27)(48–54)(59)
- Oral squamous cell cancer (55)
- Cervical cancer (56–59)
- Gastric cancer – augments cisplatin (60–61)
- Glioblastoma (12)(14–15)
- Lung cancer (28)(62)
- Medulloblastoma (63–64)
- Multiple myeloma (9)(65–66)
- Squamous cell carcinoma (23)(67–69)
- Prostate cancer (70–72)
- Pancreatic cancer (73)
- Ovarian cancer (74–75)
- Renal cell cancer (22)(24)
- Inhibits benign prostatic hyperplasia (BPH) in mice (76)

Thymoquinone Is Neuroprotective

Various studies have shown TQ protects against acute and chronic cerebral pathology, such as peripheral neuropathy, Parkinson's disease, traumatic brain injury, amyloid toxicity, and aging. (77–84)

TQ Improves Sperm Count and Quality

In young males treated with chemotherapy for cancer, a common adverse effect is testicular damage and infertility. TQ could serve to improve sperm morphology and counts in these cases. In 2014, Dr. M. Kolahdooz et al. studied the beneficial effects of TQ in 30 infertile males with low sperm counts, showing significant improvement after 2 months of 5 ml per day TQ oil:

> Results showed that sperm count, motility and morphology and semen volume, pH and round cells were improved significantly in N. sativa oil treated group compared with placebo group after 2 months. It is concluded that daily intake of 5ml N. sativa oil for two months improves abnormal semen quality in infertile men without any adverse effects. (85)

Safety and Adverse Side Effects

In 2017, Dr. Alireeza Tavakkoli et al. reviewed all clinical trials using TQ, remarking that TQ is remarkably safe with very few adverse side effects. Those adverse effects reported were considered minor. (86)

Conclusion

Thymoquinone (black seed oil) is an ancient remedy with anti-cancer activity by virtue of HIF-1 and glycolysis inhibition, inactivation of nuclear factor kappa B (NF-kB), reversal of DNA hyper-methylation, and inhibition of late-stage autophagy. Perhaps TQ may serve as replacement for the autophagy inhibitor, chloroquine. TQ is capable of modulating the epigenetic machinery of the cancer cell, inducing both P53-dependent and P53-independent apoptosis. There is synergy with melatonin and artemisinin, enhancement of host anti-cancer immunity, and inhibition of Notch signaling. Diverse medical uses include neuroprotection, improved fertility, and antiviral effects.(87-103)

References for Chapter 34:
Thymoquinone Autophagy Inhibitor

1) Padhye, Subhash, et al. "From here to eternity-the secret of Pharaohs: Therapeutic potential of black cumin seeds and beyond." Cancer therapy 6.b (2008): 495.

2) Ahmad, Anas, et al. "Thymoquinone (2-Isoprpyl-5-methyl-1, 4-benzoquinone) as a chemopreventive/anticancer agent: Chemistry and biological effects." Saudi Pharmaceutical Journal (2019).

3) Majdalawieh, Amin F., Muneera W. Fayyad, and Gheyath K. Nasrallah. "Anti-cancer properties and mechanisms of action of thymoquinone, the major active ingredient of Nigella sativa." Critical reviews in food science and nutrition 57.18 (2017): 3911-3928.

4) Khan, Md Asaduzzaman, et al. "Thymoquinone, as an anticancer molecule: from basic research to clinical investigation." Oncotarget 8.31 (2017): 51907.

5) Imran, Muhammad, et al. "Thymoquinone: A novel strategy to combat cancer: A review." Biomedicine & Pharmacotherapy 106 (2018): 390-402.

6) Mostofa, A. G. M., et al. "Thymoquinone as a potential adjuvant therapy for cancer treatment: evidence from preclinical studies." Frontiers in pharmacology 8 (2017): 295.

7) Khan, Md Asaduzzaman, Mousumi Tania, and Junjiang Fu. "Epigenetic role of thymoquinone: impact on cellular mechanism and cancer therapeutics." Drug discovery today 24.12 (2019): 2315-2322.

8) Sethi, Gautam, Kwang Seok Ahn, and Bharat B. Aggarwal. "Targeting nuclear factor-κB activation pathway by thymoquinone: role in suppression of antiapoptotic gene products and enhancement of apoptosis." Molecular cancer research 6.6 (2008): 1059-1070.

9) Siveen, Kodappully Sivaraman, et al. "Thymoquinone overcomes chemoresistance and enhances the anticancer effects of bortezomib through abrogation of NF-κB regulated gene products in multiple myeloma xenograft mouse model." Oncotarget 5.3 (2014): 634.

10) Hussain, Azhar R., et al. "Phosphorylated IκBα predicts poor prognosis in activated B-cell lymphoma and its inhibition with thymoquinone induces apoptosis via ROS release." PloS one 8.3 (2013).

11) Pang, Jiuxia, et al. "Thymoquinone exerts potent growth-suppressive activity on leukemia through DNA hypermethylation reversal in leukemia cells." Oncotarget 8.21 (2017): 34453.

12) Racoma, Ira O., et al. "Thymoquinone inhibits autophagy and induces cathepsin-mediated, caspase-independent cell death in glioblastoma cells." PLoS One 8.9 (2013).

13) Pazhouhi, Mona, et al. "Thymoquinone synergistically potentiates temozolomide cytotoxicity through the inhibition of autophagy in U87MG cell line." Iranian journal of basic medical sciences 19.8 (2016): 890.

14) Chowdhury, Fabliha Ahmed, et al. "Therapeutic potential of thymoquinone in glioblastoma treatment: targeting major gliomagenesis signaling pathways." BioMed research international 2018 (2018).

15) Singh, Davinder, et al. "Overexpression of hypoxia-inducible factor and metabolic pathways: possible targets of cancer." Cell & bioscience 7.1 (2017): 62.

16) Schito, Luana, and Gregg L. Semenza. "Hypoxia-inducible factors: master regulators of cancer progression." Trends in cancer 2.12 (2016): 758-770.

17) Semenza, Gregg L. "Regulation of cancer cell metabolism by hypoxia-inducible factor 1." Seminars in cancer biology. Vol. 19. No. 1. Academic Press, 2009.

18) Powis, Garth, and Lynn Kirkpatrick. "Hypoxia inducible factor-1α as a cancer drug target." Molecular cancer therapeutics 3.5 (2004): 647-654.

19) Melillo, Giovanni. "Inhibiting hypoxia-inducible factor 1 for cancer therapy." Molecular Cancer Research 4.9 (2006): 601-605.

20) Belozerov, Vladimir E., and Erwin G. Van Meir. "Hypoxia inducible factor-1: a novel target for cancer therapy." Anti-cancer drugs 16.9 (2005): 901-909.

21) Wong, Carmen Chak-Lui, et al. "Hypoxia-inducible factor 1 is a master regulator of breast cancer metastatic niche formation." Proceedings of the National Academy of Sciences 108.39 (2011): 16369-16374.

22) Lee, Yoon-Mi, et al. "Thymoquinone Selectively Kills Hypoxic Renal Cancer Cells by Suppressing HIF-1α-Mediated Glycolysis." International journal of molecular sciences 20.5 (2019): 1092.

23) Chu, Shu-Chen, et al. "Thymoquinone induces cell death in human squamous carcinoma cells via caspase activation-dependent apoptosis and LC3-II activation-dependent autophagy." PloS one 9.7 (2014).

24) Zhang, Yujiao, et al. "Thymoquinone inhibits the metastasis of renal cell cancer cells by inducing autophagy via AMPK/mTOR signaling pathway." Cancer science 109.12 (2018): 3865-3873

25) Aumeeruddy, M. Zakariyyah, and M. Fawzi Mahomoodally. "Combating breast cancer using combination therapy with 3 phytochemicals: Piperine, sulforaphane, and thymoquinone." Cancer 125.10 (2019): 1600-1611.

26) Alobaedi, Omar H., Wamidh H. Talib, and Iman A. Basheti. "Antitumor effect of thymoquinone combined with resveratrol on mice transplanted with breast cancer." Asian Pacific journal of tropical medicine 10.4 (2017): 400-408.

27) Odeh, Lena Hisham, Wamidh H. Talib, and Iman A. Basheti. "Synergistic effect of thymoquinone and melatonin against breast cancer implanted in mice." Journal of cancer research and therapeutics 14.9 (2018): 324.

28) Singh, Santosh Kumar, et al. "Thymoquinone enhanced the tumoricidal activity of NK Cells against Lung Cancer." (2018): 124-5.

29) Gruber, Lisa, et al. "Treatment of multidrug-resistant leukemia cells by novel artemisinin-, egonol-, and thymoquinone-derived hybrid compounds." Molecules 23.4 (2018): 841.

30) Froehlich, Tony, et al. "Synthesis of novel hybrids of thymoquinone and artemisinin with high activity and selectivity against colon cancer." ChemMedChem 12.3 (2017): 226-234.

31) Ndreshkjana, Benardina, et al. "Combination of 5-fluorouracil and thymoquinone targets stem cell gene signature in colorectal cancer cells." Cell death & disease 10.6 (2019): 1-16.

32) Wirries, André, et al. "Thymoquinone hydrazone derivatives cause cell cycle arrest in p53-competent colorectal cancer cells." Experimental and therapeutic medicine 1.2 (2010): 369-375.

33) Dastjerdi, Mehdi Nikbakht, et al. "Effect of thymoquinone on P53 gene expression and consequence apoptosis in breast cancer cell line." International journal of preventive medicine 7 (2016).

34) Arslan, Belkis Atasever, et al. "Apoptotic effect of Nigella sativa on human lymphoma U937 cells." Pharmacognosy magazine 13.Suppl 3 (2017): S628.

35) El-Mahdy, Mohamed A., et al. "Thymoquinone induces apoptosis through activation of caspase-8 and mitochondrial events in p53-null myeloblastic leukemia HL-60 cells." International journal of cancer 117.3 (2005): 409-417.

36) Roepke, Martin, et al. "Lack of p53 augments thymoquinone-induced apoptosis and caspase activation in human osteosarcoma cells." Cancer biology & therapy 6.2 (2007): 160-169.

37) Bimonte, Sabrina, et al. "Dissecting the roles of thymoquinone on the prevention and the treatment of hepatocellular carcinoma: an overview on the current state of knowledge." Infectious agents and cancer 14.1 (2019): 10.

38) Ke, Xiquan, et al. "TQ inhibits hepatocellular carcinoma growth in vitro and in vivo via repression of Notch signaling." Oncotarget 6.32 (2015): 32610.

39) Gali-Muhtasib, Hala, et al. "Thymoquinone extracted from black seed triggers apoptotic cell death in human colorectal cancer cells via a p53-dependent mechanism." International journal of oncology 25.4 (2004): 857-866.

40) Ahmad, Israr, et al. "Thymoquinone suppresses metastasis of melanoma cells by inhibition of NLRP3 inflammasome." Toxicology and applied pharmacology 270.1 (2013): 70-76.

41) Hatiboglu, Mustafa Aziz, et al. "Thymoquinone induces apoptosis in B16-F10 melanoma cell through inhibition of p-STAT3 and inhibits tumor growth in a murine intracerebral melanoma model." World neurosurgery 114 (2018): e182-e190.

42) Soltani, Amin, et al. "Antiproliferative and apoptosis-inducing activities of thymoquinone in lymphoblastic leukemia cell line." Indian Journal of Hematology and Blood Transfusion 33.4 (2017): 516-524.

43) Salim, Landa Zeenelabdin Ali, et al. "Thymoquinone induces mitochondria-mediated apoptosis in acute lymphoblastic leukaemia in vitro." Molecules 18.9 (2013): 11219-11240.

44) Abusnina, Abdurazzag, et al. "Down-regulation of cyclic nucleotide phosphodiesterase PDE1A is the key event of p73 and UHRF1 deregulation in thymoquinone-induced acute lymphoblastic leukemia cell apoptosis." Cellular signalling 23.1 (2011): 152-160.

45) Norsharina, Ismail, et al. "Thymoquinone rich fraction from Nigella sativa and thymoquinone are cytotoxic towards colon and leukemic carcinoma cell lines." Journal of Medicinal Plants Research 5.15 (2011): 3359-3366.

46) Al-Oqail, M. M., et al. "Nigella sativa seed oil suppresses cell proliferation and induces ROS dependent mitochondrial apoptosis through p53 pathway in hepatocellular carcinoma cells." South African journal of botany 112 (2017): 70-78.

47) Ashour, Abdelkader E., et al. "Thymoquinone suppression of the human hepatocellular carcinoma cell growth involves inhibition of IL-8 expression, elevated levels of TRAIL receptors, oxidative stress and apoptosis." Molecular and cellular biochemistry 389.1-2 (2014): 85-98.

48) Sutton, Kimberly M., Anna L. Greenshields, and David W. Hoskin. "Thymoquinone, a bioactive component of black caraway seeds, causes G1 phase cell cycle arrest and apoptosis in triple-negative breast cancer cells with mutant p53." Nutrition and cancer 66.3 (2014): 408-418.

49) Yegin, Z., T. Duran, and I. H. Yildirim. "Thymoquinone Down-regulates VEGFA and Up-regulates FLT1 Transcriptional Levels in Human Breast Cancer Cells." Int J Hum Genet 20.1 (2020): 19-24.

50) Yıldırım, İbrahim Halil, Ali Ahmed Azzawri, and Tuğçe Duran. "Thymoquinone induces apoptosis via targeting the Bax/BAD and Bcl-2 pathway in breast cancer cells." Dicle Tıp Dergisi 46.3 (2019): 411-417.

51) Talib, Wamidh H. "Regressions of breast carcinoma syngraft following treatment with piperine in combination with thymoquinone." Scientia pharmaceutica 85.3 (2017): 27.

52) Barkat, Md A., et al. "Insights into the targeting potential of thymoquinone for therapeutic intervention against triple-negative breast cancer." Current drug targets 19.1 (2018): 70-80.

53) Shanmugam, Muthu K., et al. "Thymoquinone inhibits bone metastasis of breast cancer cells through abrogation of the CXCR4 signaling axis." Frontiers in pharmacology 9 (2018): 1294.

54) Kabil, Nashwa, et al. "Thymoquinone inhibits cell proliferation, migration, and invasion by regulating the elongation factor 2 kinase (eEF-2K) signaling axis in triple-negative breast cancer." Breast cancer research and treatment 171.3 (2018): 593-605.

55) Ren, Xun, and Wei Luo. "Exploration of pro-apoptotic effect of Thymoquinone on oral squamous cell carcinoma cells through PI3K/Akt signaling pathway." Cellular and molecular biology (Noisy-le-Grand, France) 65.1 (2019): 61-64.

56) Butt, Ayesha Siddique, et al. "Isolation of thymoquinone from Nigella sativa L. and Thymus vulgaris L., and its anti-proliferative effect on HeLa cancer cell lines." Tropical Journal of Pharmaceutical Research 18.1 (2019): 37-42.

57) Li, Jun, et al. "Thymoquinone inhibits the migration and invasive characteristics of cervical cancer cells SiHa and CaSki in vitro by targeting epithelial to mesenchymal transition associated transcription factors Twist1 and Zeb1." Molecules 22.12 (2017): 2105.

58) Ichwan, S. J., et al. "Apoptotic activities of thymoquinone, an active ingredient of black seed (Nigella sativa), in cervical cancer cell lines." Chin J Physiol 57.5 (2014): 249-255.

59) Ng, Wei Keat, et al. "Thymoquinone-loaded nanostructured lipid carrier exhibited cytotoxicity towards breast cancer cell lines (MDA-MB-231 and MCF-7) and cervical cancer cell lines (HeLa and SiHa)." BioMed research international 2015 (2015).

60) Ma, Jingjing, et al. "Enhancing conventional chemotherapy drug cisplatin-induced anti-tumor effects on human gastric cancer cells both in vitro and in vivo by thymoquinone targeting PTEN gene." Oncotarget 8.49 (2017): 85926.

61) Feng, Li-Min, Xue-Feng Wang, and Qing-Xian Huang. "Thymoquinone induces cytotoxicity and reprogramming of EMT in gastric cancer cells by targeting PI3K/Akt/mTOR pathway." Journal of biosciences 42.4 (2017): 547-554.

62) Samarghandian, Saeed, Mohsen Azimi-Nezhad, and Tahereh Farkhondeh. "Thymoquinone-induced antitumor and apoptosis in human lung adenocarcinoma cells." Journal of cellular physiology 234.7 (2019): 10421-10431.

63) Ashour, Abdelkader E., et al. "Thymoquinone inhibits growth of human medulloblastoma cells by inducing oxidative stress and caspase-dependent apoptosis while suppressing NF-κB signaling and IL-8 expression." Molecular and cellular biochemistry 416.1-2 (2016): 141-155.

64) Farkhondeh, Tahereh, et al. "Therapeutic effects of thymoquinone for the treatment of central nervous system tumors: A review." Biomedicine & Pharmacotherapy 96 (2017): 1440-1444.

65) Li, Feng, Peramaiyan Rajendran, and Gautam Sethi. "Thymoquinone inhibits proliferation, induces apoptosis and chemosensitizes human multiple myeloma cells through suppression of signal transducer and activator of transcription 3 activation pathway." British journal of pharmacology 161.3 (2010): 541-554.

66) Badr, Gamal, Eric A. Lefevre, and Mohamed Mohany. "Thymoquinone inhibits the CXCL12-induced chemotaxis of multiple myeloma cells and increases their susceptibility to Fas-mediated apoptosis." PloS one 6.9 (2011).

67) Kwan, K., et al. "Thymoquinone Preferentially Targets Squamous Cell Carcinoma and Demonstrates Radioprotective Effects on Normal Keratinocytes." International Journal of Radiation Oncology Biology Physics 106.5 (2020): 1188.

68) Kotowski, Ulana, et al. "Effect of thymoquinone on head and neck squamous cell carcinoma cells in vitro: Synergism with radiation." Oncology letters 14.1 (2017): 1147-1151.

69) Noorwali, Abdulwahab, et al. "Thymoquinone synergizes the anticancer properties of cisplatin against head and neck squamous cell carcinoma and protects normal oral epithelial cells." (2017): 2176-2176.

70) Singh, Santosh Kumar, et al. "Docetaxel Combined with Thymoquinone Induces Apoptosis in Prostate Cancer Cells via Inhibition of the PI3K/AKT Signaling Pathway." Cancers 11.9 (2019): 1390.

71) Saffari Chaleshtori, Javad, et al. "The Effects of Thymoquinone on Viability, and Anti-apoptotic Factors (BCL-XL, BCL-2, MCL-1) in Prostate Cancer (PC3) Cells: An In Vitro and Computer-Simulated Environment Study." Advanced pharmaceutical bulletin 9.3 (2019): 490.

72) Ranjbari, Azadeh, Esfandiar Heidarian, and Keihan Ghatreh-Samani. "Effects of thymoquinone on IL-6 Gene expression and some cellular signaling pathways in prostate cancer PC3 cells." Jundishapur Journal of Natural Pharmaceutical Products 12.3 (2017).

73) Relles, Daniel, et al. "Thymoquinone promotes pancreatic cancer cell death and reduction of tumor size through combined inhibition of histone deacetylation and induction of histone acetylation." Advances in preventive medicine 2016 (2016).

74) Liu, Xiaoli, et al. "The effect of thymoquinone on apoptosis of SK-OV-3 ovarian cancer cell by regulation of Bcl-2 and Bax." International Journal of Gynecologic Cancer 27.8 (2017): 1596-1601.

75) Taha, M. M. E., et al. "Thymoquinone induces apoptosis and increase ROS in ovarian cancer cell line." Cellular and Molecular Biology 62.6 (2016): 97-101.

76) Al-Trad, Bahaa, et al. "Inhibitory effect of thymoquinone on testosterone-induced benign prostatic hyperplasia in Wistar rats." Phytotherapy Research 31.12 (2017): 1910-1915.

77) Isaev, N. K., et al. "Thymoquinone as a Potential Neuroprotector in Acute and Chronic Forms of Cerebral Pathology." Biochemistry (Moscow) 85.2 (2020): 167-176.

78) Tabeshpour, Jamshid, et al. "Neuroprotective effects of thymoquinone in acrylamide-induced peripheral nervous system toxicity through MAPKinase and apoptosis pathways in rat." Neurochemical research 44.5 (2019): 1101-1112.

79) Ebrahimi, Seyedeh Shohreh, et al. "Thymoquinone exerts neuroprotective effect in animal model of Parkinson's disease." Toxicology letters 276 (2017): 108-114.

80) Gülşen, İsmail, et al. "Neuroprotective effects of thymoquinone on the hippocampus in a rat model of traumatic brain injury." World neurosurgery 86 (2016): 243-249.

81) Farkhondeh, Tahereh, et al. "The neuroprotective effects of thymoquinone: A review." Dose-Response 16.2 (2018): 1559325818761455.

82) Alhibshi, A. H., A. Odawara, and I. Suzuki. "Neuroprotective efficacy of thymoquinone against amyloid beta-induced neurotoxicity in human induced pluripotent stem cell-derived cholinergic neurons." Biochemistry and biophysics reports 17 (2019): 122-126.

83) Saleh, Hamid A., et al. "Thymoquinone ameliorates oxidative damage and histopathological changes of developing brain neurotoxicity." Journal of histotechnology 42.3 (2019): 116-127.

84) Badibostan, Hasan, et al. "Protective Effect of Thymoquinone on D-Galactose-Induced Aging in Mice." Jundishapur Journal of Natural Pharmaceutical Products 14.1 (2019).

85) Kolahdooz, M., et al. "Effects of Nigella sativa L. seed oil on abnormal semen quality in infertile men: a randomized, double-blind, placebo-controlled clinical trial." Phytomedicine 21.6 (2014): 901-905.

86) Tavakkoli, Alireza, et al. "Review on clinical trials of black seed (Nigella sativa) and its active constituent, thymoquinone." Journal of pharmacopuncture 20.3 (2017): 179.

87) Hussain, Azhar R., et al. "Thymoquinone-mediated suppression of NF-αB activity causes inhibition of cell viability and induces apoptosis in activated B-cell sub-type of diffuse large B-cell lymphoma." (2012): 170-170.

88) Xu, Dongsheng, et al. "Thymoquinone induces G2/M arrest, inactivates PI3K/Akt and nuclear factor-κB pathways in human cholangiocarcinomas both in vitro and in vivo." Oncology Reports 31.5 (2014): 2063-2070.

89) Zhang, Lida, Yangqiu Bai, and Yuxiu Yang. "Thymoquinone chemosensitizes colon cancer cells through inhibition of NFκB.» Oncology letters 12.4 (2016): 2840-2845.

90) El Gazzar, Mohamed A., et al. "Thymoquinone attenuates proinflammatory responses in lipopolysaccharide-activated mast cells by modulating NF-kappaB nuclear transactivation." Biochimica et Biophysica Acta (BBA)-General Subjects 1770.4 (2007): 556-564.

91) Al-Malki, Abdulrahman L., and Ahmed Amir Radwan Sayed. "Thymoquinone attenuates cisplatin-induced hepatotoxicity via nuclear factor kappa-β." BMC complementary and alternative medicine 14.1 (2014): 1-8.

92) Vaillancourt, France, et al. "Elucidation of molecular mechanisms underlying the protective effects of thymoquinone against rheumatoid arthritis." Journal of cellular biochemistry 112.1 (2011): 107-117.

93) Wang, Dongyan, et al. "Thymoquinone inhibits IL-1β-induced inflammation in human osteoarthritis chondrocytes by suppressing NF-κB and MAPKs signaling pathway." Inflammation 38.6 (2015): 2235-2241.

94) Woo, Chern Chiuh, et al. "Thymoquinone: potential cure for inflammatory disorders and cancer." Biochemical pharmacology 83.4 (2012): 443-451.

95) Gökçe, Ahmet, et al. "Protective effects of thymoquinone against methotrexate-induced testicular injury." Human & experimental toxicology 30.8 (2011): 897-903.

96) Fouad, A. A., and I. Jresat. "Thymoquinone therapy abrogates toxic effect of cadmium on rat testes." Andrologia 47.4 (2015): 417-426.

97) Atta, Mustafa S., et al. "Thymoquinone defeats diabetes-induced testicular damage in rats targeting antioxidant, inflammatory and aromatase expression." International journal of molecular sciences 18.5 (2017): 919.

98) Mabrouk, Aymen, and Hassen Ben Cheikh. "Thymoquinone supplementation ameliorates lead-induced testis function impairment in adult rats." Toxicology and Industrial Health 32.6 (2016): 1114-1121.

99) Umar, S., et al. "Synergistic effects of thymoquinone and curcumin on immune response and anti-viral activity against avian influenza virus (H9N2) in turkeys." Poultry science 95.7 (2016): 1513-1520.

100) Sommer, Andrei P., Horst-Dieter Försterling, and Kurt G. Naber. "Thymoquinone: shield and sword against SARS-CoV-2." Precision Nanomedicine (2020): 541-548.

101) Zihlif, Malek A., et al. "Thymoquinone efficiently inhibits the survival of EBV-infected B cells and alters

EBV gene expression." Integrative cancer therapies 12.3 (2013): 257-263.

103) Forouzanfar, Fatemeh, Bibi Sedigheh Fazly Bazzaz, and Hossein Hosseinzadeh. "Black cumin (Nigella sativa) and its constituent (thymoquinone): a review on antimicrobial effects." Iranian journal of basic medical sciences 17.12 (2014): 929.

Chapter 35

Clarithromycin Anti-Cancer Antibiotic

Eradicating Cancer Stem Cells

IN 2015, DR. MICHAEL LISANTI'S group reported that the common antibiotics erythromycin (clarithromycin) and doxycycline can be repurposed to "eradicate cancer stem cells"(CSCs). Both antibiotics inhibit ribosomal protein production in bacteria. Likewise, they do the same for mitochondria in cancer cells that share a resemblance with bacteria. Actually, mitochondria have two ribosomes, a larger and a smaller one. Doxycycline targets the smaller ribosome, while clarithromycin targets the larger one. (1)

Note: Azithromycin (the commonly known Z-Pack) is another macrolide antibiotic chemically similar to erythromycin and clarithromycin.

Lynn Margulis and the Endosymbiont Hypothesis

In 1967, biologist Lynn Margulis revolutionized evolutionary theory by suggesting that mitochondria "evolved" from free living bacteria. Mitochondria started off when bacteria were incorporated into eukaryotic cells in a symbiotic relationship, thus the "endosymbiont hypothesis" was born. Indeed, bacteria and mitochondria have an uncanny resemblance to each other and share many other similarities, thus supporting this idea. One similarity is the ribosomes, the little protein factories are remarkably the same for bacteria and mitochondria. Another similarity is the way in which certain antibiotics act on both, inhibiting bacterial and mitochondrial ribosomes equally. This inhibits protein production for the electron transport chain ETC in the mitochondria involved in oxidative phosphorylation (OXPHOS). Thus, these antibiotics are OXPHOS inhibitors. (1–2)

Cancer Stem Cell Metabolism— Metabolic Plasticity

In 2016, Dr. Maria Peiris-Pagès et al. reviewed metabolic pathways of the CSC, writing that CSCs have "metabolic plasticity," and are able to shift back and forth between OXPHOS and GLYCOLYSIS, depending on the principle source of energy:

Cancer is now viewed as a stem cell disease. There is still no consensus on the metabolic characteristics of cancer stem cells, with several studies indicating that they are mainly glycolytic and others pointing instead to mitochondrial metabolism [OXPHOS] as their principal source of energy. Cancer stem cells also seem to adapt their metabolism to microenvironmental changes by conveniently shifting energy production from one pathway to another, or by acquiring intermediate metabolic phenotypes ... The specific elimination of CSCs may thus represent one of the most important challenges of current cancer research ... In practice, combinational treatments involving both a standard cytotoxic therapy and a CSC-targeted therapy will probably be required to ablate all cancer cells. (5)

Cancer Stem Cells Depend on Mitochondrial Biogenesis

Dr. Lisanti's group also showed that CSCs depend on "mitochondrial biogenesis." Cancer stem cells have increased mitochondrial mass and rely on mitochondrial oxidative phosphorylation (OXPHOS) for energy requirements. (1–8)

Cancer Stem Cell Plasticity

Dr. Lisanti's paper in *Oncotarget* (2017) was discussed in chapter 9, on the vitamin C and doxycycline combination. In this 2017 report, Dr. Lisanti's group explores the "metabolic plasticity of cancer stem cells", meaning that cancer cells develop resistance to antibiotic treatment by switching from an "oxidative phenotype" (OXPHOS) to a "glycolytic phenotype"(GLYCOLYSIS). The CSCs adapt by switching away from mitochondrial energy production and instead use the less efficient GLYCOLYSIS in the cytosol. These glycolytic CSCs are now sensitive to treatment with a GLYCOLYSIS inhibitor, providing "synthetic lethal synergy". Among many others, high-dose IV vitamin C (ascorbate) may serve as such a GLYCOLYSIS inhibitor. Other GLYCOLYSIS Inhibitors such as DCA, Diclofenac and Quercetin might be considered. (1–3).

Targeting Both Ribosomes

Combined use of doxycycline and clarithromycin was studied in order to target both large and small ribosomes. This provides more profound inhibition of mitochondrial protein production (involved in the ETC) in CSCs than either agent alone, amounting to OXPHOS inhibition. In 2019, the Lisanti group studied this combination of doxycycline plus azithromycin (similar to clarithromycin), showing this is indeed the case. (4)

However, the addition of vitamin C resulted in a lethal pro-oxidant effect rather than a GLYCOLYSIS inhibition effect. One might therefore speculate the addition of IV alpha lipoic acid (600mg) infused immediately after the IV vitamin C might potentiate this pro-oxidant lethal effect on CSCs, providing synergy. See chapter 7 on alpha lipoic acid for more on this topic.

Dual Inhibition Targets Cancer Stem Cells

In 2016, in *Breast Cancer Research*, Dr. Lisanti's group studied breast CSCs. Because of the metabolic plasticity of the CSC, they suggested that a dual blockade of both OXPHOS and the GLYCOLYSIS metabolic pathways would be a better way to eradicate CSCs.

[Dual Blockade] may represent a better way to eradicate CSC [Cancer Stem Cell] heterogeneity than focusing exclusively on glycolysis inhibition or suppression of mitochondrial respiration [OXPHOS]. (5)

Dual or Triple Blockade?

If this concept of a dual blockade is a good one for eradication of CSCs, then a triple blockade is even better. Why not add in autophagy inhibition? Blocking autophagy prevents the CSC from shifting into survival mode with "protective autophagy," and is included as one of the "three major pillars of cancer cell metabolism"—OXPHOS, GLYCOLYSIS and Autophagy. (5–8)

Inflammatory Cytokines in the Micro-environment

Dr. Lisanti's group also pointed out that inflammatory cytokines (IL-6, IL-8) derived from the tumor micro-environment stimulate GLYCOLYSIS and activate CSCs to proliferate, grow, and trigger metastatic behavior via activation of NF-kB and PI3K/AKT/mTOR. In highly aggressive cancers, these inflammatory cytokines are massively upregulated and feed the cancer's aggressive behavior:

> Inflammatory cytokines generated by the tumour micro-environment [such as IL-6 and IL-8] with activation of NF-κB induce glycolysis with activation of PI3K and AKT and stimulate CSC [Cancer Stem Cell] self-renewal, which then may promote tumour growth and metastasis. (5)

Clarithromycin also serves as an anti-inflammatory drug, temporarily suppressing production of the pro-inflammatory cytokines, decreasing IL-6, and inhibiting NF-kB activation. This is remarkably effective for decreasing cancer aggressivity. (9)

Clarithromycin: A Repurposed Anti-Cancer Drug

In 2015, Dr. A. M. Van Nuffell et al. suggested repurposing clarithromycin as an anti-cancer agent. In addition to mitochondrial ribosomal inhibition, clarithromycin (CAM) has other anti-cancer benefits, such as:

prolonged reduction of pro-inflammatory cytokines, autophagy inhibition, and anti-angiogenesis ... at clinically relevant concentrations [6 to 50 µg/mL] CAM inhibits lysosomal function [after fusion of the autophagosomes with the lysosomes]. (9)

In vitro animal xenograft studies and human studies using CAM have shown efficacy in multiple myeloma, lymphoma, chronic myeloid leukemia (CML), and lung cancer. (9)

Inhibits Autophagy, BCL-XL and Wnt Pathway

A few other anti-cancer benefits:

- CAM is a potent inhibitor of autophagy at clinically relevant concentrations (6–50 microgram/ml).
- CAM downregulates the anti-apoptotic protein BCL-XL.
- CAM inhibits Beta-Catenin, the signal protein for the Wnt pathway, a CSC pathway. (9)

CAM Synergy with Tyrosine Kinase Inhibitors

In 2012, Dr. A. M. Carella et al. reported improved clinical outcome of chronic leukemia (CML) patients treated with tyrosine kinase inhibitor (TKI), either dasatinib or nilotinib, when used in combination with CAM. Dr. Carella's group observed seven patients responding poorly to tyrosine kinase inhibitor (dasatinib). However, a dramatic change occurred when these same patients were treated with clarithromycin, inducing complete remission.

Dr. Carella et al. write:

The remarkable responses obtained in

these seven patients support the hypothesis that [CAM] inhibition of autophagy may make CML [chronic myelogenous leukemia] cells sensitive to killing by TKIs [Tyrosine Kinase Inhibitors]. (10)

As we have seen in the autophagy chapters, many of the autophagy inhibitors enhance the activity of TKIs (tyrosine kinase inhibitors). CAM also downregulates Bcl-xL, inhibits lysosomal function, and increases natural killer cell activity. (9–10)

CAM Inhibits Wnt /Beta-Catenin

In 2013, Dr. Cristina Semino-Mora et al. studied 48 patients with pseudomyxoma peritonei, an abdominal cancer originating from the appendix. Prior to surgical removal of the appendix, the patients were treated with a triple therapy regimen for H. pylori eradication, a regimen that includes clarithromycin (CAM). Surgical samples were studied showing reduction in Beta-Catenin levels, a signaling protein for the Wnt pathway (for CSCs), which thus served to eradicate CSCs:

> Beta-catenin levels were decreased in the cytoplasm, the cell nuclei, and the mucin-associated cells while Beta-catenin levels within membranes increased in pseudomyxoma peritonei patients after H pylori eradication treatment containing CAM, providing potential protection against cell detachment, cellular invasion, and metastasis. (11)

Note: B-Catenin is the signaling protein for the Wnt pathway, a CSC pathway. Translocation of Beta-Catenin from nucleus to the cell membrane prevents activation of the Wnt pathway.

CAM for MALT Lymphoma- Human Study – H.Pylori

MALT lymphoma is a B-cell lymphoma originating in the "mucosa-associated lymphoid tissue (MALT)," frequently involving stomach or other parts of the gastrointestinal (GI) tract. MALT Lymphoma is closely associated with H. pylori infections of the stomach and is responsive to triple therapy regimens that include the antibiotic clarithromycin. (12)

In 2017, Dr. Andrés Ferreri et al. analyzed 55 cases of MALT lymphoma treated with CAM monotherapy. Three-year survival was 96%, with no patient dying of lymphoma. Four-year progression-free survival was 60%. Dr. Ferreri and colleagues reported that CAM should be repurposed against MALT lymphoma, and that a long-term daily dose of one gram a day is safe and effective. They further suggested the combination of CAM and lenalidamide might be synergistic and more effective, writing:

> Clarithromycin is an exemplary model of a repurposing drug for lymphoma patients; a long-lasting treatment with a daily dose of 1 g is safe, active and cost-effective ... (13)

A later study by Dr. Ferreri et al. used higher doses of Clarithromycin for relapsed/refractory malt lymphoma (four courses of oral clarithromycin 2 g/day, once daily, days 1–14, every 21 days). (14)

Another MALT Lymphoma type occurs in the eye, in the orbital lymphoid tissue. In this sub-type, infection with the chlamydia organism has been implicated, and clarithromycin induces complete remission as a first-line treatment. (15)

Association of Mantle Cell Lymphoma with H. Pylori Infection

In 2000, Dr. T. G. Paglieroni et al. reported an association of Helicobacter pylori infection with mantle cell lymphoma. Dr. Paglieroni's group isolated a patient's mantle cell lymphoma cells. Even though they are cancer cells, they are still B cells and produce antibodies like other B cells. Dr. Paglieroni et al. found the lymphoma B cells produced massive amounts of antibodies against the H. pylori organism, prompting Dr. Paglieroni to recommend antibiotic treatment for H. Pylori in all mantle cell lymphoma patients:

> Consideration of antibacterial therapy as an adjunct to chemotherapy is warranted. The frequency of the association of H. pylori infection and MCL merits further study. (16)

CAM for B-Cell Lymphoma—In Vitro study

In 2004, Dr. Tadashi Ohara et al. reported in *Anti-Cancer Research* that CAM directly induces apoptosis in B-cell lymphoma cells derived from mice in vitro. Dr. Ohara's group identified downregulation of BCL-2 protein in the CAM-treated cell cultures. BCL2 is the anti-apoptotic protein, frequently upregulated in lymphoma, which "immortalizes" the cancer cells by preventing programmed cell death (apoptosis). Downregulating BCL-2 restores the cancer cells' ability to undergo apoptosis. This is immensely important in cancer cell types with upregulated BCL-2. (17)

CAM Case Report in Lymphoma

A 34-year-old male with a one-year history of B-cell lymphoma achieved complete remission after chemotherapy and allogeneic stem cell transplant. However, three months later, a PET scan detected a few active paratracheal and mediastinal lymph nodes indicating relapse. Over 6 months' time, the mediastinal mass gradually increased in size reaching the rather large size of 7 cm. diameter, at which point the oncologist prescribed ibrutinib (Bruton's tyrosine kinase inhibitor). There was no response to the tyrosine kinase inhibitor drug initially. However, about six weeks after starting the drug, the patient reported a painful throat from strep pharyngitis for which a Z-pack (azithromycin) was prescribed. The evening after starting the azithromycin, the patient experienced drenching night sweats for three nights in a row, indicating lymphoma cell lysis. A follow-up PET scan two weeks later showed complete remission, with disappearance of the mass. The azithromycin served as autophagy inhibitor, enhancing the cell-killing effect of the tyrosine kinase inhibitor drug, providing complete remission.

Clarithromycin as Autophagy Inhibitor

As mentioned in a previous chapter 33, clarithromycin is an excellent autophagy inhibitor that enhances the effect of TKIs, as reported in 2012 by Dr. A. M. Carella et al. in a study of drug-resistant chronic myeloid leukemia (CML). (10)

More CAM/Lymphoma Case reports

In 2011, Dr. Masashi Ohe from Korea reported success in four cases of various lymphoma cell types in which complete remission was achieved using CAM as monotherapy at a dosage of 400 mg twice a day, given indefinitely. (18–21)

CAM/ Spontaneous Remission of B-Cell Lymphoma of Oral Cavity

In 2015, Dr. Nobuyuki Kaibuchi et al. reported the case of an 87-year-old man with a 3-cm mass in the left side of his oral cavity. Biopsy revealed B-cell lymphoma. A CAT scan showed the enhancing mass was found near the left-lower wisdom tooth. A PET scan showed localized accumulation of radio-isotope at the mass in the left mandible. On the same day as the biopsy, the patient was started on azithromycin, routinely given to prevent infection at the biopsy site. Three weeks later, the mass had undergone "spontaneous remission" and disappeared. Repeat biopsy of the area was negative. One might speculate that the azithromycin was responsible for the "spontaneous remission." The patient was followed for 2.5 years with no recurrence. The authors reported 11 similar cases of "spontaneous disappearance" of oral lymphomas published in the medical literature. (22)

Clarithromycin for Indolent Lymphoma—Prospective Trial

In 2015, Dr. Carol Portlock et al. reported on their prospective study of advanced-stage, bulky indolent lymphoma in thirty-two patients given a 12-week course of clarithromycin, 500 mg by mouth twice daily. Seven of thirty-two patients responded at one month and two additional patients responded later during follow-up for a 28 % overall response. Survival time for responders was more than double compared to non-responders. (23)

Clarithromycin for Multiple Myeloma

Dr. Tomer Mark showed his enthusiasm for clarithromycin in multiple myeloma by adding clarithromycin to the standard regimen of revlimid and dexamethasone, finding longer remissions and ability to overcome drug-resistant cell types for patients taking the added clarithromycin. **Note:** clarithromycin is a macrolide antibiotic similar to azithromycin. (24–29)

Clarithromycin, Cancer Cell Types, and Synergy with Other Drugs:

Here is a list of studies of CAM efficacy against various cancer cell types and synergies with other drugs. CAM has:

- Synergy with bortezomib in myeloma (30)
- Synergy with TKIs in chronic myeloid leukemia (31–32)
- Modulates autophagy in leukemia (33)
- Synergy with gefitinib in lung cancer (34)
- Suppresses VEGF in lung cancer (35)
- Inhibits autophagy in colon cancer (36)
- Enhances vincristine in cervical and gastric cancer (37)

Autophagy Induced by Tyrosine Kinase Inhibitors

In 2020, Dr. Hideki Tanaka et al. studied autophagy induced by various tyrosine kinase inhibitors, and their enhanced cytotoxicity via inhibition of autophagy with azithromycin.

One of the more potent growth stimulators for the cancer cell is endothelial growth factor receptor (EGFR), located on the outer membrane of cancer cells. EGFR is a tyrosine kinase receptor that activates the PI3K-AKT-mTOR pathway, which potently inhibits autophagy. Blocking this EGFR receptor with an EGFR-TKI drug such as gefitinib (GEF) or erlotinib potently induces "protective autophagy." Macrolide antibiotics, azithromycin (AZM), and clarithromycin strongly inhibit autophagy flux and enhanced the cytotoxicity of EGFR-TKIs in non-small-cell lung cancer and pancreatic cancer, resulting in "non-apoptotic cell death." Azithromycin showed the most potent effect. Dr. Tanaka et al. write:

> The multi-kinase inhibitors appear to have a higher propensity for autophagy induction. Once autophagy was induced, blocking TKI-induced autophagy with AZM resulted in enhanced cytotoxicity via non-apoptotic cell death. These data suggested a clinical benefit in cancer therapy for the combination therapy of TKI and AZM. (38–39)

Adverse Side Effects: Neurotoxicity

Clarithromycin may cause neurotoxicity, presenting as psychiatric illness, encephalopathy, or epilepsy. Caution is advised. (40–41)

Inhibition of Liver CYP Enzyme Metabolism

Clarithromycin is a potent cytochrome P450 (CYP) 3A4 inhibitor, raising the serum level and exposure to other drugs. A number of reports of rhabdomyolysis (muscle necrosis) have been made when used in combination with statin drugs. Other CYP3A4 inhibitors include itraconazole. Caution is advised. (42–47)

Conclusion

Clarithromycin can be considered a dual OXPHOS and autophagy Inhibitor and therefore may synergize with GLYCOLYSIS inhibitors such as DCA, Diclofenac and Quercetin. Clarithromycin is also a CSC agent, since both OXPHOS and Autophagy are linked with CSCs. Clarithromycin has other favorable effects, such as downregulation of inflammatory cytokines via suppression of NF-kB and inhibition of anti-apoptosis proteins to allow apoptosis in the cancer cell. Considering the above favorable studies, one wonders why clarithromycin has not been incorporated into routine protocols for all lymphoma and myeloma patients on the oncology wards.

References for Chapter 35: Clarithromycin

1) Lamb, Rebecca, et al. "Antibiotics that target mitochondria effectively eradicate cancer stem cells, across multiple tumor types: treating cancer like an infectious disease." Oncotarget 6.7 (2015): 4569.

2) Gray, Michael W. "Lynn Margulis and the endosymbiont hypothesis: 50 years later." Molecular biology of the cell 28.10 (2017): 1285-1287.

3) De Francesco, Ernestina Marianna, et al. "Vitamin C and Doxycycline: A synthetic lethal combination therapy targeting metabolic flexibility in cancer stem cells (CSCs)." Oncotarget 8.40 (2017): 67269.

4) Fiorillo, M., et al. "Doxycycline, Azithromycin and vitamin C (DAV): a potent combination therapy for targeting mitochondria and eradicating cancer stem cells (CSCs)." Aging 11.8 (2019): 2202-2216.

5) Peiris-Pagès, Maria, et al. "Cancer stem cell metabolism." Breast Cancer Research 18.1 (2016): 55.

6) Lamb, Rebecca, et al. "Mitochondrial mass, a new metabolic biomarker for stem-like cancer cells: Understanding WNT/FGF-driven anabolic signaling." Oncotarget 6.31 (2015): 30453.

7) De Luca, Arianna, et al. "Mitochondrial biogenesis is required for the anchorage-independent survival and propagation of stem-like cancer cells." Oncotarget 6.17 (2015): 14777.

8) Chiarugi, Paola, and Persio Dello Sbarba. "Cancer stemness and progression: mitochondria on the stage." Oncotarget 6.35 (2015): 36924.

9) Van Nuffel, An MT, et al. "Repurposing Drugs in Oncology (ReDO)—clarithromycin as an anti-cancer agent." ecancermedicalscience 9 (2015).

10) Carella, A. M., et al. "Inhibition of autophagy with clarithromycin: a new strategy to enhance sensitivity of CML stem cells to tyrosine kinase inhibitors." Leukemia supplements 1.S2 (2012): S49.

11) Semino-Mora, Cristina, et al. "Antibiotic treatment decreases microbial burden associated with pseudomyxoma peritonei and affects β-catenin distribution." Clinical Cancer Research 19.14 (2013): 3966-3976.

12) Bilgilier, Ceren, et al. "Prevalence of clarithromycin-resistant Helicobacter pylori strains in gastric mucosa-associated lymphoid tissue lymphoma patients." (2016).

13) Ferreri, Andrés JM, et al. "Clarithromycin as a "repurposing drug" against MALT lymphoma." British Journal of Haematology (2017).

14) Ferreri, Andrés JM, et al. "High-dose clarithromycin is an active monotherapy for patients with relapsed/refractory extranodal marginal zone lymphoma of mucosa-associated lymphoid tissue (MALT): the HD-K phase II trial." Annals of Oncology 26.8 (2015): 1760-1765.

15) Kiesewetter, Barbara, et al. "Clarithromycin leading to complete remission in the first-line treatment of ocular adnexal mucosa-associated lymphoid tissue lymphoma." Journal of Clinical Oncology 33.35 (2014): e130-e132.

16) Paglieroni, T. G., et al. "Association of Helicobacter pylori with mantle cell lymphoma." Blood. Vol. 96. No. 11. 2000.

17) Ohara, Tadashi, et al. "Antibiotics directly induce apoptosis in B cell lymphoma cells derived from BALB/c mice." Anticancer research 24.6 (2004): 3723-3730.

18) Ohe, Masashi, and Satoshi Hashino. "A case of follicular B-cell lymphoma treated using clarithromycin." The Korean journal of hematology 46.3 (2011): 203-206.

19) Ohe, Masashi, Satoshi Hashino, and Atsuo Hattori. "Successful treatment of diffuse large B-cell lymphoma with clarithromycin and prednisolone." The Korean journal of hematology 47.4 (2012): 293-297.

20) Ohe, Masashi, and Satoshi Hashino. "Successful treatment of angioimmunoblastic T-cell lymphoma with clarithromycin." Blood research 51.2 (2016): 139-142.

21) Ohe, Masashi, and Satoshi Hashino. "Successful treatment of recurrent follicular B-cell lymphoma with clarithromycin, prednisolone, and cyclophosphamide." The Korean journal of internal medicine 28.3 (2013): 377.

22) Kaibuchi, Nobuyuki, et al. "A case of spontaneous regression of lymphoma in the mandibular gingiva after biopsy." Oral and Maxillofacial Surgery Cases 1.3 (2015): 33-37.

23) Portlock, Carol S., et al. "A Positive Prospective Trial of Antibiotic Therapy in Advanced Stage, Non-Bulky Indolent Lymphoma." Tumor microenvironment and therapy 2.1 (2015): 14-18.

24) Shaulov, Adir, et al. "Progressive refractory light chain amyloidosis and multiple myeloma patients are responsive to the addition of clarithromycin to IMiD based therapy." American journal of hematology 92.2 (2017): 131-135.

25) Ghosh, Nilanjan, et al. "Clarithromycin overcomes resistance to lenalidomide and dexamethasone in multiple myeloma." American journal of hematology 89.8 (2014).

26) Rossi, Adriana, et al. "BiRd (clarithromycin, lenalidomide, dexamethasone): an update on long-term lenalidomide therapy in previously untreated patients with multiple myeloma." Blood 121.11 (2013): 1982-1985.

27) Gay, Francesca, et al. "Clarithromycin (Biaxin)-lenalidomide-low-dose dexamethasone (BiRd) versus lenalidomide-low-dose dexamethasone (Rd) for newly diagnosed myeloma." American journal of hematology 85.9 (2010): 664.

28) Niesvizky, Ruben, et al. "BiRD (Biaxin [clarithromycin]/Revlimid [lenalidomide]/dexamethasone) combination therapy results in high complete-and overall-response rates in treatment-naive symptomatic multiple myeloma." Blood 111.3 (2008): 1101-1109.

29) Mark, Tomer M., and Morton Coleman. "It's time to take clarithromycin seriously in multiple myeloma." Acta haematologica 135.2 (2016): 101-102.

30) Moriya, Shota, et al. "Macrolide antibiotics block autophagy flux and sensitize to bortezomib via endoplasmic reticulum stress-mediated CHOP induction in myeloma cells." International Journal of Oncology 42.5 (2013): 1541.

31) Carella, Angelo Michele, et al. "Clarithromycin potentiates tyrosine kinase inhibitor treatment in patients with resistant chronic myeloid leukemia." Leukemia & lymphoma 53.7 (2012): 1409-1411.

32) Schafranek, Lisa, et al. "Clarithromycin enhances dasatinib-induced cell death in chronic myeloid leukemia cells, by inhibition of late stage autophagy." Leukemia & lymphoma 54.1 (2013): 198-201.

33) Pillozzi, S., et al. "Macrolide antibiotics exert anti-leukemic effects by modulating the autophagic flux through inhibition of hERG1 potassium channels." Blood cancer journal 6.5 (2016): e423-e423.

34) Sugita, Shohei, et al. "EGFR-independent autophagy induction with gefitinib and enhancement of its cytotoxic effect by targeting autophagy with clarithromycin in non-small cell lung cancer cells." Biochemical and biophysical research communications 461.1 (2015): 28-34.

35) Li, Fajiu, et al. "Azithromycin effectively inhibits tumor angiogenesis by suppressing vascular endothelial growth factor receptor 2-mediated signaling pathways in lung cancer." Oncology letters 14.1 (2017): 89-96.

36) Qiao, Xinran, et al. "Azithromycin enhances anticancer activity of TRAIL by inhibiting autophagy and up-regulating the protein levels of DR4/5 in colon cancer cells in vitro and in vivo." Cancer Communications 38.1 (2018): 43.

37) Zhou, Xuezhang, et al. "Azithromycin synergistically enhances anti-proliferative activity of vincristine in cervical and gastric cancer cells." Cancers 4.4 (2012): 1318-1332.

38) Tanaka, Hideki, et al. "Comparison of autophagy inducibility in various tyrosine kinase inhibitors and their enhanced cytotoxicity via inhibition of autophagy in cancer cells in combined treatment with azithromycin." Biochemistry and Biophysics Reports 22 (2020): 100750.

39) Altman, Jessica K., and Leonidas C. Platanias. "A new purpose for an old drug: inhibiting autophagy with clarithromycin." Leukemia & lymphoma 53.7 (2012): 1255.

40) Bhattacharyya, Shamik, Ryan Darby, and Aaron L. Berkowitz. "Antibiotic-induced neurotoxicity." Current infectious disease reports 16.12 (2014): 448.

41) Di Poggio, M. Bandettini, et al. "Clarithromycin-induced neurotoxicity in adults." Journal of Clinical Neuroscience 18.3 (2011): 313-318.

42) Wagner, Judith, Christine Suessmair, and Hans-Walter Pfister. "Rhabdomyolysis caused by co-medication with simvastatin and clarithromycin." Journal of neurology 256.7 (2009): 1182-1183.

43) Page, S. R., and K. C. Yee. "Rhabdomyolysis in association with simvastatin and dosage increment in clarithromycin." Internal medicine journal 44.7 (2014): 690-693.

44) Sipe, Brooke E., Ronald J. Jones, and Gordon H. Bokhart. "Rhabdomyolysis causing AV blockade due to possible atorvastatin, esomeprazole, and clarithromycin interaction." Annals of Pharmacotherapy 37.6 (2003): 808-811.

45) Liukas, Antti, et al. "Inhibition of cytochrome P450 3A by clarithromycin uniformly affects the pharmacokinetics and pharmacodynamics of oxycodone in young and elderly volunteers." Journal of clinical psychopharmacology 31.3 (2011): 302-308.

46) Hagelberg, Nora M., et al. "Clarithromycin, a potent inhibitor of CYP3A, greatly increases exposure to oral S-ketamine." European Journal of Pain 14.6 (2010): 625-629.

47) Amsden, Guy W., Olatunde Kuye, and Greg CG Wei. "A study of the interaction potential of azithromycin and clarithromycin with atorvastatin in healthy volunteers." The Journal of Clinical Pharmacology 42.4 (2002): 444-449.

Chapter 36

Itraconazole Antifungal Drug Repurposed as Anti-cancer Drug

Itraconazole, also known as Sporonox, is a common antifungal drug developed in the 1980s, usually prescribed as 100 mg or 200 mg oral capsules with daily dosage in the 100–600 mg range. Itraconazole is well tolerated when used long term to prevent or treat chronic fungal infection in immunosuppressed patients. Four hundred milligrams per day for a year is not uncommon for chronic pulmonary aspergillosis or blastomycosis, both fungal infections. Human dosage required to achieve anti-cancer levels used in animal studies is in the 600–900 mg per day range. (1–2)

Itraconazole has been in clinical use for 30 years with an established safety record. Multiple phase 2 clinical trials investigating itraconazole for non-small-cell lung cancer, prostate cancer, and basal cell carcinoma have been completed, showing an increase in progression-free and overall survival. (3–7)

Retrospective studies of patients with ovarian cancer and recurrent triple-negative breast cancer taking itraconazole revealed significant increases in overall survival, thought to be due to the anti-angiogenic effects of itraconazole. Other angiogenesis-dependent diseases such as macular degeneration and diabetic retinopathy may benefit from itraconazole, as well. (3–7)

Itraconazole for Double Hit Lymphoma

Double-hit lymphoma (DHL), having two separate harmful mutations upregulating the c-Myc and BCL pathways, is an extremely aggressive cell-type refractory to conventional chemotherapy (usually R+CHOP), and median survival is less than 1.5 years. An in vitro study by Dr. Juan Gu et al. in *Blood* (2016) using three DHL cell lines with escalating doses of itraconazole showed a strong anti-cancer synergy with "targeted" oncology drugs venetoclax, a BCL2 inhibitor; Ibrutinib, and bortezomib. Dr. Gu and colleagues write:

> Itraconazole caused G1 cell cycle arrest and decreased S-phase in DHL. Moreover, itraconazole had a strong synergistic anti-tumor effect combined with BCL-2 inhibitor ABT199 [Venetoclax], c-Myc inhibitor JQ1, bruton's kinase inhibitor ibrutinib and proteasome inhibitor [bortezomib] with loss of ATP, Caspase 3/7 activation, and loss of mitochondrial membrane potential … (2)

Disrupting Hexokinase II from Mitochondrial Membrane Enhances Chemotherapy

As discussed in chapter 4, on cancer as a metabolic disease, the key location of hexokinase II on the voltage-dependent anion channel (VDAC) pore on the outer mitochondrial membrane can be targeted as a vulnerable metabolic weakness in cancer cells. By separating the hexokinase II from the VDAC, mitochondrial apoptosis can be restored/induced in the cancer cell. In *Blood* (2016), Dr. Gu et al. studied rituximab-resistant non-Hodgkin's lymphoma (NHL) cell lines in vitro and found itraconazole disrupts hexokinase II from the mitochondria and enhances the efficacy of chemotherapy agents. Dr. Gu's group writes:

> The disruption of HKII from mitochondria following itraconazole exposure may contribute to lower the mitochondrial membrane potential and enhance the chemotherapeutic efficacy. Our finding highlights itraconazole as a potential therapeutic agent in the treatment of B-cell malignancies, and strongly supports clinical translation of its use. (3)

Many lymphoma patients have already been put on long-term antifungal prophylaxis with itraconazole by their oncologist, meaning these patients are unknowingly being given a potent anti-cancer agent synergistic with their chemotherapy.

Other antifungal "azole" drugs ketoconazole, clotrimazole, and posaconazole also target HK2 and may be useful in glioblastoma with highly expressed HK2, according to Dr. Sameer Agnihotri et al. writing in 2019. (4)

Repurposing Itraconazole as Anti-Cancer Agent

In 2017, Dr. Hiroshi Tsubamoto et al. reviewed itraconazole as an anti-cancer agent in *Oncology Letters*. Dr. Tsubamoto and colleagues note that itraconazole's anti-cancer activities include the activation of AMP-kinase and the inhibition of mTOR:

Itraconazole directly binds to the mitochondrial protein voltage-dependent anion channel 1 (VDAC1) and interferes with mitochondrial ATP production, leading to the activation of the AMP-activated protein kinase pathway and the subsequent inhibition of mTOR activity.

Its potential anti-cancer activity also includes:

Reversing chemoresistance mediated by P-Glycoprotein, modulating the signal transduction pathways of Hedgehog [Hh], mechanistic target of rapamycin [mTOR], and Wnt/β-catenin [Wnt] in cancer cells, inhibiting angiogenesis and lymphangiogenesis, and possibly interfering with cancer-stromal cell interactions. (5)

Many Successful Clinical Trials

One of the attractive features of itraconazole is that the drug has been the subject of numerous successful clinical trials, showing clinical benefit in prostate and basal cell carcinoma, as well as survival advantage with the itraconazole/chemotherapy combination for relapsed non-small-cell lung, ovarian, triple-negative breast, pancreatic, and biliary-tract cancer.(5)

Itraconazole Binds to VDAC

Perhaps the most illuminating study showing the mechanism of action of itraconazole was done in 2015 by Dr. Sarah Head et al. and published in *Proc Nat Acad Sci.* It showed that itraconazole binds directly to the VDAC on the mitochondrial membrane and modulates the AMPK/mTOR signaling pathway, a regulator of angiogenesis. Dr. Head's group synthesized a fluorescent probe of itraconazole to identify the voltage-dependent anion channel 1 (VDAC1) as a "primary binding protein of itraconazole."(6–7)

When itraconazole binds to VDAC1, this interferes with mitochondrial function, causing a reduction in cellular energy level, which in turn activates AMP-activated protein kinase (AMPK), which downregulates mTOR activity, leading to inhibition of endothelial cell proliferation (angiogenesis).(6–7)

Other substances that activate AMPK include metformin, resveratrol, pterostilbene, and berberine, which also inhibit mitochondrial function. Similar to itraconazole, curcumin also interferes with the function of the VDAC. See chapter 10 on natural substances targeting CSCs.

Important: Activation of AMP-kinase, which downregulates the mTOR pathway, inhibits angiogenesis by decreasing VEGF secretion (vascular endothelial growth factor).

Note: Angiogenesis is the formation of new blood vessels to feed the cancer. (7)

Itraconazole 1,000 times More Effective than Metformin

Dr. Head et al. compared itraconazole and metformin in their ability to activate AMP-kinase (AMPK) in human umbilical endothelial cells (HUVEC), finding itraconazole more effective by a factor of one thousand. The concentration of metformin required for AMP activation was 1,000 times higher than itraconazole. Another effect discovered by Dr. Head's group is inhibition of cholesterol trafficking by itraconazole due to the direct inhibition of the lysosomal protein NPC1. The combined simultaneous inhibition of cholesterol trafficking and AMPK activation resulted in synergistic inhibition of the mTOR pathway, which inhibits angiogenesis (8)

Cervical Cancer in Vitro – 8-Fold Downregulation

A study of cervical cancer cells in vitro in *Anti-cancer Research* (2017) by Dr. Tomoko Ueda et al. showed that itraconazole modulates Hedgehog, Wnt /Beta-catenin, as well as Akt Signaling and inhibits proliferation of cervical cancer cells. Dr. Ueda's group found

> 8-fold downregulation in the expression of GLi1 [hedgehog], Wnt 4 and Wnt 10A among itraconazole-treated CaSki [cervical cancer] cells. (9)

Dr. Ueda found itracconazole suppressed Beta-Catenin expression and blocked Akt phosphorylation. Suppression of Beta-Catenin inactivates the Wnt pathway. Blocking Akt phosphorylation inactivates the Akt pathway and its downstream PI3K (phosphoinositide 3-kinase) pathway, and inactivates the mTOR pathway. These pathways are involved in upregulating cancer-cell metabolism and proliferation.

Itraconazole Clinical Trials

As mentioned above, there are many ongoing clinical trials using Itraconazole for prostate, gastric, pancreatic, esophageal, lung, gynecologic, and basal cell cancers.

Prostate Cancer Clinical Trial

A 2013 clinical trial was published by Dr. Emmanuel Antonarakis et al. in the *Oncologist* using itraconazole in men with metastatic castration-resistant prostate cancer. Forty six men were randomized to receive either a low dose, 200 mg per day, or high-dose, 600 mg per day of itraconazole. Progression-free survival was determined by PSA. The progression-free survival for the high-dose group was 4 times greater than the low-dose group.

The PFS [progression-free survival] rates at 24 weeks were 11.8% in the low-dose arm and 48.0% in the high-dose arm. The median PFS times were 11.9 weeks and 35.9 weeks.(10)

Fifty percent of the men remained progression-free for 6 months on the 600 mg per day itraconazole.

Phase Two Clinical Trial in Prostate Cancer

In a 2019 phase two clinical trial by Dr. Mina Lee et al. for recurrent prostate cancer, nineteen men were given itraconazole 300 mg orally twice a day for 12 weeks. Of the 19, one had a greater than 50% reduction in PSA. Nine others had a (median) 25% reduction in PSA after 12 weeks of itraconazole. Adverse effects were related to mineralocorticoid effects of itraconazole with edema and hypertension. (11)

Combining Hydroxychloroquine with Itraconazole for Prostate Cancer

A new recurrent prostate cancer clinical trial (NCT03513211) studying the effect of itraconazole combined with autophagy inhibitor, hydroxychloroquine (HQ), is underway in Sydney, Australia, by Dr. Anthony Joshua et al. In this study, the addition of an autophagy inhibitor (HQ) is expected to augment the anti-cancer effect of itraconazole. We await the results. (12–13)

Immune Suppression?

The immuno-suppressive effects of itraconazole in vitro were found to be artifacts when studied in vivo. (14–17)

Anti-Inflammatory Effects, Potent Inhibitor of 5-LOX

In 1989, Dr. K. Jaschonek et al. found itraconazole a potent inhibitor of 5-lipoxygenase (5-LOX) activity at low serum concentrations in human polymorphonuclear leukocytes (PMNL). 5-LOX is an inflammatory pathway. Inhibition of 5-LOX is important because of its role in maintaining CSCs. Boswellia (Frankincense) is another 5-LOX inhibitor as discussed in Chapter 17. (18)

Wnt, Cox-2 and 5-LOX and Cancer Stem Cells

In 2016, Dr. Jessica Roos et al. studied the regulation of tumorigenic Wnt signaling by cyclo-oxygenase-2, 5-lipoxygenase and their pharmacological inhibitors (COX-2 and 5-LOX inhibitors). They reported that NSAIDs, such as the COX-2 inhibitor celecoxib, suppress Wnt signaling by targeting the pro-inflammatory enzyme 5-lipoxygenase (5-LOX). Inhibition of 5-LOX led to an impairment of Wnt-dependent myeloid leukemia stem cells (both acute and chronic types of leukemia). Dr. Roos believes that 5-lipoxygenase inhibitors might represent a novel type of Wnt inhibitor and anti-CSC agent. (19)

5-LOX inhibitors are Wnt Inhibitors

Based on the study by Dr. Jessica Roos et al., the combination of a COX-2 inhibitor (Celebrex®) with a 5-LOX inhibitor itraconazole (or Boswellia) might be synergistic, targeting CSCs through Wnt inhibition. (19–25) They write:

Our own studies have shown that nonsteroidal anti-inflammatory drugs [NSAIDS] suppress Wnt signaling by targeting the pro-inflammatory enzyme 5-lipoxygenase which is the key enzyme pathophysiologically involved in the synthesis of leukotrienes. Furthermore, we found a direct link between the 5-lipoxygenase and Wnt signaling pathways, which is essential for the maintenance of leukemic stem cells. Accordingly, genetic and pharmacological inhibition of 5-lipoxygenase led to an impairment of Wnt-dependent acute and chronic myeloid leukemia stem cells. We believe that 5-lipoxygenase inhibitors might represent a novel type of Wnt inhibitor activating a potentially naturally occurring novel mechanism of suppression of Wnt signaling that is nontoxic, at least in mice, and is potentially well tolerated in patients. (19)

5-LOX Overexpressed in MCL Cells 7-Fold

5-LOX inhibitors are a promising therapeutic strategy for mantle cell lymphoma (MCL). In his 2009 study, Dr. Robert Boyd et al. found

that aberrant 5-LOX activity is upregulated 7-fold in B-Cell lymphoma compared to normal lymphocytes:

5-lipoxygenase [5-LOX], a key enzyme in leukotriene biosynthesis, was associated with lipid rafts and was upregulated 7-fold in MCL [B-Cell Lymphoma] compared with normal B cells…. Inhibitors of 5-LOX activity induced apoptosis in MCL cell lines and primary chronic lymphocytic leukemia cells, indicating an important role for the leukotriene biosynthetic pathway in MCL and other B-cell malignancies…. this could be a promising therapeutic strategy for MCL and CLL [chronic lymphocytic lymphoma]. (22)

Dr. Yilmad Mahshid et al. found high expression of 5-LOX in malignant MCL cells. (23)

Note: Fenofibrate is another drug targeting lipid rafts. See chapter 37 for more on this.

Countering CD40 Activation of B-Cell Lymphoma with 5-LOX inhibitor

In 2005, Dr. Gudmundur Runarsson observed that treatment of B-CLL cells (chronic lymphocytic leukemia) with a 5-LOX inhibitor drug then inhibited CD-40 activation of the lymphoma cells. Dr. Runarsson writes that the 5 LOX inhibitor treatment:

counteracted CD40-dependent activation of these cells by inhibiting CD40-induced DNA synthesis and CD40-induced expression of CD23, CD54, and CD150. (24)

CD-40 is a protein on the surface of immune cells and a critical regular of the immune system typically used in the laboratory to activate B cells in vitro. B-cell malignancies are heavily

CD-40 dependent for activation, proliferation, and survival.

Note: 5-LOX inhibition by Boswellia (Frankincense) is discussed in chapter 17 in this book.

Suppressing Lymphangiogenesis

In 2015, Dr. Yunfen Wang studied malignant pleural effusion (MPE), fluid in the chest cavity in mice, showing itraconazole inhibits MPE by suppressing lymphangiogenesis, the creation of new lymph vessels by the cancer cells, which leads to growth of the tumor mass.(26)

In 2013, Dr. Song found that lenalidamide, a new oncology drug derived from thalidomide, also suppressed lymphangiogenesis in a mouse xenograft model of MCL, inhibiting networks of new lymphatics within the tumor mass.(27)

Caution: Concurrent Use of Itraconazole with Rituximab

The treatment of lymphoma was revolutionized in 1997 with FDA approval of rituximab, a monoclonal antibody targeting the B-cell surface protein CD20. Commonly given IV in combination with chemotherapy for lymphoma, rituximab stabilizes the CD20 protein on lipid rafts. This has a cytotoxic effect on the B cells, increasing remission rates and prolonging patient survival. (28)

However, concurrent use of itraconazole with rituximab is not recommended. Itraconazole is a lipid raft agent that counteracts (abrogates) the effect of rituximab. Dr. Pan Pantziarka et al. (2015) write:

> Concurrent use of ITZ [itraconazole] was shown, in vitro and in vivo using a murine

xenograft model of lymphoma, to abrogate the therapeutic effect of rituximab. (1)

Cancer Stem Cells – Hedgehog Inhibitor

In 2010, Dr. James Kim et al. screened a panel of 2400 FDA-approved drugs, identifying itraconazole as potent Hh (Hedgehog) inhibitor with suppression of Hh-dependent tumor growth in vivo at serum levels comparable to levels obtained with routine antifungal dosage (IC50 of approximately 800 nM).

The Hedgehog (Hh) pathway is a key regulator of embryonic development and tissue repair, as well as a CSC pathway. Disrupted regulation of Hh is associated with CSC formation. (29–32)

Hedgehog Pathway in Lymphoma

In 2015, Drs. Victoria Campbell and Mhairi Copland reviewed hedgehog signaling in CSCs with a focus on NHL (Non Hodgkin's Lymphoma). Dr. Campbell found the anti-apoptotic protein BCL-2 is increased by the active Hedgehog pathway signaling, while inhibition of Hh downregulates BCL-2:

> Expression of BCL-2 is increased in the presence of active Hh signaling and downregulated upon inhibition of the pathway…. Components of the Hh pathway and key downstream targets [BCL-2 and BCL-XL] are expressed in a variety of NHL [Non-Hodgkin's Lymphoma] cell lines … Burkitt's Lymphoma cells underwent apoptosis in the absence of Hh signaling both in vitro and in vivo. (32)

GLI proteins are the downstream effectors of Hh signaling. When studied by Drs. Campbell and Copland, they were found to be upregulated in mantle cell lymphoma, a rare form of B Cell Lymphoma. Inhibiting GLI in an animal xenograft model resulted in downregulation of BCL-2 and cyclin D1, decreased proliferation, and greater sensitivity to chemotherapy. They write:

> In mantle cell lymphoma, a murine model showed upregulation of the GLI transcription factors at the gene level, confirming previous work showing the GLI transcription factors to be overexpressed in mantle cell lymphoma, both in cell lines and primary lymphoma cells, compared to normal B cells. Further, targeting the GLI transcription factors with antisense oligonucleotides downregulated BCL-2 and Cyclin D1 resulting in decreased proliferation and increased susceptibility to chemotherapy. (33)

In 2008, Dr. Ganapati Hegde et al. writes that molecular targeting of the hedgehog-GLI signaling pathway in MCL improved chemotherapy drug sensitivity:

> [It] increased susceptibility to chemotherapeutic drug, doxorubicin. Also, downregulation of GLI decreased cyclin D1 and BCL2 transcript levels ... and molecular targeting of GLI is a potential therapeutic approach to improve the treatment for MCL. (34)

Itraconazole Inhibits Hh Pathway in Gastric Cancer

Gastric cancers typically exhibit upregulated Hedgehog (Hh) pathway. In 2017, Dr. Qiang Hu et al. studied the anti-cancer effect of oral administration of itraconazole on gastric cancer cell lines using in vitro and in vivo xenograft animal models, finding a remarkable inhibition of gastric cancer-cell proliferation and inhibition of the transcription of GLI, the downstream Hedgehog signaling protein. Dr. Hu et al. write:

> Itraconazole induces apoptosis and cell cycle arrest via inhibiting Hedgehog signaling in gastric cancer cells ... oral administration could inhibit the growth of cancer cell xenografts. Itraconazole synergized and enhanced efficacy of the chemotherapy drug, 5FU [5-flouro-uracil]. (35)

Itraconazole for Breast Cancer Inhibits Hedgehog (Hh) Pathway – Autophagic Cell Death

In 2017, Dr. Xiaoya Wang et al. reported in *Cancer Letters* that itraconazole has antiproliferative effects on breast cancer cell lines and the xenograft mouse model by inhibiting the Hedgehog pathway and inducing apoptosis and autophagic cell death. Dr. Wang and colleagues write:

> In breast cancer cell lines, itraconazole-induced apoptosis by altering mitochondria membrane potential, reducing BCL-2 expression and elevating caspase-3 activity. Itraconazole also induced autophagic cell death via LC3-II expression upregulation ... Itraconazole treatment inhibited hedgehog pathway key molecular expression, such as SHH and Gli1, resulting in promotion of apoptosis and autophagy. The anti-proliferation effect of itraconazole-induced apoptosis and autophagy via hedgehog pathway inhibition was confirmed ... A human xenograft nude mouse model corroborated the anti-breast cancer activity as evidenced by reduced tumor size, and increased tumor tissue apoptosis and autophagy. (36)

Hedgehog Pathway Crosstalk with Autophagy

In 2013, Dr. Ying Wang et al. studied hepatocellular cancer cell lines, showing that inhibition of Hedgehog pathway induces autophagy.

However, things are not so simple, as Drs. Xian Zeng, and Dianwen Ju in 2018 reviewed all the available studies on the association of Hedgehog signaling with autophagy, finding conflicting results. Some studies show induction (activation) of autophagy, while others show inhibition of autophagy upon applying a Hedgehog inhibitor drug such as itraconazole. Drs. Zeng and Zu write that we need more research:

> Before we can harness the Hh [Hedgehog]–Autophagy crosstalk to design improved anti-cancer strategies, considerable research efforts are needed to gain a deeper understanding of the underlying molecular mechanisms. (38)

If Dr. Zheng is confused about the role of autophagy, then you can imagine that many others are too! One of the goals of this book is to clarify these concepts for the reader and eliminate this confusion. Earlier in this book (chapters 31–34), we explained the role of "protective autophagy". Autophagy is one of the three pillars of cancer cell metabolism, along with OXPHOS and GLYCOLYSIS. Because of metabolic plasticity, simultaneous inhibition of all three pillars is necessary to eradicate CSCs and achieve durable remission.

Upregulation of Hh in Breast Cancer

In 2017, Dr. Helen Oladapo et al. studied triple-negative inflammatory breast cancer cells, reporting in *Cancer Letter* upregulation of the Hedgehog (Hh/Gli) pathway:

> Activation of the Hedgehog [Hh] pathway effector GLi1 is linked to tumorigenesis and invasiveness in a number of cancers, and pharmacological targeting of GLi1 inhibits proliferation, tumor emboli formation and in vivo tumor growth of inflammatory breast cancer cells. (39)

In 2014, Drs. Hiroshi Tsubamoto et al. reported on their study of 13 patients with Triple-Negative Breast Cancer with relapsed/refractory metastatic disease who were treated by adding itraconazole to conventional chemotherapy. Median overall survival was prolonged by 20 months when compared to similar studies using chemotherapy alone. (40)

Anti-Cancer Concentrations Similar to Antifungal

In *Cell* (2019), Dr. Riobo-Del Galdo et al. reported on itraconazole's role as a hedgehog inhibitor in breast cancer, writing that anticancer activity occurs at concentrations similar to those used for anti-fungal treatment:

> its inhibitory effect on Hh signaling is distinct and appears to be through prevention of ciliary accumulation of SMO [smoothened protein]. When administered systemically in mice, itraconazole suppressed the growth of medulloblastoma and reduced Hh activation markers at similar concentrations than required for its antifungal activity. (41)

Itraconazole as Adjuvant for Breast Cancer

Dr. Galdo's group also reports itraconazole-induced cell death in in vitro breast-cancer cell lines, reducing angiogenesis both in vitro and in vivo, and synergizing with 5-FU, a common chemotherapy agent. In concluding, Dr. Galdo et al. suggest itraconazole is a drug of choice for use as adjuvant in breast cancer treatment:

> The low cost of itraconazole and well-known safety profile makes it a possible drug of choice for use as an adjuvant in cancer treatment in developing countries or areas of socioeconomic disadvantage. (41)

Dr. Richard Kast and Itraconazole as Hh Inhibitor

Dr. Richard Kast et al., write in *Oncotarget* (2017) that itraconazole is useful in glioblastoma as a hedgehog inhibitor, which decreases the cell proliferation rate and enhances apoptosis in glioblastoma cell lines:

> The primary mode of anti-cancer action is inhibition of Hh [Hedgehog] signaling ... Itraconazole inhibits release of Gli1 thus keeping it sequestered in the cytoplasm ... In preclinical studies itraconazole inhibition of Hh signaling inhibited growth of breast cancer, melanoma, and endometrial cancer.(42)

Inhibiting AKT/mTOR in Endometrial Cancer

In 2017, Dr. Tsubamoto studied et al. the effect of itraconazole on endometrial cancer cell lines in vitro. They found that Itraconazole:

suppresses the growth of EC [endometrial cancer] cells by inhibiting AKT/mTOR signaling. (43)

In this model of EC, treatment with itraconazole inhibits the AKT/mTOR signaling pathway with activation of "protective autophagy."

Dr. Tsubamoto et al. wrote:

> Itraconazole did not suppress GLI1 or GLI2 transcription but did inhibit the expression of mammalian target of rapamycin [mTOR] signaling components in AN3-CA and HEC-1A [endometrial cancer] cells, while inducing that of microtubule-associated protein 1A/1B-light chain 3-II [LC3], a marker of autophagy [indicates induction of autophagy typical for mTOR inhibition] ... (43)

Note: mTOR is the master controller of autophagy. Inhibition of mTOR activates protective autophagy.

Simultaneous Suppression of BTK and mTOR

Dr. Jiao Li et al. In *J Cancer* (2018) reported synergistic enhancement with combination of an mTOR inhibitor drug along with Bruton's tyrosine kinase (BTK) inhibitor in B-cell lymphoma. Originally approved by the FDA in 2016 as an oral capsule, ibrutinib (Imbruvica®) BTK inhibitor, targets the B-cell receptor (BCR) signaling pathway and has revolutionized treatment of B-cell malignancies. In his 2018 study, Dr. Li et al. used a more potent tyrosine kinase inhibitor drug, "a novel irreversible BTK inhibitor, PLS-123, more potent and selective than ibrutinib." (44)

Using in vitro screening, Dr. Li's group discovered that the combination of BTK inhibitor drug and mTOR inhibitor drug (in this case, everolimus) synergistic in reducing proliferation and motility of aggressive B-cell lymphoma (Mantle Cell Lymphoma in vitro and in vivo). Dr. Li says:

> Simultaneous inhibition resulted in marked induction of apoptosis and cell cycle arrest in the G1 phase, which were accompanied by upregulation of pro-apoptotic proteins [cleaved Caspase-3, cleaved PARP and Bax], repression of anti-apoptotic proteins [Mcl-1, Bcl-xl and XIAP], and downregulation of regulators of the G1/S-phase transition [CDK2, CDK4, CDK6 and Cyclin D1]. Gene expression profile analysis revealed simultaneous treatment with these agents led to inhibition of the JAK2/STAT3, AKT/mTOR signaling pathways and SGK1 expression. Finally, the anti-tumor and pro-apoptotic activities of combination strategy have also been demonstrated using xenograft mice models. Taken together, simultaneous suppression of BTK and mTOR may be indicated as a potential therapeutic modality for the treatment of MCL. (44)

These findings suggest possible synergy of itraconazole, another potent mTOR inhibitor, with ibrutinib. Indeed, studies show such a synergy of itraconazole with ibrutinib and venetoclax (BCL2 inhibitor) as reported by Dr. Gu in 2016. (2–3)

Drug Interaction CYP Inhibitor

However, caution with dosing is advised since itraconazole inhibits the CYP enzyme system in the liver, which metabolizes drugs. The net effect is increased serum levels of ibrutinib and venetoclax, would could reach excessive levels.

Ibrutinib Resistance Reversed by mTOR Inhibitor

Although dramatic remissions can be achieved with ibrutinib in lymphoma patients, eventually an ibrutinib-resistant cell type develops, with inevitable relapse.

In 2017, Dr. Xiaohong Zhao et al. studied acquired ibrutinib resistance in mantle cell lymphoma (MCL), reporting that ibrutinib has high response rates in B-cell lymphomas; however, all patients eventually develop ibrutinib resistance with relapse and fulminant progression. This is a growing problem. Dr. Xiaohong Zhao studied the tumor micro-environment (TME) influence on ibrutinib efficacy, and acquired ibrutinib resistance and found that feedback from the TME (tumor micro-environment) was responsible for development of ibrutinib resistance with reactivation of mTOR pathway:

> MCL cells develop ibrutinib resistance through evolutionary processes driven by dynamic feedback between MCL cells and TME [tumor micro-environment], leading to kinome adaptive reprogramming, bypassing the effect of ibrutinib and reciprocal activation of PI3K-AKT-mTOR and integrin-β1 signalling. Combinatorial disruption of B-cell receptor signalling [with ibrutnib] and PI3K-AKT-mTOR axis [mTOR inhibitor such as itraconazole] leads to release of MCL cells from TME, reversal of drug resistance and enhanced anti-MCL activity in MCL patient samples and patient-derived xenograft models. (45)

Note: The term, "Kinome" was first coined in 2002 by Gerard Manning referring to the complete set of protein kinases encoded in the genome of an organism. "Kinome adaptive reprogramming" refers to the ability of the cancer cell to switch to alternate kinase pathways, overcoming a tyrosine kinase inhibitor drug such as ibrutinib. Thus, creating ibrutinib resistance.

Note: Itraconazole profoundly inhibits mTOR, so combination with ibrutinib could potentially overcome TME-acquired resistance.

Pterostilbene a Natural mTOR Inhibitor

Pterostilbene, a methylated resveratrol derivative is another mTOR inhibitor. Adding Pterostilbene, a botanical supplement derived from grapes and blueberries, might be useful in this case to overcome ibrutinib resistance. In 2018, Dr. Yu found that pterostilbene attenuates progression of mantle cell lymphoma by targeting the PI3K/Akt/mTOR signaling pathway. (46)

Ibrutinib Resistance and the Micro-environment

In 2017, Dr. D. Chiron et al. studied the micro-environment in mantle cell lymphoma (MCL) and its effect on resistance to drug treatment with ibrutinib. Dr. Chiron's group found that

> despite a significant level of the proliferation index Ki67 in LN [LN = lymph nodes containing malignant lymphoma cells], we did not detect any proliferating PB [peripheral blood] MCL cells, suggesting a major role of the tumor ecosystem.

In other words, once the MCL cells left the lymph node and appeared in circulation, they were no longer proliferating. The tumor micro-environment in the lymph node was responsible for molecular signaling with CD40L and cytokines, which upregulated genetic signatures in lymphoma cells for proliferation and migration, i.e., more aggressive behavior. (47)

Inducing Cell Cycle Progression with CD40 and Cytokine Cocktail Co-Culture Model

CD40 is a key protein that activates the dormant B cells. Once activated, the B cells are no longer dormant. They rapidly proliferate and become invasive. Dr. Chiron's lab cultured twenty-one mantle cell lymphoma (MCL) samples and found that cell cycle progression (proliferation) was induced by CD40L, which was amplified by a MCL-specific cytokine cocktail (Ck), such as cytokines IL-6, and IL-10. Dr. Chiron's lab then performed RNA sequencing in MCL cells from peripheral blood (PB) or co-cultured with CD40 and cytokine cocktail (CD40 + Ck), and then compared gene expression. They found more than 65% of genes induced in the "CD40L + Ck" co-culture model are also upregulated in the LN (lymph node), and not in PB (peripheral blood), which has no CD40 stimulus. The co-culture model revealed upregulation of molecular signatures characteristic of MCL such as cell cycle, BCR (B-Cell Receptor), nuclear factor kappa B (NF-kB), and the anti-apoptotic Bcl2 family.

Dr. Chiron's group discusses the triple-drug combination of BCL inhibitor, venetoclax, B-cell receptor inhibitor ibrutinib, and the next-generation anti-CD20 antibody, obinutuzumab, as effective for overcoming drug resistance conferred by the CD40 and cytokine cocktail released by the micro-environment.

Note: BH3 profiling assay refers to the anti-apoptotic proteins BCL-2. Dr. Chiron comments that venetoclax failed to induce apoptosis in the B-cell lymphoma cells residing in lymph nodes. The addition of Ibrutinib and obinutuzumab overcame this drug resistance conferred by the micro-environment:

Using the functional BH3-profiling assay, we demonstrated that, whereas PB [peripheral blood] MCL [lymphoma] cells are dependent on Bcl2 for survival, Bcl-xL upregulation was responsible for loss of mitochondrial priming and resistance. Consequently, whereas Bcl2 BH3-mimetic [Venetoclax] efficiently triggered apoptosis in PB MCL, cells protected by the micro-environment were resistant ... We then hypothesized that targeting Bcl-xL could increase treatment efficacy. Using our co-culture model, we developed efficient targeted strategies [i.e., BTK inhibitor ibrutinib, Type II anti-CD20 Obinutuzumab], which counteract Bcl-xL [apoptotic protein] overexpression and overcome drug resistance in primary cells ex vivo.

This is an example of using combinations of targeted drugs to overcome drug resistance induced by cytokines in the micro-environment. (47–53)

Itraconazole Cervical Cancer – 8-Fold Downregulation of Hedgehog Signals

In 2017, Dr. Tomoko Ueda et al. studied cervical cancer cells, finding that itraconazole inhibits two of the three main CSC pathways, hedgehog and Wnt, as well as the Akt signaling pathway:

[Itraconazole] modulates Hedgehog, Wnt /B-catenin, as well as Akt Signaling, and

Inhibits Proliferation ... [causing] 8-fold downregulation in the expression of GLI1 [Hedgehog], Wnt 4 and Wnt 10A among itraconazole-treated CaSki [Cervical Cancer] cells. Immunoblots showed suppression in B-catenin expression and Akt phosphorylation. (54)

Itraconazole Inhibits VEGF, Anti-Angiogenesis

As mentioned previously, VEGF stimulates growth of new blood vessels to feed the growing tumor and is upregulated in many cancers. In 2018, Dr. Benjamin Nacev reported that itraconazole has potent anti-angiogenic activity because it inhibits the binding of VEGF to its receptor. (55)

Phase 2 Trial for Basal Skin Cancer Itraconazole

In 2014, a phase two trial of oral itraconazole for basal cell carcinoma was reported by Dr. Daniel Kim et al., yielding impressive results in 19 patients placed into two groups receiving either 200 mg a day or 400 mg a day of the itraconazole drug for 1–3 months. Cancer cell proliferation was reduced by 65%, Hedgehog (Hh) activity reduced by 65%, and tumor area reduced by 24%. (56)

Both basal cell and squamous cell types of skin cancer show upregulation of the hedgehog/GLI pathway. High expression of the Hh pathway is a prognostic factor that confers a poor overall survival. The Hh/Gli pathway is inhibited by itraconazole, thus serving as an effective anti-cancer agent for basal cell and squamous cell skin cancer. (56–59)

Mebendazole Hh Inhibitor

Another Hedgehog inhibitor is mebendazole, as discussed in 2015 by Dr. Andrew Larsen et al. Thus, efficacy of mebendazole for skin cancer might be expected. One might also expect the combination of mebendazole with itraconazole to be synergistic with augmented effects in skin cancer as well as other cancers, with upregulated hedgehog signaling. The usual antiparasitic dosage for mebendazole is 100 mg caps, one cap twice a day. For more on mebendazole, see chapter 20, "Cancer as a Parasitic Disease" and chapter 24, "Mebendazole and Fenbendazole." (60)

Itraconazole as Hh Inhibitor for Basal Cell Cancer

In 2016, Dr. Mohd Wahid et al. compared three hedgehog inhibitors for treatment of basal cell cancer—vismodegib, sonidegib, and itraconazole. Both vismodegib and sonidegib are new hedgehog inhibitor drugs FDA-approved for basal cell carcinoma of the skin. Both drugs bind to the smoothened (SMO) transmembrane protein, thereby inhibiting the hedgehog pathway. Dr. Wahid's group concludes that all three drugs show positive results, to some extent but fail in the resistant tumors, suggesting the need for drug combinations to gain greater efficacy. (61)

Adding Autophagy Inhibitor Enhances Effect of Hh Inhibitor

Perhaps adding an autophagy inhibitor would enhance the anti-cancer effect of itraconazole, as reported in 2016 by Dr. Zhang, who observed that the hedgehog inhibitor erismodegib inhibited migration and adhesion of MCL. However, the cancer cells escaped the effect by stimulating "protective autophagy." The combination of Hh inhibitor, erismodegib, with autophagy inhibitors, further enhanced cancer cell death. (62)

Other autophagy inhibitors include mefloquine, chloroquine, hydroxychloroquine, clarithromycin, azithromycin, thymoquinone, loratadine, and PPIs. See chapters 31-35 for more on autophagy inhibitors.

Itraconazole for Melanoma

In 2017, Dr. Liang studied itraconazole anticancer effects on melanoma cells in vitro, finding effective inhibition of melanoma by suppression of the Hedgehog (Hh), Wnt, and PI3K-mTOR signaling pathways. The KI-67 measure of proliferation was inhibited in a dose-dependent manner. The Wnt pathway growth factor proteins declined dramatically when treated with 1-2 micromolar itraconazole. All three major signaling pathways—Hedgehog, Wnt, and PI3K/mTOR—were suppressed. Dr. Liang says:

In these cases, a high dose of itraconazole ranging from 600 to 900 mg/day can be given to patients for 3 to 16 months with close monitoring for any toxicity of this compound. (63)

FDA Boxed Warning for Itraconazole in patients with CHF

The FDA Boxed warning is as follows:

Congestive Heart Failure, Cardiac Effects and Drug Interactions: Itraconazole capsules should not be administered for the treatment of onychomycosis [nail fungus] in patients with evidence of ventricular dysfunction such as congestive heart failure [CHF] or a history of CHF. Ref: FDA Boxed Warning.

This problem is related to aldosterone-like mineralocorticoid activity of itraconazole, which causes fluid retention, a potentially dangerous condition in CHF patients who are typically treated with potent diuretics (furosemide) to eliminate excess fluid and relieve the CHF.

Itraconazole Drug Interactions CYP-450

Itraconazole inhibits the p450 enzyme system, CYP3A, in the liver which metabolizes drugs. (64)

This will increase the serum levels of other concurrent drugs metabolized by CYP3A, and dosage should be adjusted. One such itraconazole interaction is with ibrutinib, which increases exposure 10-fold. When using itraconazole concurrently with ibrutinib, dosage should be decreased to adjust for this effect. (65)

However, for poorly absorbed drugs with low serum levels, concurrent itraconazole is beneficial for increasing drug efficacy. In addition, supplements such as garlic, ginkgo biloba, echinacea, ginseng, St. John's wort , grapeseed extract, and grapefruit juice may also inhibit CYP3A and increase serum levels of various medications metabolized by CYP3A.(65–66)

Itraconazole Inhibits P-Glycoprotein Activity Drug Resistance

Since the P-glycoprotein confers multidrug resistance on the cancer cell, p-glycoprotein inhibitors re-sensitize the cancer cell type to drug treatment. In 2015, Dr. Allen Lam et al. reported that both itraconazole and clarithromycin inhibit p-glycoprotein activity in vitro, overcoming drug resistance. This is a useful feature that can be harnessed for drug-resistant cancer cell types. (67)

Adverse Side Effects of Itraconazole (ITZ)

Dr. Ke Li in et al. (2019) write:

A drug screen identified ITZ as an inhibitor of the Hh [hedgehog] pathway at a clinically relevant concentration of 800 nM (nanomolar), and at this concentration, ITZ is very safe and has little adverse effects on human beings.(68)

Most adverse effects are related to the mineralocorticoid activity of itraconazole. Dr. Antonarakis writes in 2013:

The most common adverse events were edema, fatigue, hypertension, and hypokalemia ... [thought to be related to] mineralocorticoid excess. (10)

Dr. Pan Pantziarka et al. (2015) write:

Itraconazole is a relatively safe drug with clear pharmacokinetic characteristics and minimal side effects, including neutropenia, liver failure, and heart failure. (1)

Conclusion

The old antifungal drug, itraconazole, has many attractive features as a repurposed anti-cancer drug, serving to detach HK2 from the VDAC, serving as hedgehog inhibitor, mTOR inhibitor, VEGF, and angiogenesis inhibitor. Success in many clinical trials is an added plus. Adverse effects are related to mineralocorticoid activity. Hopefully, itraconazole will be incorporated into mainstream oncology on a routine basis in the near future.

References Chapter 36: Itraconazole

1) Pantziarka, Pan, et al. "Repurposing Drugs in Oncology (ReDO)—itraconazole as an anti-cancer agent." ecancermedicalscience 9 (2015).

2) Gu, Juan J., et al. "Itraconazole, an Oral Antifungal Drug, Inhibits Tumor Growth and Enhances Therapeutic Agent Activity in Double Hit Lymphoma." (2016): 5380-5380.

3) Gu, Juan J., et al. "Itraconazole, an Oral Antifungal Drug, Is Active in Chemotherapy Resistant B-Cell Non-Hodgkin Lymphoma and Enhances the Anti-Tumor Activity of Chemotherapy Agents." Blood. (2016): 5138-5138.

4) Agnihotri, Sameer, et al. "Ketoconazole and posaconazole selectively target HK2-expressing glioblastoma cells." Clinical Cancer Research 25.2 (2019): 844-855.

5) Tsubamoto, Hiroshi, et al. "Repurposing itraconazole as an anticancer agent." Oncology Letters 14.2 (2017): 1240-1246.

6) Head, Sarah A., et al. "Antifungal drug itraconazole targets VDAC1 to modulate the AMPK/mTOR signaling axis in endothelial cells." Proceedings of the National Academy of Sciences 112.52 (2015): E7276-E7285.

7) Karar, Jayashree, and Amit Maity. "PI3K/AKT/mTOR pathway in angiogenesis." Frontiers in molecular neuroscience 4 (2011): 51.

8) Head, Sarah A., et al. "Simultaneous Targeting of NPC1 and VDAC1 by Itraconazole Leads to Synergistic Inhibition of mTOR Signaling and Angiogenesis." ACS chemical biology 12.1 (2016): 174-182.

9) Ueda, Tomoko, et al. "Itraconazole modulates hedgehog, WNT/β-catenin, as well as Akt Signalling, and inhibits proliferation of cervical Cancer cells." Anticancer research 37.7 (2017): 3521-3526.

10) Antonarakis, Emmanuel S., et al. "Repurposing itraconazole as a treatment for advanced prostate cancer: a noncomparative randomized phase II trial in men with metastatic castration-resistant prostate cancer." The oncologist 18.2 (2013): 163-173.

11) Lee, Mina, et al. "Itraconazole as a noncastrating treatment for biochemically recurrent prostate cancer: a phase 2 study." Clinical genitourinary cancer 17.1 (2019): e92-e96.

12) Clinical Trial NCT03513211. Phase I/II Study of Hydroxychloroquine With Itraconazole With Biochemically Recurrent Prostate Cancer (HITMAN-PC) Anthony Joshua, FRACP, St Vincent's Hospital, Sydney

13) Tompkins, Kenneth D., and Andrew Thorburn. "Focus: Death: Regulation of Apoptosis by Autophagy to Enhance Cancer Therapy." The Yale Journal of Biology and Medicine 92.4 (2019): 707.

14) Pawelec, G., et al. "Comparison of the immunosuppressive activities of the antimycotic agents itraconazole, fluconazole, ketoconazole and miconazole on human T-cells." International journal of immunopharmacology 13.2-3 (1991): 299-304.

15) Kim, Joung Hoon, and Young Keun Ahn. "The effects of itraconazole on the immune responses in ICR mice." The Journal of toxicological sciences 19.1 (1994): 7-15.

16) Cools, Marina, Frans Aerts, and Jean Van Wauwe. "Lack of immunosuppression by ketoconazole and itraconazole." International journal of immunopharmacology 14.6 (1992): 1011-1017.

17) Drummond, D. C., et al. "The effects of amphotericin B, fluconazole and miconazole on neutrophil and lymphocyte function in a guinea pig model." Journal of Antimicrobial Chemotherapy 36.2 (1995): 375-384.

18) Jaschonek, K., et al. "5-Lipoxygenase inhibition by antifungal azole derivatives: new tools for immunosuppression?." Eicosanoids 2.3 (1989): 189-190.

19) Roos, Jessica, et al. "Regulation of tumorigenic Wnt signaling by cyclooxygenase-2, 5-lipoxygenase and their pharmacological inhibitors: A basis for novel drugs targeting cancer cells?." Pharmacology & therapeutics 157 (2016): 43-64.

20) Sareddy, Gangadhara Reddy, et al. "Nonsteroidal anti-inflammatory drugs diclofenac and celecoxib attenuates Wnt/β-catenin/Tcf signaling pathway in human glioblastoma cells." Neurochemical research 38.11 (2013): 2313-2322.

21) Maier, Thorsten Jürgen, et al. "Targeting the beta-catenin/APC pathway: a novel mechanism to explain the cyclooxygenase-2-independent anticarcinogenic effects of celecoxib in human colon carcinoma cells." The FASEB journal 19.10 (2005): 1353-1355.

22) Boyd, Robert S., et al. "Protein profiling of plasma membranes defines aberrant signaling pathways in mantle cell lymphoma." Molecular & Cellular Proteomics 8.7 (2009): 1501-1515.

23) Mahshid, Yilmaz, et al. "High expression of 5-lipoxygenase in normal and malignant mantle zone B lymphocytes." BMC immunology 10.1 (2009): 2.

24) Runarsson, Gudmundur, et al. "Leukotriene B 4 plays a pivotal role in CD40-dependent activation of chronic B lymphocytic leukemia cells." Blood 105.3 (2005): 1274-1279.

25) deleted

26) Wang, Yunfen, et al. "Itraconazole can inhibit malignant pleural effusion by suppressing lymphangiogenesis in mice." Translational lung cancer research 4.1 (2015): 27.

27) Song, Kai, et al. "Lenalidomide inhibits lymphangiogenesis in preclinical models of mantle cell lymphoma." Cancer research 73.24 (2013): 7254-7264.

28) Feugier, Pierre. "A review of rituximab, the first anti-CD20 monoclonal antibody used in the treatment of B non-Hodgkin's lymphomas." Future oncology 11.9 (2015): 1327-1342.

29) Kim, James, et al. "Itraconazole, a commonly used antifungal that inhibits Hedgehog pathway activity and cancer growth." Cancer cell 17.4 (2010): 388-399.

30) Takebe, Naoko, et al. "Targeting Notch, Hedgehog, and Wnt pathways in cancer stem cells: clinical update." Nature reviews. Clinical oncology 12.8 (2015): 445.

31) Coni, Sonia, Paola Infante, and Alberto Gulino. "Control of stem cells and cancer stem cells by Hedgehog signaling: pharmacologic clues from pathway dissection." Biochemical pharmacology 85.5 (2013): 623-628.

32) Kim, James, et al. "Itraconazole and arsenic trioxide inhibit Hedgehog pathway activation and tumor growth associated with acquired resistance to smoothened antagonists." Cancer cell 23.1 (2013): 23-34.

33) Campbell, Victoria, and Mhairi Copland. "Hedgehog signaling in cancer stem cells: a focus on hematological cancers." Stem cells and cloning: advances and applications 8 (2015): 27.

34) Hegde, Ganapati V., et al. "Targeting of sonic hedgehog-GLI signaling: a potential strategy to improve therapy for mantle cell lymphoma." Molecular cancer therapeutics 7.6 (2008): 1450-1460.

35) Hu, Qiang, et al. "Itraconazole induces apoptosis and cell cycle arrest via inhibiting Hedgehog signaling in gastric cancer cells." Journal of Experimental & Clinical Cancer Research 36.1 (2017): 50.

36) Wang, Xiaoya, et al. "Anti-proliferation of breast cancer cells with itraconazole: Hedgehog pathway inhibition induces apoptosis and autophagic cell death." Cancer letters 385 (2017): 128-136.

37) Wang, Ying, et al. "Hedgehog signaling pathway regulates autophagy in human hepatocellular carcinoma cells." Hepatology 58.3 (2013): 995-1010.

38) Zeng, Xian, and Dianwen Ju. "Hedgehog signaling pathway and autophagy in cancer." International journal of molecular sciences 19.8 (2018): 2279.

39) Oladapo, Helen O., et al. "Pharmacological targeting of GLI1 inhibits proliferation, tumor emboli formation and in vivo tumor growth of inflammatory breast cancer cells." Cancer letters 411 (2017): 136-149.

40) Tsubamoto, Hiroshi, Takashi Sonoda, and Kayo Inoue. "Impact of itraconazole on the survival of heavily pre-treated patients with triple-negative breast cancer." Anticancer research 34.7 (2014): 3839-3844.

41) Galdo, Riobo-Del, et al. "Role of Hedgehog Signaling in Breast Cancer: Pathogenesis and Therapeutics." Cells 8.4 (2019): 375.

42) Kast, Richard E., et al. "Blocking epithelial-to-mesenchymal transition in glioblastoma with a sextet of repurposed drugs: the EIS regimen." Oncotarget 8.37 (2017): 60727.

43) Tsubamoto, Hiroshi, et al. "Itraconazole inhibits AKT/mTOR signaling and proliferation in endometrial cancer cells." Anticancer research 37.2 (2017): 515-519.

44) Li, Jiao, et al. "The mTOR kinase inhibitor everolimus synergistically enhances the anti-tumor effect of the Bruton's tyrosine kinase (BTK) inhibitor PLS-123 on Mantle Cell lymphoma." International journal of cancer 142.1 (2018): 202-213..

45) Zhao, Xiaohong, et al. "Unification of de novo and acquired ibrutinib resistance in mantle cell lymphoma." Nature Communications 8 (2017).

46) Yu, Dandan, et al. "Targeting the PI3K/Akt/mTOR signaling pathway by pterostilbene attenuates mantle cell lymphoma progression." Acta biochimica et biophysica Sinica 50.8 (2018): 782-792.

47) Chiron, D., et al. "Novel Targeted Strategies to Overcome Microenvironment-Dependent Resistance in Mantle Cell Lymphoma." Hematological Oncology 35 (2017): 258-258.

48) Chiron, David, et al. "Microenvironment-dependent proliferation and mitochondrial priming loss in mantle cell lymphoma is overcome by anti-CD20." Blood (2016): blood-2016.

49) Tessoulin, Benoit, et al. "BCL2-family dysregulation in B-cell malignancies: from gene expression regulation to a targeted therapy biomarker." Frontiers in oncology 8 (2018): 645.

50) Chiron, David, et al. "Rational targeted therapies to overcome microenvironment-dependent expansion of mantle cell lymphoma." Blood 128.24 (2016): 2808-2818.

51) Le Gouill, Steven, et al. "Ibrutinib Plus Obinutuzumab and Venetoclax in Relapsed/Refractory Mantle Cells Lymphoma Patients, Results of the OASIS Phase I Clinical Trial." (2018): 4158-4158.

52) Le Gouill, Steven, et al. "Ibrutinib, Venetoclax Plus Obinutuzumab in Newly Diagnosed Mantle Cell Lymphoma Patients." (2019): 1530-1530.

53) Papin, Antonin, Steven Le Gouill, and David Chiron. "Rationale for targeting tumor cells in their microenvironment for mantle cell lymphoma treatment." Leukemia & lymphoma 59.5 (2018): 1064-1072.

54) Ueda, Tomoko, et al. "Itraconazole Modulates Hedgehog, WNT/β-catenin, as well as Akt Signalling, and Inhibits Proliferation of Cervical Cancer Cells." Anticancer Research 37.7 (2017): 3521-3526.

55) Nacev, Benjamin A., et al. "The antifungal drug itraconazole inhibits vascular endothelial growth factor receptor 2 (VEGFR2) glycosylation, trafficking, and signaling in endothelial cells." Journal of Biological Chemistry 286.51 (2011): 44045-44056.

56) Kim, Daniel J., et al. "Open-label, exploratory phase II trial of oral itraconazole for the treatment of basal cell carcinoma." J Clin Oncol 32.8 (2014): 745-751.

57) Li, Chengxin, Sumin Chi, and Jingwu Xie. "Hedgehog signaling in skin cancers." Cellular signalling 23.8 (2011): 1235-1243.

58) Schneider, Sven, et al. "Expression of the Sonic hedgehog pathway in squamous cell carcinoma of the skin and the mucosa of the head and neck." Head & neck 33.2 (2011): 244-250.

59) Celebi, Ali Riza Cenk, Hayyam Kiratli, and Figen Soylemezoglu. "Evaluation of the 'Hedgehog' signaling pathways in squamous and basal cell carcinomas of the eyelids and conjunctiva." Oncology letters 12.1 (2016): 467-472.

60) Larsen, Andrew R., et al. "Repurposing the antihelmintic mebendazole as a hedgehog inhibitor." Molecular cancer therapeutics 14.1 (2015): 3-13.

61) Wahid, Mohd, et al. "Vismodegib, itraconazole and sonidegib as hedgehog pathway inhibitors and their relative competencies in the treatment of basal cell carcinomas." Critical reviews in oncology/hematology 98 (2016): 235-241.

62) Zhang, Han, et al. "Hedgehog inhibitors selectively target cell migration and adhesion of mantle cell lymphoma in bone marrow microenvironment." Oncotarget 7.12 (2016): 14350.

63) Liang, Guanzhao, et al. "Itraconazole exerts its anti-melanoma effect by suppressing Hedgehog, Wnt, and PI3K/mTOR signaling pathways." Oncotarget 8.17 (2017): 28510.

64) Krasulova, Kristyna, Zdenek Dvorak, and Pavel Anzenbacher. "In vitro analysis of itraconazole cis-di-astereoisomers inhibition of nine cytochrome P450 enzymes: stereoselective inhibition of CYP3A." Xenobiotica 49.1 (2019): 36-42.

65) Tapaninen, Tuija, et al. "Itraconazole increases ibrutinib exposure ten-fold and reduces inter-individual variation—A potentially beneficial drug-drug interaction." Clinical and translational science (2019).

66) Finnes, Heidi D., et al. "Pharmacovigilance during ibrutinib therapy for chronic lymphocytic leukemia (CLL)/small lymphocytic lymphoma (SLL) in routine clinical practice." Leukemia & lymphoma 58.6 (2017): 1376-1383.

67) Lam, Allen, et al. "Itraconazole and clarithromycin inhibit P-glycoprotein activity in primary human sin-onasal epithelial cells." International forum of allergy & rhinology. Vol. 5. No. 6. 2015.

68) Li, Ke, et al. "Inhibition of the hedgehog pathway for the treatment of cancer using Itraconazole." OncoTargets and therapy 12 (2019): 6875.

Chapter 37

Fenofibrate Lipid Drug

Fenofibrate, an Old Lipid Drug is also an Anti-Cancer Drug

FENOFIBRATE IS AN OLD, LIPID-LOWERING drug used since 1975 to treat hyper-triglyceridemia (high-serum triglycerides) by way of activating the peroxisome proliferator-activated receptor-alpha (PPAR-alpha), a nuclear receptor, and the master regulator of lipid metabolism. Fenofibrate has been repurposed as a potent anti-cancer drug, a dual OXPHOS and GLYCOLYSIS inhibitor.

Fenofibrate Mimics Fasting and a Ketogenic Diet

Activation of PPAR-alpha is an adaptive response to fasting, resulting in preferential metabolism of body fat stores rather than circulating glucose, which is unavailable during the fasting state. As such, fenofibrate mimics the fasting state, thought to be beneficial for the cancer patient. Similar to fenofibrate, metformin (Chapter 14) also induces a fasting-mimicking metabolic state. As a PPAR-alpha activator, fenofibrate mimics the ketogenic diet, another diet that resembles fasting. (1-10) Dr. Sander Kersten (2014) writes:

> A ketogenic diet is almost entirely devoid of carbohydrate and elicits a metabolic state of low insulin, high plasma free fatty acids, and enhanced ketogenesis that resembles fasting. (1)

Similar to the action of fenofibrate, the high-fat, low-carbohydrate ketogenic diet activates PPAR-alpha. In 2014, Dr. Kerston summarized the activities of PPAR-alpha:

> PPARα is at the center of a regulatory hub impacting fatty acid uptake, fatty acid activation, intracellular fatty acid binding, mitochondrial and peroxisomal fatty acid oxidation, ketogenesis.(1)

Fenofibrate Inactivates PDK— GLYCOLYSIS Inhibitor

In the chapter 5, on dichloroacetate (DCA), we discussed how DCA inhibits PDK and activates pyruvate dehydrogenase complex (PDH), the rate-limiting step that controls the switch from GLYCOLYSIS to OXPHOS, resulting in inhibition of GLYCOLYSIS. PPAR-alpha activators such as fenofibrate also shift cancer cell metabolism from Glycolysis to OXPHOS. The mechanism is described by Dr. Dongfen Han (2015) and Chia-Ing Jan (2016) involves altering the ratio of two isoforms of PDK [pyruvate dehydrogenase kinase], called PKM2 and PKM1, downregulating PKM2 expression, as well as upregulating PDH. This serves to shift energy production in cancer cells away from GLYCOLYSIS and towards OXPHOS.

Dr Dongfen Han et al. write (2015):

> Here we show that FF [fenofibrate] not only inhibits glucose uptake and lactate

production but also induces mitochondrial damage in human glioblastoma cells. FF also causes NF-κB/RelA-dependent down-regulation of PKM2 expression, depending on PPARα.(54)

Dr Chia-Ing Jan et al. write (2016):

Thus, fenofibrate increased the protein levels of PKM2 and pyruvate dehydrogenase may further direct the aerobic processes (Warburg effect) of cancer cells towards the TCA cycle [OXPHOS] and shift the energy production pathway. (23)

Fenofibrate is a GLYCOLYSIS inhibitor by way of PPAR-alpha activation. As we will read below, fenofibrate is also an OXPHOS inhibitor via a PPARα-independent mechanism.

Classical Fenofibrate Signaling Pathway

According to Dr. Jonathan Noonan et al. al. (2013), the classical fenofibrate signaling pathway is as follows: fenofibrate is rapidly converted to fenofibric acid, which enters the cancer cells and forms a heterodimer complex with retinoid X receptor (RXR). This complex then enters the nucleus, binds to PPAR-alpha, and activates target gene transcription involved in cellular metabolism. The retinoid receptor is a vitamin A receptor, thus the benefits of fenofibrate depend on vitamin A (or retinoids), explaining the importance of vitamin A derivatives when using fenofibrate. (11)

Fenofibrate OXPHOS Inhibitor

In 2015, Dr. Anna Wilk et al. studied the effect of fenofibrate on glioblastoma cells in vitro, finding that fenofibrate accumulates in the mitochondrial fraction and inhibits com-plex I of the electron transport chain (ETC), serving as OXPHOS inhibitor. However, the glioblastoma cells have already made the fenofibrate induced PPAR-alpha dependent switch from GLYCOLYSIS to OXPHOS. At this point the inhibition of OXPHOS is a "double whammy" resulting in "metabolic catastrophe." Dr. Anna Wilk et al. write:

Here we report a novel PPARα-independent mechanism explaining FF's [Fenofibrate's] cytotoxicity in vitro and in an intracranial mouse model of glioblastoma. The mechanism involves accumulation of FF in the mitochondrial fraction, followed by immediate impairment of mitochondrial respiration at the level of complex I of the electron transport chain. This mitochondrial action sensitizes tested glioblastoma cells to the PPARα-dependent metabolic switch from glycolysis to fatty acid β-oxidation. As a consequence, prolonged exposure to FF depletes intracellular ATP, activates the AMP-activated protein kinase–mammalian target of rapamycin–autophagy pathway [AMP/mTOR], and results in extensive tumor cell death. Interestingly, autophagy activators attenuate and autophagy inhibitors enhance FF-induced glioblastoma cytotoxicity. (12)

The work of Dr. Anna Wilk's group demonstrates dual OXPHOS and GLYCOLYSIS inhibition of fenofibrate. By adding a third agent, an Autophagy inhibitor, synthetic lethality is achieved. Thus, Dr. Wilk's work has rendered support to the central idea of this book, that inhibition of all three pillars of cancer cell metabolism are key to cracking cancer— GLYCOLYSIS, OXPHOS and Autophagy. (12–14)

Autophagy Inhibitors Enhance Fenofibrate Cytotoxicity

One might expect autophagy inhibitors such as mefloquine, chloroquine, hydroxychloroquine, clarithromycin, propranolol, niclosamide, thymoquinone, loratidine (Claritin®), PPIs, etc. to enhance the activity of fenofibrate , a dual OXPHOS and GLYCOLYSIS inhibitor, as suggested by Dr. Wilk and colleagues. We await further NIH-funded studies for confirmation. See the chapters on autophagy Inhibitors (31–34) for more on this topic.

GLYCOLYSIS Inhibition in Glioblastoma Cells

In agreement with Dr. Wilk, in 2015, Dr. Han studied the effect of fenofibrate in a glioblastoma cell line, finding inhibition of GLYCOLYSIS in a PPAR-alpha dependent manner. Both glucose uptake and lactate production were inhibited. (54)

GLYCOLYSIS Inhibition in Colorectal cells

In 2019, Dr. Quian Gou et al. studied the effect of PPAR-alpha agonist on a colorectal cell line finding inhibition of GLYCOLYSIS via inhibition of glucose transporter 1 (GLUT-1) gene transcription activity. (67)

Fenofibrate Downregulates VEGF, HIF-1, NF-kB, and PI3K/Akt.

In 2015, Dr. Tomas Koltai reviewed the main mechanisms involved in the anti-cancer activity of fenofibrate via downregulation of VEGF, HIF-1, NF-kB, and PI3K/Akt. In other words, all major growth factors and pathways of the cancer cell are inhibited:

1) Anti-Angiogenesis through downregulation of Vascular Endothelial Growth Factor [VEGF], and Receptor [VEGFR] and Hypoxia-Inducible factor-1 a [HIF-1a],

2) Inhibition of endothelial cell migration.

3) Apoptosis and cell cycle arrest mechanism include:

   a) Downregulation of nuclear factor kappa B [NF-kB] and protein kinase B [also called Akt].

   b) Decrease of cellular energy by impairing mitochondrial function.

   c) Growth impairment from downregulation of Phospho-Inositol 3 Kinase [PI3K/Akt] axis and downregulation of the p38 map kinase [MAPK] cascade.

Antimetastatic Activities of Fenofibrate:

1) Downregulation of MCP-1 [monocyte chemotactic protein]

2) Decreased Metalloprotease-9 [MMP-9] production

3) Weak downregulation of adhesion molecules like intercellular adhesion molecules [ICAM] and Vascular Endothelial Adhesion Molecules [VCAM]

4) Decreased secretion of chemokines like Interleukin-6 [IL-6], and downregulation of cyclin D-1. (15)

Angiogenesis Inhibition Potentiated by ATRA (All-Trans Retinoic Acid)

Angiogenesis inhibition is one of the main anti-tumor activities of FF and it is potentiated by vitamin A and its synthetic analogs. Dr. Koltai writes:

Treatment of human endometrial cells with

a PPARα agonist leads to reduced secretion of VEGF in addition to reduced proliferation. This was potentiated by RxR (Retinoid X receptor) agonist like ATRA. (15)

Retinoids (ATRA) and Cancer

Retinoid drugs such as Accutane (isotretinoin) are commonly used to treat acne. Another retinoid variant, ATRA, is FDA-approved for leukemia and lymphoma. ATRA is first-line treatment of acute pro-myelocytic leukemia (APL). ATRA induces complete remission in 90% of patients with APL. The combination of ATRA with chemotherapy is "curative" in 75% of patients with APL. Commonly available vitamin A is another retinoid that might be considered for potentiation of fenofibrate. Caution is advised when using vitamin A and derivatives, as excess dosage can cause toxicity. See Chapter 11 for more on ATRA. (16–20)

Combination of GLYCOLYSIS Inhibitor 2-DG and Fenofibrate

In 2016, Dr. Huaping Liu studied et al. the combination of GLYCOLYSIS inhibitor 2-DG given IV along with daily fenofibrate, which was found effective for three cancer cell models in vitro—breast carcinoma (SKBR 3), melanoma (NM2C5), and osteosarcoma. Fenofibrate was found to serve as an OXPHOS inhibitor by inhibiting complex I of the (electron transport chain (ETC).

Additionally, an in vivo study in a melanoma mouse xenograft model found the combination was safe and effective for reduction of tumor size in a synergistic manner. Fenofibrate is typically administered orally in a dosage of 40 mg to 400 mg per day, achieving plasma concentration of about 10 µM to about 50 µM. 2-De-oxy-glucose (2 DG) is a GLYCOLYSIS inhibitor. Alternatively, other GLYCOLYSIS inhibitors such as DCA (dichloroacetate), diclofenac or high-dose IV vitamin C may serve in place of 2-DG. The combination of fenofibrate (OXPHOS inhibitor) and GLYCOLYSIS inhibitor activated protective autophagy. Potential synergy with autophagy inhibitors was suggested. (21–22)

Fenofibrate Interrupts Binding of HK II to VDAC

Fenofibrate interrupts the Warburg Effect. In 2016, Dr. Jan studied fenofibrate in a mouse xenograft model of oral cancer, finding interruption of the binding of hexokinase II to the voltage-dependent anion channel (VDAC). **Note:** VDAC consists of pores (channels) in the outer mitochondrial membrane that control glucose metabolism and apoptosis. Dr. Chia-Ing Jan et al. write:

> Fenofibrate caused changes in the protein expressions of hexokinase II [HK II], pyruvate kinase, pyruvate dehydrogenase, and voltage-dependent anion channel [VDAC], which are associated with the Warburg Effect. In addition, fenofibrate reprogrammed the metabolic pathway by interrupting the binding of HK II to VDAC. (23)

Fenofibrate Destroys BCL2 Protein

One consequence of disrupting the HKII from the VDAC is the restoration of apoptosis controlled by the BCL-2 protein. In 2015, Dr. Gao found that fenofibrate destroys BCL-2 protein, thus restoring apoptosis in the cancer cell. Dr. Jiaming Gao's group found that PPAR-alpha binds to BCL-2 (anti-apoptosis protein) and promotes its degradation through ubiquitination and degradation by the proteasome, thus reducing cancer cell resistance to apoptosis and enhancing cancer cell sensitivity to chemotherapy. (24)

Fenofibrate Inhibits Fatty Acid Synthetase - Hepatoma Model

In 2019, Dr. Bang-Jau You et al. studied the effect of fenofibrate on hepatoma cells (liver cancer) in vitro, a cancer with highly expressed fatty acid synthetase (FASN) involved in generating fatty acids for tumor energy requirements. Dr. You and colleagues found that fenofibrate docked into the binding site of FASN, blocking its activity, in an effect similar to that of orlistat, an FDA-approved drug for treatment of obesity. By blocking FASN, fenofibrate produced a potent anti-cancer effect, causing apoptosis and necroptosis in a human hepatoma model in vitro. (25)

B-Cell Lymphoma Model

In 2012, Dr. Aadra Bhatt et al. studied the metabolism of PEL, primary effusion lymphoma, a cancer thought to be associated with Herpes virus infection. Dr. Bhatt's group concludes that FASN would be a suitable molecular target for treating lymphoma:

> PEL overexpress the fatty acid synthesizing enzyme, FASN, and both PEL and other B-NHL were much more sensitive to the FAS inhibitor, C75, than primary B cells.

Our findings suggest that FASN may be a unique candidate for molecular targeted therapy against PEL and other B-NHL. (26)

FASN in Mantle Cell Lymphoma

In 2012, Dr. Pascal Gelebart et al. studied mantle cell lymphoma, finding FASN to be highly expressed, while benign lymph node tissue and peripheral blood monocytes were negative. Blocking FASN with orlistat (Xenical), resulted in significant apoptosis of MCL cells. Further knockdown of FASN with short interfering RNA (SiRNA) led to a dramatic decrease in the cyclin D1 level and in Beta-catenin, a downstream signal protein in the Wnt pathway. (27)

In view of the above studies, there has been considerable interest in FASN inhibitors such as orlistat as anti-cancer agents. (28–33)

Fenofibrate Synergy with Taxanes

FASN is also involved with production of palmitate, a component in construction of microtubules, so FASN inhibition leads to microtubule disruption in the cancer cells. In 2017, Dr. Timothy Heuer et al. studied combining FASN inhibitors with a taxane, paclitaxel, or with docetaxel, a microtubule inhibitor chemotherapy agent, to enhance anti-cancer activity in xenograft models of lung, ovarian, prostate, and pancreatic cancer. Indeed, highly proliferating, invasive cancer cell types are addicted to FASN to maintain lipid rafts, microtubules, and other lipid functions in the cancer cell. FASN inhibition causes:

1) blockade of palmitate synthesis,

2) disruption of membrane-associated protein, localization and plasma membrane architecture,

3) inhibition of oncogenic signal transduction [e.g. Wnt-β-catenin and Akt],

4) gene expression reprogramming.

5) induction of tumor cell apoptosis. (34)

The studies by Dr. Heuer's group found enhanced synergy both in vitro and in vivo when FASN inhibitors (TVB-3166 and 3664) were combined with taxane drugs. Dr. Heuer et al. write that the combination of FASN inhibition and a taxane drug:

> demonstrate significantly enhanced anti-tumor efficacy when FASN inhibition is combined with paclitaxel or docetaxel in vitro and in vivo ... Impressively, the effects include induction of **near complete tumor regression** in a variety of diverse tumor cell-line-and patient-derived tumor models that include lung, ovarian, pancreatic, and prostate tumor models ... Together, these results provide **compelling mechanism- and efficacy-based evidence** for combined FASN and taxane therapy as a cancer therapy. (34)

Once might speculate on taxane synergy with other FASN inhibitors, such as orlistat, fenofibrate and quercetin. (99)

One might also speculate on synergy of fenofibrate with microtubule-disrupting agents, mebendazole, and fenbendazole. We await confirmation with NIH-funded studies of these combinations.

Fenofibrate for Lymphoma and Myeloma

High-endoplasmic reticulum activity renders multiple myeloma highly sensitive to mitochondrial inhibitors such as fenofibrate. In 2017, Dr. Leonard Schmeel et al. studied various doses of fenofibrate in vitro using seven human and two murine myeloma/lymphoma cell lines. He wrote:

> Fenofibrate significantly reduced viability due to apoptosis induction in all investigated myeloma and lymphoma cell lines in a dose-dependent manner. (35–36)

Fenofibrate Effective in Mantle Cell Lymphoma

In 2010, Dr. Z. Zak et al. studied the effect of fenofibrate in vitro against mantle cell lymphoma, a rare type of B-Cell lymphoma, reporting fenofibrate is an agonist for peroxisome proliferator-activated receptor-alpha (PPAR-alpha), inhibits NF-kB and induces apoptosis in mantle cell lymphoma cells (in vitro). (37)

Anti-Inflammatory Effects of Inhibition of NF-kB

Fenofibrate decreased the nuclear translocation of nuclear factor Kappa B p-65 protein (NF-KB)–p65, and inhibited the DNA binding of NF-kappa-B. This significantly downregulated downstream secretion of tumor necrosis factor-alpha (TNF alpha). These anti-inflammatory effects were independent of PPAR-alpha transcription. In addition, fenofibrate downregulated expression of cyclin D1, which is typically overexpressed and used as a marker for mantle cell lymphoma. Dr. Zak's group states that effective serum levels of fenofibrate can be achieved at clinically relevant doses up to 400 mg per day, taken with the evening meal, which is well tolerated without significant adverse effects. They write:

> The half-life of fenofibrate has been reported to be 20 hours in individuals with normal renal functions, and the level of fenofibrate required to achieve IC50 [concentration for 50% cancer cell death] for MCL [Mantle Cell Lymphoma] is within the therapeutic range that is used to treat hyperlipidemia. In light of the excellent safety, tolerability and affordability of fenofibrate, there is merit in investigating the possibility of extending the clinical use of fenofibrate, either as a sole agent or in combination with conventional chemotherapy, in the treatment of MCL. (37–39)

Lymphoma: Fenofibrate Regulates Lipid Metabolism

In 2013, Dr. Jianfeng Huang et al. further elucidated the effect of fenofibrate on B-cell lymphoma in a xenograft mouse model. Dr. Huang's group found that B-Cell lymphomas hijack host lipid metabolism to recruit fatty acids to fuel rapid growth. They write:

> B-cell tumors trigger systemic lipid mobilization from WAT [White Adipose Tissue] to the liver and increase VLDL/LDL [Low Density Lipoprotein Cholesterol] release from the liver to promote tumor growth.

They found that fenofibrate significantly suppressed tumor growth independent of angiogenesis and inflammation. The mechanism was related to white adipose tissue (WAT) depletion, stimulation of free fatty acid (FFA)

uptake by the liver, and restoration of hepatic fatty acid (FA) oxidation. Fenofibrate accelerated clearance of serum lipids and blocked hepatic lipid release induced by the tumor. Dr. Huang and colleagues concluded that fenofibrate-associated effects on hepatic lipid metabolism with deprivation of serum lipids suppress B-cell lymphoma growth, serving as a novel treatment strategy. (40)

Fenofibrate OXPHOS Inhibitor in Gastric Cancer

In 2020, Dr. Lulu Chen studied the anti-tumor effects of fenofibrate on gastric cancer cells via inhibition of PPAR-alpha which is highly expressed in this cancer cell type, finding inhibition of implanted xenograft tumors in mice without obvious toxicity.

Dr. Lulu Chen et al. write that fatty acid biosynthesis is a "key metabolic requirement" for many cancer cell types, suggesting its inhibition as a viable anti-cancer strategy. Dr. Chen's group found that cancer treatment with fenofibrate regulates mitochondrial function and normalizes cancer cell metabolism. Fenofibrate downregulates fatty acid synthetase (FASN), which decreased amounts of free fatty acids and triglycerides in cancer cells. As a separate mechanism, fenofibrate accumulates in mitochondria, inhibiting complex I, serving as an OXPHOS inhibitor, and inducing apoptosis. In the study by the Chen group, hexokinase II (HK2) was significantly decreased, and HKII dissociated from the VDAC on the outer mitochondria membrane. This caused release of cytochrome C with activation of caspase-9, which induced apoptosis of the cancer cells. Dr. Chen et al. write:

> In our study, damaged mitochondrial structures and released apoptotic bodies were evident, showing the pro-apoptotic potential of fenofibrate... Collectively, our results indicate that fenofibrate exhibits anti-tumor activity in vitro and in vivo via the mitochondria and metabolic reprogramming, demonstrating that mitochondrial regulation and the normalization of cancer cell metabolism are novel therapeutic strategies for cancer. (41)

Studies show efficacy of fenofibrate in the following cancer cell types:

- Glioblastoma (12)
- Oral cancer (23)
- Hepatoma (25)
- Non-Hodgkin's lymphoma (NHL) (26–27)(35)(37)(40)
- Multiple myeloma (35)
- Gastric cancer (41)
- Prostate cancer (42–48)
- Benign prostatic hypertrophy (BPH) (49)
- Breast cancer (50–52)
- Cervical cancer (53)
- Glioblastoma (12)(54–62)
- Melanoma (63–65)
- Angiosarcoma (66)
- Colorectal cancer (67)
- Mycosis fungoides (68)
- Inflammatory hepatic adenoma (69)
- Inhibition of angiogenesis and inflammation in multiple tumor cell lines (70)

Other Clinical Uses of Fenofibrate:

- Diabetic retinopathy/nephropathy (11) (71–73)
- Neuroprotection (74–87)
- Immune regulation of T Cell response (88)
- Anti-inflammatory suppression of NF-kB (37)(89–94)

Case Report: Hepatocellular Adenoma

In 2016, Dr. Poupon et al. reported a 52-year-old female who had been on oral contraceptives (OC) and presented with multiple inflammatory hepatocellular adenomas (IHCA) that regressed dramatically on treatment with fenofibrate 400 mg per day. After 6 months of fenofibrate, there was 50% regression of the lesions with no side effects. (69)

Adverse Effects of Fenofibrate – Mitochondrial Toxicity

Fenofibrate impairs complex I of the electron transport chain in the mitochondria, and therefore is considered a mitochondrial toxin. This effect may be magnified by accumulation of the drug in the mitochondria. Symptoms of mitochondrial toxicity include myalgias, muscle pain, myopathy, and muscle necrosis (rhabdomyolysis), with typical elevation of creatinine phospho-kinase CPK. Indeed, this effect may be magnified when fenofibrate is combined with statin drugs, flouro-quinolone antibiotics (ciprofloxin) or other OXPHOS inhibitors that are also mitochondrial toxins. (95–98)

Conclusion

Fenofibrate, the old lipid drug, is a PPAR-alpha agonist and repurposed anti-cancer drug, serving as glycolysis inhibitor via PPAR-alpha effects. Fenofibrate interrupts the binding of hexokinase II to the VDAC, thereby blocking the Warburg Effect and inducing apoptosis. Fenofibrate accumulates in mitochondria and inhibits complex I, serving as an OXPHOS inhibitor. Autophagy inhibitors enhance the activity of fenofibrate. Independent of PPAR-alpha, fenofibrate is a fatty acid synthetase (FASN) inhibitor and synergizes with microtubule agents such as the taxanes and mebendazole.

Fenofibrate has remarkable anti-angiogenesis and anti-inflammatory activity with potent inhibition of NF-kB, also independent of PPAR-alpha. The combination of OXPHOS inhibitor fenofibrate with a GLYCOLYSIS inhibitor (such as DCA, diclofenac or quercetin), an autophagy inhibitor (such as hydroxychloroquine, loratidine, thymoquinone, etc.) and a microtubule inhibitor (such as mebendazole) might prove synergistic. We await NIH-funded confirmatory studies.

References for Chapter 37: Fenofibrate

1) Kersten, Sander. "Integrated physiology and systems biology of PPARα." Molecular metabolism 3.4 (2014): 354-371.

2) Weng, Mei-lin, et al. "Fasting inhibits aerobic glycolysis and proliferation in colorectal cancer via the Fdft1-mediated AKT/mTOR/HIF1α pathway suppression." Nature communications 11.1 (2020): 1-17.

3) Qi, Jie, et al. "Fasting Induces Hepatocellular Carcinoma Cell Apoptosis by Inhibiting SET8 Expression." Oxidative medicine and cellular longevity 2020 (2020).

4) Di Tano, Maira, et al. "Synergistic effect of fasting-mimicking diet and vitamin C against KRAS mutated cancers." Nature communications 11.1 (2020): 1-11.

5) de Groot, Stefanie, et al. "Effects of short-term fasting on cancer treatment." Journal of Experimental & Clinical Cancer Research: CR 38 (2019).

6) Szypowska, Alicja, and Bożena Regulska-Ilow. "Significance of Low Carbohydrate Diets and Fasting in Patients with Cancer." Rocz Panstw Zakl Hig 70.4 (2019).

7) Lee, C., and V. D. Longo. "Fasting vs dietary restriction in cellular protection and cancer treatment: from model organisms to patients." Oncogene 30.30 (2011): 3305-3316.

8) Lee, Changhan, et al. "Fasting cycles retard growth of tumors and sensitize a range of cancer cell types to chemotherapy." Science translational medicine 4.124 (2012): 124ra27-124ra27.

9) Bianchi, Giovanna, et al. "Fasting induces anti-Warburg effect that increases respiration but reduces ATP-synthesis to promote apoptosis in colon cancer models." Oncotarget 6.14 (2015): 11806.

10) Cuyàs, Elisabet, et al. "Metformin induces a fasting-and antifolate-mimicking modification of systemic host metabolism in breast cancer patients." Aging (Albany NY) 11.9 (2019): 2874.

11) Noonan, Jonathan E., et al. "An update on the molecular actions of fenofibrate and its clinical effects on diabetic and other microvascular end points in patients with diabetes." Diabetes 62.12 (2013): 3968-3975.

12) Wilk, Anna, et al. "Molecular mechanisms of fenofibrate-induced metabolic catastrophe and glioblastoma cell death." Molecular and cellular biology 35.1 (2015): 182-198.

13) Nadanaciva, Sashi, et al. "Mitochondrial impairment by PPAR agonists and statins identified via immunocaptured OXPHOS complex activities and respiration." Toxicology and applied pharmacology 223.3 (2007): 277-287.

14) Scatena, Roberto, et al. "Mitochondrial dysfunction by synthetic ligands of peroxisome proliferator

activated receptors (PPARs)." IUBMB life 56.8 (2004): 477-482.

15) Koltai, Tomas. "Fenofibrate in cancer: mechanisms involved in anticancer activity." F1000Research 4 (2015).

16) Chen, Mei-Chih, et al. "Retinoic acid and cancer treatment." BioMedicine 4.4 (2014).20) Distel,

17) Tallman, Martin S., et al. "All-trans-retinoic acid in acute promyelocytic leukemia." New England Journal of Medicine 337.15 (1997): 1021-1028.

18) Fenaux, P., et al. "Long-term follow-up confirms the benefit of all-trans retinoic acid in acute promyelocytic leukemia." Leukemia 14.8 (2000): 1371-1377.

19) Emilie, et al. "Early induction of pyruvate dehydrogenase kinase 4 by retinoic acids in adipocytes." Molecular nutrition & food research 61.5 (2017): 1600920.

20) Abildgaard, Cecilie, et al. "Inhibition of retinoic acid receptor β signaling confers glycolytic dependence and sensitization to dichloroacetate in melanoma cells." Oncotarget 8.48 (2017): 84210.

21) Liu, Huaping, et al. "Combining 2-deoxy-D-glucose with fenofibrate leads to tumor cell death mediated by simultaneous induction of energy and ER stress." Oncotarget 7.24 (2016): 36461.

22) US patent: Theodore J. Lampidis. Combination therapy with fenofibrate and 2-deoxyglucose or 2-deoxymannose WO 2016065353 A1

23) Jan, Chia-Ing, et al. "Fenofibrate suppresses oral tumorigenesis via reprogramming metabolic processes: potential drug repurposing for oral cancer." International journal of biological sciences 12.7 (2016): 786.

24) Gao, Jiaming, et al. "PPARa induces cell apoptosis by destructing Bcl2." Oncotarget 6.42 (2015): 44635.

25) You, Bang-Jau, et al. "Fenofibrate induces human hepatoma Hep3B cells apoptosis and necroptosis through inhibition of thioesterase domain of fatty acid synthase." Scientific reports 9.1 (2019): 3306.

26) Bhatt, Aadra P., et al. "Dysregulation of fatty acid synthesis and glycolysis in non-Hodgkin lymphoma." Proceedings of the National Academy of Sciences of the United States of America (2012): 11818-11823.

27) Gelebart, Pascal, et al. "Blockade of Fatty Acid Synthase Triggers Significant Apoptosis in Mantle Cell Lymphoma." PLoS ONE 7.4 (2012).

28) Schcolnik-Cabrera, Alejandro, et al. "Orlistat as a FASN inhibitor and multitargeted agent for cancer therapy." Expert opinion on investigational drugs 27.5 (2018): 475-489.

29) Buckley, Douglas, et al. "Fatty acid synthase—modern tumor cell biology insights into a classical oncology target." Pharmacology & therapeutics 177 (2017): 23-31.

30) Agostini, Michelle, et al. "The fatty acid synthase inhibitor orlistat reduces the growth and metastasis of orthotopic tongue oral squamous cell carcinomas." Molecular cancer therapeutics 13.3 (2014): 585-595.

31) Dengler, Michael A., et al. "Fatty acid metabolism is a possible target for treatment of cyclin D1 over-expressing mantle cell lymphoma." (2012): 4675-4675.

32) Höring, Elisabeth, et al. "Dual targeting of MCL1 and NOXA as effective strategy for treatment of mantle cell lymphoma." British journal of haematology 177.4 (2017): 557-561.

33) Azadbakht, Leila, Zahra Jamali-Gojani, and Motahar Heidari-Beni. "Anti-obesity drug orlistat (xenical) is a novel antitumor medication." Shiraz E-Medical Journal 16.1 (2015).

34) Heuer, Timothy S., et al. "FASN inhibition and taxane treatment combine to enhance anti-tumor efficacy in diverse xenograft tumor models through disruption of tubulin palmitoylation and microtubule organization and FASN inhibition-mediated effects on oncogenic signaling and gene expression." EBioMedicine 16 (2017): 51-62.

35) Schmeel, Leonard Christopher, Frederic Carsten Schmeel, and Ingo GH Schmidt-Wolf. "In vitro apoptosis induction by fenofibrate in lymphoma and multiple myeloma." Anticancer research 37.7 (2017): 3513-3520.

36) Kurtoglu, Metin, et al. "High endoplasmic reticulum activity renders multiple myeloma cells hypersensitive to mitochondrial inhibitors." Cancer chemotherapy and pharmacology 66.1 (2010): 129-140.

37) Zak, Z., P. Gelebart, and R. Lai. "Fenofibrate induces effective apoptosis in mantle cell lymphoma

by inhibiting the TNFα/NF-κB signaling axis." Leukemia 24.8 (2010): 1476.

38) Kluin-Nelemans, H. C., P. M. Kluin, and E. Schuuring. "Cyclin D1 messenger RNA overexpression as a marker for mantle cell lymphoma." Oncogene 10.9 (1995): 1833-1840.

39) Krempf, M., et al. "Efficacy and safety of micronised fenofibrate in a randomised double-blind study comparing four doses from 200 mg to 400 mg daily with placebo in patients with hypercholesterolemia." Diabetes & metabolism 26.3 (2000): 184-191.

40) Huang, Jianfeng, et al. "The PPARa agonist fenofibrate suppresses B-cell lymphoma in mice by modulating lipid metabolism." Biochimica et Biophysica Acta (BBA)-Molecular and Cell Biology of Lipids 1831.10 (2013): 1555-1565.

41) Chen, Lulu, et al. "Fenofibrate-induced mitochondrial dysfunction and metabolic reprogramming reversal: the anti-tumor effects in gastric carcinoma cells mediated by the PPAR pathway." American Journal of Translational Research 12.2 (2020): 428.

42) Luty, Marcin, et al. "Fenofibrate Augments the Sensitivity of Drug-Resistant Prostate Cancer Cells to Docetaxel." Cancers 11.1 (2019): 77.

43) Lian, Xin, et al. "Fenofibrate inhibits mTOR-p70S6K signaling and simultaneously induces cell death in human prostate cancer cells." Biochemical and biophysical research communications 496.1 (2018): 70-75.

44) Wybieralska, Ewa, et al. "Fenofibrate attenuates contact-stimulated cell motility and gap junctional coupling in DU-145 human prostate cancer cell populations." Oncology reports 26.2 (2011): 447-453.

45) Wróbel, T., et al. "1947P Fenofibrate impairs pro-tumorigenic potential of cancer stem cell-like cells within drug-resistant prostate cancer cell populations." Annals of Oncology 30. Supplement 5 (2019): 268-074.

46) Tao, Tao, et al. "Fenofibrate inhibits the growth of prostate cancer through regulating autophagy and endoplasmic reticulum stress." Biochemical and biophysical research communications 503.4 (2018): 2685-2689.

47) Lian, Xin, et al. "Fenofibrate inhibits mTOR-p70S6K signaling and simultaneously induces cell death in human prostate cancer cells." Biochemical and biophysical research communications 496.1 (2018): 70-75.

48) Wróbel, T., et al. "1947P Fenofibrate impairs pro-tumorigenic potential of cancer stem cell-like cells within drug-resistant prostate cancer cell populations." Annals of Oncology 30.Supplement_5 (2019): mdz268-074.

49) Refaie, Marwa MM, Rehab A. Rifaai, and Nagwa M. Zenhom. "Role of PPAR-α agonist fenofibrate in the treatment of induced benign prostatic hyperplasia with dysplastic changes in rats." Fundamental & clinical pharmacology 32.6 (2018): 617-626.

50) Li, Ting, et al. "Fenofibrate induces apoptosis of triple-negative breast cancer cells via activation of NF-KappaB pathway." BMC cancer 14.1 (2014): 96.

51) Sun, Jianguo, et al. "Fenofibrate potentiates chemosensitivity to human breast cancer cells by modulating apoptosis via aKT/NF-κB pathway." OncoTargets and therapy 12 (2019): 773.

52) Nguyen, Chi Huu, et al. "Fenofibrate inhibits tumour intravasation by several independent mechanisms in a 3-dimensional co-culture model." International journal of oncology 50.5 (2017): 1879-1888.

53) Yoo, H. J. "Fenofibrate induces G0/G1 phase cell cycle arrest in cervical cancer by targeting the AMPK/mtorc pathways." Gynecologic Oncology 154 (2019): 98.

54) Han, Dongfeng, et al. "NF-κB/RelA-PKM2 mediates inhibition of glycolysis by fenofibrate in glioblastoma cells." Oncotarget 6.28 (2015): 26119.

55) Han, Dong-feng, et al. "Fenofibrate induces G 0/G 1 phase arrest by modulating the PPARα/FoxO1/p27 kip pathway in human glioblastoma cells." Tumor Biology 36.5 (2015): 3823-3829.

56) Grabacka, Maja M., et al. "Fenofibrate induces ketone body production in melanoma and glioblastoma cells." Frontiers in endocrinology 7 (2016): 5.

57) Kast, Richard E., et al. "Glioblastoma-synthesized G-CSF and GM-CSF contribute to growth and immunosuppression: Potential therapeutic benefit from dapsone, fenofibrate, and ribavirin." Tumor Biology 39.5 (2017): 1010428317699797.

58) Wilk, Anna, et al. "Fenofibrate-induced nuclear translocation of FoxO3A triggers Bim-mediated

apoptosis in glioblastoma cells in vitro." Cell cycle 11.14 (2012): 2660-2671.

59) Wilk, Anna M., et al. "Fenofibrate-mediated energy crisis and apoptotic cell death of glioblastoma." (2012): 3230-3230.

60) Wilk, Anna M., et al. "PPAR alpha independent effect of fenofibrate on glioblastoma cancer metabolism." (2013): 5431-5431.

61) Giordano, Antonio, and Marcella Macaluso. "Fenofibrate triggers apoptosis of glioblastoma cells in vitro: New insights for therapy." Cell Cycle 11.17 (2012): 3154-3154.

62) Binello, Emanuela, et al. "Characterization of fenofibrate-mediated anti-proliferative pro-apoptotic effects on high-grade gliomas and anti-invasive effects on glioma stem cells." Journal of neuro-oncology 117.2 (2014): 225-234.

63) Dana, N., S. Haghjooy Javanmard, and G. Vaseghi. "The effect of fenofibrate, a PPARα activator on toll-like receptor-4 signal transduction in melanoma both in vitro and in vivo." Clinical and Translational Oncology (2019):

64) Huang, Yu-Chun, et al. "Fenofibrate suppresses melanogenesis in B16-F10 melanoma cells via activation of the p38 mitogen-activated protein kinase pathway." Chemico-biological interactions 205.3 (2013): 157-164.

65) Grabacka, Maja, et al. "Inhibition of melanoma metastases by fenofibrate." Archives of Dermatological Research 296.2 (2004): 54-58.

1-9.

66) Majeed, Yasser, et al. "Potent and PPARα-independent anti-proliferative action of the hypolipidemic drug fenofibrate in VEGF-dependent angiosarcomas in vitro." Scientific reports 9.1 (2019): 6316.

67) Gou, Qian, et al. "PPARα agonist alleviates tumor growth and chemo-resistance associated with the inhibition of glucose metabolic pathway." European journal of pharmacology 863 (2019): 172664.

68) Steinhoff, Matthias, et al. "Complete clinical remission of tumor-stage mycosis fungoides after acute extensive skin necroses, granulomatous reaction, and fever under treatment with bexarotene, vorinostat, and high-dose fenofibrate." Journal of the American Academy of Dermatology 58.5 (2008): S88-S91.

69) Poupon, Raoul, Dominique Cazals-Hatem, and Lionel Arrivé. "Fenofibrate-induced massive regression of multiple inflammatory hepatocellular adenoma." Clinics and research in hepatology and gastroenterology 40.1 (2016): e1-e3.

70) Panigrahy, Dipak, et al. "PPARα agonist fenofibrate suppresses tumor growth through direct and indirect angiogenesis inhibition." Proceedings of the National Academy of Sciences 105.3 (2008): 985-990.

71) Cheng, Rui, et al. "Interaction of PPARalpha with the Wnt pathway, a mechanism for the therapeutic effect of fenofibrate on diabetic nephropathy." Diabetes (2016): db160426.

72) Stewart, Stephen, and Noemi Lois. "Fenofibrate for diabetic retinopathy." The Asia-Pacific Journal of Ophthalmology 7.6 (2018): 422-426.

73) Wong, Tien Yin, Rafael Simó, and Paul Mitchell. "Fenofibrate—a potential systemic treatment for diabetic retinopathy?" American journal of ophthalmology 154.1 (2012): 6-12.

74) Boese, Austin C., Jean-Pyo Lee, and Milton H. Hamblin. "Neurovascular protection by peroxisome proliferator-activated receptor α in ischemic stroke." Experimental Neurology (2020): 113323.

75) Pearsall, Elizabeth A., et al. "Neuroprotective effects of PPARα in retinopathy of type 1 diabetes." PloS one 14.2 (2019).

76) Agarwal, Swati, Anuradha Yadav, and Rajnish Kumar Chaturvedi. "Peroxisome proliferator-activated receptors (PPARs) as therapeutic target in neurodegenerative disorders." Biochemical and biophysical research communications 483.4 (2017): 1166-1177.

77) Deplanque, Dominique, et al. "Peroxisome proliferator-activated receptor-α activation as a mechanism of preventive neuroprotection induced by chronic fenofibrate treatment." Journal of Neuroscience 23.15 (2003): 6264-6271.

78) Besson, Valérie C., et al. "Fenofibrate, a peroxisome proliferator-activated receptor α agonist, exerts neuroprotective effects in traumatic brain injury." Neuroscience letters 388.1 (2005): 7-12.

79) Kreisler, Alexandre, et al. "Lipid-lowering drugs in the MPTP mouse model of Parkinson's disease:

fenofibrate has a neuroprotective effect, whereas bezafibrate and HMG-CoA reductase inhibitors do not." Brain research 1135 (2007): 77-84.

80) Bordet, R., et al. "PPARs: a new target for neuroprotection." (2006): 285-287.

81) Chen, Xiao Ru, et al. "Neurological recovery-promoting, anti-inflammatory, and anti-oxidative effects afforded by fenofibrate, a PPAR alpha agonist, in traumatic brain injury." Journal of neurotrauma 24.7 (2007): 1119-1131.

82) Ramanan, Sriram, et al. "The PPARα agonist fenofibrate preserves hippocampal neurogenesis and inhibits microglial activation after whole-brain irradiation." International Journal of Radiation Oncology* Biology* Physics 75.3 (2009): 870-877.

83) Greene-Schloesser, Dana, et al. "The peroxisomal proliferator-activated receptor (PPAR) α agonist, fenofibrate, prevents fractionated whole-brain irradiation-induced cognitive impairment." Radiation research 181.1 (2014): 33-44.

84) deleted

85) Xuan, Ai-Guo, et al. "PPARα agonist fenofibrate ameliorates learning and memory deficits in rats following global cerebral ischemia." Molecular neurobiology 52.1 (2015): 601-609.

86) Xu, Jihong, et al. "Agonists for the peroxisome proliferator-activated receptor-α and the retinoid X receptor inhibit inflammatory responses of microglia." Journal of neuroscience research 81.3 (2005): 403-411.

87) Jiang, Bo, et al. "Antidepressant-like effects of fenofibrate in mice via the hippocampal brain-derived neurotrophic factor signalling pathway." British journal of pharmacology 174.2 (2017): 177-194.

88) Bahrambeigi, Saman, et al. "Targeting PPAR ligands as possible approaches for metabolic reprogramming of T cells in cancer immunotherapy." Immunology Letters (2020).

89) Tsai, Shih-Chang, et al. "AMPK-dependent signaling modulates the suppression of invasion and migration by fenofibrate in CAL 27 oral cancer cells through NF-κ

B pathway." Environmental toxicology 31.7 (2016): 866-876.

90) Okayasu, Toshie, et al. "PPARα activators upregulate eNOS activity and inhibit cytokine-induced NF-κB activation through AMP-activated protein kinase activation." Life sciences 82.15-16 (2008): 884-891.

91) Okamoto, H., et al. "Inhibition of NF-B signaling by fenofibrate, a peroxisome proliferator-activated receptor-ligand, presents a therapeutic strategy for rheumatoid arthritis." Clin Exp Rheumatol 23 (2005): 323-30.

92) Okamoto, H., and N. Kamatani. "Successful treatment with fenofibrate, a peroxisome proliferator activated receptor α ligand, for a patient with rheumatoid arthritis." Annals of the rheumatic diseases 63.8 (2004): 1002-1003.

93) Yang, Tian-Lun, et al. "Fenofibrate decreases asymmetric dimethylarginine level in cultured endothelial cells by inhibiting NF-κB activity." Naunyn-Schmiedeberg's archives of pharmacology 371.5 (2005): 401-407.

94) Zheng, Shuang, et al. "Fenofibrate attenuates fatty acid-induced islet β-cell dysfunction and apoptosis via inhibiting the NF-κB/MIF dependent inflammatory pathway." Metabolism 77 (2017): 23-38.

95) Filippatos, Theodosios D., and Moses S. Elisaf. "Safety considerations with fenofibrate/simvastatin combination." Expert opinion on drug safety 14.9 (2015): 1481-1493.

96) Barker, Billie J., Roger R. Goodenough, and James M. Falko. "Fenofibrate monotherapy induced rhabdomyolysis." Diabetes Care 26.8 (2003): 2482-2483.

97) Motojima, Kiyoto, and Kouichi Seto. "Fibrates and statins rapidly and synergistically induce pyruvate dehydrogenase kinase 4 mRNA in the liver and muscles of mice." Biological and Pharmaceutical Bulletin 26.7 (2003): 954-958.

98) Ghosh, Bhaskar, et al. "Fenofibrate-induced myopathy." Neurology India 52.2 (2004): 268.

99) Sultan, Ahmed S., et al. "Quercetin induces apoptosis in triple-negative breast cancer cells via inhibiting fatty acid synthase and β-catenin." Int. J. Clin. Exp. Pathol 10.1 (2017): 156-172.

Chapter 38

Celecoxib COX2 Inhibitor

OUR INFLAMMATORY PATHWAYS DEFEND OUR bodies against infection and promote tissue healing. This is a good thing. However, it is not a good thing when our inflammatory pathways are hijacked and massively amplified by cancer cells via activation of the nuclear factor kappa-B pathway (NF-kB), with production of inflammatory cytokines, IL-6 and IL-8. These cytokines stimulate cancer cell growth, proliferation, and invasive behavior. In Chapter 3 we discussed inflammation as one of Drs. Hanahan and Weinberg's "ten hallmarks of cancer." Hyper inflammatory response with activation of NF-kB is also a hallmark of many pathogenic viral infections, resulting in dangerous "cytokine storm." (1–9) Pathogenic bacterial infections such as Helicobacter pylori also activate inflammatory pathways NF-kB and COX-2. (10)

Many of the repurposed anti-cancer drugs and nontoxic natural substances discussed in this book inhibit the NF-kB pro-inflammatory pathway. These include artemisinin, thymoquinone, curcumin, berberine, boswellia, sulforaphane, parthenolide, pterostilbene, fenofibrate, sulfasalazine, aspirin, statin drugs (atorvastatin), ivermectin, niclosamide, clarithromycin, azithromycin, doxycycline, etc.

The COX-2 Inflammatory Pathway

The Cyclo-Oxygenase-2 (COX-2) enzyme is a key inflammatory pathway usually upregulated along with NF-kB activation in diverse diseases such as cancer, infections, and auto-immune, post traumatic, and degenerative diseases, all of which evoke an inflammatory response. Regulation of COX-2 protein expression is downstream to, and mediated by, the Nuclear Factor Kappa B pathway. (11–14)

We are fortunate the drug industry invented a class of highly potent COX-2 inhibitor drugs—celecoxib, diclofenac, and sulindac. This chapter covers celecoxib (Celebrex®), FDA-approved in 1998 for rheumatoid arthritis and osteoarthritis; in 2005 for ankylosing spondylosis; and in 2006 for juvenile rheumatoid arthritis. Another lesser-known use of the drug is for prevention of familial adenomatous polyposis, a precursor for colon cancer. This use was approved in 1999. We make the case here for repurposing celecoxib as an anti-cancer drug.

Cancer Has High Levels of COX-2

Cancer cells frequently upregulate the COX-2 inflammatory pathway, and most cancers exhibit a high level of COX-2 protein expression. Blocking this inflammatory pathway with a COX-2 inhibitor such as celecoxib can inhibit cancer cell proliferation, tumor invasiveness, and angiogenesis. COX-2 inhibitors overcome apoptosis resistance by suppressing the BCL-2 anti-apoptosis protein, overcome P-glycoprotein/MDR drug resistance, and restore anti-tumor immune response. (15–26)

In this chapter, we examine the COX-2 inhibitor celecoxib as an anti-cancer agent. In the next chapter, we look at other NSAID COX-2 inhibitor drugs, diclofenac and sulindac.

Note: COX = Cyclo-Oxygenase, LOX = Lipo-Oxygenase, and NSAID= Nonsteroidal Anti-Inflammatory Drug.

COX-2 in Cancer Reviewed

In 2019, Dr. Nassar Hashemi Goradel et al. reviewed the role of COX-2 in cancer and the major metabolite of COX-2, prostaglandin E2, with attention on cancer-associated fibroblasts (CAFs) in the tumor micro-environment (TME), which express COX-2 protein that then "feeds back" to the cancer-inducing CSC activity. This in turn promotes:

> apoptosis resistance, proliferation, angiogenesis, inflammation, invasion, and metastasis of cancer cells…. Chemotherapeutic agents adversely induce COX-2 activity. (16A)

Upstream control of COX-2 is mediated by:

- Nuclear factor-kappa B (NF-kB)
- Mitogen-activated protein kinase (MAPK)
- Epidermal growth factor receptor (EGFR)

Downregulating Chemotherapy Induced Inflammation

In previous chapters, we discussed hyper activation of COX-2 and NF-kB inflammatory pathways as a major adverse effects of chemotherapy. Combined use of COX-2 inhibition with chemotherapy is beneficial for the cancer patient, downregulating this massive inflammation.

COX-2 Inhibition Improves Chemo/Radiotherapy

With celecoxib CO-2 inhibition, cancer cells become dramatically more sensitive to chemotherapy and radiation therapy. Dr. Hashemi Goradel and colleagues conclude that COX-2 inhibition should be used as adjuvant with chemotherapy and radiation therapy:

> Therefore, it would be advisable to **use COX-2 inhibitors as an adjuvant with chemotherapy and/or radiotherapy.** Such combination has been reported to synergistically increase the antitumoral activity for chemotherapeutic agents like sorafenib, 5-fluorouracil, bleomycin, irinotecan, cisplatin, paclitaxel, carboplatin, sunitinib, and cetuximab [an EGFR blocker] among others. This combination also improves the rate of tolerance to chemo-radiation and overall response rate for advance stages of cancers, especially when it is administered before radiotherapy. (16A)

Targeting COX2 and EGFR in Familial Polyposis

COX-2 inhibitors such as celecoxib and sulindac are useful in chemoprevention of cancer in patients with familial polyposis. Dr. Deborah Neklason (2016) et al. write:

> Familial adenomatous polyposis [FAP] is an autosomal dominant inherited disorder caused by a germline mutation in the APC gene, leading to a nearly 100% risk of colorectal cancer and a 12% lifetime risk of duodenal cancer. (29)

Note: APC= Adenomatous polyposis coli.

The standard of care for the FAP patient is a total colectomy, leaving behind the duodenum, which is at risk for duodenal polyps and duodenal cancer. The combined use of COX-2 inhibitor, sulindac, with an EGFR inhibitor (erlotinib) is effective for cancer chemoprevention in FAP. (27–32)

Targeting COX2 in B-Cell Lymphoma, Leukemia, Multiple Myeloma

The cyclo-oxygenase 2 (COX-2) inflammatory pathway is frequently overexpressed in hematologic cancers such as leukemia, lymphoma and multiple myeloma, associated with poor prognosis. Inhibition of COX-2 with celecoxib is enormously useful for hematologic cancers, as discussed in 2008 by Dr. M. P. Bernard et al., who wrote:

> Malignant B cells, namely chronic lymphocytic leukemia [CLL], highly express Cox-2, which confers increased survival. Conversely, Cox-2 selective inhibitors increased apoptosis in B-CLL cells, indicating their potential to act as anti-malignant tumor therapeutic agents. (25)

In 2008, Dr. Bernard's group summarized the anti-cancer effects of Cox2 inhibitors, such as celecoxib (Celebrex):

1) Inhibition of angiogenesis by reducing VEGF [Vascular Endothelial Growth Factor]
2) Reduced invasion by reduction in MMP [Matrix Metallo-Proteinase]
3) Inhibition of proliferation by reduction in NF-kB, STAT3, MEK and Cyclins, upregulation of p27 [tumor suppressor gene].

4) Impaired survival by downregulating BCL-2 [anti-apoptotic protein], NF-kB, Glutathione, AKT, increasing reactive oxygen species (ROS), Caspase activity.
5) Significantly attenuated Glutathione levels.
6) Enhanced host immune function.
7) Reduced T-Reg Cells [immunosuppressive cells]. (25)

In *Cancer Letter* (2005), Dr. J. Subhashini et al. reported that celecoxib had antiproliferative and apoptotic effects in leukemia cells in vitro. As mentioned above, celecoxib decreases the anti-apoptotic protein BCL-2, and inhibits NF-kB activation in a myeloid leukemia cell line. (26)

Attenuates Glutathione Levels

In 2008, Dr. Elizabeth Ryan et al. reported celecoxib 400 mg per day attenuates glutathione levels in human malignant B cells, and reduces chronic lymphocytic leukemia (B-CLL) proliferation and survival. Glutathione is the main element of the cancer cell's antioxidant system. Reducing glutathione renders the cancer cell more susceptible to damaging effects of ROS and oxidative therapies. (33)

Celecoxib Blocks the PI3K-Akt pathway

Celecoxib blocks activation of the phospho-inositol-kinase-Akt/mTOR (PI3K/Akt/mTOR) pathway, a "master regulator" for cancer cell survival, growth, and proliferation. (34–38)

In 2000, Dr. Ao-Lin Hsu et al. studied a prostate cancer-cell model, finding:

celecoxib induces apoptosis by blocking Akt [PI3K/Akt pathway] activation in human prostate cancer cells independently of Bcl-2 ... inhibition of Akt activation may play a crucial role in the induction of apoptosis by celecoxib. (34)

Note: PI3K-Akt Pathway is a growth survival pathway for cancer cells.

PI3K/Akt/mTOR Cancer Stem Cell Agent Pathway

Recent studies show the PI3K/Akt/mTOR pathway is a CSC pathway, which is inhibited by celecoxib, a potent CSC agent. (34–41)

In 2015, Dr. Pu Xia and Xiao-Yan Xu studied this topic, writing:

The PI3K/Akt/mTOR signaling pathway can be considered as a master regulator for cancer. More and more recent studies have shown the links between PI3K/Akt/mTOR signaling pathway and CSC biology.... Overall, the current available data suggest that the PI3K/Akt/mTOR signaling pathway could be a promising target for development of CSC-target drugs. (39)

Dr. Alberto Martinelli et al. (2010) write:

We present the evidence which links the signals emanating from the PI3K/Akt/mTOR cascade with the functions of cancer stem cells, both in solid and hematological tumors ... the PI3K/Akt/mTOR signaling pathways is rapidly emerging as a signaling network important for CSC survival. (40)

Colon Cancer Stem Cells

In 2017, Dr. Sugong Chen et al. studied colon CSCs in vitro using both "transcriptomic and proteomic approaches" to identify signaling pathways that control the colon cancer stem cell (CCSC) population. Dr. Chen's group found that several components of the PI3K/Akt/mTOR pathway were overexpressed in CSCs, and that treatment with PI3K inhibitor (LY294002) decreases stem cells. They write:

LY294002-treated CCSCs showed decreases in proliferation, sphere formation and self-renewal, in phosphorylation-dependent activation of Akt, and in expression of cyclin D1.... Inhibition of PI3K in vivo reduced tumorigenicity, increased detection of cleaved caspase 3, an indicator of apoptosis, and elevated expression of the inflammatory chemokine, CXCL8. Collectively, these results indicate that PI3K/Akt/mTOR signaling controls CCSC proliferation and CCSC survival. (41)

Note: LY294002 is the first research drug developed as a PI3K inhibitor, developed from and sharing structural similarity with quercetin, a commonly available plant bioflavonoid. (42–43)

Important: the PI3K/Akt/mTOR pathway is a CSC pathway. All OXPHOS inhibitors also inhibit mTOR, thus serving as CSC agents.

OXPHOS Inhibitors Inhibit Wnt Pathway

Previously, we discussed the revelation made by Dr. Roberto Costa et al. in 2019 that OXPHOS inhibition downregulates Wnt signaling, a CSC pathway. This explains why all mitochondrial OXPHOS inhibitors are also anti-CSC agents. (44)

Crosstalk Between mTOR and Wnt Signaling

Other OXPHOS inhibitors, such as metformin and itraconazole, also inhibit the mTOR pathway via activation of AMPK (AMP-kinase), which inhibits mTOR. In addition, there is considerable "crosstalk" between mTOR and Wnt, which are both CSC pathways. Wnt protein activation upregulates the mTOR pathway, stimulating cell growth and proliferation. Blocking both the Wnt and mTOR pathways yields a more robust anti-CSC effect. (45–46)

Quercetin Synergy with Celecoxib— Remarkable Anti-Cancer Effects

In 2017, Dr. C.-P. Yu et al. studied a hepatocellular cancer cell line finding that the combination of celecoxib and quercetin had synergistic anti-cancer effects. Quercetin, a natural plant flavonoid found in apples and onions, inhibits the PI3K/Akt/mTOR signaling pathway, serving as an anti-CSC agent. Quercetin also inhibits fatty acid synthetase (FASN) and the Beta-Catenin/Wnt (CSC pathway). Fisetin, another flavonoid structurally similar to quercetin, has similar anti-cancer activity. (47-53)

Note: FASN was discussed in chapter 37, on fenofibrate. (Fenofibrate, quercetin and orlistat are FASN inhibitors).

In 2019, Dr. Dharambir Kashyap et al. write:

Specifically, fisetin and quercetin, two well-studied flavonoids, have shown remarkable anti-cancer effects in multiple in vitro and in vivo systems. (51)

Celecoxib Inhibits Wnt Pathway

In 2017, Dr. Chaolin Huang et al. studied the effect of celecoxib on breast CSCs, finding downregulation of the Wnt pathway. Dr. Huang's group found that celecoxib decreases both Beta-Catenin, the main Wnt pathway protein, as well as messenger RNA (mRNA) expression levels of Wnt pathway target genes, which produce the downstream proteins cyclin-D1 and C-Myc. Their excellent study demonstrated the potent anti-CSC properties of celecoxib. (54)

Celecoxib and Conventional Chemotherapy

As mentioned in earlier chapters, a major problem encountered with conventional chemotherapy is the stimulation of inflammatory pathways that upregulate CSCs. In 2017, Dr. Pilar Jiménez et al. studied the combination of celecoxib with 5-FU chemotherapy in an esophageal cancer cell line, in vitro, finding the 5-FU resulted in increased CSC marker CD24, while the addition of celecoxib to the 5-FU reduced the CD24 stem cell marker. This type of benefit is also seen by combining chemotherapy with aspirin as discussed in chapter 13.

Dr. Pilar Jiménez and colleagues write:

Treatment with celecoxib alone or in combination with 5-FU … resulted in a reduction of CD24 expression [a CSC marker]. Moreover, celecoxib inhibited the growth of tumor spheres [a CSC marker]. These findings showing a reduction in CSC markers induced by celecoxib. (55)

Note: CD24 is a CSC marker.

Drs. Lisa Pang et al. report (2016) that COX-2 plays an important role in CSC survival and repopulation of CSCs after chemotherapy. Inhibition of COX-2 prevents this chemotherapy induced cancer stem cell survival and repopulation, potentially leading to "curative efficacy". (55A)

Celecoxib - Anti-Cancer Stem Cell Agent

In 2019, Dr. Jerry Harb et al. discussed cancer treatment with Wnt pathway signaling inhibitors. Celecoxib and pyrvinium (discussed in its own chapter 12) were prominently mentioned. Dr. Harb's group found celecoxib suppressed breast CSCs and synergized with chemotherapy agents with **"dramatically increased sensitivity."** They summarized the anti-CSC activity of celecoxib in breast and colon cancer cell studies, writing:

> Celecoxib has been shown to **suppress mammary cancer stem cell renewal,** enhance responsiveness to chemotherapeutic agents, impede epithelial to mesenchymal transition [EMT], and mitigate metastatic potential in MCF-7 and MDA-MB-231 [breast cancer] cells by inhibiting prostaglandin E2 [the COX-2 pathway] and promoting B-catenin degradation [the Wnt pathway] … combination use of both celecoxib and conventional chemotherapeutic drugs dramatically increased the chemo-sensitivity of breast cancer cells … (56)

Inhibits mTOR, Restores GSK3-B, Inhibits B-Catenin

In 2016, Dr. Beatrice Riva et al. studied a chronic myelogenous leukemia (CML) and acute lymphoblastic leukemia (ALL) cell model, showing celecoxib to be effective as anti-CSC agent. They write:

> Celecoxib rapidly activated AMP-activated protein kinase [AMPK] and the consequent inhibition of mTORC1…. Treatment with celecoxib also restored GSK3ß function and led to downregulation of ß-catenin activity

through transcriptional and post-translational mechanisms… (57)

GSK3Beta is the cytoplasmic protein that forms a "destruction complex" that degrades Beta-Catenin, thus preventing nuclear translocation and transcription, essentially turning off Wnt signaling. Restoring GSK3Beta with celecoxib downregulates Beta-Catenin, which then inhibits the Wnt pathway, a critical pathway for cancer stem cell maintenance.

Induction of Apoptosis – Downregulates BCL2

In 2011, Dr. Justine Rudner studied the mechanism of celecoxib-induced apoptosis in lymphoma cells, finding celecoxib caused the depletion of the anti-apoptotic protein Mcl-1, which was sufficient to induce apoptosis, in spite of BCL2 overexpression.

Note: Mcl-1 = Myeloid cell leukemia 1 (Mcl-1), an anti-apoptotic protein. BCL-2 is the main anti-apoptosis protein.

This means that celecoxib induces apoptosis in cancer cells independent of high BCL-2 protein levels. BCL-2 is upregulated in many cancers, conferring apoptosis resistance and cancer cell immortality. Celecoxib may be a good choice for induction of apoptosis in cancers expressing high BCL-2 protein on immunohistology. (58–60)

Cancers with Overexpressed BCL-2

Indeed, Dr. Jendrossek from Essen Germany says in *Cancer Letter* 2013:

> Celecoxib may be of specific value for the

treatment of apoptosis-resistant tumors with overexpression of Bcl-2. (61)

Celecoxib Downregulates C-Myc OncoGene

In 2011, Dr. Cyril Sobolewski studied celecoxib in a lymphoblastic leukemia cell model, finding celecoxib prevents cancer cell replication with early downregulation of c-Myc Oncogene and protein. This halts cancer cell replication in the G0 phase, a non-replicating resting phase, outside of the cell cycle. The c-Myc oncogene is a "master regulator" that controls proliferation, growth, and apoptosis. In the rapidly proliferating cancer cells, C-Myc is massively upregulated. Dr. Sobelewski writes:

> These events [celecoxib treatment] are associated with a rapid downregulation [within one hour] of c-Myc expression, accompanied by the upregulation of p27 and the downregulation of PCNA [proliferating cell nuclear antigen] and cyclin D1. (62)

Note: P27 is a tumor suppressor gene, so upregulation is a good anti-cancer strategy. PCNA promotes cell proliferation and tumorigenesis, so downregulation of PCNA is a good thing.

Celecoxib Restores Host Immune Function

In 2017, Dr. Marc Hennequart reports COX-2 stimulates tumor immune evasion via the IDO gene, and conversely, COX-2 inhibition downregulates IDO gene expression and restores immune function, a valid anticancer strategy. (63)

Inhibiting the IDO Gene – Restoring Anti-Cancer Immunity

In 2011, Dr. Cesario reviewed the preclinical studies, looking at the link between COX-2 and the IDO gene, finding that celecoxib is a potent IDO gene inhibitor, thus restoring host anti-cancer immunity:

> IDO1 is traditionally viewed as a general suppressor of T cell activation and mediator of immune escape in cancer.... Celecoxib serves as a potent IDO inhibitor thus restoring host immune function.... Thus, COX-2 inhibitors can increase the infiltration of CD4+and CD8+T cells [anti-cancer immune cells] to tumor sites, restoring immune response within the tumor micro-environment. (64)

Tumor Micro-Environment (TME) COX-2 in TAMS

In a 2015, Dr. Hongzhong Li studied breast cancer cells and the TME, finding tumor-associated macrophages (TAMS) express COX-2 protein. This stimulates the cancer cells in a positive-feedback loop between TAMs and cancer cells. The secreted COX-2 protein stimulates cancer proliferation and invasive behavior. In addition, COX-2 protein increases the anti-apoptotic protein BCL-2 and the drug-resistant protein P-gp. Dr. Li writes:

> COX-2+ TAMs promoted breast cancer cell proliferation and survival by increasing Bcl-2 and P-gp and decreasing Bax in cancer cells. (65)

Note: BCL-2 is the anti-apoptotic protein. P-gp is the P-Glycoprotein drug efflux pump, which confers drug resistance. Bax is a pro-apoptosis protein. By inhibiting COX2 secretion by TAMs in the micro-environment, celecoxib disrupts this feedback loop, preventing TAMs from supporting the cancer cell growth.

Other natural substances that increase Bax and decrease BCL-2 protein levels in cancer cells are Quercetin (66), Garlic (Allicin) (67), and Di-Indole Methane (DIM). (68–69)

Overcoming Drug Resistance and Inducing Apoptosis

As mentioned previously, conventional oncology has a thorny problem. The repeated use of chemotherapy induces a chemo-resistant cell type, rendering further chemotherapy useless. This is where COX-2 inhibitors come into play. COX-2 inhibitors enhance efficacy and restore sensitivity to chemotherapy agents. (71–73)

Restores Chemo-Sensitivity

Chemotherapy drug resistance in cancer is due to upregulation of genes controlling the MDR (Multidrug Resistance) efflux pump. This is the molecular pump located at the cancer cell outer membrane that promptly pumps out the chemotherapy drugs. Many studies show that COX-2 inhibitors downregulate the MDR gene, reducing expression of P-glycoprotein (P-gp), thus downregulating the efflux pump and increasing chemotherapy drug concentration in the cancer cells. (74–79)

Chemotherapy Enhanced Tenfold

In 2010, Dr. Roy studied the effect of celecoxib on a hepatoma cell line, finding celecoxib treatment caused a tenfold enhancement of sensitivity to the chemotherapy drugs within hepatoma cancer cells (HepG2):

> Celecoxib, a selective inhibitor of COX-2, at 25 microM concentration increased the accumulation of doxorubicin in HepG2 cells and **enhanced the sensitivity of the cells to doxorubicin by tenfold.** (75)

Causal Link Between COX2 and Drug Resistance

In 2002, Dr. Vimal Patel studied a mouse model of kidney cells genetically engineered to overexpress the COX-2 enzyme, finding the highly upregulated MDR1 gene responsible for production of the P-gp glycoprotein acting as efflux pump conferring drug resistance. Dr. Vimal Patel concluded:

> These results prove the existence of a causal link between Cox-2 and P-gp activity, which would have implications for multi-drug resistance in tumors where Cox-2 is overexpressed. (77).

P-Glycoprotein Blocks Apoptosis

The P-glycoprotein (P-gp) is also an anti-apoptotic protein which blocks release of cytochrome C from the mitochondria thus inhibiting the intrinsic pathway.

In 2007, Dr. Omella Fantappiè reported that low doses (10 micromolar/L) of celecoxib reduced P-gp levels and induced apoptosis in a multidrug-resistant (MDR) hepatocellular cancer line, writing:

> 10 micromol/L celecoxib reduced P-glycoprotein, Bcl-x(L), and Bcl-2 expression and induced translocation of Bax from

cytosol to mitochondria and cytochrome c release into cytosol in MDR-positive hepatocellular carcinoma cells. (79)

Synergy with Radiation Therapy

Cox-2 inhibitors have been shown to improve efficacy of radiotherapy by protecting normal cells and sensitizing tumor cells to the effects of radiation. This may be related to the pro-oxidant effect of the COX-2 inhibitor celecoxib as described by Dr. Ralph below. (80–89)

Celecoxib as Pro-Oxidant

In 2018, Dr. Ralph summarized anti-cancer research on celecoxib, emphasizing its "pro-oxidant" properties, and the increased ROS in the mitochondria, a form of mitochondrial toxin. Dr. Ralph writes:

1) Celecoxib combined with chemotherapy synergistically improves clinical response in preclinical animal models of advanced metastatic cancer.

2) Celecoxib combined with chemotherapy has **"curative efficacy"** in human clinical trials of advanced-stage metastatic cancer.

3) Celecoxib's main mechanism is as a **"mitochondrial toxin" and "pro-oxidant"** that sensitizes cancer stem cells to chemotherapy. (80)

Complete Regression Celecoxib and EGF inhibitor, Cetuximab

In 2008, Dr. Jalili reported the case of an 88-year-old male with advanced recurrent squamous cell cancer involving the orbit (eye socket), which was positive for expression of both EGFR (Epithelial Growth Factor Receptor) and COX-2. Cetuximab (Erbitux®) is a new drug, a humanized murine (mouse) monoclonal antibody against EGFR, approved in 2005 in Switzerland for the treatment of squamous cell carcinoma (SCC) of the head and neck. The patient was treated with intravenous Cetuximab to block EGFR, in combination with the COX 2 inhibitor Celebrex, 100 mg orally daily, with excellent results on follow-up CAT Scan. Dr. Jalili writes treatment caused complete regression of the cancer mass:

> Complete regression of the intraorbital mass as well as the submandibular metastases was observed at week 8 and confirmed at week 16 … There was no further progression of the disease for the next 7 months. The therapy was well tolerated, did not result in any noteworthy laboratory adverse events … Almost all cutaneous SCC express EGFR, which may confer metastatic potential. (91)

Celecoxib Synergy With CAR T Therapy

CAR T therapy, Chimeric Antigen Receptor-T Cell, is a new form of immunotherapy described more completely in chapter 27, "the Mouse that Killed Cancer". In 2017, Dr. Dinh suggested Celecoxib would be synergistic with CAR T therapy—for example, in B-Cell Lymphoma to sensitize resistant lymphoma cells to the apoptotic (lytic) effects of the CAR T cells. Dr. Dinh writes that in Non-Hodgkin's Lymphoma (NHL) patients treated with CAR-T Cell Therapy, the addition of celecoxib COX-2 inhibition provides augmented efficacy, potentially improving treatment outcome:

> Celecoxib is ….an effective apoptotic

inducer of B cell lymphoma... Recent modern developments... suggest a promising role of CD19 CAR T cell therapy in NHL. However, a subset of tumor cells either inherently resistant or develop resistance to CAR-mediated immunotherapy. Based on the apoptotic gene regulatory effects of celecoxib, we propose that combination of CD19 CAR T cell therapy and celecoxib can potentially improve the treatment outcome of NHL patients. (92)

Similarly, in 2018, Dr. Torres-Collado also suggested using celecoxib in combination with CD-19 CAR T therapy in NHL to overcome apoptosis resistance. (93)

Since CAR T therapy is so new, we do not yet have any studies confirming the above hypothesis suggesting synergy of celecoxib with CAR T cell therapy. We await confirmatory NIH-funded studies.

Celecoxib Synergy with Auranofin, Inhibition of HK II

In 2019, Dr. Han was interested in finding a drug to enhance the anti-cancer activity of auranofin, an old gold-based rheumatology drug. Dr. Han did a high through-put screen on a large library of drugs, identifying that celecoxib potently enhanced the activity of auranofin at routine therapeutic doses both in vitro and in vivo. The combination of celecoxib and auranofin induced:

severe oxidative stress that caused ROS-mediated inhibition of hexokinase (HK) and a disturbance of mitochondrial redox homeostasis, resulting in a significant decrease of ATP generation.... and dysfunction of the electron transport chain....

that effectively eliminates cancer cells in vivo ... the combination induced severe ROS stress leading to protein oxidation and dysfunction of mitochondrial electron transport chain, suppression of glycolysis through inhibition of hexokinase (HK) and abrogation of mitochondrial oxidative phosphorylation via oxidative damage to respiratory chain seem to be two key mechanisms by which AF [auranofin] and CE [celecoxib] induce energy crisis in cancer cells.... These results seem clinically relevant since AF concentrations of 1–3 μM in plasma are achievable without obvious side effects in patients or in volunteer subjects who received the recommended dose of 6 mg/day for rheumatoid arthritis. Similarly, plasma CE concentrations greater than 10 μM are also achievable in human receiving 400 mg/day, which seem well tolerated. (94)

In 2019, Dr. Onodera reviewed Auranofin, suggesting it may be a potent anti-cancer agent. The mechanism is inhibition of the TrxR (thioredoxin reductase system), which is a selenium based intracellular anti-oxidant system which protects the cancer cells from excess ROS (reactive oxygen species). (95–97)

Dr. Onodera writes:

Auranofin inhibits the activity of thioredoxin reductase [TrxR], an enzyme of the thioredoxin system that is important for maintaining the intracellular redox state. Particularly in cancers, TrxR inhibition leads to an increase in cellular oxidative stress and induces apoptosis. (95)

Both Celecoxib and Auranofin are included in the nine-drug protocol CUSP9 for glioblastoma recommended by Dr. Richard Kast. (98)

Although this combination looks promising in preclinical studies, future human clinical trials would be needed for confirmation of anti-cancer efficacy and tolerability. We await those studies.

COX-2 Inhibitor Synergy with CheckPoint Inhibitors

In 2017, Dr. Murphy pointed out a possible synergy of COX-2 inhibitors with immunotherapy with the new checkpoint inhibitors, as suggested by preclinical studies. (99)

In 2019, Dr. Yamaguchi explored this further, finding that celecoxib augments the effect of PD-1 blockade (checkpoint blockade) in a malignant glioma model. (100)

Case Report – Celecoxib Synergy with Lenalidamide

Lenalidamide, a new immunomodulatory drug derived from thalidomide has shown impressive results in hematologic cancers. In 2018, Dr. Garcia-Recio reported a 35-year-old female patient with NHL (non-Hodgkin's lymphoma) refractory to six lines of chemotherapy. Since chemotherapy was no longer useful, the patient was switched to a combination of lenalidamide (20 mg/d for 3 of every 4 weeks) and celecoxib (200 mg orally twice a day) achieving complete remission for 22 months. This is very impressive. (101)

Cardiovascular Adverse Effects of COX-2 Inhibitors

COX-2 inhibitors increase the risk for cardiovascular disease, and patients should be monitored closely for cardiovascular disease adverse events (chest pain, angina, myocardial infarction etc.). (102–103)

Testosterone Adverse Effects

In addition, COX-2 inhibitors reduce serum testosterone by reducing prostaglandin synthesis in testicular Leydig cells. This reduces testosterone production and may cause infertility. Inhibition of COX2 with celecoxib in an animal study decreased the number of Leydig cells and reduce testosterone levels. As such, it would be prudent to monitor Testosterone levels during long-term treatment with celecoxib as well as other NSAIDs. (104–107)

NSAIDS and Gastrointestinal Bleeding

NSAID (nonsteroidal anti-inflammatory) drugs are widely used for osteoarthritis pain relief. Unfortunately, NSAIDS are associated with gastrointestinal (GI) damage and bleeding. The newer "coxib" NSAIDS were developed to reduce GI mucosal damage and GI bleeding and are considered safer than the older NSAIDs.

Celecoxib Studied in Various Cancer Cell Types

- Colorectal adenomas and cancer (11–13)(20)(78)(94)(119–120) (150)
- Intestinal polyposis (27–32)
- Colon cancer stem cells (41)
- Endometrial cancer (14)(121)
- Glioblastoma (18)(98)(146–148)
- Prostate cancer (19)(34)
- Non-small-cell lung cancer (22)(71) (136–140)(160)

- Breast cancer (23)(37)(65)(76)(113–116)(127–135)
- Breast cancer stem cells (54)
- Morphine induced cancer growth (24)
- Chronic myeloid leukemia (25–26)(57)(62)(117)
- Leukemia (124–125) (143–144)
- B-cell lymphoma (33)(92–93)(123)(141–142)
- Gastric cancer (35)
- Hepatoma (36)(75)(118)(161)
- Esophageal cancer (55)
- Squamous cell cancer (91)
- CNS lymphoma (112)
- Pancreatic cancer (122)(159)
- Melanoma (126)
- Gastric cancer (145)
- Ewing sarcoma (151–152)
- Ovarian cancer (153–158)

Synergy with Autophagy Inhibition, Chloroquine in Osteosarcoma

In 2018, Dr. Zhou studied the effects of celecoxib on an osteosarcoma cell line, finding enhanced anti-cancer effect with addition of chloroquine for autophagy inhibition. Celecoxib-induced "protective autophagy," while chloroquine caused lysosomal dysfunction, thus inducing apoptosis. (162)

Conclusion

The COX2 Inhibitor, celecoxib has been repurposed as a potent anti-CSC agent via inhibition of inflammatory pathways that support CSCs, inhibition of p-glycoprotein efflux pump,

overcoming BCL-2 anti-apoptosis protein, restoration of anti-cancer immunity, increase in ROS, restoring drug sensitivity, and improving efficacy of radiotherapy. Dr. Ralph writes in 2018 that the combination of celecoxib with chemotherapy has shown **"curative efficacy"** in human clinical trials of advanced-stage metastatic cancer. Any time the words "curative efficacy" are mentioned, my ears perk up. Hopefully, celecoxib will soon be incorporated into routine oncology protocols. (90)

References for Chapter 38: Celecoxib COX2 Inhibitors As Anti-Cancer Agents

1) Lin, Yong, et al. "The NF-κB activation pathways, emerging molecular targets for cancer prevention and therapy." Expert opinion on therapeutic targets 14.1 (2010): 45-55.

2) Dolcet, Xavier, et al. "NF-kB in development and progression of human cancer." Virchows archiv 446.5 (2005): 475-482.

3) Serasanambati, Mamatha, and Shanmuga Reddy Chilakapati. "Function of nuclear factor kappa B (NF-kB) in human diseases-a review." South Ind. J. Biol. Sci 2 (2016): 368-387.

4) Colotta, Francesco, et al. "Cancer-related inflammation, the seventh hallmark of cancer: links to genetic instability." Carcinogenesis 30.7 (2009): 1073-1081.

5) Dep Prete, Annalisa, et al. "Molecular pathways in cancer-related inflammation." Biochemia medica: Biochemia medica 21.3 (2011): 264-275.

6) Hiscott, J., et al. "Manipulation of the nuclear factor-κ B pathway and the innate immune response by viruses." Oncogene 25.51 (2006): 6844-6867.

7) Hiscott, John, Hakju Kwon, and Pierre Génin. "Hostile takeovers: viral appropriation of the NF-kB pathway." The Journal of clinical investigation 107.2 (2001): 143-151.

8) Santoro, M. Gabriella, Antonio Rossi, and Carla Amici. "NF-κB and virus infection: who controls whom." The EMBO journal 22.11 (2003): 2552-2560.

9) Liu, Qiang, Yuan-hong Zhou, and Zhan-qiu Yang. "The cytokine storm of severe influenza and development of immunomodulatory therapy." Cellular & molecular immunology 13.1 (2016): 3-10.

10) Wu, Chun-Ying, et al. "Helicobacter pylori promote gastric cancer cells invasion through a NF-kB and COX-2-mediated pathway." World journal of gastroenterology: WJG 11.21 (2005): 3197.

11) Charalambous, M. P., et al. "Upregulation of cyclooxygenase-2 is accompanied by increased expression of nuclear factor-κ B and I κ B kinase-α in human colorectal cancer epithelial cells." British journal of cancer 88.10 (2003): 1598-1604.

12) Vandoros, Gerasimos P., et al. "PPAR-gamma is expressed and NF-kB pathway is activated and correlates positively with COX-2 expression in stromal myofibroblasts surrounding colon adenocarcinomas." Journal of cancer research and clinical oncology 132.2 (2006): 76-84.

13) Cherukuri, Durga, et al. "Selenomethionine regulates cyclooxygenase-2 (COX-2) expression through nuclear factor-kappa B (NF-kB) in colon cancer cells." Cancer biology & therapy 4.2 (2005): 183-188.

14) St-Germain, Marie-Eve, et al. "Regulation of COX-2 protein expression by Akt in endometrial cancer cells is mediated through NF-κB/IκB pathway." Molecular Cancer 3.1 (2004): 7.

15) Khan, Zakir, et al. "Biology of Cox-2: an application in cancer therapeutics." Current drug targets 12.7 (2011): 1082-1093.

16) Ghosh, Nilanjan, et al. "COX-2 as a target for cancer chemotherapy." Pharmacological reports 62.2 (2010): 233-244.

16A) Hashemi Goradel, Nasser, et al. "Cyclooxygenase-2 in cancer: A review." Journal of cellular physiology 234.5 (2019): 5683-5699.

17) Funakoshi-Tago, Megumi, et al. "Celecoxib potently inhibits TNFα-induced nuclear translocation and activation of NF-κB." Biochemical pharmacology 76.5 (2008): 662-671.

18) Sareddy, Gangadhara Reddy, et al. "The nonsteroidal anti-inflammatory drug celecoxib suppresses the growth and induces apoptosis of human glioblastoma cells via the NF-κB pathway." Journal of neuro-oncology 106.1 (2012): 99-109.

19) Huang, Huarong, et al. "Combination of Lipitor and Celebrex inhibits prostate cancer VCaP cells in vitro and in vivo." Anticancer research 34.7 (2014): 3357-3363.

20) Grosch, Sabine, et al. "COX-2 independent induction of cell cycle arrest and apoptosis in colon cancer cells by the selective COX-2 inhibitor celecoxib." The FASEB journal 15.14 (2001): 2742-2744.

21) Koki, Alane T., and Jaime L. Masferrer. "Celecoxib: a specific COX-2 inhibitor with anticancer properties." Cancer control 9.2_suppl (2002): 28-35.

22) Shishodia, Shishir, Dimpy Koul, and Bharat B. Aggarwal. "Cyclooxygenase (COX)-2 inhibitor celecoxib abrogates TNF-induced NF-κB activation through inhibition of activation of IκBα kinase and Akt in human non-small cell lung carcinoma: correlation with suppression of COX-2 synthesis." The Journal of Immunology 173.3 (2004): 2011-2022.

23) Kundu, Namita, and Amy M. Fulton. "Selective cyclooxygenase (COX)-1 or COX-2 inhibitors control metastatic disease in a murine model of breast cancer." Cancer research 62.8 (2002): 2343-2346.

24) Farooqui, Mariya, et al. "COX-2 inhibitor celecoxib prevents chronic morphine-induced promotion of angiogenesis, tumour growth, metastasis and mortality, without compromising analgesia." British journal of cancer 97.11 (2007): 1523-1531.

25) Bernard, M. P., et al. "Targeting cyclooxygenase-2 in hematological malignancies: rationale and promise." Current pharmaceutical design 14.21 (2008): 2051-2060.

26) Subhashini, J., S. V. K. Mahipal, and P. Reddanna. "Anti-proliferative and apoptotic effects of celecoxib on human chronic myeloid leukemia in vitro." Cancer letters 224.1 (2005): 31-43.

27) Neubert, Zachary S., and Mark Potter. "Attenuated Familial Adenomatous Polyposis: A Novel Treatment with Celecoxib." PRACTICAL GASTROENTEROLOGY 40.2 (2016): 64-65.

28) Delker, Don A., et al. "Chemoprevention with cyclooxygenase and epidermal growth factor receptor inhibitors in familial adenomatous polyposis patients: mRNA signatures of duodenal neoplasia." Cancer Prevention Research 11.1 (2018): 4-15.

29) Neklason, Deborah, et al. "Chemoprevention with COX2 and EGFR inhibition in familial adenomatous polyposis patients: mRNA signatures of duodenal neoplasia." (2016): 38-38.

30) Wang, Jiping, et al. "Chemopreventive efficacy of the cyclooxygenase-2 (Cox-2) inhibitor, celecoxib, is predicted by adenoma expression of Cox-2 and 15-PGDH." Cancer Epidemiology and Prevention Biomarkers 27.7 (2018): 728-736.

31) Oshima, Masanobu, et al. "Suppression of intestinal polyposis in ApcΔ716 knockout mice by inhibition of cyclooxygenase 2 (COX-2)." Cell 87.5 (1996): 803-809.

32) Khan, K. N. M., et al. "Enhanced cyclooxygenase-2 expression in sporadic and familial adenomatous polyposis of the human colon." Scandinavian journal of gastroenterology 36.8 (2001): 865-869.

33) Ryan, Elizabeth P., et al. "Cyclooxygenase-2 independent effects of cyclooxygenase-2 inhibitors on oxidative stress and intracellular glutathione content in normal and malignant human B-cells." Cancer Immunology, Immunotherapy 57.3 (2008): 347-358.

34) Hsu, Ao-Lin, et al. "The cyclooxygenase-2 inhibitor celecoxib induces apoptosis by blocking Akt activation in human prostate cancer cells independently of Bcl-2." Journal of Biological Chemistry 275.15 (2000): 11397-11403.

35) Liu, Min, et al. "Celecoxib regulates apoptosis and autophagy via the PI3K/Akt signaling pathway in SGC-7901 gastric cancer cells." International journal of molecular medicine 33.6 (2014): 1451-1458.

36) Leng, Jing, et al. "Cyclooxygenase-2 promotes hepatocellular carcinoma cell growth through Akt activation: evidence for Akt inhibition in celecoxib-induced apoptosis." Hepatology 38.3 (2003): 756-768.

37) Glynn, Sharon A., et al. "COX-2 activation is associated with Akt phosphorylation and poor survival in ER-negative, HER2-positive breast cancer." BMC cancer 10.1 (2010): 626.

38) Luo, Ji, Brendan D. Manning, and Lewis C. Cantley. "Targeting the PI3K-Akt pathway in human cancer: rationale and promise." Cancer cell 4.4 (2003): 257-262.

39) Xia, Pu, and Xiao-Yan Xu. "PI3K/Akt/mTOR signaling pathway in cancer stem cells: from basic research to clinical application." American journal of cancer research 5.5 (2015): 1602.

40) Martelli, Alberto M., et al. "The emerging role of the phosphatidylinositol 3-kinase/Akt/mammalian target of rapamycin signaling network in cancer stem cell biology." Cancers 2.3 (2010): 1576-1596.

41) Chen, Sugong, et al. "Inhibition of PI3K/Akt/mTOR signaling in PI3KR2-overexpressing colon cancer stem cells reduces tumor growth due to apoptosis." Oncotarget 8.31 (2017): 50476.

42) Ruiz, Pedro A., et al. "Quercetin inhibits TNF-induced NF-κ B transcription factor recruitment to proinflammatory gene promoters in murine intestinal epithelial cells." The Journal of nutrition 137.5 (2007): 1208-1215.

43) Walker, Edward H., et al. "Structural determinants of phosphoinositide 3-kinase inhibition by wortmannin, LY294002, quercetin, myricetin, and staurosporine." Molecular cell 6.4 (2000): 909-919.

44) Costa, Roberto, et al. "Impaired mitochondrial ATP production downregulates Wnt signaling via ER stress induction." Cell reports 28.8 (2019): 1949-1960.

45) Shi, W. Y., et al. "Therapeutic metformin/AMPK activation blocked lymphoma cell growth via inhibition of mTOR pathway and induction of autophagy." Cell death & disease 3.3 (2012): e275-e275.

46) Lu, Wenyan, Cuihong Lin, and Yonghe Li. "Rottlerin induces Wnt co-receptor LRP6 degradation and suppresses both Wnt/β-catenin and mTORC1 signaling in prostate and breast cancer cells." Cellular signalling 26.6 (2014): 1303-1309.

47) Yu, C.-P.; Qiu, R.-G.; Shi, L.; Liang, J. Celecoxib and quercetin induce apoptosis in human hepatocarcinoma. Biomed. Res. 2017, 28, 3465–3470

48) Li, Xiuli, et al. "Quercetin suppresses breast cancer stem cells (CD44+/CD24−) by inhibiting the PI3K/Akt/mTOR-signaling pathway." Life sciences 196 (2018): 56-62.

49) Granato, Marisa, et al. "Quercetin induces apoptosis and autophagy in primary effusion lymphoma cells by inhibiting PI3K/AKT/mTOR and STAT3 signaling pathways." The Journal of nutritional biochemistry 41 (2017): 124-136.

50) George, Vazhappilly Cijo. "Promising tumor inhibiting potentials of Fisetin through PI3K/AKT/mTOR pathway." American journal of translational research 8.2 (2016): 1293.

51) Kashyap, Dharambir, et al. "Fisetin and Quercetin: Promising Flavonoids with Chemopreventive Potential." Biomolecules 9.5 (2019): 174.

52) Sultan, Ahmed S., et al. "Quercetin induces apoptosis in triple-negative breast cancer cells via inhibiting fatty acid synthase and β-catenin." Int. J. Clin. Exp. Pathol 10.1 (2017): 156-172.

53) Zhang, Chunping, et al. "Quercetin suppresses the tumorigenesis of oral squamous cell carcinoma by regulating microRNA-22/WNT1/β-catenin axis." Journal of pharmacological sciences 140.2 (2019): 128-136.

54) Huang, Chaolin, et al. "Celecoxib targets breast cancer stem cells by inhibiting the synthesis of prostaglandin E2 and down-regulating the Wnt pathway activity." Oncotarget 8.70 (2017): 115254.

55) Jiménez, Pilar, et al. "CD24 Expression Is Increased in 5-Fluorouracil-Treated Esophageal Adenocarcinoma Cells." Frontiers in Pharmacology 8 (2017).

55A) Pang, Lisa Y., Emma A. Hurst, and David J. Argyle. "Cyclooxygenase-2: a role in cancer stem cell survival and repopulation of cancer cells during therapy." Stem cells international 2016 (2016).

56) Harb, Jerry, Pen-Jen Lin, and Jijun Hao. "Recent development of Wnt signaling pathway inhibitors for cancer therapeutics." Current oncology reports 21.2 (2019): 12.

57) Riva, Beatrice, et al. "Celecoxib inhibits proliferation and survival of chronic myelogeous leukemia (CML) cells via AMPK-dependent regulation of ß-catenin and mTORC1/2." Oncotarget 7.49 (2016): 81555.

58) Rudner, Justine, et al. "Anti-apoptotic Bcl-2 fails to form efficient complexes with pro-apoptotic Bak to protect from Celecoxib-induced apoptosis." Biochemical pharmacology 81.1 (2011): 32-42.

59) Rudner, Justine, et al. "Differential effects of anti-apoptotic Bcl-2 family members Mcl-1, Bcl-2, and Bcl-xL on celecoxib-induced apoptosis." Biochemical pharmacology 79.1 (2010): 10-20.

60) Johnson, Amy J., et al. "A novel celecoxib derivative, OSU03012, induces cytotoxicity in primary CLL cells and transformed B-cell lymphoma cell line via a caspase-and Bcl-2–independent mechanism." Blood 105.6 (2005): 2504-2509.

61) Jendrossek, Verena. "Targeting apoptosis pathways by Celecoxib in cancer." Cancer letters 332.2 (2013): 313-324.

62) Sobolewski, Cyril, et al. "Cox-2 inhibitors induce early c-Myc downregulation and lead to expression of differentiation markers in leukemia cells." Cell Cycle 10.17 (2011): 2978-2993.

63) Hennequart, Marc, et al. "Constitutive IDO1 expression in human tumors is driven by cyclooxygenase-2 and mediates intrinsic immune resistance." Cancer immunology research 5.8 (2017): 695-709.

64) Cesario, A., B. Rocca, and S. Rutella. "The interplay between indoleamine 2, 3-dioxygenase 1 (IDO1) and cyclooxygenase (COX)-2 in chronic inflammation and cancer." Current medicinal chemistry 18.15 (2011): 2263-2271.

65) Li, Hongzhong, et al. "Cyclooxygenase-2 in tumor-associated macrophages promotes breast cancer cell survival by triggering a positive-feedback loop between macrophages and cancer cells." Oncotarget 6.30 (2015): 29637.

66) Duo, Jian, et al. "Quercetin inhibits human breast cancer cell proliferation and induces apoptosis via Bcl-2 and Bax regulation." Molecular medicine reports 5.6 (2012): 1453-1456.

67) Verma, Sharad, Amit Singh, and Abha Mishra. "Complex disruption effect of natural polyphenols on Bcl-2-Bax: molecular dynamics simulation and essential dynamics study." Journal of Biomolecular Structure and Dynamics 33.5 (2015): 1094-1106.

68) Hong, Young-Sook, et al. "Effects of allyl sulfur compounds and garlic extract on the expression of Bcl-2, Bax, and p53 in non small cell lung cancer cell lines." Experimental & molecular medicine 32.3 (2000): 127-134.

69) Hong, Chibo, Gary L. Firestone, and Leonard F. Bjeldanes. "Bcl-2 family-mediated apoptotic effects of 3, 3'-diindolylmethane (DIM) in human breast cancer cells." Biochemical pharmacology 63.6 (2002): 1085-1097.

70) Li, Yiwei, Sreenivasa R. Chinni, and Fazlul H. Sarkar. "Selective growth regulatory and pro-apoptotic effects of DIM is mediated by AKT and NF-kappaB pathways in prostate cancer cells." Front Biosci 10 (2005): 236-243.

71) Hohenforst-Schmidt, Wolfgang, et al. "COX-2 Inhibitors, a Potential Synergistic Effect with Antineoplastic Drugs in Lung Cancer." Oncomedicine 2017; 2:28-36

72) Sobolewski, Cyril, et al. "The role of cyclooxygenase-2 in cell proliferation and cell death in human malignancies." International journal of cell biology 2010 (2010).

73) Lim, Jong Seung, et al. "Co-treatment with celecoxib or NS398 strongly sensitizes resistant cancer cells to antimitotic drugs independent of P-gp inhibition." Anticancer research 36.10 (2016): 5063-5070.

74) Xia, Wenhong, et al. "Celecoxib enhanced the sensitivity of cancer cells to anticancer drugs by inhibition of the expression of P-glycoprotein through a COX-2-Independent Manner." Journal of cellular biochemistry 108.1 (2009): 181-194.

75) Roy, Karnati R., et al. "Celecoxib inhibits MDR1 expression through COX-2-dependent mechanism in human hepatocellular carcinoma (HepG2) cell line." Cancer chemotherapy and pharmacology 65.5 (2010): 903-911.

76) Zatelli, Maria Chiara, et al. "Cyclooxygenase-2 inhibitors prevent the development of chemoresistance phenotype in a breast cancer cell line by inhibiting glycoprotein p-170 expression." Endocrine-related cancer 14.4 (2007): 1029-1038.

77) Patel, Vimal A., Michael J. Dunn, and Andrey Sorokin. "Regulation of MDR-1 (P-glycoprotein) by cyclooxygenase-2." Journal of Biological Chemistry 277.41 (2002): 38915-38920.

78) Zrieki, A., R. Farinotti, and M. Buyse. "Cyclooxygenase inhibitors down regulate P-glycoprotein in human colorectal Caco-2 cell line." Pharmaceutical research 25.9 (2008): 1991.

79) Fantappiè, Ornella, et al. "P-glycoprotein mediates celecoxib-induced apoptosis in multiple drug-resistant cell lines." Cancer research 67.10 (2007): 4915-4923.

80) Salehifar, Ebrahim, and Seyed Jalal Hosseinimehr. "The use of cyclooxygenase-2 inhibitors for improvement of efficacy of radiotherapy in cancers." Drug discovery today 21.4 (2016): 654-662.

81) Laube, Markus, Torsten Kniess, and Jens Pietzsch. "Development of Antioxidant COX-2 Inhibitors as Radioprotective Agents for Radiation Therapy—A Hypothesis-Driven Review." Antioxidants 5.2 (2016): 14.

82) Davis, Thomas W., et al. "Synergy between celecoxib and radiotherapy results from inhibition of cyclooxygenase-2-derived prostaglandin E2, a survival factor for tumor and associated vasculature." Cancer research 64.1 (2004): 279-285.

83) Davis, Thomas W., et al. "COX-2 inhibitors as radiosensitizing agents for cancer therapy." American journal of clinical oncology 26.4 (2003): S58-S61.

84) Nakata, Eiko, et al. "Potentiation of tumor response to radiation or chemoradiation by selective cyclooxygenase-2 enzyme inhibitors." International Journal of Radiation Oncology* Biology* Physics 58.2 (2004): 369-375.

85) Shin, You Keun, et al. "Radiosensitivity enhancement by celecoxib, a cyclooxygenase (COX)-2 selective inhibitor, via COX-2–dependent cell cycle regulation on human cancer cells expressing differential COX-2 levels." Cancer research 65.20 (2005): 9501-9509.

86) Davis, Thomas W., et al. "Synergy between celecoxib and radiotherapy results from inhibition of cyclooxygenase-2-derived prostaglandin E2, a survival factor for tumor and associated vasculature." Cancer research 64.1 (2004): 279-285.

87) Kishi, Kazushi, et al. "Preferential enhancement of tumor radioresponse by a cyclooxygenase-2 inhibitor." Cancer research 60.5 (2000): 1326-1331.

88) Petersen, Cordula, et al. "Enhancement of intrinsic tumor cell radiosensitivity induced by a selective cyclooxygenase-2 inhibitor." Clinical Cancer Research 6.6 (2000): 2513-2520.

89) Sminia, P., et al. "COX-2 inhibitors act as radiosensitizer in tumor treatment." Biomedicine & pharmacotherapy 59 (2005): S272-S275.

90) Ralph, Stephen John, et al. "NSAID celecoxib: a potent mitochondrial pro-oxidant cytotoxic agent sensitizing metastatic cancers and cancer stem cells to chemotherapy." J Cancer Metastasis Treat 4.49 (2018): 1-26.

91) Jalili, Ahmad, et al. "Combination of an EGFR blocker and a COX-2 inhibitor for the treatment of advanced cutaneous squamous cell carcinoma." JDDG 6 (2008): 1066-1069.

92) Dinh, Tam NM, Alexandra S. Onea, and Ali R. Jazirehi. "Combination of celecoxib (Celebrex®) and CD19 CAR-redirected CTL immunotherapy for the treatment of B-cell non-Hodgkin's lymphomas." Am J Clin Exp Immunol 6.3 (2017): 27-42.

93) Torres-Collado, Antoni, and Ali Jazirehi. "Overcoming resistance of human non-Hodgkin's lymphoma to CD19-CAR CTL therapy by celecoxib and histone deacetylase inhibitors." Cancers 10.6 (2018): 200.

94) Han, Yi, et al. "Synergy between auranofin and celecoxib against colon cancer in vitro and in vivo through a novel redox-mediated mechanism." Cancers 11.7 (2019): 931.

95) Onodera, Takefumi, Isao Momose, and Manabu Kawada. "Potential Anticancer Activity of Auranofin." Chemical and Pharmaceutical Bulletin 67.3 (2019): 186-191.

96) Yan, Xiang, et al. "Inhibition of thioredoxin/thioredoxin reductase induces synthetic lethality in lung cancers with compromised glutathione homeostasis." Cancer research 79.1 (2019): 125-132.

97) Wang, Hui, et al. "Auranofin radiosensitizes tumor cells through targeting thioredoxin reductase and resulting overproduction of reactive oxygen species." Oncotarget 8.22 (2017): 35728.

98) Kast, Richard E., Georg Karpel-Massler, and Marc-Eric Halatsch. "CUSP9* treatment protocol for recurrent glioblastoma: aprepitant, artesunate, auranofin, captopril, celecoxib, disulfiram, itraconazole, ritonavir, sertraline augmenting continuous low dose temozolomide." Oncotarget 5.18 (2014): 8052.

99) Murphy, J. "Anti-Cancer Therapy: Non-Steroidal Anti-Inflammatory Drugs (NSAIDS) in Combination with Immunotherapy." MOJ Immunol 5.3 (2017): 00156.

100) Yamaguchi, Izumi, et al. "Downregulation of PD-L1 via FKBP5 by celecoxib augments antitumor effects of PD-1 blockade in a malignant glioma model." Neuro-Oncology Advances (2019).

101) Garcia-Recio, Marta, et al. "Complete response associated with lenalidomide and celecoxib in a case of primary refractory Hodgkin lymphoma." OncoTargets and therapy 11 (2018): 6599.

102) Fanelli, Andrea, et al. "Cardiovascular and cerebrovascular risk with nonsteroidal anti-inflammatory drugs and cyclooxygenase 2 inhibitors: latest evidence and clinical implications." Therapeutic advances in drug safety 8.6 (2017): 173-182.

103) Varga, Zoltan, Syed Rafay Ali Sabzwari, and Veronika Vargova. "Cardiovascular risk of nonsteroidal anti-inflammatory drugs: an under-recognized public health issue." Cureus 9.4 (2017).

104) Jahanpour, N., Faezeh Jahanpour, and P. Azodi. "Celecoxib And Male Infertility-An Experimental Design." (2009): 43-44.

105) Kristensen, David Møbjerg, et al. "Ibuprofen alters human testicular physiology to produce a state of compensated hypogonadism." Proceedings of the National Academy of Sciences (2018): 201715035.

106) Tengstrand, B., K. Carlström, and I. Hafström. "Bioavailable testosterone in men with rheumatoid arthritis—high frequency of hypogonadism." Rheumatology 41.3 (2002): 285-289.

107) Albert, Océane, et al. "Paracetamol, aspirin and indomethacin display endocrine disrupting properties in the adult human testis in vitro." Human reproduction 28.7 (2013): 1890-1898.

108) Laine, Loren. "Gastrointestinal effects of NSAIDs and coxibs." Journal of Pain and Symptom Management 25.2 (2003): 32-40.

109) Caunedo-Alvarez, A., et al. "Macroscopic small bowel mucosal injury caused by chronic non-steroidal anti-inflammatory drugs (NSAID) use as assessed by capsule endoscopy." Revista Espanola De Enfermedades Digestivas 102.2 (2010): 80.

110) Go, Mae F. "Drug injury in the upper gastrointestinal tract: nonsteroidal anti-inflammatory drugs." Gastrointestinal Endoscopy Clinics 16.1 (2006): 83-97.

111) Tachecí, Ilja, et al. "Small intestinal injury in NSAID users suffering from rheumatoid arthritis or osteoarthritis." Rheumatology international 36.11 (2016): 1557-1561.

112) Wang, Weijun, et al. "Efficacy of celecoxib in the treatment of CNS lymphomas: an in vivo model." Neurosurgical focus 21.5 (2006): 1-8.

113) Wang, Guanying, et al. "Celecoxib induced apoptosis against different breast cancer cell lines by down-regulated NF-κB pathway." Biochemical and biophysical research communications 490.3 (2017): 969-976.

114) Regulski, Miłosz, et al. "COX-2 inhibitors: a novel strategy in the management of breast cancer." Drug discovery today 21.4 (2016): 598-615.

115) Friedrich, Michael, et al. "Effects of combined treatment with vitamin D and COX2 inhibitors on breast cancer cell lines." Anticancer research 38.2 (2018): 1201-1207.

116) Li, Jieqing, et al. "Celecoxib in breast cancer prevention and therapy." Cancer management and research 10 (2018): 4653.

117) Lu, Ying, et al. "Celecoxib suppresses autophagy and enhances cytotoxicity of imatinib in imatinib-resistant chronic myeloid leukemia cells." Journal of translational medicine 14.1 (2016): 270.

118) Tai, Yang, et al. "Suppressing growth and invasion of human hepatocellular carcinoma cells by celecoxib through inhibition of cyclooxygenase-2." Cancer management and research 11 (2019): 2831.

119) Veettil, Sajesh K., et al. "Efficacy and safety of celecoxib on the incidence of recurrent colorectal adenomas: a systematic review and meta-analysis." Cancer management and research 11 (2019): 561.

120) Ohira, Gaku, et al. "Preoperative chemoradiotherapy using S-1 combined with celecoxib for advanced lower rectal cancer: Phase I/II study." Journal of the anus, rectum and colon 3.1 (2019): 43-48.

121) Li, Nan, et al. "Celecoxib inhibits endometrial cancer cells through COX-2-dependent and non-dependent pathways." International Journal of Clicinical and Experimental Medicine 12.5 (2019): 4707.

122) Qiu, Xiaoxin, et al. "S-1 and celecoxib synergistically suppress pancreatic cancer growth by promoting apoptosis in vivo and in vitro." Int J Clin Exp Med 12.4 (2019): 3201-3213.

123) Wun, Theodore, Hayes McKnight, and Joseph Tuscano. "Increased cyclooxygenase-2 (COX-2): A potential role in the pathogenesis of lymphoma." Leukemia Research 28.2 (2004): 179-190.

124) Lu, Ying, et al. "Celecoxib exerts antitumor effects in HL-60 acute leukemia cells and inhibits autophagy by affecting lysosome function." Biomedicine & Pharmacotherapy 84 (2016): 1551-1557.

125) Lu, Ying, et al. "Celecoxib suppresses autophagy and enhances cytotoxicity of imatinib in imatinib-resistant chronic myeloid leukemia cells." Journal of translational medicine 14.1 (2016): 270.

126) Tudor, Diana Valentina, et al. "COX-2 as a potential biomarker and therapeutic target in melanoma." Cancer Biology & Medicine 17.1 (2020): 20.

127) Shaashua, Lee, et al. "Perioperative COX-2 and β-adrenergic blockade improves metastatic biomarkers in breast cancer patients in a phase-II randomized trial." Clinical Cancer Research 23.16 (2017): 4651-4661.

128) Haldar, Rita, et al. "Perioperative inhibition of β-adrenergic and COX2 signaling in a clinical trial in breast cancer patients improves tumor Ki-67 expression, serum cytokine levels, and PBMCs transcriptome." Brain, behavior, and immunity 73 (2018): 294-309.

129) Xie, WanYing, et al. "βblockers inhibit the viability of breast cancer cells by regulating the ERK/COX2 signaling pathway and the drug response is affected by ADRB2 singlenucleotide polymorphisms." Oncology reports 41.1 (2019): 341-350.

130) Regulski, Miłosz, et al. "COX-2 inhibitors: a novel strategy in the management of breast cancer." Drug discovery today 21.4 (2016): 598-615.

131) Majumder, Mousumi, et al. "COX-2 induces breast cancer stem cells via EP4/PI3K/AKT/NOTCH/WNT axis." Stem Cells 34.9 (2016): 2290-2305.

132) Xu, Han, et al. "CXCR2 promotes breast cancer metastasis and chemoresistance via suppression of AKT1 and activation of COX2." Cancer letters 412 (2018): 69-80.

133) Li, Bailong, et al. "miR-221/222 promote cancer stem-like cell properties and tumor growth of breast cancer via targeting PTEN and sustained Akt/NF-κB/COX-2 activation." Chemico-biological interactions 277 (2017): 33-42.

134) Krishnamachary, Balaji, et al. "Breast cancer cell cyclooxygenase-2 expression alters extracellular matrix structure and function and numbers of cancer associated fibroblasts." Oncotarget 8.11 (2017): 17981.

135) Xu, Feng, et al. "Clinicopathological and prognostic significance of COX-2 immunohistochemical expression in breast cancer: a meta-analysis." Oncotarget 8.4 (2017): 6003.

136) Dai, Ping, et al. "Efficacy and safety of COX-2 inhibitors for advanced non-small-cell lung cancer with chemotherapy: a meta-analysis." OncoTargets and therapy 11 (2018): 721.

137) Zhou, Yuan Yuan, et al. "Clinical profile of cyclooxygenase-2 inhibitors in treating non-small cell lung cancer: a meta-analysis of nine randomized clinical trials." PloS one 11.3 (2016).

138) Ammu, VVV Ravi Kiran, et al. "Possible role of PPAR-γ and COX-2 receptor modulators in the treatment of Non-Small Cell lung carcinoma." Medical hypotheses 124 (2019): 98-100.

139) deleted

140) Gulyas, Miklos, et al. "COX-2 expression and effects of celecoxib in addition to standard chemotherapy in advanced non-small cell lung cancer." Acta Oncologica 57.2 (2018): 244-250.

141) Gallouet, Anne-Sophie, et al. "COX-2–Independent Effects of Celecoxib Sensitize Lymphoma B Cells to TRAIL-Mediated Apoptosis." Clinical Cancer Research 20.10 (2014): 2663-2673.

142) Phipps, Richard P., Elizabeth Ryan, and Steven H. Bernstein. "Inhibition of cyclooxygenase-2: a new targeted therapy for B-cell lymphoma?" (2004): 109-111.

143) Zhang, Guang-Sen, et al. "Antitumor effects of celecoxib on K562 leukemia cells are mediated by cell-cycle arrest, caspase-3 activation, and downregulation of Cox-2 expression and are synergistic with hydroxy-urea or imatinib." American journal of hematology 81.4 (2006): 242-255.

144) Han, Seong-Su, et al. "l-ascorbic acid represses constitutive activation of NF-κB and COX-2 expression in human acute myeloid leukemia, HL-60." Journal of cellular biochemistry 93.2 (2004): 257-270.

145) Cho, Soo-Jeong, et al. "The anti-cancer effect of COX-2 inhibitors on gastric cancer cells." Digestive diseases and sciences 52.7 (2007): 1713-1721.

146) Wu, Megan, et al. "Aberrantly activated Cox-2 and Wnt signaling interact to maintain cancer stem cells in glioblastoma." Oncotarget 8.47 (2017): 82217.

147) Nam, Do-Hyun, et al. "Intracranial inhibition of glioma cell growth by cyclooxygenase-2 inhibitor celecoxib." Oncology reports 11.2 (2004): 263-268.

148) Sharma, Vivek, et al. "COX-2 regulates the proliferation of glioma stem like cells." Neurochemistry international 59.5 (2011): 567-571.

149) Xu, Kaiming, Lanfang Wang, and Hui-Kuo G. Shu. "COX-2 overexpression increases malignant potential of human glioma cells through Id1." Oncotarget 5.5 (2014): 1241.

150) GroSch, Sabine, et al. "COX-2 independent induction of cell cycle arrest and apoptosis in colon cancer cells by the selective COX-2 inhibitor celecoxib." The FASEB journal 15.14 (2001): 2742-2744.

151) Barlow, Meade, et al. "Celecoxib inhibits invasion and metastasis via a cyclooxygenase 2–independent mechanism in an in vitro model of Ewing sarcoma." Journal of pediatric surgery 47.6 (2012): 1223-1227.

152) Behr, Christopher A., et al. "Celecoxib inhibits Ewing sarcoma cell migration via actin modulation." Journal of Surgical Research 198.2 (2015): 424-433.

153) Vital-Reyes, Víctor, et al. "Celecoxib inhibits cellular growth, decreases Ki-67 expression and modifies apoptosis in ovarian cancer cell lines." Archives of medical research 37.6 (2006): 689-695.

154) Suri, Anuj, et al. "The effect of celecoxib on tumor growth in ovarian cancer cells and a genetically

engineered mouse model of serous ovarian cancer." Oncotarget 7.26 (2016): 39582.

155) Thill, Marc, et al. "Vitamin D inhibits ovarian cancer cell line proliferation in combination with cele-coxib and suppresses cyclooxygenase-2 expression." Anticancer research 35.2 (2015): 1197-1203.

156) Lin, Cassie, et al. "Inducible COX-2-dependent apoptosis in human ovarian cancer cells." Carcinogenesis 32.1 (2011): 19-26.

157) Kim, Hee Jung, et al. "Synergistic effect of COX-2 inhibitor on paclitaxel-induced apoptosis in the human ovarian cancer cell line OVCAR-3." Cancer research and treatment: official journal of Korean Cancer Association 46.1 (2014): 81.

158) Li, Wei, et al. "Effects of combining Taxol and cyclooxygenase inhibitors on the angiogenesis and apoptosis in human ovarian cancer xenografts." Oncology letters 5.3 (2013): 923-928.

159) Zuo, Chaohui, et al. "Celecoxib suppresses pro-liferation and metastasis of pancreatic cancer cells by down-regulating STAT3/NF-kB and L1CAM activities." Pancreatology 18.3 (2018): 328-333.

160) Kim, Bomi, Jayoung Kim, and Yeong Seok Kim. "Celecoxib induces cell death on non-small cell lung cancer cells through endoplasmic reticulum stress." Anatomy & cell biology 50.4 (2017): 293-300.

161) Tai, Yang, et al. "Suppressing growth and invasion of human hepatocellular carcinoma cells by celecoxib through inhibition of cyclooxygenase-2." Cancer man-agement and research 11 (2019): 2831.

162) Zhou, Pingting, et al. "Autophagy inhibition enhances celecoxib-induced apoptosis in osteosar-coma." Cell Cycle 17.8 (2018): 997-1006.

Chapter 39

Diclofenac (Voltaren®) and Sulindac

Diclofenac c-MYC and GLYCOLYSIS Inhibitor

DICLOFENAC IS ANOTHER ANTI-INFLAMMATORY COX-2 inhibitor used for decades for rheumatoid and osteo-arthritis, headache, pain and febrile illness. It is another Non-Steroidal Anti-Inflammatory Drug (NSAID) Most commonly taken orally, Diclofenac may also be applied to the skin for treatment of actinic keratosis, considered a premalignant lesion. (1)

GLYCOLYSIS Inhibitor - Blocks MCT

Of all the NSAIDS, diclofenac is the most potent GLYCOLYSIS inhibitor by virtue of its blocking monocarboxylate transport (MCT), whose function is to expel lactic acid from the cancer cell into the extracellular space. This prevents acidification of the extracellular space, which is very beneficial in restoring host immune function. This also causes a buildup of lactic acid inside the cancer cell, which inhibits GLYCOLYSIS. Thus Diclofenac is not only an anti-inflammatory COX-2 inhibitor. It also serves as a potent GLYCOLYSIS inhibitor.

Decreased c-MYC expression

In 2013, Dr. Eva Gottfried studied diclofenac's effect on tumor cells, finding diminished c-MYC expression (c-Myc Oncogene), decreased glucose uptake, and lactate secretion resulting in impaired proliferation of cancer cell lines, melanoma, leukemia and carcinoma in vitro and in vivo. Diclofenac inhibits lactate formation at the low concentration of 0.1 milli molar. (2)

Note: The c-Myc oncogene activates aerobic glycolysis (Warburg Effect) and stimulates mitochondrial biogenesis, is the "master regulator" of cancer cell proliferation and metabolism. (3–5)

Dr. Gottfried writes:

A significant intracellular accumulation of lactate by diclofenac preceded the observed effect on gene expression, suggesting a direct inhibitory effect of diclofenac on lactate efflux ... Diclofenac holds potential as a clinically applicable MYC and glycolysis inhibitor supporting established tumor therapies. (2)

Glioblastoma – Diclofenac Synergy with Metformin

We have previously discussed the "metabolic plasticity" of cancer cells and their ability to switch between GLYCOLYSIS and OXPHOS. Blocking both pathways concurrently is necessary for achieving "synthetic lethality," and apoptosis in the cancer cell.

In 2018, Dr. Valeria Gerthofer studied the combination of the GLYCOLYSIS inhibitor diclofenac with the OXPHOS inhibitor metformin in a murine glioma model. Metformin alone inhibited cancer cell oxygen consumption, as expected for an OXPHOS inhibitor, and also increased extracellular lactate levels, indicating a compensatory increase in GLYCOLYSIS, a "glycolytic rescue mechanism." Diclofenac was found to be synergistic, inhibiting the efflux of lactate from the cancer cell and enhancing the anti-cancer effect. This combination also targets CSCs. Dr. Gerthofer writes:

> Metformin inhibited cellular oxygen consumption and increased extracellular lactate levels, indicating glycolytic rescue mechanisms. Combined treatment inhibited metformin-induced lactate increase. The combination of metformin and diclofenac may represent a promising new strategy in the treatment of glioblastoma. (6–9)

Note: Another similar strategy is the synergistic combination of DCA (GLYCOLYSIS inhibitor) with metformin (OXPHOS inhibitor). See Chapter 5 on DCA for more on this topic.

Synergy with Checkpoint Inhibitors

Immunotherapy with checkpoint inhibitors has revolutionized cancer treatment for the lucky few who respond. However, the problem of non-responders has motivated a search for ways to augment checkpoint inhibitor therapy. One was found in 2019 by Dr. Kathrin Renner, who combined Diclofenac with checkpoint inhibitor therapy (anti-PD-1) in a melanoma cell model, finding augmented effects via inhibition of lactate transporters MCT1 and MCT4 in a COX-independent manner. (11)

Lactate and the Immune System

Early on, researchers thought lactate was simply a waste product of the cancer cell.

Recent work shows that lactate is a sophisticated signaling agent that shuts down the host anti-tumor immune system. By blocking lactate efflux with diclofenac and other GLYCOLYSIS inhibitors such as DCA, host immune function can be restored. Dr. Renner writes:

> The non-steroidal anti-inflammatory drug [NSAID] diclofenac lowers lactate secretion of tumor cells and improves anti-PD1-induced T cell killing in vitro... Notably, T cell activation, viability, and effector functions are preserved under diclofenac treatment and in a low glucose environment in vitro... These findings support the rationale for targeting glycolysis in patients with high glycolytic tumors together with checkpoint inhibitors in clinical trials. (11)

Immunomodulatory effects of diclofenac are related to potent GLYCOLYSIS inhibition, resulting in decreased glucose uptake and efflux of lactate via significant decreases in GLUT1, LDHA and MCT1. (12–13)

Note: GLUT1 is a glucose transporter protein, LDH is lactate dehydrogenase, and MCT (monocarboxylate transporter) is a lactate transporter protein, all involved in GLYCOLYSIS.

Synergy of Diclofenac with Metformin in AML Leukemia

If metformin combined with one NSAID is good, then perhaps two NSAIDS are better. In 2018, Dr. Renner studied the synergy of combining metformin with two NSAIDs, diclofenac and diflunisal, in an acute myelogenous leukemia (AML) model, writing:

> Low concentrations of metformin and the two NSAIDs diclofenac and diflunisal exert

a synergistic inhibitory effect on AML proliferation and induce apoptosis most likely by blocking tumor cell metabolism. Our results underline the feasibility of applying anti-metabolic drugs for AML therapy. (14)

Diclofenac Plus Curcumin Synergy for Colon Cancer

In 2015, Dr. Rana found the combination of diclofenac and curcumin synergistic in a colon cancer model, with downregulation of the PI3/Akt pathway and activation of mitochondrial apoptosis. (15)

Diclofenac for Lymphoma Induces Apoptosis via P73 and P53

We have previously discussed the P53 gene, frequently dysregulated in cancer cells, as the "Guardian of the Genome." Another under-appreciated member of the P53 family is the P73 gene, which is highly conserved and rarely mutated in cancers. In this case, the ratio of two P73 isoforms determines apoptosis independent of P53. By increasing the Tap73 isoform, apoptosis can be induced.

In 2015 and 2016, Dr. Hassan did a number of studies on the modulation of p73 isoform expression in B-Cell Lymphoma (mantle cell MCL) model, finding:

> Diclofenac induced a concentration and duration dependent increase in Tap73 [apoptosis isoform], cell cycle arrest, cell death, and inhibited MCL cell growth independent of p53 status ... Diclofenac treatment was associated with increased activity of caspases 3, 7, and 8 [mitochondrial apoptosis] and induction of p53 transcriptional target genes. These studies

demonstrate the potential for diclofenac as novel therapeutic agent in MCL independent of p53 status. (16–23)

Similar to diclofenac, celecoxib also upregulates the pro-apoptotic isoform, Tap73. The two COX2 inhibitor drugs also attenuate Wnt/Beta-Catenin signaling, a CSC pathway. (24–25)

Topical Diclofenac for Actinic Keratosis (AK)

Topical diclofenac gel (Solaraze ®) is a treatment for the common brown skin lesions known as actinic keratosis (AK). Considered a premalignant lesion, AK is very common and is usually associated with areas of sun exposure on the face, upper chest, arms and hands.

In 2019, Dr. Katrin Singer et al. studied metabolic pathways and immune cell infiltration in skin biopsies of actinic keratosis lesions in 28 patients before and after 12 weeks of topical diclofenac. Most cancers have upregulated GLYCOLYSIS pathways (the Warburg Effect). Similarly, Dr. Singer's group found accelerated GLYCOLYSIS with increased lactate and decreased glucose levels in the pretreated actinic keratosis lesions. In addition, dermal T cell function was inhibited. Treatment with topical diclofenac reduced lactate levels and restored dermal cytotoxic CD8+ T cell function, a finding usually associated with a good prognosis. Dr. Singer et al. write:

> Our study clearly demonstrated that not only cancers but also premalignant skin lesions, like AK, exhibit profound changes in metabolism, correlating with an altered immune infiltrate. Diclofenac normalizes

metabolism, immune cell infiltration and function in AK lesions. (26–29)

Safety and Adverse Effects of Diclofenac

Adverse effects of NSAIDS include gastro-intestinal, renal, liver and testicular injury which may result in GI bleeding, renal failure, hepato-toxicity and hypo-gonadism with low testosterone and impaired infertility. Like all NSAID drugs, diclofenac carries an increased risk of cardiovascular disease with myocardial infarction. These adverse effects are disturbing, and suggest that diclofenac may not be suitable as a long-term maintenance program for the cancer survivor in remission. Instead, use of diclofenac and NSAIDs in general should be reserved for selected cases with active disease after carefully weighing risks vs. benefits. If NSAIDS are used, a knowledgeable health care provider should be involved to monitor renal, hepatic, and gonadal function during treatment and should halt the drug at the earliest sign of any adverse effects. (30–40)

Diclofenac for veterinary use was banned in India, Pakistan, and Nepal in 2006 after 90% of the vulture population died of renal failure after ingesting diclofenac-treated domestic livestock. The kidneys of the dead vultures showed large urate crystal aggregates obscuring the renal architecture. (33–35) In humans, the combined use of diclofenac with acetaminophen (Tylenol) in the post-operative period is especially dangerous, with added renal toxicity and acute kidney injury. (36)

Interventions Reduce Toxicity of Diclofenac

Diclofenac toxicity may be alleviated by concurrent administration of thymoquinone, montelukast (Singulair®), silymarin, propolis, and/or vinpocetine. (41–44)

To summarize, diclofenac is a potent COX-2 inhibitor anti-inflammatory drug. COX-2-independent effects include C-Myc inhibition, GLYCOLYSIS inhibition and Induction of apoptosis via modulation of P73 gene expression. Diclofenac inhibition of lactate secretion into the extracellular space restores anti-tumor immune function, synergizing with other immune therapies such as checkpoint inhibitors drugs. Diclofenac as GLYCOLYSIS inhibitor has synergy with OXPHOS inhibitors such as metformin. Diclofenac's disturbing adverse side effects require the exercise of careful thought as to risks vs. benefits, and careful patient monitoring.

Other NSAIDS – Sulindac

In the past five years, there has been renewed interest in the combination use of NSAID COX-2 inhibitors with other anti-cancer agents. Tumors frequently show high expression of COX-2, which in turn upregulates the expression of BCL-2 (the anti-apoptotic protein), immortalizing the cancer cell by preventing apoptosis. In addition, the COX-2 inflammatory protein induces neovascularization and provides for tumor survival and proliferation. COX-2 also upregulates matrix metallo-proteinase (MMP), which promotes tumor invasion and metastatic spread. NSAIDS that inhibit COX-2 block all of these pro-tumorigenic effects. This includes downregulating epithelial growth factor (EGFR) expression.

Antiplatelet Drugs

In 2018, Dr. Zhen Zhang et al. suggested that the combination of a COX-2 inhibitor with anti-platelet drugs would be synergistic. (45–48)

In 2017, Dr. Rachidi et al. write:

> We conclude that platelets constrain T cell immunity though a GARP-TGFβ axis and suggest a combination of immunotherapy and platelet inhibitors as a therapeutic strategy against cancer. (46)

T-cell function, anti-cancer immunity, and various T cell therapies can be improved by the addition of antiplatelet agents. We discuss dipyridamole antiplatelet drugs in the next chapter. (49)

Sulindac and EGFR inhibitor for FAP

The NSAID, Sulindac, is a nonspecific COX inhibitor. Its metabolite, sulindac sulfide is a 5-LOX inhibitor. (70)

Sulindac clinical trials shows significant reduction in colonic polyps in familial adenomatous polyposis FAP. The usual treatment for FAP is surgical removal of the colon. However, these patients remain at risk for duodenal polyps, considered premalignant for duodenal cancer. Sulindac, combined with the EGFR inhibitor erlotinib, has been found successful in reducing both colonic polyps and duodenal polyp formation in FAP. (50–55)

Sulindac Binds to VDAC and Inhibits mTOR

Sulindac stands out from the other NSAIDS by its ability to target the voltage-dependent anion channel (VDAC) on the outer mitochondrial membrane. We have discussed Hexokinase II attached to the VDAC in previous chapters as an "Achilles heel" of the cancer cell.

In 2018, Dr. Yuichi Aono et al. studied the molecular targets of sulindac in a colorectal cancer model, finding sulindac sulfone directly binds to the VDAC, downregulating its function. This results in suppression of the mTOR pathway, reduction of cyclin D1, and arrested cell proliferation. (56)

Sulindac Synergy

A number of investigators found synergy of sulindac with DCA, mebendazole, vitamin C, and resveratrol (pterostilbene). (57–60)

Sulindac as Cancer Stem Cell Agent

In 2019, Dr. F. Hossain et al. found sulindac targets breast CSCs as a Notch inhibitor (a CSC pathway). (61) Sulindac also serves as an immune modulator in breast cancer models. (62–65) In addition, Sulindac suppresses Beta-Catenin expression, a major signaling protein for the Wnt pathway, a CSC pathway. (66–68)

Sulindac – Adverse Side Effects

Although considered to be safer than other NSAIDS with fewer adverse side effects, sulindac like all NSAIDs, can be associated with gastrointestinal bleeding, made worse by simultaneous alcohol or corticosteroid use. As with other NSAIDS, sulindac may also induce renal toxicity, hepatotoxicity, and Stevens-Johnson syndrome. Caution is advised. (60)

References for Chapter 39: Diclofenac, Sulindac

1) Pantziarka, Pan, et al. "Repurposing Drugs in Oncology (ReDO)—diclofenac as an anti-cancer agent." Ecancermedicalscience 10 (2016).

2) Gottfried, Eva, et al. "New aspects of an old drug—diclofenac targets MYC and glucose metabolism in tumor cells." PloS one 8.7 (2013).

3) Miller, Donald M., et al. "c-Myc and cancer metabolism." (2012): 5546-5553.

4) He, Tian-Lin, et al. "The c-Myc–LDHA axis positively regulates aerobic glycolysis and promotes tumor progression in pancreatic cancer." Medical Oncology 32.7 (2015): 187

5) Jose, Caroline, Nadège Bellance, and Rodrigue Rossignol. "Choosing between glycolysis and oxidative phosphorylation: a tumor's dilemma?" Biochimica et Biophysica Acta (BBA)-Bioenergetics 1807.6 (2011): 552-561.

6) Gerthofer, Valeria, et al. "Combined modulation of tumor metabolism by metformin and diclofenac in glioma." International journal of molecular sciences 19.9 (2018): 2586.

7) Duan, Ke, et al. "Lactic acid induces lactate transport and glycolysis/OXPHOS interconversion in glioblastoma." Biochemical and biophysical research communications 503.2 (2018): 888-894.

8) Chirasani, Sridhar R., et al. "Diclofenac inhibits lactate formation and efficiently counteracts local immune suppression in a murine glioma model." International journal of cancer 132.4 (2013): 843-853.

9) Tateishi, Kensuke, et al. "Myc-driven glycolysis is a therapeutic target in glioblastoma." Clinical Cancer Research 22.17 (2016): 4452-4465.

10) deleted

11) Renner, Kathrin, et al. "Restricting glycolysis preserves T Cell effector functions and augments checkpoint therapy." Cell Reports 29.1 (2019): 135-150.

12) Lacroix, Ruben, et al. "Targeting tumor-associated acidity in cancer immunotherapy." Cancer Immunology, Immunotherapy 67.9 (2018): 1331-1348.

13) Santos, Nuno, et al. "Lactate as a Regulator of Cancer Inflammation and Immunity." Immunometabolism 1.2 (2019).

14) Renner, Kathrin, et al. "Combined metabolic targeting with metformin and the NSAIDs diflunisal and diclofenac induces apoptosis in acute myeloid leukemia cells." Frontiers in pharmacology 9 (2018): 1258.

15) Rana, Chandan, et al. "Downregulation of PI3-K/Akt/PTEN pathway and activation of mitochondrial intrinsic apoptosis by Diclofenac and Curcumin in colon cancer." Molecular and cellular biochemistry 402.1-2 (2015): 225-241.

16) Hassan, Hesham M., et al. "Modulation of p73 isoforms expression induces anti-proliferative and pro-apoptotic activity in mantle cell lymphoma independent of p53 status." Leukemia & lymphoma 57.12 (2016): 2874-2889.

17) Hassan, Hesham M., et al. "The COX inhibitor, diclofenac induces mantle cell lymphoma apoptosis independent of p53 status." (2015): 2632-2632.

18) Hassan, Hesham, et al. "Diclofenac Induces Apoptosis and Suppresses Diffuse Large B-Cell Lymphoma Proliferation Independent of P53 Status." (2014): 5485-5485.

19) Hassan, H. M., Bhavana J. Dave, and Rakesh K. Singh. "TP73, an under-appreciated player in non-Hodgkin lymphoma pathogenesis and management." Current molecular medicine 14.4 (2014): 432-439.

20) Hassan, Hesham M., et al. "Cycloxygenase-2 inhibitor regulates p73 isoform expression pattern, inhibit growth, and induce apoptosis in NHL cell line model with 1p36 chromosomal disruption." (2013): 4353-4353.

21) Bae, Woo-Kyun, et al. "TAp73 inhibits cell invasion and migration by directly activating KAI1 expression in colorectal carcinoma." Cancer letters 415 (2018): 106-116.

22) Galtsidis, Sotiris, et al. "Unravelling a p73-regulated network: The role of a novel p73-dependent target, MIR3158, in cancer cell migration and invasiveness." Cancer letters 388 (2017): 96-106.

23) Lau, L. M. S., et al. "Cyclooxygenase inhibitors differentially modulate p73 isoforms in neuroblastoma." Oncogene 28.19 (2009): 2024-2033.

24) Sooriakumaran, P., et al. "A gene expression profiling approach assessing celecoxib in a randomized controlled trial in prostate cancer." Cancer Genomics-Proteomics 6.2 (2009): 93-99.

25) Sareddy, Gangadhara Reddy, et al. "Nonsteroidal anti-inflammatory drugs diclofenac and celecoxib attenuates Wnt/β-catenin/Tcf signaling pathway in human glioblastoma cells." Neurochemical research 38.11 (2013): 2313-2322.

26) Singer, Katrin, et al. "Topical diclofenac reprograms metabolism and immune cell infiltration in actinic keratosis." Frontiers in Oncology 9 (2019): 605.

27) Nelson, Christopher G. "Diclofenac gel in the treatment of actinic keratoses." Therapeutics and clinical risk management 7 (2011): 207.

28) de Oliveira, Erika CV, et al. "Actinic keratosis–review for clinical practice." International journal of dermatology 58.4 (2019): 400-407.

29) da Veiga Moreira, Jorgelindo, et al. "Metabolic therapies inhibit tumor growth in vivo and in silico." Scientific reports 9.1 (2019): 1-10.

30) Luo, Yuehui, and Mei Wang. "Nephrotic Syndrome and Acute Tubular Necrosis and Interstitial Nephritis Associated with Diclofenac." J Clin Nephrol Res 5.1 (2018): 1083.

31) Babladi, Vanishree Prakash, et al. "A Case Report on Diclofenac Induced Chronic Kidney." Indian Journal of Pharmacy Practice 12.2 (2019): 129.

32) Alkuraishy, Hayder M., Ali I. Al-Gareeb, and Nawar Raad Hussien. "Diclofenac induced-acute kidney injury is linked with oxidative stress and pro-inflammatory changes in Sprague Dawley rats." Journal of Contemporary Medical Sciences 5.3 (2019).

33) Nambirajan, Kanthan, et al. "Residues of diclofenac in tissues of vultures in India: a post-ban scenario." Archives of environmental contamination and toxicology 74.2 (2018): 292-297.

34) Shultz, Susanne, et al. "Diclofenac poisoning is widespread in declining vulture populations across the Indian subcontinent." Proceedings of the Royal Society of London. Series B: Biological Sciences 271.suppl_6 (2004): S458-S460.

35) Meteyer, Carol Uphoff, et al. "Pathology and proposed pathophysiology of diclofenac poisoning in free-living and experimentally exposed oriental white-backed vultures (Gyps bengalensis)." Journal of Wildlife Diseases 41.4 (2005): 707-716.

36) Zhu, Yan, et al. "Diclofenac—Acetaminophen combination induced acute kidney injury in postoperative pain relief." Journal of Pharmacy & Pharmaceutical Sciences 21 (2018): 19-26.

37) Lee, Eun-Hee, et al. "Immunogenomics reveal molecular circuits of diclofenac induced liver injury in mice." Oncotarget 7.12 (2016): 14983.

38) Mousa, Ahmed Abdelmoniem, et al. "Eucalyptus Globulus protects against diclofenac sodium induced hepatorenal and testicular toxicity in male rats." Journal of Traditional and Complementary Medicine (2019).

39) Al-Nahi, Alaa Shakir, and Afyaa Sabah Nasir. "Histopathological Changes in Testis Tissue Induced by Different Doses of Diclofenac Sodium in the Male Rats." Indian Journal of Public Health Research & Development 10.2 (2019): 849-853.

40) Schmidt, Morten, Henrik Toft Sørensen, and Lars Pedersen. "Diclofenac use and cardiovascular risks: series of nationwide cohort studies." bmj 362 (2018): k3426.

41) Aycan, İlker Öngüç, et al. "Diclofenac induced gastrointestinal and renal toxicity is alleviated by thymoquinone treatment." Food and Chemical Toxicology 118 (2018): 795-804.

42) Sahib, Hussein A., Ahmed M. Sultan, and Hussam H. Sahib. "Protective effect of montelukast against acute kidney injury in rats induced by diclofenac." Journal of Pharmaceutical Sciences and Research 10.9 (2018): 2415-2418.

43) Amin, Kamal Adel, et al. "Renoprotective and antioxidant effect of silymarin and propolis on diclofenac

sodium induced renal toxicity in rats." International Journal of Pure and Applied Biosciences 5.2 (2017): 31-42.

44) Fattori, Victor, et al. "Vinpocetine reduces diclofenac-induced acute kidney injury through inhibition of oxidative stress, apoptosis, cytokine production, and NF-κB activation in mice." Pharmacological research 120 (2017): 10-22.

45) Zhang, Zhen, Fulin Chen, and Lijun Shang. "Advances in antitumor effects of NSAIDs." Cancer management and research 10 (2018): 4631.

46) Rachidi, Saleh, et al. "Platelets subvert T cell immunity against cancer via GARP-TGFβ axis." Science immunology 2.11 (2017).

47) Zappavigna, Silvia, et al. "Anti-Inflammatory Drugs as Anticancer Agents." International Journal of Molecular Sciences 21.7 (2020): 2605.

48) Wong, Rebecca SY. "Role of nonsteroidal anti-inflammatory drugs (NSAIDs) in cancer prevention and cancer promotion." Advances in pharmacological sciences 2019 (2019).

49) Murphy, J. "Anti-cancer therapy: non-steroidal anti-inflammatory drugs (NSAIDS) in combination with immunotherapy." MOJ Immunol 5.3 (2017): 00156.

50) Labayle, Denis, et al. "Sulindac causes regression of rectal polyps in familial adenomatous polyposis." Gastroenterology 101.3 (1991): 635-639.

51) Cruz–Correa, Marcia, et al. "Long-term treatment with sulindac in familial adenomatous polyposis: a prospective cohort study." Gastroenterology 122.3 (2002): 641-645.

52) Lawrence, Leah. "Polyp Burden Drops With Sulindac/Erlotinib Combo in FAP." ONCOLOGY 34.5 (2020).

53) Ulusan, Ahmetmursel, et al. "Optimizing erlotinib plus sulindac dosing regimens in a preclinical model of FAP." (2019): 5074-5074.

54) Delker, Don A., et al. "Chemoprevention with cyclooxygenase and epidermal growth factor receptor inhibitors in familial adenomatous polyposis patients: mRNA signatures of duodenal neoplasia." Cancer Prevention Research 11.1 (2018): 4-15.

55) Samadder, N. Jewel, et al. "Effect of COX and EGFR Inhibition on Colorectal Neoplasia in Familial Adenomatous Polyposis: A Randomized Placebo Controlled Trial." Gastroenterology 152.5 (2017): S140.

56) Aono, Yuichi, et al. "Sulindac sulfone inhibits the mTORC1 pathway in colon cancer cells by directly targeting voltage-dependent anion channel 1 and 2." Biochemical and biophysical research communications 505.4 (2018): 1203-1210.

57) Ayyanathan, Kasirajan, et al. "Combination of sulindac and dichloroacetate kills cancer cells via oxidative damage." PloS one 7.7 (2012).

58) Gong, Eun-Yeung, et al. "Combined treatment with vitamin C and sulindac synergistically induces p53-and ROS-dependent apoptosis in human colon cancer cells." Toxicology letters 258 (2016): 126-133.

59) Williamson, Tara, et al. "Mebendazole and a non-steroidal anti-inflammatory combine to reduce tumor initiation in a colon cancer preclinical model." Oncotarget 7.42 (2016): 68571.

60) Pouyafar, Ayda, et al. "Treatment of cancer stem cells from human colon adenocarcinoma cell line HT-29 with resveratrol and sulindac induced mesenchymal-endothelial transition rate." Cell and tissue research 376.3 (2019): 377-388.

61) Hossain, F., et al. "Abstract P6-22-01: Repurposing sulindac sulfide as a notch inhibitor to target cancer stem-like cells in triple negative breast cancer." (2019): P6-22.

62) Hossain, Fokhrul, et al. "Abstract P5-04-19: Sulindac sulfide as a non-immune suppressive gamma secretase modifier to target triple negative breast cancer." (2020): P5-04.

63) Yin, Tao, et al. "Sulindac, a non-steroidal anti-inflammatory drug, mediates breast cancer inhibition as an immune modulator." Scientific reports 6 (2016): 19534.

64) McDonell, Shannon B., et al. "Sulindac reverses an immunosuppressive tumor microenvironment associated with obesity-driven metastatic mammary tumors in mice." (2019): 2815-2815.

65) Sui, He-Huan, et al. "Effects of sulindac sulfide on proliferation and apoptosis of human breast cancer cell." Oncology letters 15.5 (2018): 7981-7986.

66) Lee, Kevin J., et al. "Novel non-COX inhibitory sulindac derivative with β-catenin suppressing activity reduces the formation of colorectal adenomas and adenocarcinomas in the APC+/min-FCCC mouse model." (2017): 5243-5243.

67) Han, Anjia, et al. "Sulindac suppresses β-catenin expression in human cancer cells." European journal of pharmacology 583.1 (2008): 26-31.

68) Yi, Zhang, et al. "Effects of Nonsteroidal Anti-inflammatory Drugs on the Self-renewal Capacity of Blast Progenitors in Hematological Malignancies." Anticancer research 37.5 (2017): 2315-2322

69) Munjal, Akul, and Roopma Wadhwa. "Sulindac." StatPearls [Internet]. StatPearls Publishing, 2020.

70) Steinbrink, Svenja D., et al. "Sulindac sulfide suppresses 5-lipoxygenase at clinically relevant concentrations." Cellular and molecular life sciences 67.5 (2010): 797-806.

Chapter 40

Dipyridamole and Statin Drugs

Errors in Oncology-Ignoring the Role of Platelets

IF WE CUT OUR SKIN, we bleed. Platelets help to stop the bleeding by aggregating into blood clots. This is a good thing. However, it is not a good thing when platelets are recruited by cancer cells to evade the immune system, induce new blood vessels (angiogenesis), and assist cancer cell migration to distant sites, forming metastatic tumors. The circulating tumor cells cloak themselves with a layer of adherent platelets, insulating themselves from the host immune system. (1–2). In 2017, Dr. Omar Elaskalani et al. write:

> Cancer cell adhesion to platelets is vital for successful metastasis…. within the blood circulation, platelet-cloaked tumour cells can bypass natural killer cell-mediated cytotoxicity. (2)

In chapter 13, we discussed aspirin as an antiplatelet and anti-cancer drug. Here, we discuss dipyridamole (Persantine®), an old drug with a long history of safe use as a platelet inhibitor. Dipyridamole (DP) is an anti-platelet drug, a phosphodiesterase inhibitor that prevents blood clots, stroke, and heart attack by preventing platelet adhesion and activation. As you might expect, bleeding is the main adverse effect of antiplatelet drugs such as aspirin and dipyridamole.

The Role of Platelets in Cancer and Regenerative Medicine

Platelets are the "first responders" to an area of tissue injury. Tissue injury causes the platelets to stick together and form blood clots rich in fibrin, growth factors, and cytokines such as PDGF, VEGF, TGF-Beta, etc. that are fundamentally involved in repair and regeneration of injured tissues. (3)

Note: PDGF= platelet-derived growth factor, VEGF= vascular endothelial growth factor, TGF = transforming growth factor.

PRP: Platelet-Rich Plasma for Sports Injuries

Revolutionizing the field of sports medicine and orthopedics is the injection of platelet-rich plasma (PRP) into tendons and joints. This is a highly effective treatment for all types of sports injuries, degenerative joint disease (DJD), wounds, and tissue injuries. PRP induces rapid healing which, in many cases, avoids the use of reparative surgery.

Unfortunately, this healing role of platelets can be subverted by cancer. Platelets are instrumental in cancer growth and proliferation, sticking to cancer cells where they secrete growth factors and other biologically active compounds. Thus, platelets are the "good guys" for the patient with a sports injury. However, platelets are the "bad guys" for the cancer patient, because they facilitate tumor growth, progression, and metastatic disease. (4–7)

Thrombocytosis and Cancer

Over one hundred years ago, it was discovered cancer patients commonly exhibit elevated platelet counts—over 400,000 on the automated blood count test (CBC). This condition, called thrombocytosis, is associated with poor prognosis and reduced survival. About 40% of patients screened for thrombocytosis will harbor underlying malignancy. (8–9)

Platelets have a 7-day half-life and are produced by megakaryocytes in massive quantities. Platelet production by the bone marrow is increased by secretion of IL-6 by cancer cells, which stimulate the liver to produce thrombopoietin (TPO), thereby stimulating megakaryopoiesis and thrombocytosis. In 2018, Dr. Monika Haemmerle et al. write:

> We discovered that in ovarian cancer, tumor-derived interleukin 6 [IL-6] stimulated thrombopoietin [TPO] production by the liver, thereby stimulating megakaryopoiesis and thrombocytosis.... Platelets are … functional players in primary tumor growth and in all steps of the metastatic process. They infiltrate into the tumor micro-environment to directly interact with cancer cells. In the circulation, platelets protect CTCs [Circulating Tumor Cells] from the deadly attack of the immune system and other pro-apoptotic stimuli. (10)

No Man is an Island—Platelet Satellitism

If it is true that "no man is an island," the same can be said about the cancer cell. It cannot exist by itself. Not only do platelets interact with cancer cells in the tumor micro-environment (TME) to assist in growth and metastatic spread, platelets also interact with circulating tumor cells in the bloodstream. This is where platelets play the role demonstrated on routine blood smears as "platelet satellitism" in hematologic cancers, such as B-cell lymphoma. Visible on blood smear slides under the microscope, the pathologist observes platelets adhering around the cancer cell as "satellites." (10–13)

Anti-Cancer Benefits of Dipyridamole

Over the years, observational studies of patients on long-term dipyridamole (DP) have revealed striking benefits for prevention and treatment of various cancers.

Dipyridamole for Melanoma Patients

One of the first reports of DP in cancer treatment was published (1985) in *Lancet* by Dr. E. L. Rhodes et al., who treated thirty melanoma patients over 11 years with DP, 300 mg a day. Of the thirty patients, 26 had distant metastatic disease at the beginning of treatment. This group enjoyed a 77%, 5-year survival on dipyridamole compared to the more dismal 20–30% survival for others not taking the drug. (14)

Breast Cancer Patients

A 2013 study by Dr. Daniela Spano et al. showed that DP prevents progression of triple-negative breast cancer in a mouse xenograft model.

> Low dose dipyridamole significantly reduced primary tumor growth and metas-

tasis ... while high dose resulted in an almost a total reduction in primary tumor ... Dipyridamole had significant effects on Wnt, ERK1/2-MAPK and NF-kB pathways in both animal models. Moreover, dipyridamole significantly decreased the infiltration of tumor-associated macrophages and myeloid-derived suppressor cells in primary tumors (p < 0.005), and the inflammatory cytokines. (15)

Note: see glossary for definition of Wnt, ERK/MAPK and NF-kB pathways, which are major cancer cell pathways.

In 2013, Dr. Chunmei Wang used a transgenic mouse model to study breast cancer, showing dipyridamole was preventive for primary tumors and metastatic lesions, such as bone metastases. (16)

Adjunct to Chemotherapy

In 2016, Dr. Ge reported that dipyridamole is a useful adjunct to the chemotherapy drugs 5-fluorouracil, methotrexate, piperidine, and vincristine by increasing drug concentration in the cancer cells.

Dipyridamole Mechanism of Action

Dipyridamole (DP) inhibits cellular uptake of adenosine and inhibits the phosphodiesterase enzymes (PDE) that normally break down cAMP, thus increasing cellular cAMP levels, which prevents platelet activation. Other effects include inhibition of smooth muscle proliferation and lowering of pressure in pulmonary hypertension. Dr. Shu-Min Ge et al. write:

It was well known that dipyridamole inhibits the phosphodiesterase enzymes

that normally break down cAMP, increasing cellular cAMP levels and blocking the platelet response to ADP.... Dipyridamole inhibits the cellular reuptake of adenosine into platelets, red blood cells and endothelial cells leading to increased extracellular concentrations of adenosine ... In addition, dipyridamole has been shown to lower pulmonary hypertension without significant drop of systemic blood pressure ... It inhibits proliferation of smooth muscle cells in vivo. (17)

Platelet-Derived Growth Factor (PDGF) and Angiogenesis

Cancer cells use PDGF to induce new vessel formation, a process called angiogenesis. Blocking receptors for PDGF in pericytes (cells lining the blood vessels) results in loss of neovascular growth needed to sustain tumor growth in lymphoma. A new oncology drug called Gleevec® (imatinib), FDA-approved for treatment of chronic lymphocytic leukemia (CLL) is a blocker of PDGF receptors and a potent angiogenesis inhibitor in a lymphoma xenograft animal model. (18–19)

Blocking Platelet-Derived Growth Factor with Gleevec

In 2012, Dr. Daniela Laimer et al. studied anaplastic large cell lymphoma in transgenic mice and in a human case report, finding a dramatic response to blocking PDGF receptors (PDGFR) with imatinib, with rapid, sustained remission:

Therapeutic inhibition of PDGFRB [with Gleevec – imatinib], markedly prolonged survival of NPM-ALK [lymphoma] transgenic mice and increased the efficacy of an ALK-specific inhibitor in transplanted NPM-ALK tumors. Notably, inhibition of PDGFRA and PDGFRB in a patient with refractory late-stage NPM-ALK(+) ALCL resulted in rapid, complete and sustained remission. (20)

Note: PDGFR = Platelet-Derived Growth Factor Receptor A and B. NPM-ALK is a specific chromosomal translocation which produces lymphoma.

Dipyridamole Decreases Platelet Release of PDGF

According to Dr. Takehara, who studied the effect of dipyridamole on platelets in 1987 and 1990:

> Dipyridamole specifically decreases platelet-derived growth factor [PDGF] release from platelets....and decrease its serum concentration. (21–22)

This effect is not seen for other platelet inhibitors, such as aspirin, trapidil, or ticlopidine. One might therefore expect DP to have a similar therapeutic effect when compared to imatinib, as they both block PDGF, preventing angiogenesis.

Histamine as Autocrine Growth Factor

Histamine, an intracellular messenger that promotes platelet aggregation, is also an autocrine growth factor for cancer, and histamine antagonists have anti-cancer effects. (23–27)

In 1995, Dr. Cricco studied histamine as a growth factor for breast cancer in a mouse model, concluding:

> In an animal model of experimental breast carcinomas, endogenous histamine was

critical for cell proliferation.... A major effect of histamine is stimulation of cancer cell growth by activating H2 membrane receptors on the cancer cell. (28)

Histamine is discussed in more detail in chapter 28 on cimetidine as anti-cancer, histamine-blocking drug. Loratidine is also an antihistamine, discussed in chapter 33.

Platelets Involved in Metastatic Spread and Immune Evasion

Platelets play an essential role in dissemination of cancer cells to distant sites (called metastatic disease), and in cancer-cell immune evasion by impeding the anti-cancer activity of killer T cells. (29–32)

Dipyridamole inhibits these platelet activities, and has anti-inflammatory effects, inhibiting COX-2, an inflammatory pathway frequently upregulated in cancer cells. (33)

Dipyridamole Prevents Platelet Activation

Upon platelet activation, granules containing growth factors such as VEGF, PDRF and TGF (transforming growth factor beta 1) are released into the tumor micro-environment, feeding and stimulating cancer cells. Dipyridamole blocks platelet activation by increasing cAMP (cyclic AMP) inside platelets, thus blocking release of growth factors. (2)(34)

In 2017, Dr. Omar Elaskalani et al. write:

> Platelets are the major storage site for TGFβ1 [transforming growth factor beta 1] within the blood circulation, which is released from α-granules [platelet-derived granules] upon activation.... platelet-de-

rived TGFβ1 … induce(s) a phenotypic conversion in cancer cells, from epithelial to mesenchymal-like cells [EMT], capable of invading extracellular matrices, migrating and surviving in the blood circulation … Soluble platelet-derived factors [mainly TGFβ1] and direct physical contact with tumour cells activating NF-κB pathway work synergistically to induce EMT and subsequent migration and metastasis. (2)

Platelet-Derived TGF-Beta Is an Immune Modulator

In 2018, Dr. Min Soon Cho et al. studied a murine model of ovarian cancer, finding that platelet inhibition restores anti-tumor immune response and could be used as adjunct to checkpoint inhibitors and other immunotherapies. (36)

Dipyridamole prevents metastasis in these cancer cell models:

- Pancreatic cancer with metastasis to liver (35)
- Ovarian cancer (36)

DP—More on Mechanism of Action

Dipyridamole (DP) inhibits the uptake of adenosine by red blood cells by greater than 90 per cent and increases plasma levels of adenosine by 60 percent. DP inhibits phosphodiesterase, which prevents adenosine degradation, thus increasing intracellular adenosine and cyclic AMP (cAMP) levels in platelets. This prevents platelet activation and aggregation. Thus, DP is useful in preventing thrombotic disease, stroke, and deep venous thrombosis. DP is a phosphodiesterase inhibitor (PDE5 and PDE6),

in the same family as theophylline, caffeine, and Viagra-type drugs used for erectile dysfunction. DP relaxes smooth muscle and is a vasodilator. DP has anti-inflammatory effects by inhibiting lymphocyte recruitment and preventing secretion of inflammatory cytokines. (37–38)

Nine-Fold Upregulated Phosphodiesterase in Lymphoma

In 2011, Dr. Lingzhi Zhang et al. studied 85 patients with CLL and compared them to 35 normal controls, finding greater than 9-fold elevation in phosphodiesterase 7B messenger RNA (PDE7B mRNA) expression in the top quartile of CLL patients, which predicted more aggressive disease with shorter time to treatment (36 months vs. 77 months). (39)

In 2013, Dr. Cheng Fang et al. found higher expression of phosphodiesterase messenger RNA (PDE7B), indicating poor prognosis in B-cell lymphoma. (40)

In 2016, Drs. Jeffrey Ricardo and Aguiar Cooney studied phosphodiesterase (PDE4 type 4) inhibitors in B-cell lymphoma, finding that PDE4 inhibition downregulates the B-cell receptor related kinase (similar to the kinase inhibitor drug ibrutinib), the PI-3K pathway, and VEGF, inducing apoptosis and blocking angiogenesis. In lymphoma cells, cAMP is inhibitory. PDE abrogates this effect by converting cAMP to inactive AMP, allowing higher PI3K/AKT-driven VEGF expression in the lymphoma cell. Thus, PDE inhibition with dipyridamole increases Cyclic AMP inside the lymphoma cell, which induces cell death. (41–47)

Other Phosphodiesterases as Anti-Cancer Drugs

Second-generation phosphodiesterase inhibitors (PDEs) have been developed for nine of the eleven families of phosphodiesterases. PDE5 inhibitors sildenafil (Viagra®), vardenafil (Levitra®) and tadalafil (Cialis®) are very effective for erectile dysfunction and pulmonary hypertension (ED). Recently, these same PDE5 drugs have been repurposed as anti-cancer agents. (48–49)

In 2003, Dr. Sarfati demonstrated that phosphodiesterase types including PDE4, PDE5, and PDE6, induce caspase-dependent apoptosis in B-Cell CLL in vitro. Levitra ® was the most effective at lower concentrations.

Note: "caspase dependent" means involving the mitochondrial apoptosis mechanism.

Dr. Marika Sarfati et al. reported a patient with CLL who, upon treatment for erectile dysfunction with sildenafil 50 mg per week, showed significant clinical improvement in his CLL. (49–50)

Dipyridamole with Chemotherapy

In 2010, Dr. Y. J. Jiang et al. observed that DP is beneficial in lymphoma patients by preventing platelet activation during chemotherapy. Dr. Jiang and colleagues write:

> It is concluded that the patients with malignant lymphoma usually accompany with platelet activation and hyperfibrinogenemia in peripheral blood. Applying dipyridamole routine dosage in chemotherapy can efficiently restrain platelet activation. (51)

DP—Synergy with Chemotherapy

Dipyridamole (DP) synergy combined with imatinib (Gleevac®), bortezomib, and chemotherapy drugs, vincristine, etoposide, and 5FU has been demonstrated. (52–57)

DP as an Autophagy Inhibitor

Throughout this book, we have discussed autophagy as one of the three pillars of cancer-cell metabolism, and the benefits of blocking all three pillars concurrently. In 2019, Dr. Marcos Thomé et al. studied DP's effect on autophagy flux in prostate cancer cells, finding increased intracellular cAMP (cyclic AMP) levels induced by DP blocks autophagic flux resulting in increased number of autophagosomes and autolysosomes accumulating in the cancer cells. Dr. Thomé and colleagues found DP as autophagy inhibitor synergizes with chemotherapy, writing:

> Treatment with DP presented antiproliferative effects in vitro alone and in combination with chemotherapy drugs. Collectively, these data demonstrate that DP can impair autophagic degradation, by preventing the normal autophagosome maturation, and might be useful in combination anti-cancer therapy. (58)

Natural PDE4 Inhibitors—Pterostilbene

A methylated resveratrol derivative, pterostilbene, a nontoxic anti-cancer agent obtained from blueberries, was discussed in chapter 16. Resveratrol and pterostilbene are also PDE4 inhibitors. (59)

DP Neuroprotective Effects

A number of investigators have shown DP has neuroprotective effects. (60–63)

Platelets Inhibit Anti-Cancer Immunity

In 2017, Dr. Saleh Rachidi et al. showed that platelets are the main culprits for impairing anti-cancer T cell immunity and that platelet inhibition is beneficial in restoring T cell function and anti-cancer immunity and synergizing with immunotherapies. Dr. Rachidi's group writes:

> Transforming growth factor β [TGFβ] and lactate [are] the major platelet-derived soluble factors to obliterate CD4+ and CD8+ T cell functions [anti-cancer immunity] … platelets are the dominant source of functional TGFβ systemically as well as in the tumor micro-environment through constitutive expression of TGFβ-docking receptor Glycoprotein A Repetitions Predominant (GARP) … T cell therapy of cancer can be substantially improved by concurrent treatment with … antiplatelet agents. We conclude that platelets constrain T cell immunity though a GARP-TGFβ axis and suggest a combination of immunotherapy and platelet inhibitors as a therapeutic strategy against cancer. (64–66)

DP Antiviral Effects

Repurposing dipyridamole (DP) as an antiviral drug has been suggested, based on studies showing antiviral effects. (68–69)

Investigators have shown that DP:

- Inhibits reactivation of Herpes Simplex (70–71)
- Prevents Epstein Barr Reactivation (72)
- Is active against Influenza A (73)
- Inhibits Vaccinia replication (74)
- Is active against Rhinovirus (75)
- Is potentially therapeutic in Covid-19 (76)

Aspirin as Antiplatelet Agent

In chapter 13, we briefly discussed aspirin's antiplatelet activities, revisited here. (77–80)

In 2017, Dr. L. M. Lichtenberger et al. studied the effects of aspirin in a mouse model of colon cancer in vitro and in vivo, finding that aspirin's ability to irreversibly inhibit COX-1 mediated platelet activation confers its remarkable anti-cancer efficacy. (77)

Similarly, in 2019, Dr. Serena Lucotti et al. studied the effect of aspirin for preventing lung metastasis in a mouse model of melanoma, finding inhibition of COX-1 derived thromboxane A2 (TXA2). They write:

> Inhibition of the COX-1/TXA2 pathway in platelets decreased aggregation of platelets on tumor cells, endothelial activation, tumor cell adhesion to the endothelium, and recruitment of metastasis-promoting monocytes/macrophages, and diminished the formation of a premetastatic niche. (78–80)

Synergy of Statins with Dipyridamole— Statin Pleotropic Effects

Although statins were developed as cholesterol-reducing drugs, it was later discovered that they have pleiotropic effects, meaning anti-inflammatory, antimicrobial, and anti-cancer effects. Statins inhibit NF-kB activation and prevent release of inflammatory cytokines, such as IL-6, which are typically hijacked by cancer cells to stimulate growth and proliferation. Statins kill bacteria and may serve as novel antimicrobial agents. (81–83)

Statins Inhibit Feedback Loop

Statin drugs block the mevalonate pathway by inhibiting HMG-CoA reductase, the rate-limiting enzyme. However, upon inhibition, this pathway undergoes compensatory upregulation as a feedback loop. Dipyridamole inhibits this "feedback loop" by preventing upregulation of the mevalonate pathway to compensate for statin inhibition. In 2014, Dr. Aleksandra Pandyra et al. studied dipyridamole and atorvastatin synergy in AML (acute myelogenous leukemia) and in MM (multiple myeloma), finding that there is an augmented effect when the two are used together. Dr. Pandyra et al. write:

> Statins block HMG-CoA reductase [HMGCR], the rate-limiting enzyme of the mevalonate [MVA] pathway. Dipyridamole blunted the feedback response, which upregulates HMGCR and HMG-CoA synthase 1 following statin treatment. We further show that dipyridamole inhibited the cleavage of the transcription factor required for this feedback regulation... simultaneously targeting the MVA pathway and its restorative feedback loop **is preclinically effective against hematologic malignancies.** (84)

Simvastatin Inhibits Actin Polymerization

Blocking the mevalonate pathway with a statin drug blocks the Rho protein, thus inhibiting actin polymerization that is fundamental for the actin filament system. Actin filaments are the contractile elements in muscle cells. This inhibition of actin filaments in muscle cells is thought to cause muscle pain, a commonly reported statin-drug adverse effect.

Inhibiting Actin Filaments in Cancer cells

In cancer cells, the actin filament system makes up the cytoskeleton that regulates movement, migration, and cell adhesion via "filopodia, lamellipodia and invadopodia" formation—pod-like extensions of the cell body. Statin drugs destabilize the cytoskeleton of the cancer cells. In 2017, Dr. Rosarita Tatè et al. observed how the statin drug simvastatin:

> induces a destruction/restructuration of the cytoskeleton that decreases mechanical strain transfer to the nuclei, inducing the loss of transmission of regulatory signals from the cytoskeleton to the nucleoskeleton.... inhibits the metastatic invasion of human cancer cells via destruction of the cytoskeleton.... and ... induces a destructuration of the cytoskeleton, and that it is the destabilized cytoskeleton that results in the inhibition of stemness gene expression and lamellipodia and filopodia formation. (85)

Several of the Rho family GTP-ase proteins are located at the Golgi apparatus, which is responsible for sorting and moving proteins to the correct location in the cell. Dr. Maeve Long and Jeremy Simpson (2017) write:

> The Golgi complex is the central unit of the secretory pathway, modifying, processing and sorting proteins and lipids to their correct cellular localization. (86)

Rho proteins also play a role in protein

trafficking to the cell membrane. Statin drugs severely hamper this protein trafficking by inhibition of the RhoD proteins. Dr. Magdalena Blom et al. (2015) write:

> Vesicle trafficking from the endoplasmic reticulum to the plasma membrane via the Golgi apparatus measured by the VSV-G protein is severely hampered by manipulation of RhoD. (87)

Statins as Anti-Cancer Drugs

As mentioned above, the anti-cancer effects of statin drugs are related to inhibition of the HMG-CoA, the rate-limiting step in the mevalonate pathway, upregulated in cancer cells, and needed for production of key metabolites, sterols, and isoprenoids required for tumor growth and progression. Statin-drug inhibition of the mevalonate pathway causes depletion of isoprenoids in cancer cells, inducing the intrinsic apoptosis pathway (mitochondria-mediated cell death). This is correlated with downregulation of BCL-2, the anti-apoptosis protein. (88–94)

Statins for Cancer Stem Cells

In 2019, Dr. Xiao Ding et al. summarized the anti-CSC effect of statin drugs by blocking the production of isoprenoids:

> The therapeutic effects of statins have been observed in several cancers, including prostatic, gastric, esophageal, and hepatic cancer. Statins inhibit tumor growth, invasion and metastasis by blocking the production of isoprenoids, which are necessary for the post-translational modifi-

cations of many proteins.... Protein geranylgeranylation, which is a branch of the cholesterol synthesis pathway, is critical for breast CSC maintenance. (95)

The mevalonate pathway is critical for CSC function and considerable research attention has been devoted to statin drugs as anti-CSC agents. Bergamot, a natural product that targets the mevalonate pathway, also eradicates CSCs. (96–108)

Statins and Embryonic Stem Cells

Cancer cells share many similarities with embryonic stem cells, making them a useful model for cancer research. One of the Ten Hallmarks of Cancer (see chapter 3) is immortality, the ability of the cancer cell to self-renew indefinitely. Like cancer cells, embryonic stem cells (ESCs) also have immortality. (109)

Other remarkable similarities involve gene expression, cell-signaling pathways, and cell markers, as discussed in chapter 25, on the trophoblastic theory of cancer. (110–112)

In 2007, Dr. Mi-Hee Lee et al. studied the effect of simvastatin on mouse embryonic stem cells, finding suppression of self-renewal—that is, the cells were no longer immortal, due to inhibition of RhoA geranylgeranylation. Dr. Lee writes that simvastatin is the most effective statin, causing loss of self-renewal and marked downregulation of stem cell markers

> due to depletion of intracellular pools of geranylgeranyl pyrophosphate (GGPP), the substrate required for the geranylgeranylation. (109)

Zolendronic Acid for Breast Cancer Bone Metastasis

In 2013, Drs. C. Riganti and M. Massaia noted that the bisphosphonate family of drugs for osteoporosis (such as Zoledronic acid) also inhibit the mevalonate pathway, similar to simvastatin, causing depletion of intracellular pools of isoprenoids. The bisphosphonates:

> cause the deprivation of intracellular isoprenoids, farnesyl pyrophosphate (FPP) and geranylgeranyl pyrophosphate (GGPP)... Isoprenoids are critical for the post-translational modification of proteins that are essential for both cell proliferation and differentiation. (114)

Zolendronic Acid and Doxycycline Synergy

Drs. Reganti and Massaia think the bisphosphonate drugs are superior to the statins for this purpose because, in addition to blocking mevalonate, they override multidrug resistance (MDR) and restore immunogenic cell death (ICD) mechanisms. This is fortuitous because Zolendronic acid is commonly given IV monthly as a bone agent for breast cancer bone involvement (bone metastasis). Without realizing it, oncologists using Zolendronic acid have been blocking the mevalonate pathway, as statins do, thus having an anti-CSC effect. (114)

In this case, these patients benefit by adding doxycycline, which has synergy with Zoledronic acid. There may be a combined benefit with use of all three—statins, Zoledronic acid, and doxycycline—in breast cancer. (115–116)

Preclinical Studies (in vitro and in vivo xenografts) show statin drugs effective in the following cancer cell lines:

- Lymphoma (117–118)
- Breast cancer (119–120)
- Endometrial cancer (121)
- Ovarian cancer (122–123)
- Glioblastoma and medulloblastoma (124–127)
- Hepatocellular carcinoma (128)
- Lung cancer (129)
- Rhabdomyosarcoma (130)
- Melanoma (131)
- Colon cancer (132)

Chinese Skullcap (Baicalein) Synergy with Statin

In 2019, Dr. Palko-Łabuz studied the effect of simvastatin on human colon adenocarcinoma cells. The authors observed changes in the shape of the cancer cells related to alteration of the actin filaments, as noted by others above. Pro-apoptotic effects were augmented 30–50 fold by additional use of the flavone Chinese skullcap (baicalein), discussed more completely in chapter 10, on natural substances for CSCs. (132)

Statins for Endometriosis

Although not officially classified as cancer, endometriosis shares many features of a neoplastic process, such as activation of inflammatory pathways (NF-kB, and IL-6), with stimulation of angiogenesis, upregulation of VEGF and PDGF. In addition, the endometrial implants stimulate neurogenesis, the growth of new nerve fibers accounting for increased pain sensations. The endometrial implants may cause false positive PET scans related to increased glucose uptake. (133–134)

Statin Drugs for Endometriosis

Since statins are anti-cancer agents, you may not be surprised to learn that statin drugs are beneficial for endometriosis, with its many cancer-like features. (135–138) Similarly, two other repurposed anti-cancer drugs mentioned in this book are shown to be useful in endometriosis, fenofibrate and niclosamide. (139–140)

Caution with Use of Statins

Adverse side effects of statins include muscle pain, neuropathy, loss of cognitive function, neuropsychiatric disorder, depression etc., and require oversight by a knowledgeable physician.

Use of statins may impair glucose uptake in cancer cells, rendering a false negative report on a PET Scan. (141)

In patients receiving treatment with rituximab given IV for lymphoma, statins will interfere with efficacy of the drug. Concomitant use of statins with rituximab is not recommended. Similarly, another drug mentioned in this book, itraconazole, should not be used with rituximab, as recruitment of the CD20 marker is inhibited. (142–143)

Case Reports of Muscle Necrosis on Statins

Statin drugs are mitochondrial toxins that deplete coenzyme Q10 and inhibit mitochondrial respiration, thus serving as OXPHOS inhibitors. As such, adverse effects of statin drugs may include muscle pain, muscle breakdown, myopathy, neuropathy, and cognitive impairment. (154–156)

Combined use of ketoconazole with statin drugs resulted in cumulative mitochondrial toxicity with muscle necrosis (rhabdomyolysis) in two case reports in 2007 and 2011. (144–145)

Combination Regimes— Statins Deplete CoQ-10

Co-Q10 is a downstream product of the mevalonate pathwy inhibited by statin drugs. Indeed, Co-Q10 depletion induced mitochondrial toxicity is thought to be the main anti-cancer mechanism of statin drugs by Dr. Grace McGregor et al. (2020), who studied the effect of statin drugs on cancer cells using mass spectrometry and isotope tracing, finding

> that statins only modestly affected cancer cholesterol homeostasis. Instead, they significantly reduced synthesis and levels of another downstream product, the mitochondrial electron carrier coenzyme Q-10, both in cultured cancer cells and tumors. This compromised oxidative phosphorylation, causing severe oxidative stress. (157)

Dr. McGregor and colleagues found that cancer cells compensate for this oxidative stress by upregulating anti-oxidant pathways. In chapter 11, on sulfasalazine and other repurposed drugs, we discussed downregulation of cancer cell anti-oxidant capacity by blocking the xCT cystine transporter, starving the cancer cell of glutathione. Dr. McGregor et al. take a similar approach:

Targeting cystine import with an xCT transporter–lowering MEK inhibitor, in combination with statins, caused profound tumor cell death. Thus, statin-induced ROS production in cancer cell scan be exploited in a combinatorial regimen. (157)

Synergy with dual OXPHOS and glycolysis inhibition, or a statin plus another OXPHOS inhibitor have been described as lethal combinations. (158–160)

Statins for Immune Surveillance

The mevalonate pathway, upregulated in cancer, is also involved in cancer immune evasion. Downregulating mevalonate with a statin drug restores the host immune system by enhancing the CD8+ T cell response to cancer. (146–149)

Conclusion

The old antiplatelet drug, dipyridamole (DP) inhibits platelet activation, preventing release of platelet-derived growth factors used to stimulate growth and proliferation of the cancer. Platelet inhibition restores anti-tumor immunity. There may be synergy with aspirin. Dipyridamole also serves as an autophagy inhibitor. Statins block the mevalonate pathway, serving to destabilize the cancer cell cytoskeleton and eradicate CSCs. The statin and dipyridamole combination is synergistic and looks promising for our *Cracking Cancer Toolkit*. (150–153)

References for Chapter 40: Dipyridamole and Statins

1) Palumbo, Joseph S., et al. "Platelets and fibrin (ogen) increase metastatic potential by impeding natural killer cell–mediated elimination of tumor cells." Blood 105.1 (2005): 178-185.

2) Elaskalani, Omar, et al. "Targeting Platelets for the Treatment of Cancer." Cancers 9.7 (2017): 94.

3) Menter, David G., et al. "Platelet "first responders" in wound response, cancer, and metastasis." Cancer and Metastasis Reviews 36.2 (2017): 199-213.

4) Alves, Rubina, and Ramon Grimalt. "A review of platelet-rich plasma: history, biology, mechanism of action, and classification." Skin appendage disorders 4.1 (2018): 18-24.

5) Carrillo-Mora, Paul, et al. "Platelets-rich plasma: a versatile tool for regenerative medicine." Cir Cir 81.1 (2013): 74-82.

6) Mishra, Allan, et al. "Sports medicine applications of platelet rich plasma." Current pharmaceutical biotechnology 13.7 (2012): 1185-1195.

7) In't Veld, Sjors GJG, and Thomas Wurdinger. "Tumor-educated platelets." blood 133.22 (2019): 2359-2364.

8) Levin, Jack and C. Lockard Conley. "Thrombocytosis associated with malignant disease." Archives of internal medicine 114.4 (1964): 497-500.

9) Bailey, Sarah ER, et al. "How useful is thrombocytosis in predicting an underlying cancer in primary care? A systematic review." Family practice 34.1 (2017): 4-10.

10) Haemmerle, Monika, et al. "The platelet lifeline to cancer: challenges and opportunities." Cancer Cell 33.6 (2018): 965-983.

11) Yan, MengJie, and Paul Jurasz. "The role of platelets in the tumor microenvironment: From solid tumors to leukemia." Biochimica et Biophysica Acta (BBA)-Molecular Cell Research 1863.3 (2016): 392-400.

12) Cesca, Christine, Jonathan Ben-Ezra, and Roger S. Riley. "Platelet satellitism as presenting finding in mantle cell lymphoma: a case report." American journal of clinical pathology 115.4 (2001): 567-570.

13) Gatignol, Anne, et al. "B-cell non-Hodgkin lymphoma discovery after observation of a platelet

satellitism around atypical lymphocytes." Annales de biologie clinique. Vol. 77. No. 2. 2019.

14) Rhodes, E. L., et al. "Dipyridamole for treatment of melanoma." The Lancet 325.8430 (1985): 693.

15) Spano, Daniela, et al. "Dipyridamole prevents triple-negative breast-cancer progression." Clinical & experimental metastasis 30.1 (2013): 47-68.

16) Wang, Chunmei, et al. "Chemoprevention activity of dipyridamole in the MMTV-PyMT transgenic mouse model of breast cancer." Cancer Prevention Research 6.5 (2013): 437-447.

17) Ge, Shu-Min, et al. "Reverse screening approach to identify potential anti-cancer targets of dipyridamole." American journal of translational research 8.12 (2016): 5187.

18) Ruan, Jia, et al. "Imatinib disrupts lymphoma angiogenesis by targeting vascular pericytes." Blood 121.26 (2013): 5192-5202.

19) Chute, John P., and Heather A. Himburg. "Imatinib tackles lymphoma via the PDGFRβ+ pericyte." Blood 121.26 (2013): 5107-5108.

20) Laimer, Daniela, et al. "PDGFR blockade is a rational and effective therapy for NPM-ALK–driven lymphomas." Nature medicine 18.11 (2012): 1699.

21) Takehara, Kazuhiko, Atsuyuki Igarashi, and Yasumasa Ishibashi. "Dipyridamole specifically decreases platelet-derived growth factor release from platelets." Pharmacology 40.3 (1990): 150-156.

22) Takehara, Kazuhiko, et al. "Dipyridamole decreases platelet-derived growth factor levels in human serum." Arteriosclerosis: An Official Journal of the American Heart Association, Inc. 7.2 (1987): 152-158.

23) Saxena, Satya P., et al. "Histamine is an intracellular messenger mediating platelet aggregation." Science 243.4898 (1989): 1596-1600.

24) Masini, E., et al. "The role of histamine in platelet aggregation by physiological and immunological stimuli." Inflammation Research 47.5 (1998): 211-220.

25) Blaya, Bruno, et al. "Histamine and histamine receptor antagonists in cancer biology." Inflammation & Allergy-Drug Targets (Formerly Current Drug Targets-Inflammation & Allergy) 9.3 (2010): 146-157.

26) Rivera, Elena S., et al. "Histamine as an autocrine growth factor: an unusual role for a widespread mediator." Seminars in cancer biology. Vol. 10. No. 1. Academic Press, 2000.

27) Medina, Vanina A., and Elena S. Rivera. "Histamine receptors and cancer pharmacology." British journal of pharmacology 161.4 (2010): 755-767.

28) Cricco, G. P., et al. "Histamine as an autocrine growth factor in experimental mammary carcinomas." Agents and actions 43.1-2 (1994): 17-20.

29) Leblanc, Raphael, and Olivier Peyruchaud. "Metastasis: new functional implications of platelets and megakaryocytes." Blood 128.1 (2016): 24-31.

30) Menter, David G., et al. "Platelets and cancer: a casual or causal relationship: revisited." Cancer and Metastasis Reviews 33.1 (2014): 231-269.

31) Amo, Laura, et al. "Involvement of Platelet–Tumor Cell Interaction in Immune Evasion. Potential Role of Podocalyxin-Like Protein 1." Frontiers in oncology 4 (2014): 245.

32) Nieswandt, Bernhard, et al. "Lysis of tumor cells by natural killer cells in mice is impeded by platelets." Cancer research 59.6 (1999): 1295-1300.

33) Chen, Yen-Cheng, et al. "Dipyridamole inhibits lipopolysaccharide-induced cyclooxygenase-2 and monocyte chemoattractant protein-1 via heme oxygenase-1-mediated reactive oxygen species reduction in rat mesangial cells." European journal of pharmacology 650.1 (2011): 445-450.

34) Catani, Maria Valeria, et al. "The "Janus face" of platelets in Cancer." International Journal of Molecular Sciences 21.3 (2020): 788.

35) Tzanakakis, George N., Kailash C. Agarwal, and Michael P. Vezeridis. "Prevention of human pancreatic cancer cell-induced hepatic metastasis in nude mice by dipyridamole and its analog RA-233." Cancer 71.8 (1993): 2466-2471.

36) Cho, Min Soon, et al. "The Inhibition of Platelets Restore Anti-Tumor Immune Response to Ovarian Cancer and Its Therapeutic Implication." Blood 132. Supplement 1 (2018): 3698-3698.

37) Gamboa, Alfredo, et al. "Role of adenosine and nitric oxide on the mechanisms of action of dipyridamole." Stroke 36.10 (2005): 2170-2175.

38) Kim, Hyung-Hwan, and James K. Liao. "Translational therapeutics of dipyridamole." Arteriosclerosis, thrombosis, and vascular biology 28.3 (2008): s39-s42.

39) Zhang, Lingzhi, et al. "Cyclic nucleotide phosphodiesterase 7B mRNA: An unfavorable characteristic in chronic lymphocytic leukemia." International Journal Of Cancer 129.5 (2011): 1162-1169.

40) Fang, Cheng, et al. "High expression of cyclic nucleotide phosphodiesterase 7B mRNA predicts poor prognosis in mantle cell lymphoma." Leukemia research 37.5 (2013): 536-540.

41) Cooney, Jeffrey D., and Ricardo CT Aguiar. "Phosphodiesterase 4 inhibitors have wide-ranging activity in B-cell malignancies." Blood, The Journal of the American Society of Hematology 128.25 (2016): 2886-2890.

42) Suhasini, Avvaru N., et al. "A phosphodiesterase 4B-dependent interplay between tumor cells and the microenvironment regulates angiogenesis in B-cell lymphoma." Leukemia 30.3 (2016): 617-626.

43) Murray, F., and P. A. Insel. "Targeting cAMP in chronic lymphocytic leukemia: a pathway-dependent approach for the treatment of leukemia and lymphoma." Expert opinion on therapeutic targets 17.8 (2013): 937.

44) Suhasini, Avvaru N., et al. "A phosphodiesterase 4B-dependent interplay between tumor cells and the microenvironment regulates angiogenesis in B-cell lymphoma." Leukemia 30.3 (2016): 617-626.

45) Coffino, Philip, Henry R. Bourne, and G. M. Tomkins. "Mechanism of lymphoma cell death induced by cyclic AMP." The American journal of pathology 81.1 (1975): 199.

46) Nam, Jehyun, et al. "Disruption of the Myc-PDE4B regulatory circuitry impairs B-cell lymphoma survival." Leukemia 33.12 (2019): 2912-2923.

47) Kelly, Kevin, et al. "Safety and pharmacodynamics of the PDE4 inhibitor roflumilast in advanced B-cell malignancies." Clinical Cancer Research 23.5 (2017): 1186-1192.

48) Maurice, Donald H., et al. "Advances in targeting cyclic nucleotide phosphodiesterases." Nature reviews Drug discovery 13.4 (2014): 290-314.

49) Pantziarka, Pan, et al. "Repurposing drugs in oncology (ReDO)—selective PDE5 inhibitors as anti-cancer agents." ecancermedicalscience 12 (2018).

50) Sarfati, Marika, et al. "Sildenafil and vardenafil, types 5 and 6 phosphodiesterase inhibitors, induce caspase-dependent apoptosis of B-chronic lymphocytic leukemia cells." Blood 101.1 (2003): 265-269.

51) Jiang, Y. J., et al. "Influence of dipyridamole on expression of PAC-1 and CD62p in patients with malignant lymphoma." Zhongguo shi yan xue ye xue za zhi 18.4 (2010): 923-926.

52) Hirose, M., et al. "Synergistic inhibitory effects of dipyridamole and vincristine on the growth of human leukaemia and lymphoma cell lines." British journal of cancer 56.4 (1987): 413-417.

53) Howell, Stephen B., et al. "Dipyridamole enhancement of etoposide sensitivity." Cancer research 49.15 (1989): 4147-4153.

54) Grem, Jean L., and P. H. Fischer. "Enhancement of 5-fluorouracil's anticancer activity by dipyridamole." Pharmacology & therapeutics 40.3 (1989): 349-371.

55) Grem, Jean L., and Paul H. Fischer. "Augmentation of 5-fluorouracil cytotoxicity in human colon cancer cells by dipyridamole." Cancer research 45.7 (1985): 2967-2972.

56) Goda, Ahmed E., et al. "Preclinical evaluation of bortezomib/dipyridamole novel combination as a potential therapeutic modality for hematologic malignancies." Molecular oncology 9.1 (2015): 309-322.

57) El-Sisi, Alaa E., et al. "Enhanced anticancer activity of combined treatment of imatinib and dipyridamole in solid Ehrlich carcinoma-bearing mice." Naunyn-Schmiedeberg's Archives of Pharmacology (2020): 1-17.

58) Thomé, Marcos P., et al. "Dipyridamole impairs autophagic flux and exerts antiproliferative activity on prostate cancer cells." Experimental cell research 382.1 (2019): 111456.

59) Zhao, Peng, et al. "The molecular basis for the inhibition of phosphodiesterase-4D by three natural

resveratrol analogs. Isolation, molecular docking, molecular dynamics simulations, binding free energy, and bioassay." Biochimica et Biophysica Acta (BBA)-Proteins and Proteomics 1834.10 (2013): 2089-2096.

60) Farinelli, Stephen E., Lloyd A. Greene, and Wilma J. Friedman. "Neuroprotective actions of dipyridamole on cultured CNS neurons." Journal of Neuroscience 18.14 (1998): 5112-5123.

61) Blake, Allan D. "Dipyridamole is neuroprotective for cultured rat embryonic cortical neurons." Biochemical and biophysical research communications 314.2 (2004): 501-504.

62) Sloka, Scott, et al. "Reduction of microglial activity in a model of multiple sclerosis by dipyridamole." Journal of neuroinflammation 10.1 (2013): 1-11.

63) Lana, Daniele, et al. "The neuron-astrocyte-microglia triad in a rat model of chronic cerebral hypoperfusion: protective effect of dipyridamole." Frontiers in aging neuroscience 6 (2014): 322.

64) Rachidi, Saleh, et al. "Platelets subvert T cell immunity against cancer via GARP-TGFβ axis." Science immunology 2.11 (2017).

65) Xu, Xiaohong Ruby, George M. Yousef, and Heyu Ni. "Cancer and platelet crosstalk: opportunities and challenges for aspirin and other antiplatelet agents." Blood 131.16 (2018): 1777-1789.

66) Contursi, Annalisa, et al. "Platelets as crucial partners for tumor metastasis: from mechanistic aspects to pharmacological targeting." Cellular and Molecular Life Sciences 74.19 (2017): 3491-3507.

67) Gurevich, K. G., and I. D. Surkina. "A Pharmacokinetic Model of the Antiviral Action of Dipyridamole." Pharmaceutical Chemistry Journal 35.12 (2001): 643-646.

69) Mastikova, Margarita, et al. "Antiviral Activity of Dipyridamole in Experimental Viral Infections in Mice." Acta Microbiologica Bulgarica: 46.Vol 35/2 (2019)

70) Hay, Kathleen A., Andrew Gaydos, and Richard B. Tenser. "Inhibition of herpes simplex virus reactivation by dipyridamole in a mouse model." Journal of medical virology 50.2 (1996): 198-203.

71) Tenser, Richard B., Andrew Gaydos, and Kathleen A. Hay. "Inhibition of herpes simplex virus reactivation by dipyridamole." Antimicrobial agents and chemotherapy 45.12 (2001): 3657-3659.

72) Thomé, Marcos P., et al. "Dipyridamole as a new drug to prevent Epstein-Barr virus reactivation." Antiviral Research 172 (2019): 104615.

73) Tonew, E., M. K. Indulen, and D. R. Dzeguze. "Antiviral action of dipyridamole and its derivatives against influenza virus A." Acta virologica 26.3 (1982): 125-129.

74) Korbecki, M., et al. "Dipyridamole as an inhibitor of vaccinia virus replication." Molekuliarnaia genetika, mikrobiologiia i virusologiia 1 (1985): 29-32.

75) Oehring, H., and J. Schmidt. "The antiviral action of dipyridamole on rhinoviruses." Zeitschrift fur Attgemeine Mikrobiologie, Morphologic, Physiologic, Genetik und Okologie der Microorganismen 24.6 (1978): 447-449.

76) Liu, Xiaoyan, et al. "Potential therapeutic effects of dipyridamole in the severely ill patients with COVID-19." Acta Pharmaceutica Sinica B (2020).

77) Lichtenberger, L. M., et al. "Unlocking Aspirin's Chemopreventive Activity: Role of Irreversibly Inhibiting Platelet Cyclooxygenase-1." Cancer prevention research (Philadelphia, Pa.) 10.2 (2017): 142-152.

78) Lucotti, Serena, et al. "Aspirin blocks formation of metastatic intravascular niches by inhibiting platelet-derived COX-1/thromboxane A 2." The Journal of clinical investigation 129.5 (2019).

80) Huong, Phung Thanh, et al. "The role of platelets in the tumor-microenvironment and the drug resistance of cancer cells." Cancers 11.2 (2019): 240.

81) Lazzerini, P. E., et al. "Simvastatin inhibits cytokine production and nuclear factor-kB activation in interleukin 1 beta-stimulated synoviocytes from rheumatoid arthritis patients." Clinical and experimental rheumatology 25.5 (2007): 696.

82) Hölschermann, Hans, et al. "Statins prevent NF-κB transactivation independently of the IKK-pathway in human endothelial cells." Atherosclerosis 185.2 (2006): 240-245.

83) Hennessy, Emma, et al. "Is there potential for repurposing statins as novel antimicrobials?." Antimicrobial agents and chemotherapy 60.9 (2016): 5111-5121.

84) Aleksandra Pandyra et al. "Immediate utility of two approved agents to target both the metabolic mevalonate pathway and its restorative feedback loop." Cancer research 74.17 (2014): 4772-4782.

85) Tatè, Rosarita, et al. "Simvastatin inhibits the expression of stemness-related genes and the metastatic invasion of human cancer cells via destruction of the cytoskeleton." International journal of oncology 51.6 (2017): 1851-1859.

86) Long, Maeve, and Jeremy C. Simpson. "Rho GTPases operating at the Golgi complex: implications for membrane traffic and cancer biology." Tissue and Cell 49.2 (2017): 163-169.

87) Blom, Magdalena, et al. "RhoD is a Golgi component with a role in anterograde protein transport from the ER to the plasma membrane." Experimental cell research 333.2 (2015): 208-219.

88) Iannelli, Federica, et al. "Targeting mevalonate pathway in cancer treatment: repurposing of statins." Recent patents on anti-cancer drug discovery 13.2 (2018): 184-200.

89) Matusewicz, Lucyna, et al. "The effect of statins on cancer cells." Tumor Biology 36.7 (2015): 4889-4904.

90) Mullen, Peter J., et al. "The interplay between cell signalling and the mevalonate pathway in cancer." Nature Reviews Cancer 16.11 (2016): 718.

91) Zahra Bathaie, Seyedeh, et al. "Mevalonate pathway and human cancers." Current molecular pharmacology 10.2 (2017): 77-85.

92) Alizadeh, Javad, et al. "Mevalonate cascade inhibition by simvastatin induces the intrinsic apoptosis pathway via depletion of isoprenoids in tumor cells." Scientific reports 7 (2017): 44841.

93) Spampanato, Carmine, et al. "Simvastatin inhibits cancer cell growth by inducing apoptosis correlated to activation of Bax and down-regulation of BCL-2 gene expression." International journal of oncology 40.4 (2012): 935-941.

94) Kubatka, Peter, et al. "Statins in oncological research: from experimental studies to clinical practice." Critical reviews in oncology/hematology 92.3 (2014): 296-311.

95) Ding, Xiao, et al. "The role of cholesterol metabolism in cancer." American journal of cancer research 9.2 (2019): 219.

96) Kim, Woo-Young. "Therapeutic targeting of lipid synthesis metabolism for selective elimination of cancer stem cells." Archives of pharmacal research 42.1 (2019): 25-39.

97) Choi, Seok Gyeong, et al. "Clinical and biochemical relevance of monounsaturated fatty acid metabolism targeting strategy for cancer stem cell elimination in colon cancer." Biochemical and biophysical research communications 519.1 (2019): 100-105.

98) Zhao, Guangyuan, Horacio Cardenas, and Daniela Matei. "Ovarian Cancer—Why Lipids Matter." Cancers 11.12 (2019): 1870.

99) Gauthaman, Kalamegam, Chui-Yee Fong, and Ariff Bongso. "Statins, stem cells, and cancer." Journal of cellular biochemistry 106.6 (2009): 975-983.

100) Thurnher, Martin, and Georg Gruenbacher. "Mevalonate Metabolism Promotes Cancer Stemness and Immunity via EMT-like Reverse Differentiation." Frontiers in Oncology 8 (2018): 394.

101) Ginestier, Christophe, Emmanuelle Charafe-Jauffret, and Daniel Birnbaum. "p53 and cancer stem cells: the mevalonate connexion." (2012): 2583-2584.

102) Ginestier, Christophe, et al. "Mevalonate metabolism regulates Basal breast cancer stem cells and is a potential therapeutic target." Stem cells 30.7 (2012): 1327-1337.

103) Likus, Wirginia, et al. "Could drugs inhibiting the mevalonate pathway also target cancer stem cells?." Drug resistance updates 25 (2016): 13-25.

104) Rennó, André Lisboa, et al. "Decreased Expression of Stem Cell Markers by Simvastatin in 7, 12-dimethyl-benz (a) anthracene (DMBA)–induced Breast Cancer." Toxicologic pathology 43.3 (2015): 400-410.

105) Likus, Wirginia, et al. "Could drugs inhibiting the mevalonate pathway also target cancer stem cells?" Drug resistance updates 25 (2016): 13-25.

106) Brandi, Jessica, et al. "Proteomic analysis of pancreatic cancer stem cells: Functional role of fatty acid synthesis and mevalonate pathways." Journal of proteomics 150 (2017): 310-322.

107) Gruenbacher, Georg, and Martin Thurnher. "Mevalonate metabolism in cancer stemness and trained immunity." Frontiers in oncology 8 (2018).

108) Fiorillo, Marco, et al. "Bergamot natural products eradicate cancer stem cells (CSCs) by targeting mevalonate, Rho-GDI-signalling and mitochondrial metabolism." Biochimica et Biophysica Acta (BBA)-Bioenergetics 1859.9 (2018): 984-996.

109) Lee, Mi-Hee, Yee Sook Cho, and Yong-Mahn Han. "Simvastatin suppresses self-renewal of mouse embryonic stem cells by inhibiting RhoA geranylgeranylation." Stem Cells 25.7 (2007): 1654-1663.

110) Dreesen, Oliver, and Ali H. Brivanlou. "Signaling pathways in cancer and embryonic stem cells." Stem cell reviews 3.1 (2007): 7-17.

111) Ben-Porath, Ittai, et al. "An embryonic stem cell–like gene expression signature in poorly differentiated aggressive human tumors." Nature genetics 40.5 (2008): 499.

112) Schoenhals, Matthieu, et al. "Embryonic stem cell markers expression in cancers." Biochemical and biophysical research communications 383.2 (2009): 157-162.

113) Mathieu, Julie, et al. "HIF induces human embryonic stem cell markers in cancer cells." Cancer research 71.13 (2011): 4640-4652.

114) Riganti, C., and M. Massaia. "Inhibition of the mevalonate pathway to override chemoresistance and promote immunogenic cell death in cancer cells: hitting two birds with one stone. ONCOIMMUNOLOGY (2013) 2." (2019).

115) Duivenvoorden, W. C. M., et al. "Effect of zoledronic acid on the doxycycline-induced decrease in tumour burden in a bone metastasis model of human breast cancer." British journal of cancer 96.10 (2007): 1526.

116) Göbel, Andy, et al. "Combined inhibition of the mevalonate pathway with statins and zoledronic acid potentiates their anti-tumor effects in human breast cancer cells." Cancer letters 375.1 (2016): 162-171.

117) Qi, X. F., et al. "HMG-CoA reductase inhibitors induce apoptosis of lymphoma cells by promoting ROS generation and regulating Akt, Erk and p38 signals via suppression of mevalonate pathway." Cell death & disease 4.2 (2013): e518.

118) van de Donk, Niels WCJ, et al. "Protein geranylgeranylation is critical for the regulation of survival and proliferation of lymphoma tumor cells." Clinical cancer research 9.15 (2003): 5735-5748.

119) Wang, Tingting, et al. "Simvastatin-induced breast cancer cell death and deactivation of PI3K/Akt and MAPK/ERK signalling are reversed by metabolic products of the mevalonate pathway." Oncotarget 7.3 (2016): 2532.

120) Sethunath, Vidyalakshmi, et al. "Targeting the mevalonate pathway to overcome acquired anti-HER2 treatment resistance in breast cancer." Molecular Cancer Research 17.11 (2019): 2318-2330.

121) Schointuch, Monica N., et al. "Simvastatin, an HMG-CoA reductase inhibitor, exhibits anti-metastatic and anti-tumorigenic effects in endometrial cancer." Gynecologic oncology 134.2 (2014): 346-355.

122) Kobayashi, Yusuke, et al. "Drug repositioning of mevalonate pathway inhibitors as antitumor agents for ovarian cancer." Oncotarget 8.42 (2017): 72147.

123) Jones, Hannah M., et al. "Atorvastatin exhibits anti-tumorigenic and anti-metastatic effects in ovarian cancer in vitro." American journal of cancer research 7.12 (2017): 2478.

124) Seliger, Corinna, et al. "Use of statins or NSAIDs and survival of patients with high-grade glioma." PloS one 13.12 (2018): e0207858.

125) Yanae, Masashi, et al. "Statin-induced apoptosis via the suppression of ERK1/2 and Akt activation by inhibition of the geranylgeranyl-pyrophosphate biosynthesis in glioblastoma." Journal of Experimental & Clinical Cancer Research 30.1 (2011): 74.

126) Wang, Xiuxing, et al. "MYC-regulated mevalonate metabolism maintains brain tumor–initiating cells." Cancer research 77.18 (2017): 4947-4960.

127) Sheikholeslami, Kimia, et al. "Simvastatin induces apoptosis in medulloblastoma brain tumor cells via mevalonate cascade prenylation substrates." Cancers 11.7 (2019): 994

128) Kim, Gyuri, and Eun Seok Kang. "Prevention of Hepatocellular Carcinoma by Statins: Clinical Evidence

and Plausible Mechanisms." Seminars in liver disease. Vol. 39. No. 02. Thieme Medical Publishers, 2019.

129) Hassanabad, Ali Fatehi, and Fady Mina. "Targeting the Mevalonate Pathway for Treating Lung Cancer." American Journal of Clinical Oncology 43.1 (2020): 69-70.

130) Araki, Makoto, Masatomo Maeda, and Kiyoto Motojima. "Hydrophobic statins induce autophagy and cell death in human rhabdomyosarcoma cells by depleting geranylgeranyl diphosphate." European journal of pharmacology 674.2-3 (2012): 95-103.

131) Zanfardino, Mario, et al. "Simvastatin reduces melanoma progression in a murine model." International journal of oncology 43.6 (2013): 1763-1770.

132) Palko-Łabuz, Anna, et al. "MDR reversal and pro-apoptotic effects of statins and statins combined with flavonoids in colon cancer cells." Biomedicine & Pharmacotherapy 109 (2019): 1511-1522.

133) Varma, Rajesh, et al. "Endometriosis and the neoplastic process." Reproduction 127.3 (2004): 293-304.

134) Jeffry, Louis, et al. "Endometriosis with FDG uptake on PET." European Journal of Obstetrics & Gynecology and Reproductive Biology 117.2 (2004): 236-239.

135) Piotrowski, Piotr C., et al. "Statins inhibit growth of human endometrial stromal cells independently of cholesterol availability." Biology of reproduction 75.1 (2006): 107-111.

136) Nasu, Kaei, et al. "Simvastatin inhibits the proliferation and the contractility of human endometriotic stromal cells: a promising agent for the treatment of endometriosis." Fertility and sterility 92.6 (2009): 2097-2099.

137) Yilmaz, Bulent, et al. "Atorvastatin causes regression of endometriotic implants in a rat model." Reproductive biomedicine online 20.2 (2010): 291-299.

138) Bruner-Tran, Kaylon L., Kevin G. Osteen, and Antoni J. Duleba. "Simvastatin protects against the development of endometriosis in a nude mouse model." The Journal of Clinical Endocrinology & Metabolism 94.7 (2009): 2489-2494.

139) Fertil Steril. 2009 Dec;92(6):2100-2. Fenofibrate causes regression of endometriotic implants: a rat model. Onalan G1, Zeyneloglu HB, Bayraktar N.

140) Prather, Genna R., et al. "Niclosamide as a potential nonsteroidal therapy for endometriosis that preserves reproductive function in an experimental mouse model." Biology of reproduction 95.4 (2016): 74-1.

141) Malenda, Agata, et al. "Statins impair glucose uptake in tumor cells." Neoplasia (New York, NY) 14.4 (2012): 311.

142) Winiarska, Magdalena, et al. "Statins impair antitumor effects of rituximab by inducing conformational changes of CD20." PLoS medicine 5.3 (2008): e64.

143) Ringshausen, Ingo, et al. "Antifungal therapy with itraconazole impairs the anti-lymphoma effects of rituximab by inhibiting recruitment of CD20 to cell surface lipid rafts." Cancer research 70.11 (2010): 4292-4296.

144) Stein, C. A., Sanjay Goel, and Reza Ghavamian. "Hepatitis and rhabdomyolysis in a patient with hormone refractory prostate cancer on ketoconazole and concurrent lovastatin therapy." Investigational new drugs 25.3 (2007): 277-278.

145) Watkins, Jack L., Bradley J. Atkinson, and Lance C. Pagliaro. "Rhabdomyolysis in a prostate cancer patient taking ketoconazole and simvastatin: case report and review of the literature." Ann Pharmacother 45.2 (2011): e9.

146) Gruenbacher, Georg, and Martin Thurnher. "Mevalonate metabolism governs cancer immune surveillance." Oncoimmunology 6.10 (2017): e1342917.

147) Moon, Sung-Hwan, et al. "p53 represses the mevalonate pathway to mediate tumor suppression." Cell 176.3 (2019): 564-580.

148) Burn, Olivia K., et al. "Abstract B103: Altering the mevalonate pathway to enhance CD8+ T-cell responses." (2019): B103-B103.

149) Ahmadi, Yasin, Amir Ghorbanihaghjo, and Hassan Argani. "The balance between induction and inhibition of mevalonate pathway regulates cancer suppression by statins: A review of molecular mechanisms." Chemico-biological interactions 273 (2017): 273-285.

150) Gruenbacher, Georg, and Martin Thurnher. "Mevalonate metabolism in immuno-oncology." Frontiers in immunology 8 (2017): 1714.

151) Wei, Shupei, et al. "Artesunate inhibits the mevalonate pathway and promotes glioma cell senescence." Journal of cellular and molecular medicine 24.1 (2020): 276-284.

152) Pirmoradi, Leila, et al. "Targeting cholesterol metabolism in glioblastoma: a new therapeutic approach in cancer therapy." Journal of Investigative Medicine 67.4 (2019): 715-719.

153) Gong, Li, et al. "The mevalonate coordinates energy input and cell proliferation." Cell death & disease 10.4 (2019): 327.

154) Eghbal, Mohammad Ali, Narges Abdoli, and Yadollah Azarmi. "Efficiency of hepatocyte pretreatment with coenzyme Q10 against statin toxicity." Archives of Industrial Hygiene and Toxicology 65.1 (2014): 101-108.

155) Kaufmann, P., et al. "Toxicity of statins on rat skeletal muscle mitochondria." Cellular and Molecular Life Sciences CMLS 63.19-20 (2006): 2415-2425.

156) Sadighara, Melina, et al. "Protective effects of coenzyme Q10 and L-carnitine against statin-induced pancreatic mitochondrial toxicity in rats." Research in Pharmaceutical Sciences 12.6 (2017): 434.

157) McGregor, Grace H., et al. "Targeting the metabolic response to statin-mediated oxidative stress produces a synergistic antitumor response." Cancer Research 80.2 (2020): 175-188.

158) Huang, Jiangrong, et al. "Inhibiting prenylation augments chemotherapy efficacy in renal cell carcinoma through dual inhibition on mitochondrial respiration and glycolysis." Biochemical and biophysical research communications 493.2 (2017): 921-927.

159) Senkowski, Wojciech, et al. "Mitochondrial inhibitors and statins: a lethal combination for metabolically stressed cancer cells." (2016): 213-213.

160) Feng, Jiao, et al. "Simvastatin re-sensitizes hepatocellular carcinoma cells to sorafenib by inhibiting HIF-1α/PPAR-γ/PKM2-mediated glycolysis." Journal of Experimental & Clinical Cancer Research 39.1 (2020): 1-18.

Chapter 41

Tocotrienol Vitamin E

ALTHOUGH THE OLDER TOCOPHEROL FORM of vitamin E has been available and studied for decades, the tocotrienol form with its unsaturated side chain is a relatively recent discovery. A method for mass production was discovered by Dr. Barrie Tan in 1990 while on a trip to the Amazon Rain Forest. During the trip, Dr. Tan found a suitable source in the Annato plant (Bixa Orellana) useful for his Tocotrienol extraction process patented in 2002.(75-76) Health benefits of tocotrienols are quite diverse including anti-cancer, neuroprotective, cardio-protective, and renal-protective. (1-4)

Four Isoforms

Of the four isoforms, delta and gamma appear to have the most potent anti-cancer activity, displaying antiproliferative, and apoptotic activity. In addition, studies show reversal of EMT (epithelial-to-mesenchymal transition) in breast cancer models in-vitro at concentrations having no adverse effects on normal cells. (1-4)

In vivo and in vitro studies using gamma-tocotrienol have shown anticancer activity against leukemia, breast, colon, prostate, pancreatic and lung cancers. In-vivo studies have shown suppression of angiogenesis, suppression of metastasis, and targeting of CSCs (5-9)

Myeloid Leukemia

In 2019, Dr. Ghanem studied the anticancer effects of gamma tocotrienol in-vitro in a myeloid leukemia cell model finding "profound apoptotic response" via activation of the intrinsic pathway (mitochondria mediated apoptosis). (5-6)

Prostate Cancer

Tocotrienol vitamin E is only one of many natural compounds targeting prostate cancer discussed by Dr. Fontana in 2020, writing:

> Among these naturally occurring molecules, quercetin, fisetin, luteolin, apigenin, curcumin, resveratrol, genistein, silibinin, kaempferol, epigallocatechin-3-gallate [EGCG], tocotrienols, sulforaphane, ginsenosides, ursolic acid, berberine, honokiol, xanthoumol, oridonin, and tannic acid have shown outstanding potential as anti-PCa [anti-prostate cancer] agents in in vitro and preclinical experiments. (7-9)

Dr. Fontana found that Delta Tocotrienol impaired mitochondrial respiration, induced apoptosis and endoplasmic stress which induced "protective autophagy" in prostate cancer cell models. (7-9)

Exact Mechanisms Are Largely Unknown

In 2019, Dr. Tang studied Gamma-Tocotrienol's anti-cancer effects in a prostate cancer model in vitro and in vivo, writing:

Despite its promising anti-cancer potential, the exact mechanisms responsible for the effects of γ-T3 [Gamma-Tocotrienol] are still largely unknown. (9-12)

In 2020, Dr. Szulczewska-Remi Studied Tocotrienol's anticancer effects in Liver Cancer writing:

The exact reasons for the sensitivity of liver cancer cells to tocotrienols are unknown. (20)

Although Tocotrienol research is immature relative to other anti-cancer drugs and natural substances, current preclinical studies have shed light on mechanisms of anti-cancer activity, as discussed below.

Pancreatic Cancer

In 2017, Dr. Husain studied Delta-Tocotrienol in a transgenic mouse model of PDAC (pancreatic ductal carcinoma) finding inhibition of cancer cell migration, invasion, EMT, angiogenesis, and inhibition of CSCs. (13)

Anti-Cancer Efficacy of Tocotrienol has been found in preclinical studies in various cancer cell types:

- Prostate Cancer (7-12) (21) (35)
- Pancreatic Cancer (13) (33)
- Colon Cancer (14-15) (22)
- Cervical Cancer (16-17) (41)
- Gastric Cancer (18) (37) (40)
- Lung Cancer (19)
- Liver Cancer (Hepatoma) (20)
- Breast Cancer (23-32) (42-43) (74)
- Leukemia/Lymphoma (5-6) (44-50)
- Melanoma (51-56)

Tocotrienol Effects on Various Molecular Pathways in Cancer Cells:

- Down-Regulation of COX-2 (15) (18)
- Inhibition of NF-kB (19) (36-38) (74)
- GLYCOLYSIS Inhibitor, Reversal of Warburg Effect (24-26)
- Suppression of C-Myc Protein Levels (27)
- Suppression of Wnt and Hedgehog Signaling. (28-29)
- OXPHOS Inhibitor Complex I ETC (39-41)
- Disruption of Lipid Rafts (30-32)
- Estrogen Receptor Beta Signalling (42-52)
- Cleavage of PARP (PolyADP-Ribose Polymerase) (74)

Tocotrienol Synergy with Other Agents

- Synergy with Metformin in Prostate and Colon Cancer (21-22)
- Synergy with Pterostilbene in Breast Cancer (23) (38)
- Synergy with Celecoxib (COX-2 Inhibitor) (34)
- Synergy with Statins/ Suppression of Mevalonate Pathway (57-58)

Tocotrienol as GLYCOLYSIS Inhibitor, Reverses Warburg Effect

In previous chapters, we discussed that many of repurposed anti-cancer drugs MOA (mechanism of action) involves activation of AMPK, which then inhibits mTOR, which then induces "protective autophagy". In a mechanism similar to Itraconazole and metformin, Gamma-Tocotrienol also activates AMPK. In

2020, Dr. Paul Sylvester studied anticancer effects of Gamma Tocotrienol on breast cancer cell models finding reversal of Warburg Effect (inhibition of GLYCOLYSIS) with cancer cell reduction in glucose consumption, and reduction in expression of glycolytic enzymes. Dr. Sylvester writes:

> these findings indicate that gamma-tocotrienol-induced reversal of the Warburg effect in breast cancer cells is directly associated with an increase in AMPK activation. (24-26)

Note: AMPK activation inhibits the PI3K/Akt/mTOR pathway, thus suppressing EGF signaling (as seen below).

Tocotrienol as Wnt, Hedgehog Pathway Inhibitors

In 2018, Dr. Rayan Ahmed studied effects of tocotrienol in a breast cancer cell model finding reversal of EMT was caused by inhibition of Wnt and Hedgehog pathways (CSC pathways). Dr. Ahmed writes:

> Specifically, tocotrienols have been found to suppress EGF-[Epithelial Growth Factor] dependent mitogenic [Pro-Cancer] signaling…….by significantly inhibiting activity of the…[PI3K/Akt] pathway. (28-29)

Dr. Ahmed summarizes the molecular pathways targeted by Tocotrienols:

1) PI3K/Akt

2) MAPK

3) Cell cycle

4) Mevalonate pathway

5) GLYCOLYSIS

6) Angiogenesis

7) EMT

8) Lipid rafts (28-29)

Tocotrienols Disrupt Lipid Rafts

Lipid rafts are involved in various cell functions such as receptor signaling, endocytosis (membrane transport), and the actin cytoskeleton. In 2019, Dr. Paul Sylvester studied anticancer effects of Gamma Tocotrienols in a breast cancer cell model finding anti-cancer effects are associated with accumulation in lipid rafts in the cancer cell outer membrane with interference with the Tyrosine Kinase receptor, HERS2 (human epithelial growth factor receptor 2). These are key receptors for transmitting growth signals into the cancer cell. (30-33)

Tocotrienols Inhibit NF-kB, Anti-inflammatory Effects

In 2018, Dr. Sun studied anti-cancer effects of gamma tocotrienol in a gastric cancer cell model and in-vivo xenograft animal model, finding inhibition of cancer cell proliferation by inhibition of NF-kB, the master inflammatory controller. This was done by "significantly increasing" Protein Phosphatase 2A (PP2A), a tumor suppressor protein. Dr. Sun writes:

> Our findings showed that γ-T3 [gamma tocotrienol] significantly increased the activity of PP2A and its protein expression in gastric cancer cells and a nude mouse model of implanted human gastric cancer cells. These results indicate that increasing PP2A activity contributes to the inhibition of cell proliferation and NF-κB activity in cancer cells. (36-38)

Tocotrienol is OXPHOS Inhibitor

A number of studies using gastric and cervical cancer cell models showed that gamma tocotrienol inhibits mitochondrial complex I of the ETC (similar to metformin) thereby inhibiting OXPHOS and triggering mitochondrial mediated apoptosis. Remember, all OXPHOS inhibitors are also Wnt inhibitors as discussed in a previous chapter. (39-41)

Tocotrienol Estrogen Receptor Beta Agonist

In a previous chapter we discussed usefulness of Exemestane, an irreversible aromatase inhibitor drug, for preventing cancer cells from making their own estrogen for growth stimulation (called incrine stimulation). There is more to the story. There are actually two estrogen receptors. The Alpha receptors are the growth stimulators, while the Beta receptors inhibit growth and have anticancer effects. Tocotrienol has a high affinity for the ER-Beta receptor, but not for ER-Alpha, making Tocotrienol an ER-Beta Agonist, which inhibits cancer cell growth and induces apoptosis.

In 2010, Dr. Comitato studied tocotrienols in breast cancer cell models proposing the anti-cancer (apoptotic) activity is due to ER-Beta signaling. Dr. Comitato found Tocotrienol (TTRF= Tocotrienol rich fraction) treatment of the breast cancer cells increased ER-Beta nuclear translocation, and profoundly inhibited ER-Alpha expression (459 fold) with complete disappearance of ER-Alpha from the cancer cell nucleus. **Note:** TTRF contains both Delta and Gamma Isoforms. (42-43)

Estrogen Receptor Beta in Hematologic Malignancies

As we saw in the discussion of Exemestane which is useful not only in breast cancer, but also for other epithelial cancers, the use of ER-Beta agonists such as tocotrienols extends to hematologic B-Cell malignancies, shown to possess mainly ER-Beta receptors, while normal B cells have both sub-types. This explains why B-cell malignancies predominate in males, with much fewer cases in females. In B-cell malignancies, estrogen is protective by activating ER-Beta which then inhibits cancer cell growth, vascularization and dissemination (metastatic disease). (44-46)

Alternatively blocking estrogen with an aromatase inhibitor drug stimulated B Cell Lymphoma growth in a mouse xenograft model by Dr. Talaber in 2016, "highlighting a protective role for estrogens in lymphoma pathogenesis". (47-50)

Melanoma and ER-Beta Agonists

Melanoma is another cell type found to have predominantly ER-Beta receptors sensitive to growth inhibition by ER-Beta agonists. A number of studies have found Delta and Gamma Tocotrienols exhibit considerable anti-cancer activity against melanoma, via targeting CSCs, triggering ER stress, inducing apoptosis, cell cycle arrest and suppressing invasion. (51-56)

Suppression of Mevalonate Pathway

Similar to statin drugs, Tocotrienols attenuate HMG-CoA reductase which suppresses the mevalonate pathway, albeit by different mechanisms. The two (statins and tocotrienol) demonstrate anti-cancer synergy when combined. (57-59)

Tocotrienol Safety and Lack of Toxicity

No toxicities were found in a clinical trial in humans given 800 mg per day for several months. (59-62)

Protective Effects

In 2016, Dr. Nakaso studied Gamma and Delta Tocotrienol in a mouse model of Parkinson's disease (a neurodegenerative disease involving the Basal Ganglia with characteristic pill-rolling tremor and rigidity), finding Tocotrienols cytoprotective, preventing neurotoxicity and motor deficit. This cytoprotection was mediated through the estrogen receptor Beta-PI3K/Akt pathway, with the Tocotrienol binding directly to the ER-Beta receptor. (64-65)

Others have found Tocotrienol protective in renal ischemia/injury, drug induced liver injury, diabetic neuropathy, and ulcerative colitis models. (66-70)

Adverse Effects of Vitamin E

The main adverse effect of Vitamin E supplements, including tocotrienol, is a blood thinning effect with increased risk for bleeding. This is especially true for elective surgical procedures. Discontinuing all vitamin E products as well as other blood thinners a week prior to elective surgical procedures is recommended by most anesthesiologists. (71-73)

Conclusion

The case for Tocotrienol Vitamin E as anti-cancer agent is quite strong in preclinical studies. Unfortunately, research in still in its infancy regarding human clinical trials. We await data from future human clinical trials and hope they will prove favorable. In the meantime, lack of toxicity as well as cytoprotective benefit make tocotrienols an attractive addition to our *Cracking Cancer Toolkit*.

References for Chapter 41
Tocotrienol Vitamin E

1) Aggarwal, Vaishali, et al. "Molecular mechanisms of action of tocotrienols in cancer: Recent trends and advancements." International journal of molecular sciences 20.3 (2019): 656.

2) Meganathan, Puvaneswari, and Fu Ju Yen. "Tocotrienols: Emerging Evidence of Health Benefits from Clinical Trials." Palm Oil Developments 69 (2018): 16-19.

3) Meganathan, Puvaneswari, and Ju-Yen Fu. "Biological properties of tocotrienols: evidence in human studies." International journal of molecular sciences 17.11 (2016): 1682.

4) Springett, Gregory M., et al. "A phase I safety, pharmacokinetic, and Pharmacodynamic Presurgical trial of vitamin E δ-tocotrienol in patients with pancreatic ductal neoplasia." *EBioMedicine* 2.12 (2015): 1987-1995.

5) Ghanem, Paola, et al. "The Vitamin E Derivative Gamma Tocotrienol Promotes Anti-Tumor Effects in Acute Myeloid Leukemia Cell Lines." Nutrients 11.11 (2019): 2808.

6) Ng, K. L., A. K. Radhakrishnan, and K. R. Selvaduray. "Gamma-Tocotrienol Inhibits Proliferation of Human Chronic Myeloid Leukemic Cells via Activation of Extrinsic and Intrinsic Apoptotic Pathways." J. Blood Disord. Ther 1640 (2016): 1-11.

7) Fontana, Fabrizio, et al. "Natural compounds in prostate cancer prevention and treatment: mechanisms of action and molecular targets." Cells 9.2 (2020): 460.

8) Fontana, Fabrizio, et al. "Mitochondrial functional and structural impairment is involved in the antitumor activity of δ-tocotrienol in prostate cancer cells." Free Radical Biology and Medicine (2020).

9) Fontana, Fabrizio, et al. "δ-Tocotrienol induces apoptosis, involving endoplasmic reticulum stress and autophagy, and paraptosis in prostate cancer cells." Cell proliferation 52.3 (2019): e12576.

10) Tang, Kai Dun, et al. "Gamma-Tocotrienol Induces Apoptosis in Prostate Cancer Cells by Targeting the Ang-1/Tie-2 Signalling Pathway." International journal of molecular sciences 20.5 (2019): 1164.

11) Huang, Ying, et al. "A naturally occurring mixture of tocotrienols inhibits the growth of human prostate tumor, associated with epigenetic modifications of cyclin-dependent kinase inhibitors p21 and p27." The Journal of Nutritional Biochemistry 40 (2017): 155-163.

12) Asay, Spencer, et al. "γ-Tocotrienol and α-Tocopheryloxyacetic Acid Increase the Effectiveness of Docetaxel Treatment of PC-3 Prostate Cancer Cells and Docetaxel-resistant PC-3 Cells." The FASEB Journal 33.S1 (2019): 647-2.

13) Husain, Kazim, et al. "δ-Tocotrienol, a natural form of vitamin E, inhibits pancreatic cancer stem-like cells and prevents pancreatic cancer metastasis." Oncotarget 8.19 (2017): 31554.

14) Husain, Kazim, et al. "Vitamin E delta-tocotrienol targets human colon cancer stem cells and inhibits colon cancer metastasis and induces apoptosis." (2016): 3839-3839.

15) Wada, S., et al. "δ-Tocotrienol suppresses tumorigenesis by inducing apoptosis and blocking the COX-2/PGE2 pathway that stimulates tumor–stromal interactions in colon cancer." Journal of Functional Foods 35 (2017): 428-435.

16) Xu, Weili, et al. "γ-Tocotrienol inhibits proliferation and induces apoptosis via the mitochondrial pathway in human cervical cancer HeLa cells." Molecules 22.8 (2017): 1299.

17) Comitato, Raffaella, et al. "Tocotrienols induce endoplasmic reticulum stress and apoptosis in cervical cancer cells." Genes & nutrition 11.1 (2016): 1-15.

18) Zhang, Ya Hui, et al. "γ-tocotrienol inhibits the invasion and migration of human gastric cancer cells through downregulation of cyclooxygenase-2 expression." Oncology reports 40.2 (2018): 999-1007.

19) Rajasinghe, Lichchavi D., Rohini H. Pindiprolu, and Smiti Vaid Gupta. "Delta-tocotrienol inhibits non-small-cell lung cancer cell invasion via the inhibition of NF-κB, uPA activator, and MMP-9." OncoTargets and therapy 11 (2018): 4301.

20) Szulczewska-Remi, Aleksandra, and Małgorzata Nogala-Kalucka. "Studies on the growth inhibiting and non-cytotoxic effects of tocotrienols on selected cancer cell lines." Acta Scientiarum Polonorum Technologia Alimentaria 19.2 (2020)

21) Moore, Christine A., et al. "γ-Tocotrienol and metformin are cytotoxic to prostate cancer cell lines and exhibit synergy." (2018): 3977-3977.

22) Balagoni, Harika, et al. "Cytotoxic Effects of Metformin and Gamma-Tocotrienol on Colon Cancer Cells: 153." American Journal of Gastroenterology 112 (2017): S77.

23) Algayadh, Ibrahim G., and Paul William Sylvester. "Synergistic anticancer effects of combined γ-tocotrienol and pterostilbene is associated with a suppression in Rac1/WAVE 2 signaling in highly malignant breast cancer cells." (2017): 1053-1053.

24) Sylvester, Paul William, and Venkateshwara Dronamraju. "γ-Tocotrienol reversal of the Warburg effect in breast cancer cells is associated with 5'-AMP-activated kinase activation." Molecular Nutrition. Academic Press, 2020. 387-407.

25) Dronamraju, Venkateshwara, et al. "γ-Tocotrienol suppression of the Warburg effect is mediated by AMPK activation in human breast cancer cells." Nutrition and cancer 71.7 (2019): 1214-1228.

26) Parajuli, Parash, Roshan Vijay Tiwari, and Paul William Sylvester. "Anticancer effects of γ-Tocotrienol are associated with a suppression in aerobic glycolysis." Biological and Pharmaceutical Bulletin 38.9 (2015): 1352-1360.

27) Parajuli, P., R. V. Tiwari, and P. W. Sylvester. "Antiproliferative effects of γ-tocotrienol are associated with suppression of c-Myc expression in mammary tumour cells." Cell proliferation 48.4 (2015): 421-435.

28) Ahmed, Rayan, and Paul W. Sylvester. "γ-Tocotrienol Reversal of Epithelial-to-Mesenchymal Transition in Human Breast Cancer Cells is Mediated through a Suppression of Canonical Wnt and Hedgehog Signaling." Vitamin E in Health and Disease (2018): 83.

29) Ahmed, R. A., O. A. Alawin, and P. W. Sylvester. "γ-Tocotrienol reversal of epithelial-to-mesenchymal transition in human breast cancer cells is associated with inhibition of canonical Wnt signalling." Cell proliferation 49.4 (2016): 460-470.

30) Alawin, Osama A., et al. "Antiproliferative effects of γ-tocotrienol are associated with lipid raft disruption in HER2-positive human breast cancer cells." The Journal of nutritional biochemistry 27 (2016): 266-277.

31) Alawin, Osama A., et al. "γ-Tocotrienol-induced disruption of lipid rafts in human breast cancer cells is associated with a reduction in exosome heregulin content." The Journal of Nutritional Biochemistry 48 (2017): 83-93.

32) Sylvester, Paul W. "The Role of Lipid Rafts in Mediating the Anticancer Effects of γ-Tocotrienol." Vitamin E in Human Health. Humana Press, Cham, 2019. 125-140.

33) Palau, Victoria E., et al. "γ-Tocotrienol induces apoptosis in pancreatic cancer cells by upregulation of ceramide synthesis and modulation of sphingolipid transport." BMC cancer 18.1 (2018): 1-14.

34) Shirode, Amit B., and Paul W. Sylvester. "Mechanisms mediating the synergistic anticancer effects of combined γ-tocotrienol and celecoxib treatment." Journal of bioanalysis & biomedicine 3 (2011): 001.

35) Yap, W. N., et al. "γ-Tocotrienol suppresses prostate cancer cell proliferation and invasion through multiple-signalling pathways." British journal of cancer 99.11 (2008): 1832-1841.

36) Sun, Wen-Guang, et al. "γ-Tocotrienol-Inhibited Cell Proliferation of Human Gastric Cancer by Regulation of Nuclear Factor-κB Activity." Journal of agricultural and food chemistry 67.1 (2018): 441-451.

37) Yang, Chao, and Qing Jiang. "Vitamin E δ-tocotrienol inhibits TNF-α-stimulated NF-κB activation by up-regulation of anti-inflammatory A20 via modulation of sphingolipid including elevation of intracellular dihydroceramides." The Journal of nutritional biochemistry 64 (2019): 101-109.

38) Yang, Chao. Mechanistic Investigation of Resveratrol-, Pterostilbene-, and δ-Tocotrienol-Mediated Anti-Nf-κb Activity and the Effect of δ-Tocotrienol on Colitis-Promoted Colon Tumorigenesis in Mice. Diss. Purdue University, 2017.

39) Wang, HaiXia, et al. "γ-Tocotrienol inhibits oxidative phosphorylation and triggers apoptosis by inhibiting mitochondrial complex I subunit NDUFB8 and complex II subunit SDHB." Toxicology 417 (2019): 42-53.

40) Sun, Wenguang, et al. "γ-Tocotrienol induces mitochondria-mediated apoptosis in human gastric adenocarcinoma SGC-7901 cells." The Journal of nutritional biochemistry 20.4 (2009): 276-284.

41) Xu, Weili, et al. "γ-Tocotrienol inhibits proliferation and induces apoptosis via the mitochondrial pathway in human cervical cancer HeLa cells." Molecules 22.8 (2017): 1299..

42) Comitato, Raffaella, et al. "Tocotrienols activity in MCF-7 breast cancer cells: Involvement of ERβ signal transduction." Molecular nutrition & food research 54.5 (2010): 669-678.

43) Comitato, Raffaella, et al. "A novel mechanism of natural vitamin E tocotrienol activity: involvement of ERβ signal transduction." American Journal of Physiology-Endocrinology and Metabolism 297.2 (2009): E427-E437.

44) Ladikou, Eleni-Eirini, and Eva Kassi. "The emerging role of estrogen in B cell malignancies." Leukemia & Lymphoma 58.3 (2017): 528-539.

45) Yakimchuk, Konstantin, et al. "Inhibition of lymphoma vascularization and dissemination by estrogen receptor β agonists." Blood, The Journal of the American Society of Hematology 123.13 (2014): 2054-2061.

46) Roemer, Klaus, and Michael Pfreundschuh. "How do estrogens control lymphoma?." Blood, The Journal

of the American Society of Hematology 123.13 (2014): 1980-1981.

47) Talaber, Gergely, et al. "Inhibition of estrogen biosynthesis enhances lymphoma growth in mice." Oncotarget 7.15 (2016): 20718.

48) Rota, Sarah-Grace, et al. "Estrogen receptor β is a novel target in acute myeloid leukemia." Molecular Cancer Therapeutics 16.11 (2017): 2618-2626.

49) Ladikou, Eleni-Eirini, and Eva Kassi. "The emerging role of estrogen in B cell malignancies." Leukemia & Lymphoma 58.3 (2017): 528-539.

50) Rudelius, Martina, et al. "The G protein-coupled estrogen receptor 1 (GPER-1) contributes to the proliferation and survival of mantle cell lymphoma cells." haematologica 100.11 (2015): e458.

51) Marzagalli, Monica, et al. "Estrogen receptor β agonists differentially affect the growth of human melanoma cell lines." PLoS One 10.7 (2015): e0134396.

52) Marzagalli, Monica, et al. "Estrogen receptor β in melanoma: from molecular insights to potential clinical utility." Frontiers in endocrinology 7 (2016): 140.

53) Marzagalli, Monica, et al. "Targeting melanoma stem cells with the Vitamin E derivative δ-tocotrienol." Scientific reports 8.1 (2018): 1-13.

54) Marelli, Marina Montagnani, et al. "Vitamin E δ-tocotrienol triggers endoplasmic reticulum stress-mediated apoptosis in human melanoma cells." Scientific reports 6.1 (2016): 1-14.

55) Chang, Piek Ngoh, et al. "Evidence of γ-tocotrienol as an apoptosis-inducing, invasion-suppressing, and chemotherapy drug-sensitizing agent in human melanoma cells." Nutrition and cancer 61.3 (2009): 357-366.

56) Fernandes, Nicolle V., Praveen K. Guntipalli, and Huanbiao Mo. "d-δ-Tocotrienol-mediated cell cycle arrest and apoptosis in human melanoma cells." Anticancer research 30.12 (2010): 4937-4944.

57) Wali, Vikram B., Sunitha V. Bachawal, and Paul W. Sylvester. "Suppression in mevalonate synthesis mediates antitumor effects of combined statin and γ-tocotrienol treatment." Lipids 44.10 (2009): 925.

58) Wali, Vikram B., Sunitha V. Bachawal, and Paul W. Sylvester. "Combined treatment of γ-tocotrienol with statins induce mammary tumor cell cycle arrest in G1." Experimental Biology and Medicine 234.6 (2009): 639-650.

59) Eitsuka, Takahiro, et al. "Synergistic anticancer effect of tocotrienol combined with chemotherapeutic agents or dietary components: a review." International journal of molecular sciences 17.10 (2016): 1605.

60) Montagnani Marelli, Marina, et al. "Anticancer properties of tocotrienols: A review of cellular mechanisms and molecular targets." Journal of cellular physiology 234.2 (2019): 1147-1164.

61) Ismail, Maznah, et al. "Safety and Neuroprotective Efficacy of Palm Oil and Tocotrienol-Rich Fraction from Palm Oil: A Systematic Review." Nutrients 12.2 (2020): 521.

62) Kanchi, Madhu M., et al. "Tocotrienols: the unsaturated sidekick shifting new paradigms in vitamin E therapeutics." Drug Discovery Today 22.12 (2017): 1765-1781.

63) Mishra, B. P., et al. "Tocotrienols as Potential Therapeutic Supplement." Indian Journal of Medical & Health Sciences 3.1 (2016): 51.

64) Nakaso, Kazuhiro, et al. "The estrogen receptor β-PI3K/Akt pathway mediates the cytoprotective effects of tocotrienol in a cellular Parkinson's disease model." Biochimica et Biophysica Acta (BBA)-Molecular Basis of Disease 1842.9 (2014): 1303-1312.

65) Nakaso, Kazuhiro, et al. "Estrogen receptor-mediated effect of δ-tocotrienol prevents neurotoxicity and motor deficit in the MPTP mouse model of Parkinson's disease." Neuroscience letters 610 (2016): 117-122.

66) Nowak, Grazyna, Judit Megyesi, and Yingni Che. "γ-Tocotrienol Protects Against Mitochondrial Dysfunction, Energy Deficits, Tissue Damage, and Decreases in Renal Functions After Renal Ischemia." The FASEB Journal 34.S1 (2020): 1-1.

67) Ng, Yeek Tat, et al. "The Effects of Tocotrienol-Rich Vitamin E (Tocovid) on Diabetic Neuropathy: A Phase II Randomized Controlled Trial." Nutrients 12.5 (2020): 1522.

68) Tan, Gerald Chen Jie, et al. "Tocotrienol-rich vitamin E improves diabetic nephropathy and persists 6–9 months after washout: a phase IIa randomized

controlled trial." Therapeutic advances in endocrinology and metabolism 10 (2019): 2042018819895462.

69) Saw, Tzuen Yih, et al. "Oral supplementation of tocotrienol-rich fraction alleviates severity of ulcerative colitis in mice." Journal of nutritional science and vitaminology 65.4 (2019): 318-327.

70) Tan, Cheau Yih, et al. "Comparative hepatoprotective effects of tocotrienol analogs against drug-induced liver injury." Redox biology 4 (2015): 308-320.

71) Beoy, Lim Ai, Wong Jia Woei, and Yuen Kah Hay. "Effects of tocotrienol supplementation on hair growth in human volunteers." Tropical life sciences research 21.2 (2010): 91.

72) Schauss, Alexander G., John R. Endres, and Amy Clewell. "Safety of unsaturated vitamin e tocotrienols and their isomers." Tocotrienols: Vitamin E beyond tocopherols (2013).

73) Meganathan, Puvaneswari, and Ju-Yen Fu. "Biological properties of tocotrienols: evidence in human studies." International journal of molecular sciences 17.11 (2016): 1682.

74) Loganathan, R., et al. "Tocotrienols promote apoptosis in human breast cancer cells by inducing poly (ADP-ribose) polymerase cleavage and inhibiting nuclear factor kappa-B activity." Cell proliferation 46.2 (2013): 203-213.

75) Tan, Barrie, and John Foley. "Tocotrienols and geranylgeraniol from Bixa orellana byproducts." U.S. Patent No. 6,350,453. 26 Feb. 2002.

76) Tan, Barrie, Ronald Ross Watson, and Victor R. Preedy, eds. Tocotrienols: vitamin E beyond tocopherols. CrC press, 2012.

Chapter 42

Final Words

THE GOAL OF *CRACKING CANCER Toolkit* is to provide a basic understanding of metabolic pathways in cancer cells, and the repurposed drugs and supplements targeting them. In this journey, we have identified the three pillars of cancer cell metabolism, OXPHOS, GLYCOLYSIS and Autophagy. Blocking all three concurrently results in "synthetic lethality" and our best chance to eradicate cancer stem cells, thus providing long term durable remission. We have also identified additional anti-cancer targets; detaching HKII from VDAC, restoring anti-cancer immunity, downregulating inflammation, and preventing platelet activation, etc.

Why Hasn't My Doctor Told Me About This?

One might then ask the next obvious question: "Why hasn't my doctor already told me about repurposed anticancer drugs?" The answer becomes obvious if we look at a different disease, viral disease. The fact that repurposed drugs exist for highly effective treatment of viral disease has been recently highlighted by the COVID-19 pandemic. Indeed, many of the drugs repurposed for cancer treatment, have anti-viral activity, especially in the category of autophagy inhibitors.

Repurposed Drugs for Highly Effective Anti-Viral Treatment

I would like you to read this quote from Lee Merritt, MD (2020). "The Treatment of Viral Diseases: Has the Truth Been Suppressed for Decades?" J Amer Phys and Surg 25.3. In your mind, while reading this quote, replace the word "virus", with the word "cancer", and replace the word "vaccine" with the word "chemotherapy ", and voila, everything becomes clear. In many ways, repurposing drugs for anti-viral treatment is analogous to repurposing drugs for anti-cancer treatment.

The Untreatable Viral Diseases

Dr. Merritt writes about her early medical school days in 1976, indoctrinated in the medical dogma that viral diseases are "untreatable". Dr. Merritt believed this for many years until the recent COVID-19 pandemic made her aware of old research showing Hydroxychloroquine, Azithromycin and Zinc highly effective for treatment of viral disease:

> Since I started medical school in 1976, until 2020, I have heard the dogma that viral diseases are not treatable….certainly not with antimicrobials…. Since viral diseases are not treatable, our only weapon is vaccination…. Consider that the entire $69 billion-per-year vaccine industry is based on "preventing" viral diseases that are otherwise "untreatable"—like viral influenza

A, measles, etc. If a cheap and effective treatment is available for these illnesses, **the entire vaccine industry crashes down like a house of cards** [emphasis mine]…

Based on the currently available science, it is probable that treatment with HCQ [Hydroxychloroquine] in patients with severe influenza and ILI [Influenza like Illness] could have saved millions of Americans from dying. And people within the inner circle of pharmaceutical research **must have known this** [emphasis mine]. Pharmaceutical firms employ thousands of virologists and infectious disease experts. Are we to believe they failed to read and pursue the relevant viral research?… How could all our medical education "overlook" this basic science? It may be difficult for non-physicians to appreciate the magnitude of this world-shaking scientific omission—and probable cover-up. It is the pharmaceutical equivalent of being told for 40 years the world is flat—only to have it conclusively exposed overnight to be round. This idea that viruses—like the current pandemic SARS-CoV-2 virus—can be killed by commonly used drugs—antibiotics, antimalarial, or antiparasitic agents—profoundly changes the practice of medicine…

The COVID-19 pandemic is calling attention to the potential for treating viral diseases with currently available drugs, and exposing long-available but ignored research. The implications of all this are very disturbing. Where have the virologists been, and the CDC "experts" who claim to care about influenza deaths? Has the burgeoning nearly trillion-dollar vaccine industry been built at the expense of patients' lives?

[Endquote Lee Merritt, MD]

Crashing Down Like a House of Cards

The extraordinary thing about Dr. Merritt's testimony is the astonishing fact she was kept in the dark for decades (most of her medical career), with no knowledge of repurposed drugs as highly effective antiviral treatment. This suppression of knowledge, and even government interference with prescribing repurposed drugs for anti-viral treatment is not an isolated event, and happens in other fields of medicine, particularly oncology and cancer treatment.

So-called "untreatable" viral diseases can be treated with highly effective repurposed drugs. The same can be said for "incurable" cancers, now made treatable and perhaps "curable" with repurposed drugs. Now you know why your doctor has not told you about repurposed drugs for cancer treatment. They just don't know about it. The knowledge has been suppressed.

As Dr. Merritt points out, should knowledge and use of repurposed drugs for viral disease become widespread in the medical community, the vaccine industry is at risk, since many vaccines target viral disease, and vaccine use depends on having "no other effective treatment."

Similarly, should knowledge and widespread use of repurposed drugs for cancer become widespread in the medical community, the chemotherapy paradigm and chemotherapy drug industry is at risk.

What happens next? As Dr. Merritt so eloquently stated: "the entire industry crashes down like a house of cards."

Join the Revolution in Medicine

By reading this book, you are taking part in a revolution in medicine happening right now. To make this revolution succeed, give a copy of this book to your oncologist, and friends and family members who have cancer. My hope is that *Cracking Cancer Toolkit* will illuminate the path toward improved outcomes for the 2 million new cancer patients annually.

Do you have a success story using repurposed drugs? We want to hear about it. You are invited to visit us at www.crackingcancertoolkit.com and www.jeffreydachmd.com. There you will find links to join our *Cracking Cancer Toolkit* social media community and share your stories with others.

Jeffrey Dach MD
Davie, Florida

Quick Reference Guide

Glycolysis Inhibitors

2DG 2-De-Oxy-Glucose

Alpha Lipoic Acid (ALA) Increases PDC activity.

Aspirin

Auranofin Dual GLYCOLYSIS and OXPHOS Inhibitor

Betulinic Acid

Clotrimazole

Curcumin

DCA Dichloroacetate

Diclofenac

EGCG Epigallocatechin Gallate Green Tea

Fenbendazole

Melatonin

Poly-MVA Palladium, ALA and Thiamine

Quercetin Inhibits PDK.

Thiamine Increases PDC activity.

Thymoquinone HIF1 and Glycolysis Inhibitor

Tocotrienol Vitamin E

Vitamin C Intravenous

HKII – VDAC Inhibitors- Detach HK2 from VDAC

3Bromo-Pyruvate 3BP, Research only

Aspirin Detaches HK2 from VDAC

Baicalin Skull Cap, Oroxylin A

CBD Cannabidiol

Chrysin

Clotrimazole

Curcumin

Fenbendazole

Fenofibrate Lipid Lowering

Itraconazole Anti-fungal

Lithium Orotate or Lithium Carbonate

Methyl Jasmonate

Pterostilbene Resveratrol

Sulindac

OXPHOS Inhibitors – (all inhibit Wnt pathway, cancer stem cell agents)

Atovaquone Inhibits Complex II and III of ETC.

Auranofin Dual GLYCOLYSIS and OXPHOS Inhibitor

Berberine Inhibits Complex I of ETC.

Clarithromycin (Azithromycin) Inhibits large mitochondrial ribosome. Also Inhibits Autophagy.

Doxycycline Inhibits small mitochondrial ribosome.

Fenofibrate Inhibits Complex I of ETC.

Ivermectin Inhibits Complex I ETC.

Metformin Inhibits Complex I of ETC.

Niclosamide Dual OXPHOS and Autophagy inhibitor

Propranolol Dual OXPHOS and Autophagy Inhibitor

Pterostilbene

Pyrvinium pamoate Inhibits Complex I and II of ETC.

Sulforaphane Depletes Glutathione, Increases ROS.

Tocotrienol Vitamin E Inhibits Complex I and II of ETC.

Autophagy Inhibitors

Chloroquine Antimalarial

Clarithromycin Potently blocks late stage autophagy.

Dipyridamole Anti-Platelet Agent

Doxycycline Down-regulates autophagy Marker LC3B.

Hydroxychloroquine Anti-Malarial

Loratidine Claritin® CAD Antihistamine

Mefloquine Anti-Malarial

Niclosamide Anti-parasitic, inhibits mTOR, induces protective autophagy, yet, strongly blocks late stage autophagy by inducing lysosomal dysfunction.

Omeprazole Prilosec® PPI Proton Pump Inhibitor

PPI's Proton Pump Inhibitors

Propranolol Beta-Blocker, Both OXPHOS and Autophagy Inhibitor, Synergy with Glycolysis Inhibitors such as DCA

Pyrvinium Anti-parasitic, suppresses transcription of autophagy genes.

Thymoquinone Black Seed, inhibition of auto-phagy at the gene transcriptional level, induces lysosomal dysfunction.

Restores Anti-Tumor Immunity

AHCC Beta-Glucans

Artemisinin Artesunate

ATRA All-Trans Retinoic Acid, Vesinoid®

Celecoxib Cox-2 Inhibitor

Coley's Toxins

Cimetidine Antihistamine, Antacid

DCA By inhibiting lactate in the microenvironment.

Diclofenac

Dipyridamole

Glycolysis Inhibitors Reduces lactate production in TME.

Iodine molecular

Mebendazole

Metformin

Mifepristone (RU-486) Blocks PIBF.

Probiotics

Propranolol

Retinoids Vitamin A, Synthetic Derivatives, ATRA, Accutane

Vitamin D3

Topo-Isomerase Inhibitors

Boswellia (Frankincense)

Fluoroquinolone Antibiotics

Etoposide

Microtubule Inhibitors

Fenbendazole Synergy with DCA

Mebendazole Synergy with Autophagy Inhibitors

Mifepristone RU-486

Statin Drugs Destabilize Cytoskeleton

Taxane Chemotherapy Drugs

DNA Methylation Inhibitors (Inhibits DNMT)

Thymoquinone

Curcumin

Berberine

Cancer Stem Cell Agents

ATRA Vitamin A Derivatives

Chloroquine

Clarithromycin Dual OXPHOS and Glycolysis Inhibitor

Combination of IV Vitamin C, Doxycycline

Curcumin

DCA Combined with Melatonin

Doxycycline

Ivermectin

Melatonin

Niclosamide

Pyrvinium

Sulforaphane

Downregulating Antioxidant Protection Depleting Glutathione

Auranofin Inhibits thioredoxin reductase system.

Celecoxib Cox-2 Inhibitor

Parthenolide (Feverfew)

PQQ PyrroloQuinoline-Quinine

Solomon's seal PCL

Sulfasalazine Blocks Xct system for cysteine uptake.

Sulforaphane Downreglulates intracellular glutathione.

Tumor Micro Environment (TME)

Aspirin (ASA) Decreases inflammatory cytokines in TME.

Metformin Decreases inflammatory cytokines in TME.

Pyrvinium Blocks energy and glutathione transfer from stromal cells to cancer cells.

Sulfasalazine Prevents cysteine uptake by CAFs, cancer associated fibroblasts, in TME.

Blocking Growth Factors

Dipyridamole Blocks PDGF, Platelet Derived Growth Factor.

Exemestane Irreversible aromatase inhibitor blocks local estrogen production incrine by cancer cells.

LDN-OGF Opiate Growth Factor, Low Dose Naltrexone binds to OGF Receptor and inhibits tumor growth.

Solomon's Seal Blocks EGFR, Epithelial Growth Factor Receptor.

VEGF inhibitors (Vascular Endothelial Growth Factor)

Itraconazole

Propranolol

Sulforaphane

Thymoquinone

HIF-1 Inhibitor (inhibits angiogenesis)

Curcumin

DCA

EGCG epigallocatechin

Quercetin

Resveratrol/Pterostilbene

Sulforaphane

Thymoquinone Leader

MMP inhibition- Matrix Metallo Proteinase

Alpha Lipoic Acid

Doxycycline

Fenofibrate

Mebendazole

Parthenolide (Feverfew)

Sulforaphane

Blocking NF-kB Inflammatory Pathway

Artemisinin Artesunate

Aspirin

Azithromycin

Baicalein Oroxylin A, Chinese Skullcap

Berberine

Boswellia (Frankincense)

CBD Cannabidiol

Clarithromycin

Curcumin

Doxycycline Potent Inhibitor

Fenofibrate

Ivermectin

Mefloquine

Niclosamide

Parthenolide (Feverfew)

Pterostilbene

Statin Drugs (Atorvastatin)

Sulfasalazine Potent Inhibitor

Sulforaphane

Thymoquinone

COX Inhibitors

Aspirin Irreversible Inhibitor of COX-1 and COX-2

Celecoxib COX-2 Inhibitor

Diclofenac Nonspecific COX Inhibitor

Dipyridamole

Sulindac Nonspecific COX inhibitor, suppresses 5-LOX.

5-LOX Inhibitors:

Allicin Active Ingredient in Garlic

Boswellia Frankincense

Itraconazole Potent 5-LOX Inhibitor

Sulindac NSAID

Thymoquinone Black Seed Nigella Sativa

WNT Pathway inhibitors

Artemisinin Artesunate

Curcumin

ECGC (Green Tea)

Itraconazole

Ivermectin Blocks TCF gene expression perfectly.

Melatonin

Niclosamide Inhibits co-receptor LRP6.

OXPHOS Inhibitors are all Wnt inhibitors.

Pyrvinium

Pterostilbene Resveratrol

Retinoids Vitamin A Derivatives

Silybin (Milk Thistle) Also Inhibits LRP6.

Sulforaphane

Tocotrienol Vitamin E

Hedgehog Pathway Inhibitors

Chloroquine

Curcumin

Itraconazole

Mebendazole

Sulforaphane

Tocotrienol Vitamin E

Notch Pathway Inhibitors

Curcumin

Niclosamide

Sulindac

Downregulate BCL-2 Restoring Apoptosis
All agents which detach HKII from VDAC, and OXPHOS agents down regulate BCL2.

Alpha Lipoic Acid

Curcumin

Fenofibrate

Itraconazole

Ivermectin

LDN (Low Dose Naltrexone)

Mebendazole

Drugs Independent of Mutated P53

Alpha Lipoic Acid

Metformin Plus Curcumin

Niclosamide

Thymoquinone

Angiogenesis Inhibitors

Cimetidine

Itraconazole

Fenofibrate

Propranolol

Antihistamines

Loratidine (Claritin®) H1 Receptor Blocker

Cimetidine H2 Receptor Blocker

FASN inhibitor Fatty Acid Synthetase (Orlistat)

Fenofibrate

Quercetin

Reduce P-Glycoprotein (Multi Drug Resistance)

Itraconazole

Clarithromycin

Ivermectin

Depends on Functioning P53

Fenbendazole

Androgen Receptor Blocker

Pyrvinium (potent blocker)

PI3K/Akt/mTOR inhibitors – all activate protective autophagy

Boswellia

Ivermectin PAK1 Inhibitor-mTOR

Itraconazole Also autophagy inhibitor by inhibition of NPC1 (Niemann-Pick C1) a lysosomal membrane protein.

Propranolol

Pterostilbene

Quercetin

Solomon's seal

C-Myc Inhibitors
(Note C-Myc is downstream from Wnt, so all Wnt inhibitors are also c-Myc inhibitors)

Artesunate Degrades c-Myc.

Celecoxib Cox-2 Inhibitor

Diclofenac NSAID

Nitazoxanide (Alinia) (Top Hit)

Pterostilbene

Sulforaphane

Glossary Terms in Alphabetical Order

Aerobic Glycolysis (Warburg Effect)

is the metabolic alteration of the cancer cell using massive amounts of glucose in the cytoplasm to support rapid growth and proliferation. This is called the Warburg Effect, and allows visualization of cancer on the PET scan using a radio-labeled isotope of glucose (fluorodeoxyglucose, 18 F-FDG or FDG). Aerobic glycolysis means the cancer cells upregulate GLYCOLYSIS in the cytoplasm while downregulating, or inhibiting OXPHOS (oxidative phosphorylation) in the mitochondria. Aerobic glycolysis (the Warburg Effect) is associated with high lactate generation and low glucose oxidation despite normal levels of oxygen. The expelled lactate extruded by cancer cells into the extra-cellular space inhibits the host immune system. In this book, we refer to aerobic glycolysis simply as GLYCOLYSIS, a term referring to the metabolism of glucose by cancer cells (the Warburg Effect). (1-2)

Anaerobic Glycolysis

Takes place in normal cells under hypoxic conditions in which glucose is metabolized in the cytoplasm to carbon dioxide and water with production of lactate. For example hypoxic skeletal muscle cells in marathon runners use anaerobic glycolysis.

AIF (Apoptosis-Inducing Factor)

is a small protein located in mitochondria, which triggers apoptosis when released into the cytosol, and ultimately reaches the cell nucleus (nuclear translocation) where AIF triggers DNA fragmentation. For example, metformin and cisplatin induce apoptosis in cancer cells via nuclear translocation of AIF. (3-4)

Akt Oncogene (Protein Kinase B)

Akt is activated by phosphorylation (adding a phosphate group), and Akt is the main effector of PI3K pathway, which strongly promotes cancer cell metabolism, proliferation, survival by stimulating GLYCOLYSIS. This is done by increasing Glucose transporters, and activating the pro-cancer mTOR pathway, turning on angiogenesis, increased metabolic activity, growth, proliferation, survival, protein synthesis, transcription, and preventing apoptosis. (5-6)

AMPK (5' adenosine monophosphate-activated protein kinase)

is the main fuel (energy) sensor in cancer cells. Activation of AMPK inhibits the PI3K/Akt/mTOR pathway which induces "protective autophagy", suppresses tumor growth and helps reverse the Warburg Effect. AMP-K is activated by Metformin, Berberine, Fenofibrate, Itraconazole, Tocotrienol (Vitamin E), intermittent fasting, caloric restriction (CR), etc. (7-8)

Angiogenesis

is the induction and ingrowth of new blood vessels which provide nutrients for a growing cancer mass. Growth factors such as VEGF (vascular endothelial growth factor) and PDGF (platelet derived growth factor) are potent stimulators of angiogenesis. (9)

Antegrade Lysosomal Trafficking

is a function controlled by mTOR in which lysosomes migrate along the cytoskeleton system to the cell periphery near the cell membrane in preparation for invasive, aggressive behavior. Once located at the cell membrane, the lysosomes are now in position for releasing enzymes for digestion and degradation of the extracellular tissues in preparation for tumor invasion, as well as for taking up nutrients from the microenvironment to feed the cancer mass. The opposite of antegrade trafficking is "Peri-Nuclear Clustering" of lysosomes, in which lysosomes migrate to the center of the cell near the nucleus. "Perinuclear Clustering" indicates a dormant, benign state called "protective autophagy". For example, Niclosamide inhibits antegrade lysosomal trafficking. (10- 12)

Apoptosis (Intrinsic and Extrinsic)

is programmed cell death normally invoked when cells are damaged by the aging process. The goal of *Cracking Cancer Toolkit* is to gently push the cancer cell over the "Apoptotic Threshold". This triggers mitochondrial apoptosis, also called the intrinsic pathway, a form of programmed cell death initiated by increased MMP (mitochondrial membrane permeability) with leakage of cytochrome C into the cytoplasm. Cytochrome C is a protein found in the ETC, the electron transport chain. This release of Cytochrome C from the VDAC at the outer membrane into the cytosol activates the caspase 9 enzyme cascade culminating in DNA fragmentation and cell death. The process is controlled by the pro-apoptotic Bax proteins and the anti-apoptotic BCL-2 and Bcl-XL family of proteins located on the outer mitochondrial membrane. The BCL-2 inhibitor drug Venetoclax, FDA approved drug for hematologic malignancy, induces apoptosis by disrupting the interaction of BCL-2 with the VDAC.

The Extrinsic Pathway is initiated by cell membrane death receptors such as TNF (tumor necrosis factor) receptor ultimately leading to activation of caspase 8, and cell death.

Apoptosis results in an orderly process of cell death with little inflammatory response, unlike cell necrosis caused by chemotherapy which spills cell contents freely into the extra-cellular space, causing an undesirable massive inflammatory reaction. The inflammatory reaction induced by chemotherapy is a growth stimulator for cancer stem cells, and a direct cause of cancer relapse with a more aggressive, now drug resistant cell type. Thus, apoptotic death of cancer cells is preferable to necrotic death induced by chemotherapy. (13-15)

Apoptotic Threshold

The point at which cancer cells spontaneously undergo apoptosis, usually induced by simultaneous inhibition of the "Three Pillars of Cancer Cell Metabolism", GLYCOLYSIS, OXPHOS and AUTOHAGY. Additional anti-cancer interventions include detachment of Hexokinase II from the VDAC, restoration of the host immune system, and downregulation of inflammatory cytokines.

Atovaquone (Mepron®)

Is an FDA approved antimalarial, antiparasitic drug used for pneumocystis prophylaxis, also repurposed as anti-cancer drug as OXPHOS inhibitor via inhibition of mitochondrial ETC Complex II and III. Atovaquone is an analog of ubiquinone, and also inhibits Coenzyme Q10 (Ubiquinone) synthesis. Thus, taking a Co-Q10 supplement simultaneously with atovaquone reduces its efficacy. (16-18)

ATPase Adenylpyrophosphatase (ATP hydrolase)

is the enzyme which splits ATP into ADP and P- (free phosphate ion), thus liberating energy. ATPase is inhibited by Propranolol, thus inhibiting

mitochondrial OXPHOS activity. (see Dr. Wei, 1985) Quercetin also inhibits plasma membrane Calcium-ATPase (PMCA). (152)

ATP Synthase (Complex V of the ETC)

Unlike ATPase which splits ATP, ATP Synthase goes in the opposite direction, and forms ATP from ADP by catalyzing the reaction of ADP to ATP. ATP Synthase is mitochondrial complex V of the ETC (electron transport chain) inhibited by Bedaquiline (antibiotic for Tuberculosis) and Mefloquine.

ATRA (All Trans Retinoic Acid – Vesinoid®)

Is a retinoid, a synthetic version of vitamin A, FDA approved for treatment of lymphoma and leukemia, and actually "curative" for promyelocytic leukemia. ATRA regulates miRNA and augments anti-tumor immunity by reducing the population of MDSC's (Myeloid Derived Suppressor Cells). This improves efficacy of CAR-T therapy and anti-angiogenesis therapy. Retinoids (Vitamin A derivatives) are synergistic with the PPAR agonist drugs such as Fenofibrate, improving anti-cancer efficacy. The anti-acne drug, Accutane® (isotretinoin) and many other Vitamin A derivatives (retinoids) are repurposed as anti-cancer drugs. (19-23)

Auranofin (AF)

Is an old gold-containing, FDA approved, rheumatology drug used for arthritis, repurposed as anticancer drug via inhibition of the thioredoxin reductase anti-oxidant system (TrxR), thus sensitizing cancer cells to oxidative therapies. Auranofin (AF) inhibits the PI3K/AKT/mTOR pathway and has been repurposed for treatment of P53 mutated and PTEN-deleted refractory B Cell Lymphoma, and enhances activity of Ibrutinib in EGFR mutant Lung Cancer. Auranofin has potent preclinical activity in CLL (chronic lymphocytic leukemia). Auranofin was found surprisingly effective against B Cell lymphoma (Mantle Cell) mouse xenografts, overcoming drug resistance in the stromal microenvironment. Apparently, TrxR is upregulated in lymphoma located in the stromal microenvironment, where AF transforms the TrxR system into an ROS generating anti-cancer weapon. However, the main AF anticancer mechanism of action (MOA) is independent of the TrxR system, found to be dual GLYCOLYSIS and OXPHOS inhibition with suppression of FTC Complex II activity, and inhibition of GAPDH (glyceraldehyde phosphate dehydrogenase), a key Glycolytic enzyme, with reduction in cellular ATP. Normal cells were able to compensate and were unaffected. Recent studies show triple combination of AF, Vitamin C (ascorbate) and Vitamin K (Menadione) synergistic against TNBC (triple negative breast cancer) in vitro and in vivo. Similarly, the combination of Auranofin and anti-PD-L1 checkpoint inhibitor drug is synergistically effective for TNBC. Auranofin has antiviral activity, inhibits corona virus replication (SARS-COV-2), as well as anti-inflammatory and antibacterial effects against MERSA and Clostridia. (24-31)

Autophagy

In 2020 Dr. Gewirtz defined "Autophagy", a Greek word meaning "self-eating", as a cell process in which the cell eats its own organelles in response to nutrient deprivation, anoxia, chemotherapy, radiation and other stressful conditions. The first step is autophagosome formation. These are double membraned vacuoles containing the cellular cargo later to be fused with lysosomes, small vesicles containing acid and enzymes, to form autolysosomes, in which the cargo is degraded in preparation for recycling by the cell. Autophagy is controlled by the AMPK/mTOR pathway. Inhibition of mTOR activates "protective autophagy", a dormant state with perinuclear clustering of lysosomes. Activation of mTOR activates antegrade lysosomal tracking, and aggressive, proliferative cancer behavior. For use in the lab, the accumulation of LC-II, LC3-II (light chain microtubule associated protein) and p62 protein are the two markers indicating successful inhibition of autophagy. Lysosomal function is dependent on acid pH produced by the V-ATPase proton pump in membrane wall of the lysosome. For example, Niclosamide blocks late stage autophagy. See the autophagy chapters 31-35 for more on this topic. (32-33)

Bax Protein

is the pro-apoptosis protein triggered by P53, which causes cancer cells to undergo apoptosis.

BCL-2 Protein

Is the anti-apoptosis protein upregulated in many aggressive cancers, and is a major player preventing apoptosis, thus "immortalizing" the cancer cell. A valid anti-cancer strategy is downregulation of BCL2 with various natural substances and repurposed drugs mentioned in this book. A new drug, venetoclax (ABT-199) is a selective inhibitor of BCL2, allowing the cancer cells to undergo apoptosis. Detachment of HK II from the VDAC is another strategy which decreases BCL-2 and restores apoptosis to the cancer cell. The BCL-2 protein regulates release of Cytochrome C by the VDAC on the outer mitochondrial membrane, thus preventing apoptosis. (34)

Beta Catenin Protein

is the key signaling protein for the Wnt cancer stem cell pathway. When Beta-Catenin is degraded in the cytoplasm or translocated to the cell membrane, Wnt is turned off. However, when Beta Catenin is translocated to the cell nucleus, this turns on TCF/LEF for nuclear transcription of downstream mediators c-Myc and Cyclin D1.

Betulinic Acid (BET)

Is a Glycolysis Inhibitor, and natural supplement first isolated in 1788 from white birch tree bark. In addition to anti-cancer properties, BET has anti-bacterial, anti-malarial, anti-inflammatory, anti-parasitic, and anti-viral activities. (35-36)

BH3 Mimetic

is B-cell lymphoma 2 (Bcl-2) Homology 3 mimetic, a small orally available molecule (Venetoclax®) which inhibits the anti-apoptotic Bcl-2 protein family, including Bcl-2, Bcl-xl and Bcl-w. Thus restoring apoptosis in cancer cells.

Bleeding (Adverse Side Effect)

Allicin from Garlic, and thiosulfinates, are potent platelet inhibitors which can aggravate bleeding, so caution is advised when used with other platelet inhibitors such as Feverfew, Aspirin, Vitamin E, Fish Oil, Gingko, and Ibrutinib (Imbruvica – Bruton's-Kinase Inhibitor).

CAD (Cationic Amphiphilic Drug)

are drugs such as Loratadine (Claritin®), an H1 receptor blocker antihistamine, which accumulate in lysosomes 1,000 fold, causing lysosomal dysfunction and inhibition of autophagy. This drug family includes diverse drugs such as antihistamines (loratadine), antimalarials (mefloquine), antipsychotics, cardiac antiarrhythmic drugs (amiodorone), and tranquilizers. Many viruses replicate within lysosomes, a process blocked by CAD drugs. Thus many CAD drugs are excellent anti-viral agents. (37-38)

CAFs Cancer Associated Fibroblasts

are the stromal fibroblasts in the tumor microenvironment (TME) surrounding the tumor mass which are recruited to provide nutrients and growth factors to feed the cancer.

Cancer as a Metabolic Disease

proposed by Thomas N. Seyfried as alternative to the prevailing dogma that cancer is a result of somatic mutations, Dr. Seyfried proposed that alterations in metabolic pathways in the mitochondria, specifically the Warburg Effect, and relocation of HKII to the VDAC, are defining features which can be exploited as the "Achilles Heel" of the cancer cell. (39)

Cancer as a Parasitic Disease

This is the theory that cancer resembles a parasitic disease, supported by animal models in which parasitic diseases closely resemble lymphoma and other cancers. This theory is also supported by the sheer fact that many anti-parasitic and anti-fungal drugs are effective repurposed anti-cancer drugs. (40)

Cancer as a Trophoblastic Disease

This is the theory that cancer is a form of "placental cell" or "germ cell" which uses many of the same molecular circuits as trophoblast cells use, to invade locally, induce its own blood supply, and evade the immune system of the host. The trophoblast is the Placental Cell of Pregnancy. Both cancer cells and trophoblast cells secrete HCG (human chorionic gonadotropin) and PIBF (progesterone induced blocking factor). (41)

Cancer Screening for the Population

Includes the detection of breast cancer with mammography, prostate cancer with PSA, thyroid nodule screening with ultrasound, colon cancer with colonoscopy, and cervical cancer with PAP smears. This has not been discussed in the book up to this point.

To summarize my opinion: with the exception of colonoscopy for detection and removal of pre-malignant colon polyps, and PAP smears for detection of cervical cancer, the other three cancer screening programs (breast, thyroid, prostate) are a disappointment and should be discontinued. These three cancer screening programs have resulted in overdiagnosis and harm associated with unnecessary procedures, and have failed to reduce national mortality for these three cancers. (200-205)

Cancer Stem Cell Pathways Wnt, Hh and Notch

Are Wnt (Wingless Integrative), Hedgehog (Hh) and Notch, all three forming a network with considerable crosstalk. Inhibition of all three pathways eradicates cancer stem cells. (42-43)

Cancer Stem Cells

Also called "tumor initiating cells" (TICs), these cancer stem cells are dormant, not actively replicating, and not visible on PET scans because they do not avidly take up glucose. Induction of "Protective Autophagy" plays a role in maintaining dormancy of cancer stem cells. Cancer stem cells remain in the body after a course of chemotherapy, and then, after a variable length of time (called a temporary remission), the cancer stem cells become active and repopulate the tumor mass. This process is accelerated by the massive inflammation induced by chemotherapy. The cancer stem cells represent only a small fraction of the tumor mass, and are capable of inducing new tumors when transplanted into immunodeficient mice.

Cancer stem cells are chemo-resistant (MDR multi drug resistant), and have metabolic plasticity with ability to switch back and forth between Glycolysis to OXPHOS phenotype. Cancer stem cells are resistant to apoptosis and ROS (reactive oxygen species) and have a high capacity for DNA damage repair, etc. When activated, cancer stem cells become aggressive, circulate freely in the blood stream (CTC circulating tumor cells), and have the capacity for colonizing distant sites causing metastatic disease. (44-46)

Cardiac Glycosides (CG)

Is a family of cardiac drugs including digitoxin, digitalis, ouabain, strophanthidin, peruvoside, lanatoside, etc. Originally derived from the foxglove plant and used for centuries in treatment of heart disease (congestive heart failure and atrial fibrillation), CG drugs have been repurposed as anti-cancer and anti-viral drugs. These drugs all possess a steroidal ring chemical structure similar to endogenous CG produced by the adrenal gland. The MOA (mechanism of action) is suppression of the Na+/k+-ATPase, thus decreasing the intracellular Potassium (K+) and increasing Sodium (Na+) and Calcium (Ca2+). Lung cancer (with STK11 mutation), glioma, melanoma and renal cancer are known to have over-expressed Na+/k+-ATPase and are especially sensitive to the anticancer effects of CG. Additional anti-cancer mechanisms of CG include inhibition of IL-8 production (Interleukin 8) a key inflammatory cytokine, and inhibition of DNA topoisomerase I and II. Digitoxin is a potent inhibitor of NF-κB, blocking production of pro-inflammatory cytokines. As of 2020, there are four clinical trials underway. Digitoxin has more potent anticancer effects compared to digoxin. (47-54)

Catecholamines

are epinephrine and norepinephrine, stress hormones secreted by the adrenal glands in response to beta-adrenergic stimulation from the autonomic nervous system, the "fight or flight" response. Catecholamines are cancer growth factors which promote tumor progression by stimulating the secretion of VEGF, MMP, IL-6 and IL-8. Propranolol and other Beta Blocker drugs are useful as anticancer agents by inhibiting catecholamine secretion. (55)

Cathepsins

are proteolytic enzymes contained within lysosomes used by the autophagy process to digest and recycle organelles. Cathepsins promote tissue invasion when released by cancer cells into the micro-environment. When released into the cytosol, cathepsins trigger apoptosis.

CBD Cannabidiol

the major non-psychoactive component of the cannabis plant which binds to the VDAC, causing separation of HKII from the VDAC, a valid anti-cancer strategy. (56)

CD40 activation

Located at the cell surface membrane, CD40 is a TNF (tumor necrosis factor) receptor expressed on cell surface of B Cells, T-Cells (immune cells) and many cancer cell types. B cell malignancies (lymphoma) are heavily CD-40 dependent for activation, proliferation and survival. CD-40 activation is prevented by inhibiting the 5-LOX inflammatory pathway (with Boswellia and Itraconazole, for example).

CD80 Surface Protein

Is a protein on the cancer cell membrane which blocks cytotoxic T cells from killing the cancer cell. The CD80 protein plays a major role in defeating anti-tumor immune surveillance.

Cell Cycle Arrest

Cell cycle arrest means arresting cell division, also called cell replication, or mitosis. One way to accomplish this is inhibition of the spindle formation needed for cell division with a microtubule inhibitor drug such as taxol, vincristine or mebendazole. COX-2 inhibitors such as celecoxib downregulate c-Myc, which halts cancer cell replication in the G0 phase, a non-replicating resting phase.

Checkpoint Inhibitor Drugs

are immunotherapy drugs which restore immune cancer surveillance. One class of drugs target PD-1 (Programmed Death-1) including: Pembrolizumab (Keytruda). Nivolumab (Opdivo) and Cemiplimab (Libtayo). Another class of drugs block CTLA-4 (cytotoxic T-lymphocyte antigen 4), such as Ipilimumab (Yervoy) a monoclonal antibody used for advanced melanoma.

Chemokines

are signaling chemicals that orchestrate immune cell migration. Both cancer cells, and stromal cells in the TME (tumor microenvironment) secrete an array of chemokines which regulate tumor cell proliferation, cancer stem cell properties, cancer invasiveness and metastasis. (57)

Chemotherapy

A family of anti-cancer drugs widely used in conventional oncology which target rapidly replicating cells, while sparing cancer stem cells. Chemotherapy typically induces massive cancer cell necrosis, with spillage of cell contents into the extracellular space. This evokes a massive inflammatory response which actually stimulates the cancer stem cells, a harmful outcome. A preferable method of cancer cell death is apoptosis, programmed cell death, in which cell contents are recycled in an orderly fashion and do not evoke an inflammatory response, the main subject of this book. Cancer chemotherapy is considered possibly curative in some cases of lymphoma, acute lymphoblastic and acute myelogenous leukemia, germ cell (testicular) cancer, ovarian cancer, choriocarcinoma, and small cell lung cancer.

Children with Burkitt's lymphoma, Wilm's tumor, and embryonal rhabdomyosarcoma are sometimes cured with chemotherapy. The adverse side effects of chemotherapy may be quite serious. (58)

Chemotherapy Paradigm

Perpetuation of the chemotherapy paradigm by conventional oncology is a financial necessity for the pharmaceutical industry. With the FDA approval and introduction into mainstream oncology of new targeted pathway and immuno-therapy drugs, there has been gradual erosion of the chemotherapy paradigm. Alternate anti-cancer treatments with repurposed drugs or botanicals such as those mentioned in this book are regarded as a financial threat to the industry, and usually ignored or bitterly opposed by mainstream oncology. (59-61)

Clotrimazole

Clotrimazole is a Glycolysis Inhibitor which separates HKII from the VDAC in preclinical research cancer models. This is a popular anti-fungal drug available commercially as a topical cream, vaginal suppository and oro-pharyngeal troche. However, use as an anti-cancer agent is limited since Clotrimazole is only poorly water soluble, and no bioavailable oral version has been marketed. (62-65)

Chemotherapy Concession

A form of financial kickback to oncologists for using chemotherapy. A Harvard study showed that when oncologists had a choice between a low-cost and a high-cost drug treatment, they preferred the more expensive option to maximize profit margin. Thus, the chemotherapy concession provides an obvious incentive to choose the more intensive high dose chemotherapy regimen, with higher toxicity and adverse side effects, while having a similar efficacy to a low dose regimen. (66-67)

Chrysin

Is a plant flavonoid which inhibits tumor GLYCOLYSIS and induces apoptosis by targeting hexokinase II (HKII). (68)

Complex I of the ETC, Electron Transport Chain

is also called NADH: ubiquinine oxidoreductase and is involved in energy production at the inner mitochondrial membrane, a metabolic pathway called OXPHOS (oxidative phosphorylation).

Drugs which inhibit Complex I are OXPHOS inhibitors, such as Metformin, Berberine, Pyrvinium, Fenofibrate and Ivermectin.

COX-2 inflammatory Pathway

COX-2 is Cyclo-Oxygenase 2, an inflammatory pathway activated by NF-kB (Nuclear Factor Kappa B), involved in making cancer more aggressive, stimulating proliferation and metastatic spread. Blocking this inflammatory pathway with the COX-2 inhibitor, Celecoxib is enormously useful.

Curcumin

Age-Old Glycolysis Inhibitor and anti-inflammatory, anti-cancer food supplement. (69-71)

Cyclin D1

Is an oncogene which regulates cell cycle progression (cell replication), a target gene for the Wnt and MAPk pathways. Upregulated Cyclin D1 makes the cells replicate faster, a poor prognostic feature in cancer. Downregulation of Cyclin D1 is a valid anti-cancer strategy. Nuclear staining and detection of Cyclin D1 on immunohistochemistry is common in Mantle Cell Lymphoma. (72-73)

CYP-450 Enzyme System

is a major drug detoxification system in the liver. When the patient is taking a drug which inhibits CYP-450, other drugs may then achieve dangerously high concentrations in the blood stream. This is one of the main ways in which dangerous drug interactions can occur, and requires close monitoring with adjustment of drug dosages any time these types of drug combinations are used. Drugs which inhibit CYP450 (CYP3A) are: Itraconazole, Cimetidine. CYP3A is inhibited by these supplements: garlic, ginkgo biloba, Echinacea, ginseng, St. John's Wort, grape seed extract and grapefruit juice.

Cystine/Glutamate Antiporter System (system xc– or xCT)

is an amino acid transport system involved in transport of cystine into the cancer cell for production of glutathione, the major intracellular anti-oxidant. xCT is blocked by sulfasalazine (Azulfidine®). Blocking cysteine uptake to the cancer cell renders it more susceptible to damaging effects of ROS (reactive oxygen species) and oxidative therapies such as Artesunate (artemisinin).

Dichloroacetate (DCA)

Is an old off-patent drug serving as Glycolysis Inhibitor which reverses the Warburg Effect by inactivating PDK (pyruvate dehydrogenase kinase), thus freeing PDH (pyruvate dehydrogenase) to feed OXPHOS. DCA shows synergy with OXPHOS inhibitors such as metformin. DCA activates mTOR and induces "protective autophagy". DCA is usually given in combination with Poly-MVA to prevent adverse effects of neuropathy.

Diet/Lifestyle Modifications

are undoubtably important for both prevention and treatment of cancer. I apologize that due to time and space limitations, this is discussed in only a limited fashion in this book. This topic deserves an entire book or multiple books, which are already readily available, to which the reader is referred. Max Gerson Therapy, Nicholas Gonzalez Diet Therapy, Ann Wigmore Wheatgrass Diet, Intermittent Fasting, Fasting Mimicking Diet, Ketogenic Diet, and Low Carbohydrate Diet have been touched on briefly. (195-199)

Disulfiram (Antabuse®) DSF

Is a dithiocarbamate which binds readily to metals such as copper, zinc, molybdenum, iron, copper, silver, gold, and zinc. DSF is an old drug used for treating alcohol addiction, repurposed as an anti-cancer stem cell drug which inhibits aldehyde dehydrogenase, associated with cancer stem cells. Anti-cancer efficacy is enhanced with addition of copper and autophagy inhibitor drugs. Considerable anticancer synergy was found combining Disulfiram with Auranofin. Recently, Disulfiram has been repurposed as an anti-obesity drug. (74-80)

DNA Hypermethylation

Methylation of DNA is an epigenetic control mechanism. Cancers such as leukemia have upregulated DNMT (DNA methyltransferase) which "hypermethylate" the DNA, meaning most of the DNA is covered up by methyl groups, which render those sections of the DNA unreadable. Thymoquinone suppresses DNMT and reverses hypermethylation, thereby restoring a more normal ability to read cellular DNA. Curcumin and berberine also inhibit DNMT.

EGCG (Epigallocatechin Gallate Green Tea)

EGCG an extract of Green Tea, is a Glycolysis inhibitor by downregulating genetic expression of Glycolytic Enzymes, inhibition of HIF-1, and Inhibition of VEGF. EGCG also has anti-viral activity (81-83)

EGFR (Epithelial Growth Factor Receptor)

is a tyrosine kinase receptor attached to the cell membrane which transmits growth signals from EGF into the interior of the cancer cell. This activates the PI3K-AKT-mTOR pathway which potently stimulates aggressive cancer behavior. The new anti-EGFR drugs are cetuximab, panitumumab, gefitinib and osimertinib. These are EGFR TKI's (EGFR Epithelial Growth Factor Receptor, TKI Tyrosine Kinase Inhibitor). Plant lectins such as Solomon's Seal block the active site on EGFR by competitive binding, thus blocking the EGF growth factor. Anti-Cancer effects of most tyrosine kinase inhibitors are augmented by autophagy inhibitors such as hydroxychloroquine, azithromycin and clarithromycin.

Electron Transport Chain (ETC) (see OXPHOS)

Located at the inner mitochondrial membrane, a series of proteins which transfer electrons along a chain to produce a proton gradient which makes energy in the form of ATP. Cytochrome C is one of the mitochondrial ETC proteins, which triggers apoptosis when released freely through the VDAC out to the cytosol.

Embryonic Stem Cells (mESCmouse) (hESChuman)

Are stem cells obtained from early pre-implantation embryos from a mouse (mESC) which have many similarities to cancer cells, and therefore useful in the study of cancer. Both have a glycolytic metabolic profile, maintained by upregulated PDK. Both have no Hayflick Limit, as telomerase enzyme expression prevents Telomere shortening, making possible indefinite cell replication. The use of hESC (human embryonic stem cells) for medical research is controversial because of moral, ethical and political considerations. However, no restrictions on using mice.

EMT Epithelial to Mesenchymal Transition

Activation of EMT induces the transformation of the sedentary well-behaved cancer cell into a more aggressive cell type capable of metastasizing throughout the body. EMT is closely linked to cancer stem cell pathways, Wnt and Hedgehog, as well as activation by various growth factors, the most potent being TGF-Beta (a growth factor found in platelets). Platelets are a major storage site for TGF-Beta, and play a key role in EMT. Paradoxically, EMT is activated by common cytotoxic chemotherapy, and EMT is reversible with use of Tocotrienol Vitamin E, and platelet inhibitors such as dipyridamole and aspirin. (84-87)

Epigenetic Machinery

includes modifying histone acetylation and deacetylation, DNA methylation and demethylation, and genetic expression of noncoding RNAs, such as miRNA and lncRNA.

Endosymbiont Hypothesis of Lynn Margulis, PhD.

Lynn Margulis was an evolutionary biologist married to Carl Sagan who proposed the theory that mitochondria evolved from bacteria which were incorporated into eukaryotic cells millions of years ago. Thus, explaining the many similarities in structure and function when comparing bacteria to mitochondria. For example, antibiotics (Doxycycline and Clarithromycin) which target bacterial ribosomes, also target mitochondrial ribosomes in cancer cells. (88)

FASN (Fatty Acid Synthetase)

Is an enzyme frequently upregulated in cancer cells (such as hepatoma and B-Cell Lymphoma) involved in generating fatty acids for tumor energy requirements. FASN is blocked by Fenofibrate, Orlistat® and Quercetin. Blocking FASN is a valid anti-cancer strategy. FASN inhibition also leads to microtubule disruption and synergizes with other microtubule drugs such as mebendazole, and taxol (taxanes).

Fasting Mimicking Diet

or intermittent fasting, is a popular anti-cancer diet which starves the cancer of glucose, activates AMP-kinase which inhibits mTOR, a valid anti-cancer strategy. Fenofibrate and Metformin induce a metabolic profile which mimics the fasting state.

FDG, 18F-FDG

also known as fluorine-18 fluoro-2-deoxy-glucose (18F-FDG), is the radioisotope glucose imaging agent used in visualize cancer in the body on PET scans (PET Positron Emission Tomography). Compared to normal tissue, cancer cells have dramatically increased glucose uptake because of the metabolic derangement called the Warburg Effect (aerobic glycolysis), denoted in this book as GLYCOLYSIS (in caps). This dramatically increased glucose uptake by the cancer cells makes the cancer visible on PET scan imaging.

Febrile Neutropenia

Is a common adverse effect of chemotherapy. Firstly, chemotherapy causes a low white count from bone marrow suppression rendering the patient immunosuppressed. Secondly, chemotherapy damages the lining the GI tract, causing "leaky gut". This means gram negative bacteria in the gut leak freely into the blood stream. The net effect is lethal gram negative septicemia, a form of infection in the blood. If not treated promptly with IV antibiotics and Neupogen® shot, this leads rapidly to fatal outcome.

Ferroptosis – Iron mediated cell death

is a form of apoptosis in cancer cells which contain large amounts of iron used for rapid cell growth and proliferation. The reaction of iron with oxygen, the Fenton Reaction, results in massive production of damaging ROS (reactive oxygen species) which then induces apoptosis. This is called Ferroptosis, which can be induced with Artesunate (artemisinin) or other oxidative drug treatments. The effect is enhanced by down regulating the anti-oxidant defense of the cancer cell with Sulforaphane or Sulfasalazine. (89-91)

FOXP3 protein

Is an immunosuppressive protein secreted by cancer cells which bind to a receptor on the T cell, which then converts the T cell into an immunosuppressive T-Reg cell, thus leading to tumor induced immunosuppression which allows the cancer mass to evade host immune surveillance. (92-93)

GARP-TGFβ axis

in platelets turns off anti-cancer T cell immunity, also called cancer immune surveillance. (GARP) stands for Glycoprotein A Repetitions Predominant and (TGFβ) stands for Transforming Growth Factor βeta. Antiplatelet agents such as aspirin and dipyridamole are useful here.

G-CSF (Granulocyte Colony-Stimulating Factor)

also called Neupogen®, the trademark for filgrastim, is an injectable drug which stimulated the bone marrow to produce white blood cells, useful in prevention of febrile neutropenia after chemotherapy.

Glioblastoma

is a highly aggressive brain tumor, invariably fatal in spite of best conventional treatment with neurosurgery, chemotherapy, and radiation. Average life expectancy remains 15-16 months despite treatment. Using a cocktail of repurposed anti-cancer drugs combined with conventional treatments, Ben Williams is one of the few people to ever survive Glioblastoma, a story told in his book, *Surviving Terminal Cancer.*

Glutathione (GSH)

is the main anti-oxidant system protecting cancer cells from ROS (reactive oxygen species). GSH is synthesized from cysteine, glutamate, and glycine. Cysteine is taken up by the cystine/glutamate antiporter, xCT, the rate limiting step in glutathione synthesis. The xCT antiporter is blocked by sulfasalazine, resulting in reduced glutathione levels, and greater sensitivity to oxidative therapies. Glutathione is depleted by Sulforaphane, rendering the prostate cancer cell more susceptible to oxidative damage from ROS, which leads to apoptosis. (94)

Glycolysis (Aerobic Glycolysis – Warburg Effect)

is one of the three pillars of cancer cell metabolism utilizing massive amounts of glucose, accounting for the increased uptake on the PET scan showing the cancer mass in the body. In the Warburg Effect, the main metabolic pathway is altered, glucose metabolism is shunted away from OXPHOS in the mitochondria and towards the less efficient GLYCOLYSIS in the cytoplasm where massive amounts of glucose are metabolized to serve the replicative and proliferative activities of the cancer cell.

Greek Test

A blood test for CTC's (circulating tumor cells) offered by Research Genetics Cancer Center (RGCC) Group, established in 2004 by Dr. Ioannis Papasotiriou. Testing results provide information about number of CTC's, their surface markers and cell type, and their sensitivity or resistance to various chemotherapy agents, repurposed drugs, and botanicals used in cancer treatment. This can be enormously useful in selecting treatment options.

GSK3-Beta (Glycogen Synthase Kinase-3-Beta)

is the cytoplasmic protein which together with APC (adenomatous polyposis coli) and AXIN (axis inhibitor) forms a "destruction complex" which phosphorylates cytosolic Beta-Catenin, allowing its degradation. Thus preventing nuclear translocation and transcription, essentially turning off Wnt signaling. Restoring GSK3-Beta downregulates Beta-Catenin, which then inhibits the WNT pathway, a critical pathway for cancer stem cell maintenance. For example, melatonin and celecoxib restore GSK3-Beta function which down-regulates Beta-Catenin activity.

High Through-Put Drug Screening

is a new technology for screening a library of thousands of drugs for anticancer activity, or activity against a specific metabolic pathway in cancer cells.

Hsp90 (heat shock protein 90) is a "chaperone protein" involved in housekeeping functions that assists cytosolic proteins to fold properly, and stabilize against heat stress. Hsp90 inhibitors are anti-cancer drugs.

HR Hazard Ratio

HR Hazard Ratio the ratio of risk of outcome in treatment group vs. control group. If the hazard ratio is 0.5, then the rate of deaths in one treatment group is HALF the rate in the other group. If the hazard ratio is 2.0, then the rate of deaths in one treatment group is TWICE the rate in the other group.

Hayflick Limit

In 1961, Leonard Hayflick discovered cultured fibroblast cells replicate approximately 50 times, after which they undergo senescence and apoptosis. This is called the Hayflick Limit, a process later discovered to be controlled by Telomere shortening. In 2009, Drs. Greider, Blackburn and Szostak received the Nobel Prize in Physiology and Medicine for discovery and further work on Telomeres. Telomeres are snippets of DNA attached to the ends of the chromosomes. They shorten with each cell replication until the Hayflick Limit is reached triggering senescence and cell death. Telomeres can be lengthened with an enzyme called Telomerase. Having no Hayflick limit, embryonic stem cells and cancer cells express Telomerase, and replicate indefinitely. The use of Telomerase inhibition as an anticancer strategy has been suggested, however, critics have argued normal human stem cells express telomerase, and any attempt to inhibit telomerase would be harmful to normal stem cells producing serious adverse effects. In spite if these concerns, a number of natural supplements in wide use are telomerase inhibitors. (95-96)

(HDAC) Histone Deacetylase Inhibitors

are drugs such as phenylbutyrate (butyrate) and valproic acid, involved in coiling or uncoiling of the DNA, having anti-cancer effects based on epigenetic mechanisms.

Hedgehog Pathway (Hh)

First identified in mutant fruit flies in 1980, the Hedgehog signaling pathway is a cancer stem cell pathway. The GLI protein is the downstream effector. Normally Hh is used for embryonic development, however upregulation is commonly seen in cancer cells. In the growing embryo, Hh controls the differentiation of cells into organs, cell proliferation, stem cell maintenance, and regulation of growth factors. Inhibition of Hh causes decrease in BCL2 and Cyclin D1 in lymphoma, and targets cancer stem cells.

HKII – Hexokinase II

Cancer cells replace normal hexokinase with an embryonic form called hexokinase II, the first step in metabolism of glucose. In normal cells Hexokinase is located in the cell cytoplasm. However, in cancer cells, HKII is upregulated over 100 times by genetic amplification, and is relocated to the VDAC on the outer mitochondrial membrane. Metformin, Itraconazole and Fenofibrate are three repurposed drugs which detach HKII from VDAC. There are many others mentioned in this book.

HIF – Hypoxia Inducible Factor Gene

is expressed in response to hypoxia in the microenvironment, resulting in the activation of mTOR and MAPK (mitogen activated protein kinase), promoting the Warburg Effect in cancer cells. HIF upregulates Glycolytic enzymes, Glucose transporters, enhances Glycolysis in the cytoplasm and inhibits OXPHOS in the mitochondria. Blocking HIF-1 is a valid anti-cancer strategy.

High Throughput Screening

A new technique in medical science for screening a large library of drugs for the most promising anti-cancer candidate.

HMG-CoA reductase (HMGCR)

is the rate-limiting enzyme of the MVA (mevalonate) pathway for cholesterol, Rho proteins, and CO-Enzyme Q-10 synthesis and is blocked by statin drugs, resulting in mitochondrial toxicity and cytoskeleton disorganization at the cellular level.

hTERT (Human Telomerase Reverse Transcriptase Gene and Enzyme)

is responsible for production of Telomerase, the reverse transcriptase enzyme which immortalizes both cancer cells and embryonic stem cells by lengthening Telomeres, thus preventing shortening. Cancer cells and Embryonic Stem cells express Telomerase, having no "Hayflick Limit", thus are able to replicate indefinitely. Suppression of telomerase activity can be done with a large variety of natural products and may be useful as an anticancer strategy. Critics are concerned about adverse effects on embryonic stem cells which also express Telomerase. Natural telomerase inhibitors include: Quercetin, Resveratrol/Pterostilbene, Indole-3-Carbinol, EGCG (from Green Tea), Curcumin, Mistletoe, Garlic (Allicin), Panax Ginseng, Scutellaria Baicalensis (Chinese Skullcap), Sulforaphane, Berberine, and Silymarin. (188-191) (95-96)

HUVEC (Human Umbilical Vein Endothelial Cells)

are endothelial cells from the veins from the umbilical cord.

Ibrutinib

is Bruton's Tyrosine Kinase Inhibitor, a targeted pathway drug which inhibits the B-Cell Receptor, and has revolutionized treatment of B Cell Lymphoma. Although dramatic remissions can be obtained, benefits are temporary with eventual development of drug resistance after 12-18 months in all cases, thought related to survival of mutant cancer cell clones which have resistance to the drug. These mutant clones rely on "Adaptive Kinome Reprogramming" to resist Ibrutinib. Unfortunately, Ibrutinib activates the Wnt cancer stem cell pathway, and promotes cancer stem cell survival, another possible explanation for its long-term failure.

IDO gene (indoleamine 2, 3-oxygenase)

This gene suppresses T cell activation resulting in cancer escape from immune surveillance. Silencing the IDO gene is a form of immunotherapy, beneficial as an anti-cancer strategy. Cox-2 inhibitors, such as celecoxib, are potent IDO inhibitors, thus restoring immune response within tumor microenvironment.

IL-6 (Interleukin 6) The Main Inflammatory Cytokine

IL-6 is the main downstream inflammatory cytokine induced by activation of NF-kB (Nuclear Factor Kappa B), commonly upregulated in many aggressive cancers, especially B cell lymphoma in which IL-6 is responsible for maturation of B cells into antibody producing cells. IL-6 is a cancer growth factor. A round of chemotherapy causes massive elevation of IL-6, which is responsible for cancer relapse with a more aggressive drug resistant cell type. IL-6 chemical structure and genes are similar to G-CSF (Filgrastim, Neupogen®) suggesting some overlap in function. (97)

IL-12 (Interleukin 12) IL-12–IFN-gamma pathway

is a cytokine which exerts potent anti-tumor effects by enhancing anti-tumor immunity via the IL-12–IFN-gamma pathway which upregulates NK cell and T cell immune response. DCA, for example, increases IL-12. (192-193)

IL-18 (Interleukin 18)

is an immunostimulatory cytokine secreted by T Helper (Th1) cells (white blood cells also called leukocytes or monocytes) which works in combination with IL-12 to expand and activate NK Natural Killer Cells enhancing the cell mediated anti-tumor immunity, as well as anti-viral and antimicrobial immunity. IL-18 is useful when added to PDL1 Checkpoint Inhibitor Immunotherapy and CAR-T cell therapy. IL-18 is induced by the over the counter antacid drug, Cimetidine (Tagamet®). (98-102)

Immunogenic Cell Death (ICD)

is a form of cancer cell death which stimulates an anti-cancer immune response. For example, ICD is induced by Ivermectin.

Inflammatory Pathways

such as NF-kB, COX-2 and 5-LOX are upregulated in cancer and stromal cells of the TME (tumor microenvironment). Inflammation represents one of the "Hallmarks of Cancer", promoting tumor growth, proliferation, and metastasis. Upregulated Inflammation inhibits host T cell anti-cancer immunity and hinders efficacy of immune therapies. Therefore, blocking inflammatory pathways with Aspirin, Celecoxib, Curcumin and Boswellia and many other agents (listed in the Quick Reference Guide), is a top priority for any anti-cancer program. (103-105)

IFN-γ Interferon Gamma

Is a cytokine involved in anticancer immunity increased by DCA, LDN, and Cimetidine.

Iodine

is an essential mineral found in sea weed avidly taken up by the thyroid gland for production of thyroid hormone. Iodine also accumulates in breast tissue and gastric mucosa. Iodine deficiency is associated with increased risk for thyroid, gastric and breast cancer. Testing for iodine level, and supplementation when low is part of our cancer prevention program. Iodine has anti-cancer activity in breast cancer and other cancers. Because iodine deficiency is a major cause of mental retardation and low IQ in babies born from iodine deficient mothers, many countries including the US have introduced iodized salt, effectively providing iodine supplementation to the entire population. After iodized salt was introduced in the US in 1924, IQ levels of newborns increased by 15%. (106-108)

IPT Insulin Potentiated Therapy

Insulin treatment causes hypoglycemia which starves the cancer cell of glucose, and also renders the cancer cell more sensitive to the effects of chemotherapy which is now more avidly taken up into cancer cells. IPT allows smaller dosages of chemotherapy to be used without the toxic side effects of conventional dosing. (109)

LC-II, LC3-II (Light Chain Microtubule Associated Protein)

is a protein on autophagic structures such as the autophagosome, useful as a marker for monitoring autophagy. Induction of autophagy is indicated by appearance of LC3-positive puncta visible on Immunofluorescent or GFP-based microscopy. (Note: GFP Green Fluorescent Protein). Observing massive accumulation of LC3 -II and P62 protein after drug treatment (for example, with thymoquinone or PPI drug treatment) confirms inhibition of autophagy. (110-111)

Ki-67 Proliferation Marker

Is a clinically predictive proliferation marker routinely used by pathologists when reviewing histology slides of cancer biopsies. Low Ki-67, below 30% indicates less aggressive cancers. High Ki-67, greater than 30% indicates more rapidly proliferating, more aggressive cancers, predictive of poor prognosis. (112-114)

5-LOX

5 lipoxygenase is an inflammatory pathway inhibited by Boswellia (Frankincense). (115)

LDN Low Dose Naltrexone

Is an opiate receptor blocker drug with anticancer activity when taken at night before sleep. This upregulates endogenous opiate production (endorphins) and binds to the OGFR (Opiate Growth Factor Receptor), having an anti-cancer effect. LDN shows clinical benefit in auto-immune diseases such as Multiple Sclerosis, Rheumatoid Arthritis, IBD Inflammatory Bowel Disease, Hashimoto's and Graves's autoimmune thyroid disease. A similar opiate blocking drug called Narcan is used by para-medics and rescue workers to rapidly reverse the respiratory depression in the overdosed drug addict, thus miraculously restoring life to the dying patient. (116-118)

Lipid Rafts

(also known as lipid microdomains) are discrete sections of the outer cell membrane enriched with lipids such as cholesterol, glycosphingolipids, and GPI (glycosyl-phosphatidylinositol). Lipid rafts are involved in various cell functions such as receptor signaling, endocytosis (membrane transport), and the actin cytoskeleton. Lipid rafts are disrupted by tocotrienol vitamin E, and Itraconazole. (119)

Lonidamine (LON) – This is a research drug with no currently available version on the market. LON is a potent GLYCOLYSIS Inhibitor, an old drug abandoned years ago after failed clinical trials. Recently there is renewed interest in pursuing preclinical research in combination with inhibitor of glutamine metabolism (6-diazo-5-oxo-L-norleucine), and Orlistat®, an Inhibitor of fatty acid metabolism. (120)

Lysosomal Trafficking (Antegrade Lysosomal Trafficking)

Is the antegrade movement of lysosomes from the perinuclear area of the cancer cell outward to a position at the outer cell membrane. When mTOR is activated, this triggers movement of lysosomes to the cell periphery at the plasma membrane ready for Macropinocytosis, an aggressive behavior in which the cancer cells absorb and digest surrounding tissues, degrading the microenvironment in preparation for cancer invasion. For example, Antegrade Lysosomal Trafficking is inhibited by Niclosamide, or many other drugs which induce "perinuclear clustering". (10-12)

Macropinocytosis

An autophagy related function in which pseudopods or folds in the outer cell membrane engulf nutrients in the extracellular space, taken up and digested by the cancer cell. mTOR activation promotes antegrade lysosome trafficking, a preliminary step for Macropinocytosis and aggressive cell behavior. mTOR inactivation promotes lysosomal perinuclear clustering and activation of "protective autophagy" a dormant state.

MAP1 (microtubule-associated protein light chain3 (MAP1-LC3)-binding protein SQSTM1 (also known as p62)

MAPK/Erk signaling pathway

mitogen-activated protein kinases (MAPK) and extracellular signal-related kinases (ERK) pathway turn on genes which stimulate cancer growth, proliferation and migration, and orchestrates the Warburg Effect. MAPK is associated with the microtubule cytoskeleton and regulates cancer cell motility during invasive behavior. (206-208)

Matrix Metallo Proteinase (MMP)

These are proteolytic enzymes secreted by the cancer usually carried in lysosomes or vesicles released into the microenvironment which digest the extracellular matrix in preparation for local cancer invasion, and metastatic spread. This release of MMP into the extracellular space is facilitated by antegrade lysosome trafficking which shuttles the lysosomes to a peripheral location at the cell membrane ready to release the enzymes outside the cancer cell into the TME (tumor micro environment). (121-122)

Melatonin

is a naturally occurring hormone produced by the pineal gland which regulates the sleep/wake cycle. Melatonin is also synthesized in mitochondria and is a Glycolysis inhibitor (via inhibition of PDK), redirecting glucose metabolism to mitochondria, reversing the Warburg Effect. (123-127)

Metabolic Plasticity

Is the ability of cancer stem cells to switch among the three major metabolic pathways OXPHOS, Glycolysis and Autophagy, depending on nutrient levels, metabolic needs, and drug treatment. Metabolic plasticity is the reason for failure of drug treatment blocking only one metabolic pathway. The cancer cell will easily adapt to another readily available metabolic pathway to continue growth and proliferation.

MCT (MonoCarboxylate Transport)

expels lactic acid from the cancer cell. Blocking MCL with Diclofenac prevents acidification of the extracellular space, and causes buildup of lactic acid in the cancer cell which halts GLYCOLYSIS. (128)

MDR

Multi Drug Resistance makes cancer cells resistant to chemotherapy, as the chemotherapy drug is promptly pumped out by the P-Glycoprotein efflux pump. A number of drugs such as the COX-2 inhibitor (celecoxib) downregulate the P-Glycoprotein gene restoring drug sensitivity.

MicroRNAs (miRNAs)

a class of noncoding RNA molecules involved in posttranscriptional regulation of protein expression.

Microtubule System

a scaffold system inside cells made of micro-tubules, also called spindles, able to assemble and disassemble quickly, providing shape and structure, used by the cell to transfer lysosomes, mitochondria and other organelles around the cell to their proper location, sort of like a railway system. Cell replication is considered the most important function of the microtubule system. In a dividing cell, the two nuclei are pulled apart by the spindle system. Mebendazole and Taxanes are microtubule inhibitor drugs which block cancer cell replication by preventing spindle formation.

Mitochondrial Apoptosis

is the main form of programmed cell death in the cancer cell which centers on the mitochondria, usually induced by release of cytochrome C (of the ETC) from the mitochondria into the cytosol which triggers the caspase cascade, culminating in apoptosis. Another strategy which induces mitochondrial apoptosis is detachment of HKII from the VDAC at the outer mitochondrial membrane, which downregulates BCL-2 (anti-apoptotic protein), upregulates BAX (pro-apoptotic protein). A number of drugs such as Itraconazole, Fenofibrate, Cannabidiol and Methyl Jasmonate are useful here.

mRNA (Messenger RNA)

contains the coded instruction set for specific proteins (such as hexokinase II or pyruvate dehydrogenase PDH) , and is the intermediary messenger which transmitted the original code residing in the nuclear DNA to the ribosomes which manufacture the proteins. The study of mRNA in cancer cells is useful because the upregulation of specific mRNAs reveals which metabolic pathways are upregulated. It is also useful to study mRNA output from cancer cell cultures (in vitro) after drug treatment, thus revealing drug efficacy or sensitivity.

MTA1 (Metastasis Associated Protein1)

is an essential downstream effector of the c-Myc oncoprotein, regulates EMT (epithelial-to-mesenchymal transition) and metastatic progression. MTA1 also inhibits p53-induced apoptosis by deacetylation of p53. MTA1 is widely up-regulated in many cancer cell types including most lymphomas, breast, endometrial, colorectal, gastric, esophageal, pancreatic, ovarian, non–small cell lung, prostate, and hepatocellular carcinomas. MTA1 is widely up-regulated in human B-cell lymphomas. Mice genetically modified to over-express MTA1 have a very high rate of spontaneous B cell lymphoma. Pterostilbene Resveratrol, Curcumin and Diascorea inhibit MTA1, useful in prostate cancer, chemoprevention and treatment. (182-187)

mTOR Pathway

also known as Phosphatidylinositol 3-kinase (PI3K)/Akt/mammalian target of rapamycin (mTOR) is a major cancer pathway, and controller of Autophagy. mTOR activation (by Akt) results in antegrade lysosomal tracking towards the cell periphery to the cell membrane, and transforms the cancer cell into a highly aggressive cell type with local invasion and metastatic potential. mTOR inhibition (by AMPk activation) results in "protective autophagy " with peri-nuclear clustering of lysosomes, a dormant quiescent state for the cancer cell in which proliferation is halted.

MYC oncogene and protein (c-Myc) (Avian myelocytomatosis viral oncogene homolog)

The c-Myc Oncogene is a "master regulator" which controls cancer cell metabolism, growth, proliferation, apoptosis, and drives either Glycolysis (Warburg Effect) or OXPHOS in the cancer cell depending on metabolic plasticity. C-Myc inhibitors such as Nitazoxanide (Alinia®), Diclofenac and Artesunate are enormously useful in cancer treatment. (128)

Myeloid Derived Suppressor Cells (MDSC)

myeloid-derived suppressor cells (MDSCs) allow cancer cells to evade the immune system. Reduction of MDSCs is a viable anti-cancer strategy. (129)

Neupogen® Filgrastim Human Granulocyte Colony-Stimulating Factor (G-CSF)

is an FDA approved drug used to stimulate the bone marrow to make more white blood cells, thus increasing the white blood cell count, and preventing chemotherapy induced neutropenia. (130)

Nitazoxanide (Alinia)

Is an antiparasitic drug which is top hit as C-Myc Inhibitor.

NLRP3 inflammasome

was discovered by the team of Dr. Jürg Tschopp, at the University of Lausanne in 2002 which mediates pro-inflammatory responses and pyroptotic cell death. This is an immunostimulatory form of programmed cell death in which the cell releases its cytoplasmic content to induce pro-inflammatory signaling. Niclosamide activates the NLRP3 inflammasome, inducing immunostimulatory cell death.

Notch Pathway

is a Cancer Stem Cell pathway involved in tumor initiation and progression. (131)

NPC1 (Niemann-Pick C1)

is a lysosomal membrane protein which is key to egress of cholesterol from lysosomes. Inhibition of this protein (for example, by itraconazole) results in inhibition of cholesterol trafficking, accumulation of cholesterol in lysosomes, rendering them non-functional.

NF-kB (Nuclear Factor Kappa B)

Also called nuclear factor kappa-light-chain-enhancer of activated b cells (NF-kb) is the master controller of the inflammatory response, (and immune response) consisting of a protein in the cytoplasm and transcription factors in the nucleus. The IkB kinase (IKK) family of proteins sequester the NF-kB protein in the cytoplasm, preventing translocation to the nucleus and thereby blocking gene expression. Degradation of the IkB kinase protein leads to activation and translocation of the NF-kB protein to the nucleus turning on transcription of 400 genes involved in cell survival, immune response, drug resistance. Perhaps the most important are IL-6 cytokine. NF-kB activation can be induced by many agents such as endotoxin (LPS), stress, tissue injury, viral, bacterial and fungal infection, toxic chemicals etc. NF-kB gene expression is present in many inflammatory diseases and results in production of a constellation of inflammatory proteins such as COX-2, cytokines IL-6 and TNF alpha, chemokines, and many others involved in cell to cell adhesion, cell cycle regulation, angiogenesis, and drug resistance. NF-kB signaling plays a crucial role in oncogenesis and cancer progression. As mentioned in Weinberg's Ten Hallmarks of Cancer, aggressive cancers hijack the inflammatory pathways to their advantage by activating NF-kB. Obviously, downregulating the NF-KB pathway is enormously useful in cancer treatment. Many of the drugs and natural substances mentioned in this book inhibit or block the NF-kB pathway and are listed in the Quick Reference Guide. NF-kB is sometimes written as NF-kappa Beta in the medical literature. We use both interchangeably. (132-135)

Off-Label Prescription

Roughly 20 per cent of prescriptions are written off-label, meaning the drug is prescribed for a different medical indication, not the FDA approved indication.

OGF Met-enkephalin, Opiate Derived Growth Factor

inhibits cancer and its receptor is OGFR. Paradoxically, OGF inhibits cell replication, and inhibits tumor growth, by increasing p21 (cyclin-dependent kinase inhibitor), and decreasing BCL-2, thus has an anti-cancer effect. LDN (low dose naltrexone) increases endogenous OGF production, and may serve in place OGF, providing a similar function as an anti-cancer agent. (136)

OR Odds Ratio

The numerator is the odds in the intervention arm. The denominator is the odds in the control or placebo arm Odds Ratio (OR).

OXPHOS (Oxidative Phosphorylation)

is an efficient metabolic pathway in the mitochondria utilizing the mitochondrial electron transport chain (ETC) to oxidize carbon (obtained from glucose) with release of energy in the form of ATP. Energy is stored in the chemical bonds between carbon atoms of the glucose molecule. This energy is released as ATP via an oxidation reaction within the mitochondria. The actual machinery of this oxidation reaction is called the ETC (Electron Transport Chain) located at the inner mitochondrial membrane. The main metabolic derangement in cancer is the downregulation of OXPHOS in the mitochondria, and the upregulation of GLYCOLYSIS in the cytoplasm (Warburg Effect).

PAMPs

Is pathogen associated molecular patterns such as Beta Glucans (AHCC) having molecular structures which "mimic" pathogenic organisms. PAMP recognition and upregulation of the immune system is beneficial for host immune defense against cancer as well as viral, bacterial and fungal infection.

PD-1 Receptor Programmed Death-1 Receptor

Is an immune checkpoint **receptor** located on the surface of immune cells (white cells) such as T cells (CD4+ and CD8+), B cells, monocytes, natural killer (NK) cells, and dendritic cells (DCs). PD-L1 is the ligand which attaches to this PD-1 receptor, causing inhibition of host anticancer immune response by inhibiting T-cell proliferation, activation, and cytokine production.

PD-L1 Programmed Death Ligand

Is an immune checkpoint **inhibitor**, a glyco-protein that inhibits the immune system by inhibiting T-cell proliferation, activation, and cytokine production. PD-L1 binds to two receptors, PD-1 and to CD80. Many cancer cell types express PD-L1 on the outer membrane, thus suppressing T-cell mediated destruction of the cancer cells. Immunotherapy drugs are monoclonal antibodies that block PD-1 or PD-L1, restoring anti-cancer immunity.

P21

also called cyclin-dependent kinase inhibitor 1 (CDK-1). P21 inhibits cell proliferation, and promotes cell cycle arrest. p21 is major target of p53 activity, linking DNA damage to cell cycle arrest. P21 is also target for OGF (Opiate Growth Factor/ LDN).

P53 Gene and Protein "Guardian of the Genome"

In normal cells which have undergone irreparable genetic damage, the P53 Gene senses the damaged state and triggers mitochondrial (intrinsic) apoptosis, a normal process in which senescent or damaged cells are removed. Many cancers have a mutated or dysfunctional P53 gene which prevents apoptosis in spite of massive genetic mutations and alterations. Restoring P53 induced apoptosis is a valid anti-cancer strategy.

p73 isoform

also called Tap73 is a pro-apoptotic gene upregulated by Cox-2 inhibitors, celecoxib and diclofenac.

PAK1 (p21 (RAC1) activated kinase 1)

regulates structure in the cytoskeleton, and promotes cell motility, tumor cell proliferation, and progression. PAKs serve as messengers which transduce growth and proliferation signals originating from the cell membrane into the cancer cell. The PAK1 gene is frequently amplified in cancer, particularly breast cancer. PAK1 inhibition is a valid anti-cancer strategy, for example by Ivermectin which degrades the P21-activated kinase (PAK) protein, thus inhibiting mTOR, activating protective autophagy.

PARP (poly (ADP-ribose) polymerase-1)

cleaved PARP is used as a marker for apoptosis in laboratory studies using in vitro cancer cultures.

PDC Pyruvate Dehydrogenase Complex

Is the primary gateway for carbon (derived from glucose) to enter mitochondria where OXPHOS takes place. Inhibition of PDC by upregulation of PDK (pyruvate dehydrogenase kinase) is a central element of cancer cell metabolism which induces GLYCOLYSIS in the cytoplasm, the Warburg Effect.

PDGF Platelet Derived Growth Factor

is released by histamine activated platelets, serving to stimulate cancer growth. Platelet activation and release of PDGF and VEGF (Vascular Endothelial Growth Factor) can be blocked by the antihistamine Cimetidine, Dipyridamole and Aspirin.

PDI protein disulfide isomerase

is a cellular enzyme in the endoplasmic reticulum (ER) involved in protein folding. Inhibition of PDI (with Boswellia or Nitazoxanide Alinia® for example) causes ER stress and Unfolded Protein Response (UPR) with accumulation of unfolded or misfolded proteins resulting in cell death. PDI is overexpressed in ovarian cancer where inhibition of PDI has been useful in animal cancer models.

PET Scan

Positron Emission tomography using 18-FDG, an isotope of glucose which emits radiation, useful for imaging areas in the body which have high glucose uptake such as actively metabolizing cancer deposits. PET is useful for evaluating response to anti-cancer drug treatment. The main pitfall is the PET scan cannot show cancer stem cells because they are dormant and not actively metabolizing glucose. Unfortunately, cancer stem cells do not show up on the PET scan.

P-Glycoprotein MDR

This is the protein involved in the cancer cell "drug efflux pump" conferring MDR (multi drug resistance, chemotherapy resistance). Inhibiting P-glycoprotein (with Itraconazole or Clarithromycin for example) restores chemotherapy drug sensitivity.

PI3 kinase/Akt signal pathway, phosphoinositide 3 kinase (PI3K)/Akt/mammalian target of rapamycin (mTOR) pathway

The PI3K/AKT signaling pathway controls cell growth, migration, proliferation, and metabolism. Also called the PI3K/AKT/mTOR pathway.

PIBF Progesterone Induced Blocking Factor

is a protein secreted by both trophoblast cells and cancer cells which turns off the host immune system and allows the pregnancy or cancer to grow without interference from the host immune system. PIBF also induces aggressive cancer behavior. Blocking PIBF with Mifepristone is a valid anti-cancer strategy.

Pillars of Cancer Cell Metabolism

The Three Pillars of Metabolism are GLYCOLYSIS (Warburg Effect), OXPHOS and Autophagy. One might argue detaching HKII from VDAC, restoring immune surveillance and blocking inflammation are also important here.

Plant Lectin (PL)

Plant lectins such as Solomon's Seal and Mistletoe bind to aberrant glycoproteins (mannose), on the surface of cancer cells. PL's are useful as tools for cancer diagnosis, prognosis and therapy.

Platelet Satellitism

Observed on microscopic examination of routine blood smears, platelets are found adhering to B cell lymphoma cells, cloaking the cancer cells and shielding them from host immune system attack. Antiplatelet drugs such as aspirin and dipyridamole are useful for preventing this.

Poly-MVA

a nutritional supplement developed by Merrill Garnet containing a liquid polymer of palladium, alpha lipoic acid and thiamine. Commonly used together with DCA for neuroprotection, and for increasing electron flow through the mitochondria.

PPAR-alpha (Peroxisome Proliferator-Activated Receptor)

is a nuclear receptor, and master regulator of lipid metabolism. PPAR-alpha activation is an adaptive response to intermittent fasting, ketogenic diet, metformin and fenofibrate. Activation of PPAR alpha requires Vitamin A as a cofactor, resulting in inhibition of GLYCOLYSIS by inactivation of PDH, similar to the mechanism of action DCA. PPAR alpha also induces degradation of BCL2, the apoptosis protein, thus restoring apoptosis (and drug sensitivity) to the cancer cells.

Procrit (epoetin alfa)

A synthetic form of erythropoietin, a discredited oncology drug, previously used to increase the red blood cell count in patients rendered anemic from chemotherapy. After many years of oncology use, the drug was discontinued when found it stimulates cancer growth.

Preclinical Research Study Types

In Vitro – cancer cells are cultured in a petri dish and studied in the lab.

In Vivo – mouse xenograft studies. Cancer cells are injected into mice.

In Silico – studied by computer simulation. Silico is Latin for silicon (meaning a computer chip).

Protective Autophagy

is a state of dormancy, or hibernation, enabling cancer cell survival against chemotherapy drugs, hypoxia, glucose starvation and other stresses. Inhibition of mTOR activates protective autophagy characterized by "perinuclear clustering " of lysosomes in the cancer cell, i.e. the opposite of antegrade lysosomal trafficking.

Purinergic P2X Receptors (ATP sensitive receptors)

are a family of ATP-gated cation channels upregulated in the cancer cell membrane. These open in response to ATP in the microenvironment. Ivermectin and gensenoside (Ginseng) sensitize the cation channels to ATP, further opening the channel pores, allowing influx of large cations which activate the caspase cascade leading to apoptosis.

PTEN Tumor Suppressor Gene (Phosphatase and tensin homolog)

PTEN acts as a tumor suppressor gene, down-regulating the PI3K/AKT/mTOR pathway, thus suppressing cancer growth and proliferation. Inactivation of the PTEN Gene is usually present in most cancers. PTEN is part of the PTEN/AKT/NF-κB/ survivin signaling pathway. Restoring PTEN activity (with Aspirin, or other NSAIDS) is a valid anticancer strategy. Loss of PTEN gene sensitizes B-Cell lymphoma to the cytotoxic effects of Auranofin, thioreductase inhibitor. (137-139)

Quercetin

Is a dietary flavanol found in red onions which suppresses GLYCOLYSIS by binding to and inhibiting PDK (Pyruvate Dehydrogenase Kinase), decreasing protein levels of HK2 and suppressing the AKT/ mTOR pathway thus, inducing protective autophagy. Quercetin also inhibits membrane bound ATPase, (also inhibited by propranolol). Quercetin is a FASN (Fatty Acid Synthetase), Beta-Catenin and BCL-2 inhibitor. (140-143)(152)(194)

RAB 7 protein (Ras-related in brain 7)

is the key protein regulating endosomal/ lysosomal trafficking and perinuclear clustering. Upregulation of RAB7 protein is associated with increased extra-cellular vesicle secretion and invasive behavior of the cancer cells. The RAB 7 protein is targeted by Mefloquine. (144-146)

RAS Oncogene (kRas) and Protein

Extracellular growth factors attach to tyrosine kinase receptors on the cancer cell membrane. These turn on intracellular RAS proteins which orchestrate metabolic reprogramming of the cancer cell (i.e. the "Warburg Effect"), many of the "Hallmarks of Cancer", and upregulate aggressive lysosomal functions such as macropinocytosis used by cancer to digest and absorb nutrients in the microenvironment. Macropinocytosis can be blocked with Autophagy Inhibitor drugs.

T-Reg Cells (Regulatory T Cells)

are immunosuppressive T Cells, increased by secretion of histamine by cancer cells, inducing a state of immune tolerance (host immune evasion).

Reverse Warburg Effect

CAFs (cancer associated fibroblasts) in the tumor microenvironment are recruited to provide nutrients to the cancer mass. This is done by "turning on" aerobic glycolysis (Warburg Effect) in the CAFs which then secrete energy rich nutrients, pyruvate and lactate, which are shuttled back, and metabolized in mitochondria of the cancer cells using OXPHOS. The Reverse Warburg Effect is blocked by Glycolysis Inhibitors such as DCA (Dichloroacetate) and 2-DG (2-De-Oxy-Glucose).

(147-149)

ROS Reactive Oxygen Species

are harmful by products of oxidative phosphorylation (OXPHOS) such as peroxides, superoxide, and hydroxyl radicals. These are normally rendered harmless by intracellular anti-oxidant systems, glutathione peroxidase and thioreductase. ROS attack biomembranes with lipid peroxidation, leading to DNA damage and mitochondrial apoptosis. "Ferroptosis" is the oxidation of Iron to produce massive amounts of ROS in the cancer cell which then induces apoptosis. Increasing ROS simultaneous with downregulation of antioxidant system in cancer cells is a valid anti-cancer strategy.

Selenium

Is a mineral obtained in the diet from food grown on selenium rich soils. At the cellular level, selenium is incorporated into seleno-proteins, involved in cancer immune surveillance. Selenium deficiency is associated with increased cancer risk, and testing for and supplementing with selenium when deficient, reduces risk for cancer. Selenium is part of our cancer prevention program. (150-151)

Silybin (Silymarin, Milk Thistle)

Is an extract from the Milk Thistle plant with antiproliferative and apoptotic effects, especially useful in prostate and ovarian cancer. Inhibits Wnt signaling. (153-156)

SR/CR Mouse Spontaneous Regression/Complete Resistance

is a genetic trait in mice rendering them resistant to implanted cancer cells. In xenograft experiments using these mice, T cells of their immune system kill the implanted cancer cells before they can grow. The anti-cancer immunity of the SR/CR mice can be transferred to plain mice (wild type) by transfusing the T cells from a SR/CR mouse to the wild type mouse. This was the first pioneering, immunotherapy experiment.

STAT3 (Signal Transducer and Activator of Transcription 3)

regulates oncogenes which promote tumor progression, and anti-tumor immune suppression. STAT3 is activated by cytokines such as IL-6 expressed by lymphocytes. AHCC and Niclosamide downregulate STAT3 signaling. STAT3 considered a cancer stem cell pathway.

Starvation

Nutrient or glucose starvation activates AMPK (AMP Kinase), and downregulates (inactivates) mTOR, resulting in slowing of cancer cell metabolism.

Synthetic Lethality

A term originally derived from research in fruit flies involving mutations in two or more pathways which is lethal to the fly. This has been extended to cancer cells where synthetic lethality refers to blocking two or more metabolic pathways to achieve lethal endpoint, also called cancer cell apoptosis.

TAM Tumor Associated Macrophages

secrete inflammatory cytokines such as IL-6 in the tumor microenvironment, inducing aggressive cancer behavior, proliferation, migration, angiogenesis, metastasis, and suppression of anti-tumor immunity.

TCF Gene (TCF T-Cell Factor /LEF leukemia enhancer factor)

Is the target gene of the Wnt pathway (cancer stem cell pathway) perfectly blocked by the anti-parasitic drug Ivermectin. Blocking the Wnt pathway eradicates cancer stem cells.

Telomerase

See: hTERT (Human Telomerase Reverse Transcriptase Gene and Enzyme)

Telomere

A small portion of genetic material located at the ends of the chromosome which shortens with each cell replication, controlling aging and the Hayflick limit.

Testicular Cancer

One of the few cancers in which chemotherapy can be curative, because the cancer stem cells of this cell type are exquisitely sensitive to chemotherapy.

TME Tumor Micro-Environment

Is the space surrounding the tumor which contains supporting cells such as adipocytes (fat cells), fibroblasts (interstitial cells), muscle, and endothelial cells (inner lining of blood vessels, immune cells (lymphocytes, macrophages, B cells, T Cells), and platelets, all of which can be recruited by the cancer to supply nutrients, growth factors, and inflammatory cytokines to "feed" and stimulate the growing tumor mass.

TCA cycle Tricarboxylic acid cycle

also called Krebs cycle is essentially OXPHOS which takes place in the matrix of the mitochondria using the ETC, electron transport chain.

TGF-Beta – Transforming Growth Factor Beta

Is a growth factor found in platelets recruited by cancer cells to induce EMT (epithelial to mesenchymal transition) and promote invasive behavior. (87)

Tocotrienols (Vitamin E)

A newer, more biologically active form of Vitamin E compared to the older Tocopherols, having various anticancer effects including AMPK activation with suppression of Warburg Effect, suppression of c-Myc oncogene, inhibition of Wnt and Hedgehog signaling pathways and prevention, disruption of lipid rafts, and reversal of EMT (epithelial to mesenchymal transition). Efficacy against Prostate Cancer Stem Cells has been suggested. (157-171)

Topo Isomerase I and II

topo-isomerase enzymes are involved in repairing breaks and fixing tangled DNA related to unwinding and over-winding of the double helix during DNA replication. Inhibition of topoisomerase leads to permanent breaks and damage in DNA, causing apoptosis, and cell death. Boswellia, fluoroquinolone antibiotics, and chemotherapy agents etoposide and doxorubicin are all Topoisomerase inhibitors.

Triple Therapy refers to using all three agents to block cancer cell metabolism:

1) OXPHOS inhibitor
2) Glycolysis Inhibitor
3) Autophagy Inhibitor

Trophoblast Theory of Cancer

First proposed by John Beard in 1906, the Trophoblast Theory of Cancer sees the cancer cell as a "germ cell" similar to a trophoblast cell of the placenta. Trophoblast cells form the placenta of the growing embryo. Both cell types, cancer cells and trophoblast cells, produce HCG (Human Chorionic Gonadotropin) and PIBF (progesterone induced blocking factor), and share much of the same molecular circuitry for proliferation and invasion.

TrxR thioredoxin reductase system,

a selenium based intracellular anti-oxidant system which protects the cancer cells from excess ROS (reactive oxygen species). TrxR is inhibited by an old gold containing rheumatology drug, Auranofin, thus sensitizing cancer cells to oxidative therapies. (21) Auranofin has been repurposed to treat P53-mutated or PTEN deficient B cell lymphoma. (172)

Tumor Cell Dormancy

A stable, non-proliferative cellular state with reduced PI3K–AKT-mTOR signaling, associated with cancer stem cells. "Protective Autophagy" plays an important role in maintaining dormant state. (173)

UPR (unfolded protein response)

Is caused by endoplasmic stress induced by Boswellia or Silver particles. When proteins cannot be properly folded, this creates a cell crisis triggering apoptosis.

V-ATPase (Vacuolar ATPase) molecular acid pump

Is a proton pump which produces acid within lysosomes and secretory vesicles, inhibited by PPI drugs (proton pump inhibitors), CADs and autophagy inhibitors. The Wnt and Notch cancer stem cell pathways are dependent on V-ATPase function. Blocking V-ATPase with PPI drugs eradicates cancer stem cells. Cancer cells have V-ATPase on the outer cell membrane for secreting acid to degrade and digest the tissues of the extracellular space. (174-175)

VDAC -Voltage Dependent Anion Channel

VDAC is a specialized channel on the outer mitochondrial membrane providing a route for shuttling molecules in and out of the mitochondria. Attachment of HKII to the VDAC facilitates GLYCOLYSIS by using mitochondrial ATP to phosphorylate glucose. HKII attached to the VDAC also prevents mitochondrial apoptosis, immortalizing the cancer cell. Separating HKII from the VDAC restores apoptosis, a valid anti-cancer strategy. Venetoclax, a new anti-cancer drug induces apoptosis by interfering with the interaction of BCL2 with the VDAC. (176)

VEGF Vascular Endothelial Growth Factor

Is a growth factor secreted by activated platelets which stimulates new blood vessel formation providing blood flow and nutrients to the growing tumor mass. Inhibition of platelet activation with Dipyridamole and Aspirin prevents release of VEGF from platelets and is enormously useful as an anti-cancer strategy. The antihistamine, Cimetidine is useful in blocking platelet release of VEGF and PDGF. (177-178)

War Against Cancer

This is a slogan for the 1971 National Cancer Act, a massive boondoggle which wasted billions of taxpayer dollars on government funded research projects mostly supported the chemotherapy paradigm, the discredited theory that cancer is caused by somatic mutations in nuclear DNA, and failed to improve national cancer mortality. Cancer research spending by the NCI (National Cancer Institute) totaled over $100 billion from 1971 to 2008, averaging 2.7 billion per year. Paradoxically, the "War Against Cancer" funded massive volumes of basic science, in vitro and in vivo preclinical animal studies leading to numerous scientific breakthroughs which have made this book possible. (179)

Warburg Effect

Typically, rapidly proliferating tumor cells have increased glycolytic rates up to 200 times higher than those of their normal tissue of origin, even in the presence of oxygen. This is due to the Warburg effect, also called aerobic glycolysis, which utilizes massive amounts of glucose to support cancer cell growth and proliferation. The main metabolic alterations which produce the Warburg Effect are upregulation of Glycolysis in the cytoplasm, downregulation of mitochondrial OXPHOS, and relocation of Hexokinase II (HKII) to the VDAC on the outer mitochondrial membrane.

Statistics for Cancer

It has been estimated that around 13.2 million people will die of cancer annually by the year 2030, worldwide.

Venetoclax (ABT-199)

Is a new FDA approved drug, a selective BCL-2 inhibitor which restores apoptosis in hematologic cancers.

Wnt/ßeta-Catenin/TCF/LEF Pathway (T-Cell Factor/Lymphoid Enhancing Factor)

Wnt is an acronym derived from two proto-oncogenes wingless and intel 1. First described in wingless fruitflies, Wnt stands for Wingless-related integration site, regulating stem cells during embryonic development. In adults, the Wnt pathway is inactivated or silent. The main signal protein for the Wnt pathway is Beta-Catenin which is normally degraded by glycogen synthase kinase 3ß (GSK-3β) in the cytoplasm. However, in cancer stem cells Beta-Catenin is not degraded, enters the nucleus and binds to target genes, the TCF/LEF (T-cell factor/lymphoid enhancing factor), leading to expression of c-Myc, cyclin D1, COX2, MMP and VEGF. These are pro-cancer proteins which enhance proliferation and aggressive behavior, including EMT (epithelial to mesenchymal transition). Cancer stem cells typically have amplified Wnt signaling, necessary for cancer stem cell maintenance. Inhibition of Wnt signaling is a valid anti-cancer strategy which eradicates cancer stem cells. (180-181)

References for Glossary

1) Liberti, Maria V., and Jason W. Locasale. "The Warburg effect: how does it benefit cancer cells?" Trends in biochemical sciences 41.3 (2016): 211-218.

2) Chen, Xi-sha, et al. "Anticancer strategies based on the metabolic profile of tumor cells: therapeutic targeting of the Warburg effect." Acta Pharmacologica Sinica 37.8 (2016): 1013-1019.

3) Jang, Ji Hoon, et al. "Metformin induces caspase-dependent and caspase-independent apoptosis in human bladder cancer T24 cells." Anti-cancer drugs 31.7 (2020): 655.

4) Zhang, Wenguang, and Kethandapatti C. Balaji. "Role of apoptosis inducing factor in prostate cancer cell apoptosis induced by cisplatin." (2006): 126-127.

5) Liao, Yong, and Mien-Chie Hung. "Physiological regulation of Akt activity and stability." American journal of translational research 2.1 (2010): 19.

6) Hart, Jonathan R., and Peter K. Vogt. "Phosphorylation of AKT: a mutational analysis." Oncotarget 2.6 (2011): 467.

7) Faubert, Brandon, et al. "AMPK is a negative regulator of the Warburg effect and suppresses tumor growth in vivo." Cell metabolism 17.1 (2013): 113-124.

8) Faubert, Brandon, et al. "AMPK is a negative regulator of the Warburg effect and suppresses tumor growth in vivo." Cell metabolism 17.1 (2013): 113-124.

9) Anan, Keisei, et al. "Vascular endothelial growth factor and platelet-derived growth factor are potential angiogenic and metastatic factors in human breast cancer." Surgery 119.3 (1996): 333-339.

10) Saric, Amra, et al. "mTOR controls lysosome tubulation and antigen presentation in macrophages and dendritic cells." Molecular biology of the cell 27.2 (2016): 321-333.

11) Grahammer, Florian, et al. "mTOR regulates endocytosis and nutrient transport in proximal tubular cells." Journal of the American Society of Nephrology 28.1 (2017): 230-241.

12) Circu, Magdalena L., et al. "A novel high content imaging-based screen identifies the anti-helminthic niclosamide as an inhibitor of lysosome anterograde trafficking and prostate cancer cell invasion." PloS one 11.1 (2016): e0146931.

13) Campbell, Kirsteen J., and Stephen WG Tait. "Targeting BCL-2 regulated apoptosis in cancer." Open biology 8.5 (2018): 180002.

14) Tsujimoto, Y., and S. Shimizu. "VDAC regulation by the Bcl-2 family of proteins." Cell Death & Differentiation 7.12 (2000): 1174-1181.

15) Zhang, Qi, et al. "Inhibiting Mitochondria Function by Bcl-2 Inhibitor Venetoclax and Complex I Inhibitor Iacs-010759 Eliminate Leukemia Cells in Pre-Clinical AML Models." (2019): 3927-3927.

16) Fiorillo, Marco, et al. "Repurposing atovaquone: targeting mitochondrial complex III and OXPHOS to eradicate cancer stem cells." Oncotarget 7.23 (2016): 34084.

17) Stevens, Alexandra M., et al. "Atovaquone is active against AML by upregulating the integrated stress pathway and suppressing oxidative phosphorylation." Blood advances 3.24 (2019): 4215-4227.

18) Kaneshiro, Edna S., et al. "Ubiquinone synthesis and its regulation in Pneumocystis carinii." Journal of Eukaryotic Microbiology 53.6 (2006): 435-444.

19) Ni, Xiaoling, Guohua Hu, and Xun Cai. "The success and the challenge of all-trans retinoic acid in the treatment of cancer." Critical reviews in food science and nutrition 59.sup1 (2019): S71-S80.

20) Tripathi, Surya Kant, et al. "The potential of retinoids for combination therapy of lung cancer: updates and future directions." Pharmacological research 147 (2019): 104331.

21) Long, Adrienne H., et al. "Reduction of MDSCs with all-trans retinoic acid improves CAR therapy efficacy for sarcomas." Cancer immunology research 4.10 (2016): 869-880.

22) Bauer, Raimund, et al. "Blockade of myeloid-derived suppressor cell expansion with all-trans retinoic acid increases the efficacy of antiangiogenic therapy." Cancer research 78.12 (2018): 3220-3232.

23) Saidi, Samir A., et al. "In vitro and in vivo effects of the PPAR-alpha agonists fenofibrate and retinoic acid

in endometrial cancer." Molecular cancer 5.1 (2006): 13.

24) Wang, Jeffrey, et al. "Repurposing auranofin to treat TP53-mutated or PTEN-deleted refractory B-cell lymphoma." Blood cancer journal 9.12 (2019): 1-6.

25) Hu, Jing, et al. "Auranofin enhances Ibrutinib's anticancer activity in EGFR-mutant lung adenocarcinoma." Molecular cancer therapeutics 17.10 (2018): 2156-2163.

26) Fiskus, Warren, et al. "Auranofin induces lethal oxidative and endoplasmic reticulum stress and exerts potent preclinical activity against chronic lymphocytic leukemia." Cancer research 74.9 (2014): 2520-2532.

27) Raninga, Prahlad V., et al. "Therapeutic cooperation between auranofin, a thioredoxin reductase inhibitor and anti-PD-L1 antibody for treatment of triple-negative breast cancer." International Journal of Cancer 146.1 (2020): 123-136.

28) Yang, Mengqi, et al. "Effective Elimination of Lymphoma Cells in Stromal Microenvironment by Double Impact on ROS and ATP Metabolism Using Auranofin." (2020).

29) Bajor, Malgorzata, et al. "Triple Combination of Ascorbate, Menadione and the Inhibition of Peroxiredoxin-1 Produces Synergistic Cytotoxic Effects in Triple-Negative Breast Cancer Cells." Antioxidants 9.4 (2020): 320.

30) Rothan, Hussin A., et al. "The FDA-approved gold drug Auranofin inhibits novel coronavirus (SARS-COV-2) replication and attenuates inflammation in human cells." Virology (2020).

31) Fuchs, Beth Burgwyn, et al. "Inhibition of bacterial and fungal pathogens by the orphaned drug auranofin." Future medicinal chemistry 8.2 (2016): 117-132.

32) Onorati, Angelique V., et al. "Targeting autophagy in cancer." Cancer 124.16 (2018): 3307-3318.

33) Levy, Jean M. Mulcahy, Christina G. Towers, and Andrew Thorburn. "Targeting autophagy in cancer." Nature Reviews Cancer 17.9 (2017): 528-542.

34) Shimizu, Shigeomi, Masashi Narita, and Yoshihide Tsujimoto. "Bcl-2 family proteins regulate the release of apoptogenic cytochrome c by the mitochondrial channel VDAC." Nature 399.6735 (1999): 483-487.

35) Moghaddam, Mansour Ghaffari, Faujan Bin H. Ahmad, and Alireza Samzadeh-Kermani. "Biological activity of betulinic acid: a review." (2012).

36) Jiao, Lin, et al. "Betulinic acid suppresses breast cancer aerobic glycolysis via caveolin-1/NF-κB/c-Myc pathway." Biochemical pharmacology 161 (2019): 149-162.

37) Salata, Cristiano, et al. "Antiviral activity of cationic amphiphilic drugs." Expert review of anti-infective therapy 15.5 (2017): 483-492.

38) Ellegaard, Anne-Marie, et al. "Repurposing cationic amphiphilic antihistamines for cancer treatment." EBioMedicine 9 (2016): 130-139.

39) Seyfried, Thomas N. "Cancer as a mitochondrial metabolic disease." Frontiers in cell and developmental biology 3 (2015): 43.

40) Guilford, Frederick T., and Simon Yu. "Antiparasitic and Antifungal Medications for Targeting Cancer Cells Literature Review and Case Studies." synthesis 9 (2019): 11.

41) Piechowski, Jean. "Plausibility of trophoblastic-like regulation of cancer tissue." Cancer Management and Research 11 (2019): 5033.

42) Chatterjee, Sharmistha, and Parames C. Sil. "Targeting the crosstalks of Wnt pathway with Hedgehog and Notch for cancer therapy." Pharmacological research 142 (2019): 251-261.

43) Roma, Josep, et al. "Notch, wnt, and hedgehog pathways in rhabdomyosarcoma: from single pathways to an integrated network." Sarcoma 2012 (2012).

44) Smith, Alexandra G., and Kay F. Macleod. "Autophagy, cancer stem cells and drug resistance." The Journal of pathology 247.5 (2019): 708-718.

45) Ayob, Ain Zubaidah, and Thamil Selvee Ramasamy. "Cancer stem cells as key drivers of tumour progression." Journal of biomedical science 25.1 (2018): 1-18.

46) Papaccio, Federica, et al. "Concise review: cancer cells, cancer stem cells, and mesenchymal stem cells: influence in cancer development." Stem cells translational medicine 6.12 (2017): 2115-2125.

47) Reddy, Dhanasekhar, et al. "Anticancer and Antiviral Properties of Cardiac Glycosides: A Review to

Explore the Mechanism of Actions." Molecules 25.16 (2020): 3596.

48) Khan, Haroon, et al. "Glycosides from medicinal plants as potential anticancer agents: Emerging trends towards future drugs." Current medicinal chemistry 26.13 (2019): 2389-2406.

49) Johan, H. "Digitoxin has Specific Properties for Potential use to Treat Cancer and Inflammatory Diseases." Res & Rev Health Care Open Acc J 2.3 (2018).

50) Diederich, Marc, Florian Muller, and Claudia Cerella. "Cardiac glycosides: From molecular targets to immunogenic cell death." Biochemical pharmacology 125 (2017): 1-11.

51) Schneider, Naira Fernanda Zanchett, et al. "Anticancer and immunogenic properties of cardiac glycosides." Molecules 22.11 (2017): 1932.

52) Felippe Gonçalves-de-Albuquerque, Cassiano, et al. "Na/K Pump and Beyond: Na/K-ATPase as a Modulator of Apoptosis and Autophagy." Molecules 22.4 (2017): 578.

53) Newman, Robert A., et al. "Cardiac glycosides as novel cancer therapeutic agents." Molecular interventions 8.1 (2008): 36.

54) Stenkvist, B. J. Ö. R. N. "Is digitalis a therapy for breast carcinoma?" Oncology reports 6.3 (1999): 493-499.

55) Yang, Eric V. "Role for catecholamines in tumor progression: Possible use for ß-blockers in the treatment of cancer." Cancer biology & therapy 10.1 (2010): 30-32.

56) Magrì, Andrea, Simona Reina, and Vito De Pinto. "VDAC1 as pharmacological target in cancer and neurodegeneration: focus on its role in apoptosis." Frontiers in chemistry 6 (2018): 108.

57) Nagarsheth, Nisha, Max S. Wicha, and Weiping Zou. "Chemokines in the cancer microenvironment and their relevance in cancer immunotherapy." Nature Reviews Immunology 17.9 (2017): 559.

58) DeVita, Vincent T., and Edward Chu. "A history of cancer chemotherapy." Cancer research 68.21 (2008): 8643-8653.

59) Schneider, Christof, Daniela Steinbrecher, and Stephan Stilgenbauer. "Targeted therapy in CLL: Changing the treatment paradigm." Oncotarget 10.40 (2019): 4002.

60) Jain, Nitin, and Susan O'Brien. "The Shifting Paradigm in Chronic Lymphocytic Leukemia: Is Chemotherapy Still Relevant?." The Cancer Journal 25.6 (2019): 374-377.

61) Lord, Kevin. "Reports of the Demise of Chemotherapy Have Been Greatly Exaggerated." Am J Manag Care 25.6 (2019): 270-272.

62) Kadavakollu, S., et al. "Clotrimazole as a cancer drug: a short review." Medicinal chemistry 4.11 (2014): 722.

63) Coelho, Raquel Guimarães, et al. "Clotrimazole disrupts glycolysis in human breast cancer without affecting non-tumoral tissues." Molecular genetics and metabolism 103.4 (2011): 394-398.

64) Furtado, Cristiane M., et al. "Clotrimazole preferentially inhibits human breast cancer cell proliferation, viability and glycolysis." PloS one 7.2 (2012).

65) Meira, Débora Dummer, et al. "Clotrimazole decreases human breast cancer cells viability through alterations in cytoskeleton-associated glycolytic enzymes." Molecular genetics and metabolism 84.4 (2005): 354-362.

66) Newcomer, Lee N. "Changing physician incentives for cancer care to reward better patient outcomes instead of use of more costly drugs." Health Affairs 31.4 (2012): 780-785.

67) Malin, Jennifer L., et al. "Medical oncologists' perceptions of financial incentives in cancer care." Journal of clinical oncology 31.5 (2013): 530.

68) Xu, Dong, et al. "Chrysin inhibited tumor glycolysis and induced apoptosis in hepatocellular carcinoma by targeting hexokinase-2." Journal of Experimental & Clinical Cancer Research 36.1 (2017): 1-11.

69) Fadus, Matthew C., et al. "Curcumin: An age-old anti-inflammatory and anti-neoplastic agent." Journal of traditional and complementary medicine 7.3 (2017): 339-346.

70) Wang, Ke, et al. "Curcumin inhibits aerobic glycolysis and induces mitochondrial-mediated apoptosis through hexokinase II in human colorectal cancer cells in vitro." Anti-cancer drugs 26.1 (2015): 15-24.

71) Imran, Muhammad, et al. "Curcumin, anticancer, & antitumor perspectives: A comprehensive review." Critical reviews in food science and nutrition 58.8 (2018): 1271-1293.

72) Tashiro, Etsu, Ayako Tsuchiya, and Masaya Imoto. "Functions of cyclin D1 as an oncogene and regulation of cyclin D1 expression." Cancer science 98.5 (2007): 629-635.

73) Zukerberg, Lawrence R., et al. "Cyclin D1 expression in non-Hodgkin's lymphomas: detection by immunohistochemistry." American journal of clinical pathology 103.6 (1995): 756-760.

74) Li, Hong, et al. "The combination of disulfiram and copper for cancer treatment." Drug Discovery Today (2020).

75) Yao, W., et al. "Stem cell and EMT features of HNSCC-lines are reversed by the aldehyde hydrogenase inhibitor Disulfiram (Antabuse®)." Laryngo-Rhino-Otologie 98.S 02 (2019): 11415.

76) Jin, Na, et al. "Disulfiram/copper targets stem cell-like ALDH+ population of multiple myeloma by inhibition of ALDH1A1 and Hedgehog pathway." Journal of Cellular Biochemistry 119.8 (2018): 6882-6893.

77) Omran, Ziad, et al. "Repurposing Disulfiram as an Anti-Obesity Drug: Treating and Preventing Obesity in High-Fat-Fed Rats." Diabetes, Metabolic Syndrome and Obesity: Targets and Therapy 13 (2020): 1473.

78) Viola-Rhenals, Maricela, et al. "Recent advances in Antabuse (disulfiram): the importance of its metal-binding ability to its anticancer activity." Current medicinal chemistry 25.4 (2018): 506-524.

79) Wu, Xi, et al. "Suppressing autophagy enhances disulfiram/copper-induced apoptosis in non-small cell lung cancer." European Journal of Pharmacology 827 (2018): 1-12.

80) Huang, Hongbiao, et al. "Two clinical drugs deubiquitinase inhibitor auranofin and aldehyde dehydrogenase inhibitor disulfiram trigger synergistic anti-tumor effects in vitro and in vivo." Oncotarget 7.3 (2016): 2796.

81) Gao, Feng, et al. "Epigallocatechin gallate inhibits human tongue carcinoma cells via HK2-mediated glycolysis." Oncology reports 33.3 (2015): 1533-1539.

82) Wei, Ran, et al. "Suppressing glucose metabolism with epigallocatechin-3-gallate (EGCG) reduces breast cancer cell growth in preclinical models." Food & function 9.11 (2018): 5682-5696.

83) Mahmood, Muhammad Shahid, et al. "Antiviral effects of green tea (Camellia sinensis) against pathogenic viruses in human and animals (a mini-review)." African Journal of Traditional, Complementary and Alternative Medicines 13.2 (2016): 176-184.

84) Shah, Parag P., et al. "Common cytotoxic chemotherapeutics induce epithelial-mesenchymal transition (EMT) downstream of ER stress." Oncotarget 8.14 (2017): 22625.

85) Ahmed, R. A., O. A. Alawin, and P. W. Sylvester. "γ-Tocotrienol reversal of epithelial-to-mesenchymal transition in human breast cancer cells is associated with inhibition of canonical Wnt signalling." Cell Proliferation 49.4 (2016): 460-470.

86) Elaskalani, Omar, et al. "Targeting platelets for the treatment of cancer." Cancers 9.7 (2017): 94.

87) Guo, Yi, et al. "Platelets promote invasion and induce epithelial to mesenchymal transition in ovarian cancer cells by TGF-β signaling pathway." Gynecologic oncology 153.3 (2019): 639-650.

88) Gray, Michael W. "Lynn Margulis and the endosymbiont hypothesis: 50 years later." Molecular biology of the cell 28.10 (2017): 1285-1287.

89) Shen, Zheyu, et al. "Emerging strategies of cancer therapy based on ferroptosis." Advanced Materials 30.12 (2018): 1704007.

90) Wang, Ning, et al. "Artesunate activates the ATF4-CHOP-CHAC1 pathway and affects ferroptosis in Burkitt's Lymphoma." Biochemical and biophysical research communications 519.3 (2019): 533-539.

91) Mou, Yanhua, et al. "Ferroptosis, a new form of cell death: opportunities and challenges in cancer." Journal of hematology & oncology 12.1 (2019): 34.

92) Deng, Guoping, Xiaomin Song, and Mark I. Greene. "FoxP3 in Treg cell biology: a molecular and structural perspective." Clinical & Experimental Immunology 199.3 (2020): 255-262.

93) Huang, Jingyao, et al. "Targeting FOXP3 complex ensemble in drug discovery." Advances in Protein

Chemistry and Structural Biology. Vol. 121. Academic Press, 2020. 143-168.

94) Singh, Shivendra V., et al. "Sulforaphane-induced cell death in human prostate cancer cells is initiated by reactive oxygen species." Journal of Biological Chemistry 280.20 (2005): 19911-19924.

95) Suda, Yoko, et al. "Mouse embryonic stem cells exhibit indefinite proliferative potential." Journal of cellular physiology 133.1 (1987): 197-201.

96) Rubin, Harry. "The disparity between human cell senescence in vitro and lifelong replication in vivo." Nature biotechnology 20.7 (2002): 675-681.

97) Kishimoto, Tadamitsu. "The biology of interleukin-6." Blood 74.1 (1989): 1-10.

98) Dixon, Karen O., and Vijay K. Kuchroo. "IL-18: throwing off the shackles to boost anti-tumor immunity." Cell Research (2020): 1-2.

99) Zhou, Ting, et al. "IL-18 pathway agonism expands intratumoral PD1+ Tcf1+ stem-like CD8+ cells and their polyfunctional effector progeny to promote anti-tumor immunity." (2020): 2156-2156.

100) Senju, Hiroaki, et al. "Effect of IL-18 on the expansion and phenotype of human natural killer cells: application to cancer immunotherapy." International journal of biological sciences 14.3 (2018): 331.

101) Xiong, Donglan, et al. "Antitumor activity of interleukin-18 on A549 human lung cancer cell line." Journal of Cancer Research and Therapeutics 15.7 (2019): 1635.

102) Weizman, Orr-El, et al. "IL-18 immunotherapy is efficacious against checkpoint-immunotherapy refractory tumors by promoting the maturation of highly proliferative, polyfunctional NK cells." (2020): 3424-3424.

103) Colotta, Francesco, et al. "Cancer-related inflammation, the seventh hallmark of cancer: links to genetic instability." Carcinogenesis 30.7 (2009): 1073-1081.

104) Ritter, Birgit, and Florian R. Greten. "Modulating inflammation for cancer therapy." Journal of Experimental Medicine 216.6 (2019): 1234-1243.

105) Wattenberg, Max M., and Gregory L. Beatty. "Overcoming immunotherapeutic resistance by targeting the cancer inflammation cycle." Seminars in Cancer Biology. Academic Press, 2020.

106) Feyrer, James, Dimitra Politi, and David N. Weil. The Cognitive Effects of Micronutrient Deficiency: Evidence from Salt Iodization in the United States. No. w19233. National Bureau of Economic Research, 2013.

107) Shrivastava, Ashutosh, et al. "Molecular iodine induces caspase-independent apoptosis in human breast carcinoma cells involving the mitochondria-mediated pathway." Journal of Biological Chemistry 281.28 (2006): 19762-19771.

108) Aceves, Carmen, et al. "Antineoplastic effect of iodine in mammary cancer: participation of 6-iodolactone (6-IL) and peroxisome proliferator-activated receptors (PPAR)." Molecular Cancer 8.1 (2009): 33.

109) Ayre, S. G., D. Perez Garcia y Bellon, and D. Perez Garcia Jr. "Insulin potentiation therapy: a new concept in the management of chronic degenerative disease." Medical Hypotheses 20.2 (1986): 199-210.

110) Holt, Sarah V., et al. "The development of an immunohistochemical method to detect the autophagy-associated protein LC3-II in human tumor xenografts." Toxicologic pathology 39.3 (2011): 516-523.

111) Aoki, Hiroshi, et al. "Monitoring autophagy in glioblastoma with antibody against isoform B of human microtubule-associated protein 1 light chain 3." Autophagy 4.4 (2008): 467-475.

112) Zhu, Xiuzhi, et al. "The prognostic and predictive potential of Ki-67 in triple-negative breast cancer." Scientific reports 10.1 (2020): 1-10.

113) Mudassar, Muhammad, et al. "Ki-67 Proliferative Index in The Non-Hodgkin's Lymphoma and Its Clinical Significance." Annals of Punjab Medical College (APMC) 13.2 (2019): 108-112.

114) Kasajima, Atsuko, et al. "Clinicopathological Profiling of Lung Carcinoids with a Ki67 Index> 20%." Neuroendocrinology 108.2 (2019): 109-120.

115) Efferth, Thomas, and Franz Oesch. "Anti-inflammatory and anti-cancer activities of frankincense: Targets, treatments and toxicities." Seminars in cancer biology. Academic Press, 2020.

116) Zagon, Ian S., and Patricia J. McLaughlin. "Opioid growth factor and the treatment of human pancreatic

cancer: a review." World Journal of Gastroenterology: WJG 20.9 (2014): 2218.

117) Li, Zijian, et al. "Low-dose naltrexone (LDN): A promising treatment in immune-related diseases and cancer therapy." International immunopharmacology 61 (2018): 178-184.

118) Donahue, Renee N., Patricia J. McLaughlin, and Ian S. Zagon. "The opioid growth factor (OGF) and low dose naltrexone (LDN) suppress human ovarian cancer progression in mice." Gynecologic oncology 122.2 (2011): 382-388.

119) Okamura, Naoka, et al. "Antitumor effect of itraconazole on hematological malignant cells by suppression of Hedgehog signal transduction via inhibition of lipid raft formation." (2012): 149-149.

120) Cervantes-Madrid, Diana, Yair Romero, and Alfonso Dueñas-González. "Reviving lonidamine and 6-diazo-5-oxo-L-norleucine to be used in combination for metabolic cancer therapy." BioMed research international 2015 (2015).

121) Huang, Hao. "Matrix metalloproteinase-9 (MMP-9) as a cancer biomarker and MMP-9 biosensors: recent advances." Sensors 18.10 (2018): 3249.

122) Winer, Arthur, Sylvia Adams, and Paolo Mignatti. "Matrix metalloproteinase inhibitors in cancer therapy: turning past failures into future successes." Molecular cancer therapeutics 17.6 (2018): 1147-1155.

123) Hevia, David, et al. "Melatonin decreases glucose metabolism in prostate cancer cells: a 13C stable isotope-resolved metabolomic study." International journal of molecular sciences 18.8 (2017): 1620.

124) Reiter, Russel J., et al. "Inhibition of mitochondrial pyruvate dehydrogenase kinase: a proposed mechanism by which melatonin causes cancer cells to overcome cytosolic glycolysis, reduce tumor biomass and reverse insensitivity to chemotherapy." Melatonin Research 2.3 (2019): 105-119.

125) Reiter, Russel J., et al. "Melatonin inhibits Warburg-dependent cancer by redirecting glucose oxidation to the mitochondria: a mechanistic hypothesis." Cellular and Molecular Life Sciences (2020): 1-16.

126) Tan, Dun-Xian, and Russel J. Reiter. "Mitochondria: the birth place, battle ground and the site of melatonin metabolism in cells." Melatonin Research 2.1 (2019): 44-66.

127) Mayo, Juan C., et al. "Understanding the role of melatonin in cancer metabolism." Melatonin Research 2.3 (2019): 76-104.

128) Gottfried, Eva, et al. "New aspects of an old drug—diclofenac targets MYC and glucose metabolism in tumor cells." PloS one 8.7 (2013): e66987.

129) Katoh, Hiroshi, and Masahiko Watanabe. "Myeloid-derived suppressor cells and therapeutic strategies in cancer." Mediators of inflammation 2015 (2015).

130) Cornes, Paul, et al. "Systematic review and meta-analysis of short-versus long-acting granulocyte colony-stimulating factors for reduction of chemotherapy-induced febrile neutropenia." Advances in therapy 35.11 (2018): 1816-1829.

131) Meisel, Christian T., Cristina Porcheri, and Thimios A. Mitsiadis. "Cancer Stem Cells, Quo Vadis? The Notch Signaling Pathway in Tumor Initiation and Progression." Cells 9.8 (2020): 1879

132) Serasanambati, Mamatha, and Shanmuga Reddy Chilakapati. "Function of nuclear factor kappa B (NF-kB) in human diseases-a review." South Indian Journal of Biological Sciences 2.4 (2016): 368-387.

133) Labbozzetta, Manuela, Monica Notarbartolo, and Paola Poma. "Can NF-κB Be Considered a Valid Drug Target in Neoplastic Diseases? Our Point of View." International Journal of Molecular Sciences 21.9 (2020): 3070.

134) Zinatizadeh MR et al., The Nuclear Factor Kappa B (NF-kB) signaling in cancer development and immune diseases, Genes & Diseases, https://doi.org/10.1016/j.gendis.2020.06.00

135) Soleimani, Atena, et al. "Role of the NF-κB signaling pathway in the pathogenesis of colorectal cancer." Gene 726 (2020): 144132.

136) Jaglowski, Jeffrey R., et al. "Opioid growth factor enhances tumor growth inhibition and increases the survival of paclitaxel-treated mice with squamous cell carcinoma of the head and neck." Cancer chemotherapy and pharmacology 56.1 (2005): 97-104.

137) Jin, Mingji, et al. "Effects of aspirin on proliferation, invasion and apoptosis of Hep-2 cells via the PTEN/AKT/NF-κB/survivin signaling pathway." Oncology letters 15.6 (2018): 8454-8460.

138) Wang, Yunjiao, et al. "Aspirin inhibits adipogenesis of tendon stem cells and lipids accumulation in rat injury tendon through regulating PTEN/PI3K/AKT signalling." Journal of cellular and molecular medicine 23.11 (2019): 7535-7544.

139) Chu, Eric C., Jianyuan Chai, and Andrzej S. Tarnawski. "NSAIDs activate PTEN and other phosphatases in human colon cancer cells: novel mechanism for chemopreventive action of NSAIDs." Biochemical and biophysical research communications 320.3 (2004): 875-879.

140) Jia, Lijun, et al. "Quercetin suppresses the mobility of breast cancer by suppressing glycolysis through Akt-mTOR pathway mediated autophagy induction." Life sciences 208 (2018): 123-130.

141) Wu, Hongyan, et al. "Quercetin inhibits the proliferation of glycolysis-addicted HCC cells by reducing hexokinase 2 and Akt-mTOR pathway." Molecules 24.10 (2019): 1993.

142) Reyes-Farias, Marjorie, and Catalina Carrasco-Pozo. "The anti-cancer effect of quercetin: Molecular implications in cancer metabolism." International journal of molecular sciences 20.13 (2019): 3177.

143) Dahiya, Rashmi, et al. "Investigation of inhibitory potential of quercetin to the pyruvate dehydrogenase kinase 3: Towards implications in anticancer therapy." International journal of biological macromolecules 136 (2019): 1076-1085.

144) Suwandittakul, Nantana, et al. "Disruption of endocytic trafficking protein Rab7 impairs invasiveness of cholangiocarcinoma cells." Cancer Biomarkers 20.3 (2017): 255-266.

145) Liu, Huiyong, et al. "Rab7 Is Associated with Poor Prognosis of Gastric Cancer and Promotes Proliferation, Invasion, and Migration of Gastric Cancer Cells." Medical Science Monitor: International Medical Journal of Experimental and Clinical Research 26 (2020): e922217-1.

146) Guerra, Flora, et al. "Modulation of RAB7A protein expression determines resistance to cisplatin through late endocytic pathway impairment and extracellular vesicular secretion." Cancers 11.1 (2019): 52.

147) Pavlides, Stephanos, et al. "The reverse Warburg effect: aerobic glycolysis in cancer associated fibroblasts and the tumor stroma." Cell cycle 8.23 (2009): 3984-4001.

148) Lee, Minjong, and Jung-Hwan Yoon. "Metabolic interplay between glycolysis and mitochondrial oxidation: The reverse Warburg effect and its therapeutic implication." World journal of biological chemistry 6.3 (2015): 148.

149) Bonuccelli, Gloria, et al. "The reverse Warburg effect: glycolysis inhibitors prevent the tumor promoting effects of caveolin-1 deficient cancer associated fibroblasts." Cell cycle 9.10 (2010): 1960-1971.

150) Zeng, Huawei, and Gerald F. Combs Jr. "Selenium as an anticancer nutrient: roles in cell proliferation and tumor cell invasion." The Journal of nutritional biochemistry 19.1 (2008): 1-7.

151) Davis, Cindy D., Petra A. Tsuji, and John A. Milner. "Selenoproteins and cancer prevention." Annual review of nutrition 32 (2012): 73-95.

152) Ontiveros, M., et al. "Natural flavonoids inhibit the plasma membrane Ca2+-ATPase." Biochemical pharmacology 166 (2019): 1-11.

153) Delmas, Dominique, et al. "Silymarin and Cancer: A Dual Strategy in Both in Chemoprevention and Chemosensitivity." Molecules 25.9 (2020): 2009.

154) Kacar, Sedat, Nuriye Ezgi Bektur Aykanat, and Varol Sahinturk. "Silymarin inhibited DU145 cells by activating SLIT2 protein and suppressing expression of CXCR4." Medical Oncology 37.3 (2020): 1-9.

155) Snima, K. S., et al. "Silymarin encapsulated poly (D, L-lactic-co-glycolic acid) nanoparticles: a prospective candidate for prostate cancer therapy." Journal of biomedical nanotechnology 10.4 (2014): 559-570.

156) Fan, Li, et al. "Silymarin induces cell cycle arrest and apoptosis in ovarian cancer cells." European journal of pharmacology 743 (2014): 79-88.

157) Dronamraju, Venkateshwara, et al. "γ-Tocotrienol suppression of the Warburg effect is mediated by AMPK activation in human breast cancer cells." Nutrition and cancer 71.7 (2019): 1214-1228.

158) Parajuli, Parash, Roshan Vijay Tiwari, and Paul William Sylvester. "Anticancer effects of γ-Tocotrienol are associated with a suppression in aerobic glycolysis." Biological and Pharmaceutical Bulletin 38.9 (2015): 1352-1360.

159) Parajuli, P., R. V. Tiwari, and P. W. Sylvester. "Antiproliferative effects of γ-tocotrienol are associated with suppression of c-Myc expression in mammary tumour cells." Cell proliferation 48.4 (2015): 421-435.

160) Ahmed, R. A., O. A. Alawin, and P. W. Sylvester. "γ-Tocotrienol reversal of epithelial-to-mesenchymal transition in human breast cancer cells is associated with inhibition of canonical Wnt signalling." Cell proliferation 49.4 (2016): 460-470.

161) Sylvester, Paul W., Sumit J. Shah, and Ganesh V. Samant. "Intracellular signaling mechanisms mediating the antiproliferative and apoptotic effects of γ-tocotrienol in neoplastic mammary epithelial cells." Journal of plant physiology 162.7 (2005): 803-810.

162) Sylvester, Paul W., et al. "Tocotrienol combination therapy results in synergistic anticancer response." Front Biosci 17 (2011): 3183-3195.

163) Shirode, Amit B., and Paul W. Sylvester. "Mechanisms mediating the synergistic anticancer effects of combined γ-tocotrienol and celecoxib treatment." Journal of bioanalysis & biomedicine 3 (2011): 001.

164) Ahmed, Rayan, and Paul W. Sylvester. "γ-Tocotrienol Reversal of Epithelial-to-Mesenchymal Transition in Human Breast Cancer Cells is Mediated through a Suppression of Canonical Wnt and Hedgehog Signaling." Vitamin E in Health and Disease (2018): 83.

165) Montagnani Marelli, Marina, et al. "Anticancer properties of tocotrienols: A review of cellular mechanisms and molecular targets." Journal of cellular physiology 234.2 (2019): 1147-1164.

166) Tham, Shiau-Ying, et al. "Tocotrienols modulate a life or death decision in cancers." International journal of molecular sciences 20.2 (2019): 372.

167) Aggarwal, Vaishali, et al. "Molecular mechanisms of action of tocotrienols in cancer: Recent trends and advancements." International journal of molecular sciences 20.3 (2019): 656.

168) Fontana, Fabrizio, et al. "Tocotrienols and cancer: From the state of the art to promising novel patents." Recent patents on anti-cancer drug discovery 14.1 (2019): 5-18.

169) Sylvester, Paul William, and Venkateshwara Dronamraju. "γ-Tocotrienol reversal of the Warburg effect in breast cancer cells is associated with 5'-AMP-activated kinase activation." Molecular Nutrition. Academic Press, 2020. 387-407.

170) Fontana, Fabrizio, et al. "Natural compounds in prostate cancer prevention and treatment: mechanisms of action and molecular targets." Cells 9.2 (2020): 460.

171) Luk SU, Yap WN, Chiu YT, et al. Gamma-tocotrienol as an effective agent in targeting prostate cancer stem cell-like population. Int J Cancer, 2011. 128(9):2182-91.

172) Zhang, Xiaonan, et al. "Repurposing of auranofin: thioredoxin reductase remains a primary target of the drug." Biochimie 162 (2019): 46-54.

173) Sosa, María Soledad, Paloma Bragado, and Julio A. Aguirre-Ghiso. "Mechanisms of disseminated cancer cell dormancy: an awakening field." Nature Reviews Cancer 14.9 (2014): 611-622.

174) Pamarthy, Sahithi, et al. "The curious case of vacuolar ATPase: regulation of signaling pathways." Molecular cancer 17.1 (2018): 41.

175) Whitton, Bradleigh, et al. "Vacuolar ATPase as a potential therapeutic target and mediator of treatment resistance in cancer." Cancer medicine 7.8 (2018): 3800-3811.

176) Shoshan-Barmatz, Varda, et al. "Voltage-dependent anion channel 1 as an emerging drug target for novel anti-cancer therapeutics." Frontiers in oncology 7 (2017): 154.

177) Wartiovaara, Ulla, et al. "Peripheral blood platelets express VEGF-C and VEGF which are released during platelet activation." Thrombosis and haemostasis 80.07 (1998): 171-175.

178) Banks, R. E., et al. "Release of the angiogenic cytokine vascular endothelial growth factor (VEGF) from platelets: significance for VEGF measurements and cancer biology." British journal of cancer 77.6 (1998): 956-964.

179) Rehemtulla, Alnawaz. "The war on cancer rages on." Neoplasia 11.12 (2009): 1252-1263.

180) Lecarpentier, Yves, et al. "Multiple Targets of the Canonical WNT/β-Catenin Signaling in Cancers." Frontiers in oncology 9 (2019).

181) Herbst, Andreas, and Frank Thomas Kolligs. "Wnt signaling as a therapeutic target for cancer." Target Discovery and Validation Reviews and Protocols. Humana Press, 2007. 63-91.

182) Levenson, Anait S. "Metastasis-associated protein 1-mediated antitumor and anticancer activity of dietary stilbenes for prostate cancer chemoprevention and therapy." Seminars in Cancer Biology. Academic Press, 2020.

183) Moon, Hyo-Eun, Hwanju Cheon, and Myung-Shik Lee. "Metastasis-associated protein 1 inhibits p53-induced apoptosis." Oncology reports 18.5 (2007): 1311-1314.

184) Rachaiah, Kavitha, Divya Keshavan, and Bharathi P. Salimath. "Anti-Neoplastic Activity of Dioscorea Extracts by Targeting MTA1." (2019). Life Science Informatics Publication Jan–Feb Page No.549.

185) Zhang, Xiao-yong, et al. "Metastasis-associated protein 1 (MTA1) is an essential downstream effector of the c-MYC oncoprotein." Proceedings of the National Academy of Sciences 102.39 (2005): 13968-13973.

186) Bagheri-Yarmand, Rozita, et al. "Metastasis-associated protein 1 transgenic mice: a new model of spontaneous B-cell lymphomas." Cancer Research 67.15 (2007): 7062-7067.

187) Malisetty, Vijaya Lakshmi, et al. "MTA1 expression in human cancers–Clinical and pharmacological significance." Biomedicine & Pharmacotherapy 95 (2017): 956-964.

188) Avci, Cigir Biray, et al. "Quercetin-induced apoptosis involves increased hTERT enzyme activity of leukemic cells." Hematology 16.5 (2011): 303-307.

189) Misiti, Silvia, et al. "Induction of hTERT expression and telomerase activity by estrogens in human ovary epithelium cells." Molecular and cellular biology 20.11 (2000): 3764-3771.

190) Counter, Christopher M., et al. "Telomerase activity is restored in human cells by ectopic expression of hTERT (hEST2), the catalytic subunit of telomerase." Oncogene 16.9 (1998): 1217-1222.

191) Ganesan, Kumar, and Baojun Xu. "Telomerase inhibitors from natural products and their anticancer potential." International journal of molecular sciences 19.1 (2018): 13.

192) Tahara, H., and M. T. Lotze. "Antitumor effects of interleukin-12 (IL-12): applications for the immunotherapy and gene therapy of cancer." Gene therapy 2.2 (1995): 96.

193) Wang, Pengju, et al. "Re-designing Interleukin-12 to enhance its safety and potential as an anti-tumor immunotherapeutic agent." Nature communications 8.1 (2017): 1-15.

194) Sultan, Ahmed S., et al. "Quercetin induces apoptosis in triple-negative breast cancer cells via inhibiting fatty acid synthase and β-catenin." Int. J. Clin. Exp. Pathol 10.1 (2017): 156-172.

195) Kanarek, Naama, Boryana Petrova, and David M. Sabatini. "Dietary modifications for enhanced cancer therapy." Nature 579.7800 (2020): 507-517.

196) Caffa, Irene, et al. "Fasting-mimicking diet and hormone therapy induce breast cancer regression." Nature 583.7817 (2020): 620-624.

197) Wei, Min, et al. "Fasting-mimicking diet and markers/risk factors for aging, diabetes, cancer, and cardiovascular disease." Science translational medicine 9.377 (2017): eaai8700.

198) Schwedhelm, Carolina, et al. "Effect of diet on mortality and cancer recurrence among cancer survivors: a systematic review and meta-analysis of cohort studies." Nutrition reviews 74.12 (2016): 737-748.

199) Donaldson, Michael S. "Nutrition and cancer: a review of the evidence for an anti-cancer diet." Nutrition journal 3.1 (2004): 19.

200) Welch, H. Gilbert. "Cancer screening, overdiagnosis, and regulatory capture." JAMA Internal Medicine 177.7 (2017): 915-916.

201) Esserman, Laura, Yiwey Shieh, and Ian Thompson. "Rethinking screening for breast cancer and prostate cancer." Jama 302.15 (2009): 1685-1692.

202) Welch, H. Gilbert, Lisa M. Schwartz, and Steven Woloshin. "Prostate-specific antigen levels in the

United States: implications of various definitions for abnormal." Journal of the National Cancer Institute 97.15 (2005): 1132-1137.

203) Andriole, Gerald L., et al. "Mortality results from a randomized prostate-cancer screening trial." New England Journal of Medicine 360.13 (2009): 1310-1319.

204) Davies, Louise, and H. Gilbert Welch. "Current thyroid cancer trends in the United States." JAMA otolaryngology–head & neck surgery 140.4 (2014): 317-322.

205) Cronan, John J. "Thyroid nodules: is it time to turn off the US machines?" Radiology 247.3 (2008): 602-604.

206) Reszka, Alfred A., et al. "Association of mitogen-activated protein kinase with the microtubule cytoskeleton." Proceedings of the National Academy of Sciences 92.19 (1995): 8881-8885.

207) Klemke, Richard L., et al. "Regulation of cell motility by mitogen-activated protein kinase." The Journal of cell biology 137.2 (1997): 481-492.

208) Rudzka, Dominika A., et al. "Migration through physical constraints is enabled by MAPK-induced cell softening via actin cytoskeleton re-organization." Journal of cell science. 132.11 (2019).

Made in the USA
Las Vegas, NV
16 February 2024

85860297R10319